The Mechanism and Applications of Leão's Spreading Depression of Electroencephalographic Activity

The Mechanism and Applications of Leão's Spreading Depression of Electroencephalographic Activity

JAN BUREŠ
OLGA BUREŠOVÁ
JIŘÍ KŘIVÁNEK

ACADEMIA
Publishing House
of the Czechoslovak Academy
of Sciences
Prague

1974

ACADEMIC PRESS, INC.
New York and London
A Subsidiary of Harcourt
Brace Jovanovich'
Publishers

Distribution throughout the world with the exception of socialist countries:
Academic Press, Inc., 111 Fifth Avenue, New York, New York 10003

For Academic Press, Inc.:
Library of Congress Catalog Card No. ~~73-172 981~~
I. S. B. N.: 0—12—142960—1

Printed in Czechoslovakia

Contents

Preface

The effort of the human brain to understand its own function is one of the most fundamental problems of science. Having been the domain of philosophers for centuries and the subject of physiology and psychology for the last hundred years, it is now a point of convergence for a wide spectrum of scientific disciplines ranging from mathematics, electronics, and molecular biology to psychiatry, linguistics, and sociology. The history of neuroscience and its present state offers a dramatic spectacle: old ideas are being continuously abandoned in favor of new ones, theoretical approaches disappear and reappear with astonishing regularity, solutions borrowed from other fields are advertized with messianic zeal. Disappointments are hardly compensated for by modest successes but failures only stimulate more effort and attract better brains. All this accounts for the rapidly accelerating growth of neuroscience, characterized by increasing diversity based on different theoretical concepts and highly specialized research techniques.

The dynamic state of brain research makes it extremely difficult to follow all the new important developments and to fit the ever-increasing stream of data into the unifying framework of a theory. What seems to be beyond the powers of an individual is often expected from the collective effort of a group of scientists. Multidisciplinary symposia and conferences flourish nowhere more than in the neurosciences and form indispensable links ensuring the integrity of the field. Whereas conferences represent a verbal level of "multidisciplinarity" — often hampered by semantic difficulties, lack of mutual understanding, and wide gaps between the available pieces of evidence — the more desirable level of complex cooperation is represented by multidisciplinary research teams gathered around well-defined projects, cutting across different methods and approaches, exploiting different concepts and hypotheses. There are many areas of brain research in which results of various disciplines are mutually complementary and equally contribute to the understanding of the problem. In only a few cases has the analysis-synthesis sequence been completed by an hypothesis that accounts for all the available evidence and can serve as a solid departure point for further research. The aim of the present book is to describe a neurophysiological phenomenon, spreading depression, the exploration of which may be approaching this stage.

Spreading depression (SD) probably confused investigators in early experiments with electrical brain stimulation and recording in the second half of the nineteenth century. It was identified as such only in 1944 by the Brazilian physiologist A. A. P. Leão, who demonstrated that intense focal stimulation of the rabbit cerebral cortex causes local disappearance of spontaneous and evoked EEG activity, spreading at an unusually slow rate of 3 mm/min over the cortical surface. The reliability with which it was possible to reproduce the remarkable properties of this phenomenon helped from the very beginning to define SD as a separate entity, clearly distinct from other brain activities. This was doubtless one of the reasons why SD research remained over the next 25 years an easily surveyable, selfcontained area with well-developed internal linkages and a high level of information exchange. The four laboratories systematically engaged in SD investigation were able to absorb all the scattered information from isolated studies and to connect it with their own research. Useful contacts between the research centres in Rio de Janeiro, Bethesda, Pasadena, and Prague became the central links of an information network including other investigations concerned with SD in a less systematic way.

Spreading depression was discovered as an electrophysiological phenomenon and the first decade of research concentrated on electrophysiological investigations revealing other striking features of the process (slow potential change, impedance increase). The second decade marked a rapid expansion of SD investigations prompted by attempts to analyze the mechanism of SD. Neurochemical and histochemical techniques combined with methods of functional morphology were employed to substantiate different interpretations of the electrophysiological findings. The physiological analysis was extended to the cellular level and the neurohumoral hypothesis of SD proposed by Grafstein (1956a) rapidly gained support. The relationship of SD to epilepsy, concussion, anoxia, and brain metabolism was explored and the list of brain structures susceptible to SD was enlarged. Simultaneously SD started to be employed as a tool in behavioral studies (functional ablation technique) and in research into the functional organization of the brain (inhibitory neuronography). This development aroused more interest in SD which became indirectly related to problems of learning, memory, and motivation, functional organization of the brain, neuropharmacology, and neuroendocrinology. Whereas the first analysis of the phenomenon had been satisfactorily completed, the exploitation of SD as an experimental method still awaits technical improvements, new application fields, and unconventional interpretations.

The present book is mainly intended for those who want to use SD as a research tool and who are interested in the general physiology and pathophysiology of the brain. The first part of the book reviews systematically different aspects of SD using chronological ordering of data whenever possible but pointing out the evidence supporting the neurohumoral hypothesis of the phenomenon, which is discussed in detail in the last chapter of Part I. Since SD has been covered from a similar point of view in the earlier reviews by Roitbak (1955), Marshall (1959), Ochs (1962), Brinley (1963), and Van Harreveld (1966), the main stress is laid on new data, evidence unnoticed by the previous reviewers, and on the personal experience of the authors.

The second part of the book, extending and up-dating earlier reviews by Bureš (1962), Bureš and Burešová (1962, 1968c, 1970, 1972), Olds (1962), and Russell (1969), is the first attempt to survey the growing field of SD applications in neurophysiological and behavioral research. It concentrates on the theoretical principles and technical prerequisites of the proper use of the method, and describes in detail the results obtained and the interpretations suggested. Since the wide range of SD studies precludes a thorough discussion of the particular problems and favours descriptive rather than analytic approach, the reader is advised to consult the cited original publications and review articles for further information.

The experimental evidence reviewed in Part II raises more problems than it answers. Such a situation is typical for new areas of research, where well-reproducible facts have not yet been separated by systematic repetition from random observations and experimental mistakes. This is why we attempt to point out existing agreements and disagreements whenever possible. Still more striking is the fact of interpretational diversity, leaving many alternative explanations of the observed phenomena unnoticed and untested. Only in the last few years has it been attempted to explain some of the basic CSD findings on new assumptions (Schneider's generalization decrement hypothesis, Freedman's suggestion that residual learning proceeds in the depressed cortex). Even if not correct, challenging thoughts help to find the truth. It is obvious that many CSD features established by electrophysiological, biochemical, and morphological research are not adequately used to explain behavioral findings, the interpretation of which usually follows the most parsimonious and straightforward course. Another limiting factor is the novelty of the experimental possibilities offered by the reversibility of CSD. They cannot be fully exploited by investigators who are not prepared to deal with phenomena unprecedented in normal brain functions (for example parallel acquisition of engrams and transfer from decorticate to intact brain).

For all these reasons it can be expected that in the coming decade interest in the CSD technique and in other functional ablation procedures will grow, and that with further improvement such techniques may become important not only for research but perhaps also for diagnostic and therapeutic purposes.

The bulk of the original research described in this volume was completed in the Institute of Physiology of the Czechoslovak Academy of Sciences in Prague. We take this opportunity to thank all our former and present co-workers and colleagues who helped so much in preparing this book. We are particularly grateful to O. Benešová, V. Beran, Z. Bohdanecký, G. Brožek, E. Fifková, M. Janebová, P. Mareš, M. Rustová, J. Syka, T. Weiss, A. Záhorová, and D. Zacharová for important research contributions, to P. Hirš and V. Tůma for construction of electronic apparatus, and to J. Dufková, L. Jeřábková, V. Karpašová, V. Šilling and V. Vaněčková for expert technical assistance.

Many of our research projects were carried out with the participation of foreign visiting scientists. We wish to express our deep appreciation of the benefits derived from working with J. Aquino-Cias, H. Balinska, S. Belcheva, N. Freedman, L. Gaete Avaria, L. K. Gerbrandt, D. Goldowitz, W. Gutmann, G. Hartman, J. P. Huston, Kh. S. Koshtoyants, O. Kh. Koshtoyants, A. Koreli, I. B. Kozlovskaya, G. D. Kuznetsova, I. Lukaszewska, L. D. Lukyanova, A. M. Marusyeva, T. Matsuura, D. Megirian, K. K. Monakhov, L. Nadel, T. Ookawa, N. S. Popova, G. Rabending, E. Roldán,

R. B. Ross, W. Rüdiger, M. Shibata, I. Shima, V. B. Sokolov, B. F. Tolkunov, and C. D. Woody.

Throughout our work we profited very much from the stimulating contacts with the pioneers of SD research, A. A. P. Leão, W. H. Marshall, and A. Van Harreveld. We are also much indebted to V. L. Bianki, H. Caspers, G. Gerstein, C. Giurgea, B. Grafstein, A. V. Kholopov, M. Kukleta, H. Martins-Ferreira, S. Ochs, J. Olds, S. Norton, M. Petráň, A. I. Roytbak, M. Ruščák, I. S. Russell, A. M. Schneider, J. Sedláček, L. Sokoloff, F. D. Walker, and J. Zachar for stimulating discussion, valuable suggestions, technical advice, priority access to new information, or permission to use illustrations. Our special thanks are due to A. L. Hodgkin for the kind permission to reproduce his mathematical analysis of the SD phenomenon.

We are obliged to Academic Press, American Physiological Society, Editors of Brain, Elsevier Publishing Company and Wistar Press for the permission to reproduce figures from their publications; to Burroughs Welcome and Co., and UCB-DIPHA for supplying special drugs used in some of our experiments. Also the SD bibliography prepared by the UCLA Brain Information Service was of considerable help. Two of the research projects described in this book were partly supported by Foundations' Fund for Research in Psychiatry (Grants G 69-453 and 65-316).

Finally we should like to thank to the scientific editors, J. Myslivеček and Z. Servít, who carefully read the whole manuscript and gave invaluable advice, to the language editor J. Cort for correcting our English, to H. A. Buchtel and S. Rothenberg for efficient help with proof-reading, to V. Karpašová for most of the original illustrations and to E. Vojtášková for preparing the manuscript for the press.

Part I

Manifestations and Mechanism of Spreading Depression

Chapter 1

Electrical Properties of Spreading Depression

Spreading depression (SD) affects all basic types of electrical activity of the brain: spike activity of single neurons, synchronized synaptic potentials, and steady potentials generated by neurons or glia. The following paragraphs deal systematically with different electrical manifestations of SD stressing mainly recent findings, controversial problems, and interpretation of experimental evidence.

1. Spontaneous Electroencephalographic Activity

Depression of spontaneous electroencephalographic (EEG) activity, spreading at a rate of 3 mm/min across the cortical surface, accounts for the descriptive name of the phenomenon. At each cortical point the EEG decreases over approximately 30 sec to a level of maximum depression, which is maintained for 2 to 3 min. Recovery proceeds more slowly, the predepression amplitude of the EEG being asymptotically attained after 5 to 10 min. In Leão's (1944a) classical paper the EEG was recorded with a row of bipolar electrodes applied to the exposed pia-arachnoid surface of the rabbit brain but essentially similar results were also obtained in rats (Fig. 1.1) and in other animals and other neural structures (see Chap. 6). The EEG depression is most pronounced when recorded with electrode pairs, the interelectrode distance of which does not exceed the wavelength of SD (duration times velocity) and which are parallel to the front of the SD wave. In monopolar recording the depression is less pronounced because potentials are picked up from wider areas.

Typical EEG depression is obtained in animals under moderate barbiturate anesthesia, characterized by high-amplitude EEG and occasional "barbiturate spindles." During very deep anesthesia, or in unanesthetized aroused animals, the EEG amplitude is so low that it is not much affected by SD. This phenomenon can be detected by other signs, however.

Depression of the EEG is never complete. Some activity remains even at the height of the process and is probably due to (a) remote potentials from subcortical generators, (b) impulses coming through corticopetal pathways, and (c) in some cases incomplete depression of activity in deep cortical layers.

In addition to amplitude, the shape and frequency of the EEG is also affected by SD. The latter changes may occur in cortical regions not yet invaded by the actual depression, when elimination of a substantial part of the cortex affects the activity of the subcortical pacemaker and energizing centers and thus indirectly influences the remaining intact cortical regions. These mediated remote effects (see Chap. 8), usually characterized in anesthetized animals by a slowing of the EEG and suppression of spindling, can be easily differentiated from the local direct effects consisting of various signs of hyperactivity in the intervals immediately preceding and following the depression. Under certain conditions these symptoms are so enhanced that EEG depression is fully substituted by paroxysmal activity, which spreads over the cortical surface at the same rate (3 mm/min) as SD. Spreading depression may gradually change into "spreading convulsion" when repeatedly evoked at brief intervals (Whieldon and Van Harreveld 1950). Convulsion instead of depression appears in cortical regions topically treated with acetylcholine or pilocarpine (Van Harreveld and Stamm 1953c) when they are invaded by SD. Hypercapnia (7 to 15 % CO_2) has a similar effect. Al-

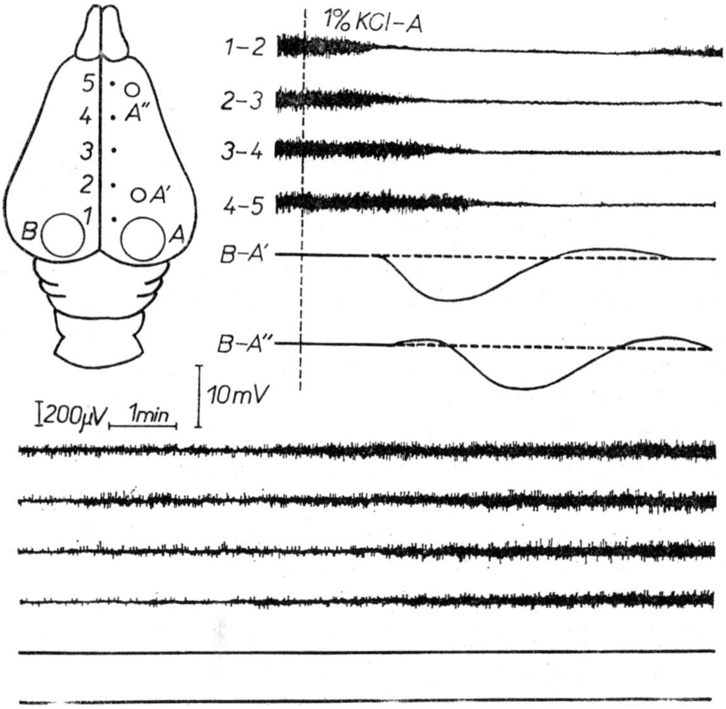

Fig. 1. 1. Cortical spreading depression in the rat. Position of electrodes indicated on the brain diagram. (1, 2, 3, 4, 5) Steel needle electrodes for EEG recording. *(A', A")* Trephine openings for application of wick calomel cell electrodes for slow potential recording. (A) Large trephine opening for application of KCl solution. (1—2, 2—3, 3—4, 4—5) Bipolar EEG recordings with the respective electrode pairs. *(B—A', B—A")* Slow potential recording from electrodes *(A')* and *(A")* against the common reference electrode situated in the contralateral hemisphere *(B)*. The upper and lower recordings are continous. Note that the onset of the negative SPC coincides with the onset of the EEG depression in the respective areas.

though the exact mechanism of spreading convulsions is not fully understood, it is obvious that the activity of some neural elements, especially in deep cortical layers, is not blocked. Selective depression of upper cortical layers may evoke transcortical steady potential gradients generating the convulsive activity.

2. Evoked Potentials

Whereas the variability of the spontaneous EEG prevents exact evaluation of depression, evoked potentials offer a better opportunity for quantitative measurement. Since these potentials are generated in circumscribed cortical areas, they have known afferent pathways and reproducible waveforms corresponding to definite intracortical dipoles.

Severe reduction or complete abolition of sensory evoked potentials and callosal responses during SD were first described by Leão (1944a). Both positive and negative components of the evoked responses are depressed for 2 to 3 min and recover predepression amplitudes by 5 to 7 min. The surface negative component of the response, representing the activity of the most superficial cortical layers, is usually the slowest to recover. The less regular late components of the evoked response appearing in unanesthetized animals are influenced for a longer period. When the averaging technique is used for their evaluation, complete recovery is often seen only after 20 to 30 min. In some evoked potentials it is possible to separate from the initial positivity a brief spikelike potential corresponding to the arrival of a highly synchronized volley of afferent impulses into the subcortical white matter and into the deep cortical layers. This potential, particularly prominent in cortical responses to single-shock stimulation of the optic nerve or optic radiation in the cat, is usually resistant to SD which abolishes all later components of the response (Marshall 1950). This component is also reduced by SD, however, when the cat cortex has been exposed for several hours to a Tyrode solution with K^+ concentration increased to 27 mEq/1 and when several SD waves have passed through the area of recording (Freygang and Landau 1955, Marshall 1959).

In a slightly different way SD affects the direct cortical response evoked by electrical stimulation of an adjacent cortical area (Grafstein 1956a, Ochs 1958, Ochs and Hunt 1960). The surface positive component of the response is usually depressed longer than the negative one, full recovery being attained after approximately 5 min in the isolated cortical slab in the cat (Grafstein 1956a) and after approximately 10 min in the intact rabbit cortex (Ochs 1958). The early spikelike component of the direct cortical response, which is believed to be generated by activation of afferent fibers, was also briefly depressed at the height of SD (Ochs, Hunt, and Booker 1961). The direct cortical response is affected by CSD not only at the recording site but also in the stimulated region. Ichijo and Ochs (1970) succeeded in separating both effects by surgical and pharmacological means. When CSD was confined to the area of stimulation, block of axons directly affected by the electrical stimulus lasted for 2 min. Cortical SD restricted to the responding region caused a more prolonged suppression (3 to 13 min),

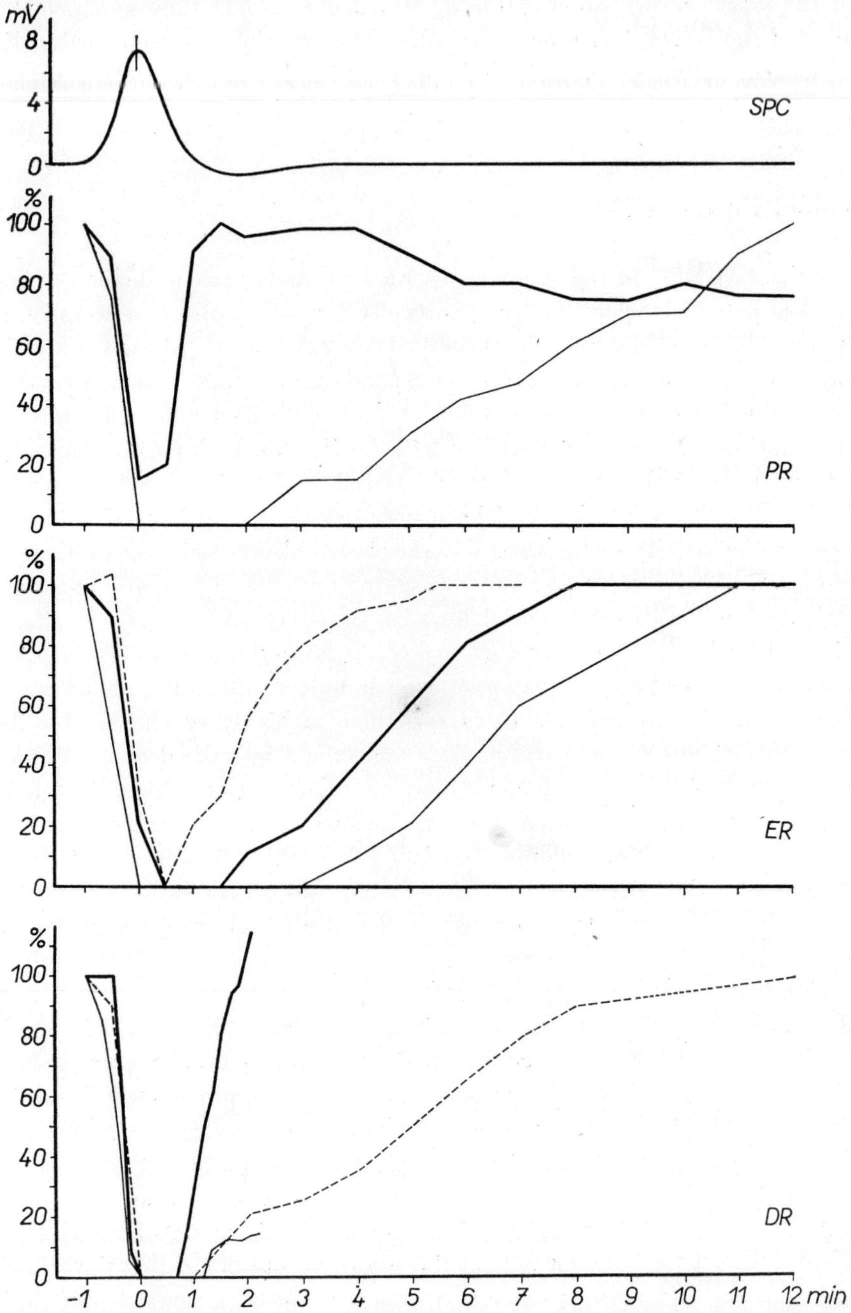

Fig. 1. 2. The effect of CSD on cortical evoked potentials. Zero of the time scale corresponds to the maximum negativity of the schematic SPC in the area of recording. Amplitude of the respective component of the evoked potential expressed as percentage of the predepression amplitude. *(PR)*

probably due to interference with the function of dendrites. Evoked responses in the motor cortex elicited by antidromic stimulation of the pyramidal tract were shown to be depressed by mechanical stimulation of the cortex, which evidently elicited SD (Chang 1955). This finding was confirmed by Bureš, Hartman and Lukyanova (1967) who recorded the antidromically evoked pyramidal responses in the motor cortex of rats. The time course of the above changes is summarized in Fig. 1. 2.

3. Slow Potentials

In 1947 Leão described the most characteristic sign of SD, the slow potential change (SPC) accompanying the advancing front of EEG depression. This consists of a surface negative wave attaining 5 to 15 mV in amplitude, followed after 1 to 2 min by a less pronounced, but longer lasting positivity (Fig. 1.1). Sometimes a small positive wave may precede the negative potential, thus completing a triphasic waveform typical for a moving dipole in a volume conductor. Recording from different depths of the cortex by semimicroelectrodes indicated (Leão 1961, Grafstein 1956b, Monakhov, Fifková, and Bureš 1962a, Ichijo and Ochs 1970) that the negative slow potential invaded all cortical layers, the superficial ones about 20 sec earlier than the deep ones. The amplitude of the intracortical SPC depended on the size of the capillary electrodes. With fine tips it may reach 30 to 40 mV. Positivity in deep cortical layers accompanying the main negative wave at the surface was found only exceptionally in cats (Muñoz-Martinez 1970). The large positive slow potentials (up to 250 mV) recorded under similar conditions with platinized indium electrodes (Rosenblueth, Garcia Ramos, and Nims 1967) are due to the electrochemical properties of the metal electrode (Garcia Ramos and Pradáč 1968) and reflect changes in the local concentration of metabolic products (Huizar Sánchez and Garcia Ramos 1969) rather than field potentials. It appears that the current source corresponding to the focal negativity in the cortex must be sought in distant parts of the corticofugal axons (Marshall 1959, Monakhov, Fifková, and Bureš 1962a, Collewijn and Van Harreveld 1966) which give rise to a widely distributed electric field that easily escapes detection. Small intracortical neurons with short axons are less important for slow potential generation because they only form short lasting weak dipoles of random orientation. A possible role of glia in the slow potential generation is discussed elsewhere (p. 147).

Responses evoked in the rabbit motor cortex by antidromic stimulation of the bulbar pyramids. Heavy line is the surface positive component; thin line is the late negative component (Chang 1955). *(ER)* Responses evoked in the rat somatosensory cortex by sciatic shocks (heavy line is the surface positive; thin line is the surface negative component) or in the cat visual cortex by flashes (dashed line is total response amplitude; Freygang and Landau 1955). *(DR)* Responses evoked by direct electrical stimulation in isolated slab of cat cortex (heavy line is the surface negative; thin line is the surface positive component; Grafstein 1956a) or in the intact rabbit cortex (dashed line; Ochs 1962).

The negative SPC also accompanies SD evoked in other structures (see Chap. 6). At all sites it has approximately the same spatiotemporal characteristics, indicating a remarkable uniformity of the underlying mechanisms.

4. Unit Activity

Grafstein (1956a) using semimicroelectrodes demonstrated that the onset of EEG depression is accompanied by a discharge of unit activity lasting for a few seconds and followed by prolonged inhibition. More systematic studies using extracellular recording from well-isolated units in the cerebral cortex of rats (Burešová, Shima, Bureš, and Fifková 1963), cats (Morlock, Mori, and Ward 1964), rabbits (Johnson, Goldring, and O'Leary 1965) and in the striatum of pigeons (Burešová, Shima, Bureš, and Fifková 1963) essentially confirmed Grafstein's results: a burst of high-frequency impulse activity lasting for 2 to 5 sec abruptly changed into complete silence lasting for 1 to 2 min and followed by slow recovery to the predepression firing rate, which was usually attained after 5 to 7 min (Fig. 1.3). The initial discharge is often preceded by short reduction of activity (Morlock, Mori, and Ward 1964) due to elimination of an excitatory influx from the cortical areas already depressed and/or to the decreased effectiveness of presynaptic structures slightly depolarized by the approaching SD wave. The striking silence accompanying SD was also reported by Krnjevič, Randič, and Straughan (1966), Dubner and Brown (1968), Gartside (1968), Li and Salmoiraghi (1963), Rosenblueth and García (1966), Goldensohn, Escueta, and Runk (1967) and can be considered a well-established fact. It seems that not a single neuron remains active in the area invaded by SD during the height of the negativity. In deep layers of cat cerebral cortex (Muñoz-Martinez 1970) which are not invaded by the SPC, depression of unit activity becomes less prominent, whereas the initial acceleration of firing rate is markedly prolonged.

Slightly different results were obtained with evoked unit activity. Whereas responses to an orthodromic input were blocked with a similar time course as the spontaneous activity, antidromically activated Betz cells displayed a steady attenuation of both the initial segment and somatodendritic spikes up to complete blockade persisting for 10 to 20 sec. The initial segment spike then started to recover and was followed by intermittent and considerably delayed somatodendritic invasion (Morlock, Mori, and Ward 1964). The changes were completed within 1 min and closely corresponded to the time course of the SPC. Reversible blockade of the antidromically activated Betz cells by CSD was confirmed by Ichijo and Ochs (1967, 1970) who found the response depressed for 1.5 min on the average.

Krnjević and Randić (1965) and Phillis and Ochs (1971) tested the response of nerve cells to microelectrophoretically administered glutamate during different phases of the SD effect. The unit was unresponsive to the amino acid during the silent interval following the initial burst but could be activated in a nearly normal manner after

1 to 2 min, that is, at a time when its spontaneous activity was still markedly depressed. The slow recovery of spontaneous unit activity is not due, therefore, to slow restitution of the postsynaptic threshold, but rather to changes in the presynaptic structures. Krnjević, Randić, and Straughan (1966) suggested that the late phase of unit activity blockade is at least partly due to a hyperpolarizing type of inhibition, perhaps due to conversion of glutamic acid, released during SD, into the depressant gamma-aminobutyric acid (Phillis and Ochs 1971).

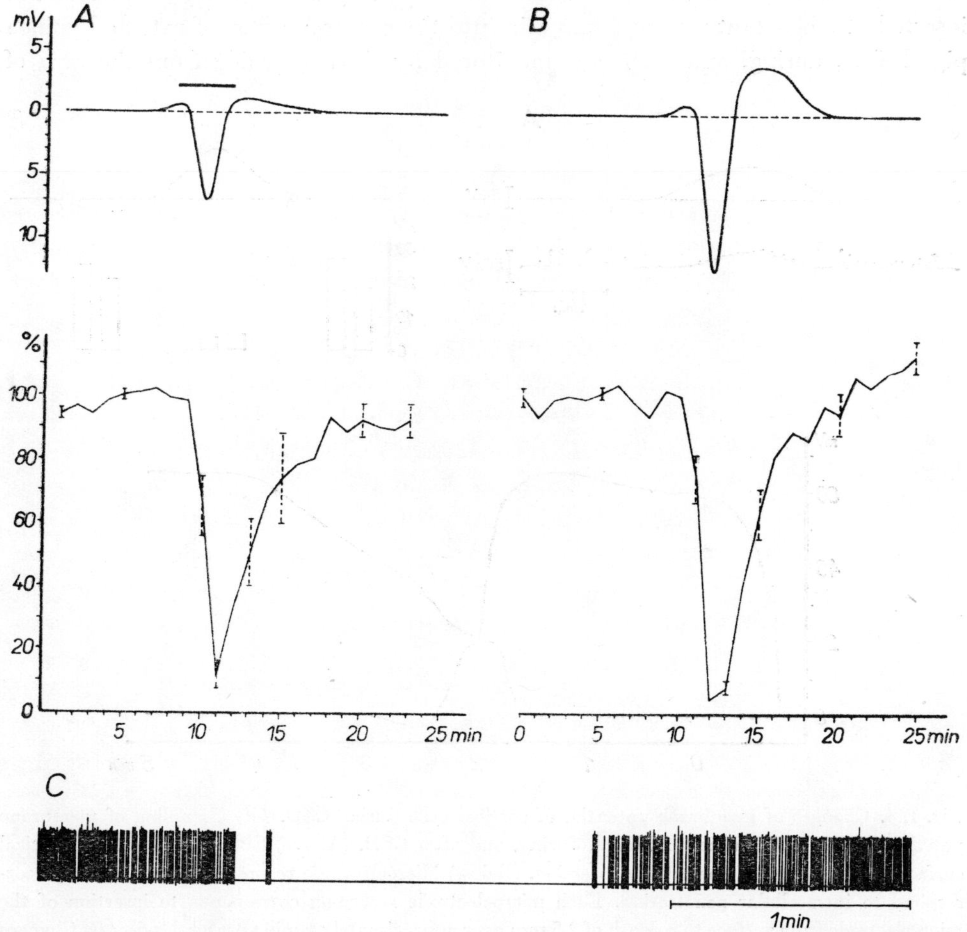

Fig. 1. 3. Changes of spontaneous unit activity during spreading depression. Average change of firing rate in 11 neurons in rat cerebral cortex *(A)* and 15 neurons in pigeon striatum *(B)*. Individual recordings are synchronized with respect to the maximum negativity of the simultaneously recorded SPC (above). The changes are expressed in percentages of the predepression activity (below). The integration interval is 1 min. Vertical dotted bars indicate the standard errors of the mean values (Burešová, Shima, Bureš, and Fifková 1963). *(C)* Typical example of changes of cortical unit activity during CSD. Horizontal bar above the SPC recording in *(A)* indicates the location of the sample. Note the brief initial silence preceding the burst.

5. Membrane Potentials

Whereas the experimental evidence reviewed in the preceding paragraphs indicates a widespread depolarization of neural elements during the negative SPC of SD, technical difficulties delayed a direct proof of this assumption. Brožek (1966) used the sampling method of membrane-potential measurement, developed by Li and McIlwain (1957), to avoid problems connected with prolonged intracellular recording. He measured all penetration potentials encountered by the capillary microelectrode inserted at a constant rate of 2 mm/min into the cerebral cortex of rats and guinea pigs before, during, and after SD, monitored by SPC recording from the area of

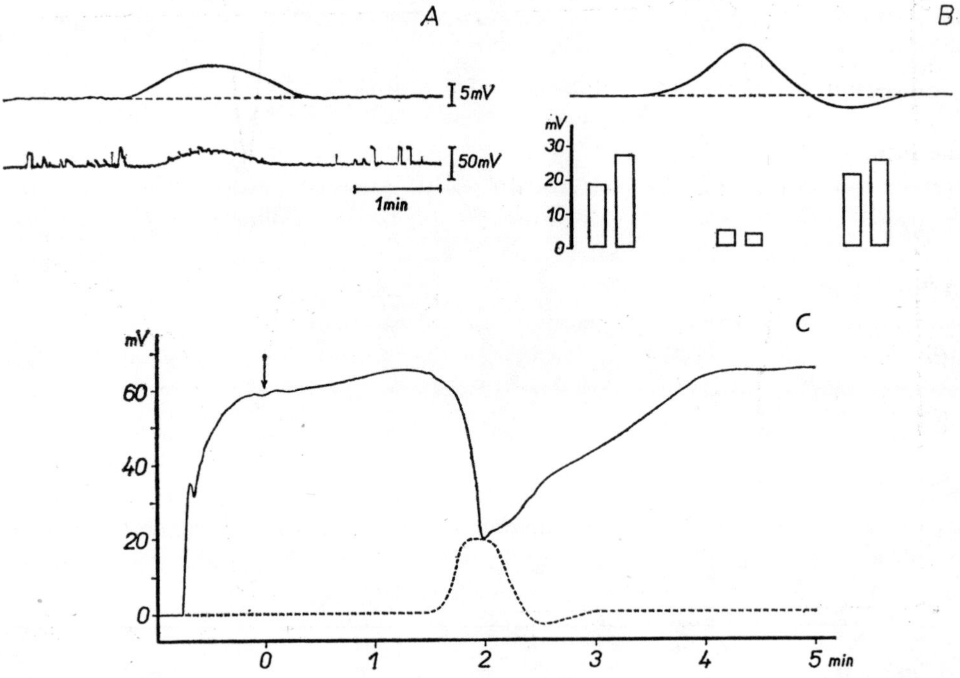

Fig. 1. 4. Changes of membrane potential of cortical cells during CSD. *(A)* Sampling of membrane potentials in rat cerebral cortex before, during, and after CSD. (Above) SPC recording from cortical surface at the site of microelectrode insertion. (Below) Microelectrode recording; potential jumps correspond to intracellular penetration. Each microelectrode recording corresponds to insertion of the microelectrode from surface to a depth of 2.5 mm over approximately 1 min (Brožek 1966). *(B)* Changes of the average membrane potential of cortical cells in rats (left columns) and guinea pigs (right columns) during CSD. The mean values were corrected by taking into account the number of cells depolarized below 5 mV. (Above) Cortical SPC (Brožek 1966). (C) Rabbit cerebral cortex. Solid line shows the intracellular potential variation in a soma during passage of SD that was initiated at a distance of 3 mm from the microelectrode at time 0 (arrow). Dotted line shows the potential changes just outside this cell during a second SD. The intra- and extracellular potentials (mV) are plotted on the ordinate as negativity with respect to the indifferent electrode. Abscissa: time in min (Collewijn and Van Harreveld 1966).

penetration. Although the method cannot distinguish between neurons and glial cells, the average membrane potential was found to be reduced during the negative potential of SD to about 20 % of control values (Fig. 1.4).

Collewijn and Van Harreveld (1966) succeeded in recording membrane potentials in 14 cortical cells throughout the period of depression. The mean membrane potential dropped to 35 % of the original value during maximum depolarization. As the membrane potential was measured against a remote referent electrode, the measurements have to be corrected for the extracellular SPC (Fig. 1.4), which is picked up by the microelectrode even when it enters the cell and causes an apparent hyperpolarization. The corrected membrane potentials were considerably lower, approaching zero in most cases. The change of the membrane potential has a different time course than the extracellular SPC: abrupt depolarization is followed by a prolonged plateau and slow recovery.

Karahashi and Goldring (1966) succeeded to hold 6 "idle" cells (probably glia) in the cat cerebral cortex during the negative SPC. Spreading depression shifted the intracellular potential by 20 to 40 mV positive, but no attempt was made to correct this change for the extracellular SPC. Assuming extracellular negativity of approximately 30 mV, intracellular recording indicates an almost complete depolarization. Higashida, Miyake, Tarao, and Watanabe (1971) obtained similar results in 11 neuroglial cells in the rabbit cortex.

Intracellular recording in the cat cerebral cortex during SD was also reported by Rosenblueth and Garcia-Rámos (1966). As their membrane potentials were small (around 20 mV) and the extracellular SPC in the superficial layers relatively high (negativity up to 25 mV), the statement that "the responses recorded intracellularly had usually the same sign as, and were smaller than those recorded extracellularly" indicates considerable depolarization at least in the upper cortical layers. Depolarization of cortical neurons was demonstrated by Goldensohn and Walsh (1968) who found a rough correlation between intracellularly recorded SPC and the changes of excitability, synaptic potentials, and frequency of firing.

6. Impedance Changes

Besides affecting active electrogenesis, SD also influences the passive electrical properties of the depressed neural tissue. Increase of cortical impedance during SD in the rabbit was first described by Leão and Martins-Ferreira (1953). Using a bridge arrangement and sinusoidal measuring current in the range of 0.05 to 10 kHz and with a platinum electrode applied to pia and the referent electrode on bone, they found an impedance increase from 2070 to 2940 ohms when the active electrode region was invaded by SD (Fig. 1.5). The impedance change closely followed the slow potential variation. Van Harreveld and Ochs (1957) measured cortical impedance between two Ag - AgCl discs (1 to 2 mm in diameter) placed on the rabbit cortex

3 to 4 mm apart. At 1000 Hz, SD decreased cortical conductivity by 17 % (Fig. 1. 5). Weiss, Kado, and Adey (1966) obtained a slightly higher change using smaller electrodes in the rat. In all these studies both the resistive and capacitive components of impedance increased but the former influenced the overall change in a decisive way. Sometimes SPC was observed without the corresponding impedance shift indicating the possible dissociation of the two phenomena. Although the bridge method gives reproducible relative data, the complex current path involving both cortex and subcortical structures prevents a more accurate interpretation of results.

Changes of specific impedance were studied by Freygang and Landau (1955) who used constant current pulses to generate a field with parallel lines of flux normal

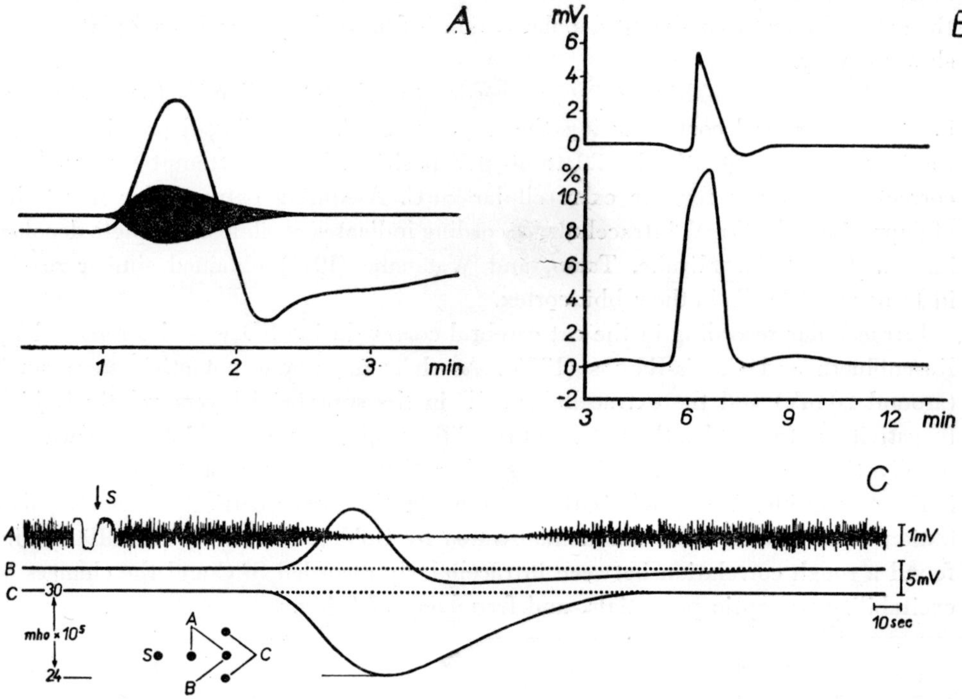

Fig. 1. 5. Impedance changes accompanying CSD. *(A)* Simultaneous recording of impedance change and of SPC during CSD in the rabbit. The bridge circuit equilibrium, established before CSD onset, was disturbed during SPC as indicated by the measuring frequency appearing across the bridge terminals. Abscissa: time from CSD initiation in min (Leão and Martins-Ferreira 1953). *(B)* Transcortical SPC (above) and percent increase in transcortical resistivity (below) during CSD in cat. Abscissa: time after CSD initiation (Freygang and Landau 1955). *(C)* Electrocorticogram (*A*), SPC record *(B)*, and conductivity change *(C*; mho · 10^5*)* during CSD in the rabbit. The cortex is stimulated at *S* (4 Volts dc). In the inset are the positions of the stimulating electrode *(S)*, the electrodes for leading off the electrocorticogram *(A)*, and the slow potential change *(B)* as well as the electrodes for resistance measurement *(C)*. Calibration: 1 mV for ECoG; 5 mV for SPC; conductivity scale from 24 to 30 mho · 10^5 (Van Harreveld and Ochs 1957).

to the cerebral surface and measured potential differences in this field between two capillary electrodes inserted to different depths of the cortex. The specific resistance of the cat cortex (222 ohm cm) increased during SD by 10 to 20 % (Fig. 1. 5), the increase being most marked in the superficial cortical layers. Impedance of the subcortical white matter decreased at the same time by approximately 5 %. Ranck (1964) established the specific impedance of rabbit cerebral cortex by passing sinusoidal currents (5 to 50 000 Hz) between a platinum electrode on the cortical surface and a remote indifferent electrode. The potential difference of two similar electrodes placed within 1.3 mm of the current electrode was recorded and displayed together with current in the form of Lissajous figures on a cathode-ray oscilloscope. During SD specific impedance increased from 250 to 400 ohm cm and the phase angle from 3.5 to 7.0 degrees at 5000 Hz, whereas at 50 Hz a similar impedance increase (from 300 to 500 ohm cm) was accompanied by a phase angle decrease from 6 to 0 degrees. Asynchronous changes of impedance and phase angle during SD in the cat cerebral cortex were reported by Wong (1969).

Chapter 2

Initiation of Spreading Depression

1. Electrical Stimuli

In the classical experiments by Leão (1944a) cortical spreading depression (CSD) was evoked in the rabbit by 1 to 5 sec of faradic stimulation of the cerebral cortex. Impulse trains lasting for 5 to 10 sec at rates from 10/sec to 50/sec were also used by Marshall (1950), Grafstein (1956a), and Ochs, Hunt, and Booker (1961). Cortical SD was usually evoked at stimulus intensities just subthreshold for eliciting an afterdischarge. Since the possible spread of convulsive activity from the stimulated area may considerably complicate the evaluation of results, most authors prefer to elicit CSD by dc stimuli (Leão and Morrison 1945, Van Harreveld and Stamm 1953a, Bureš 1954a,b, Ochs 1962). The threshold current levels vary between 0.1 and 3.0 mA and the cathode is slightly more effective than the anode. Since galvanic stimuli produce no afterdischarge, their effect can be explained in different ways. Surface negative polarization evokes asymmetric changes of membrane potentials in the radially oriented cortical elements characterized by depolarization of apical dendrites and a resulting release of K^+. Surface positive polarization causes hyperpolarization of apical dendrites, but the current entering the neuron at this level leaves it again through its deeper parts, that is, through the soma or axon-hillock area. Depolarization of this region generates intense activity (Purpura and McMurtry 1965, Gorman 1967). Higher densities of direct current cause injury irrespective of polarity.

Application of dc stimuli for exact threshold estimation has many drawbacks. The effect depends not on current intensity but on current density in the stimulated cortical region. When using wick Ag-AgCl electrodes, the contact surface is often poorly defined. The varying layer of cerebrospinal fluid, the conductivity of which exceeds the conductivity of cortical tissue several times, also contributes to the high variability of dc thresholds.

2. Mechanical Stimuli

The possibility of evoking CSD by mechanical stimuli was also reported by Leão (1944a). Stroking of the cortical surface with a blunt instrument, or even slightly touching the sensitive cortex during application of electrodes or drugs, may elicit

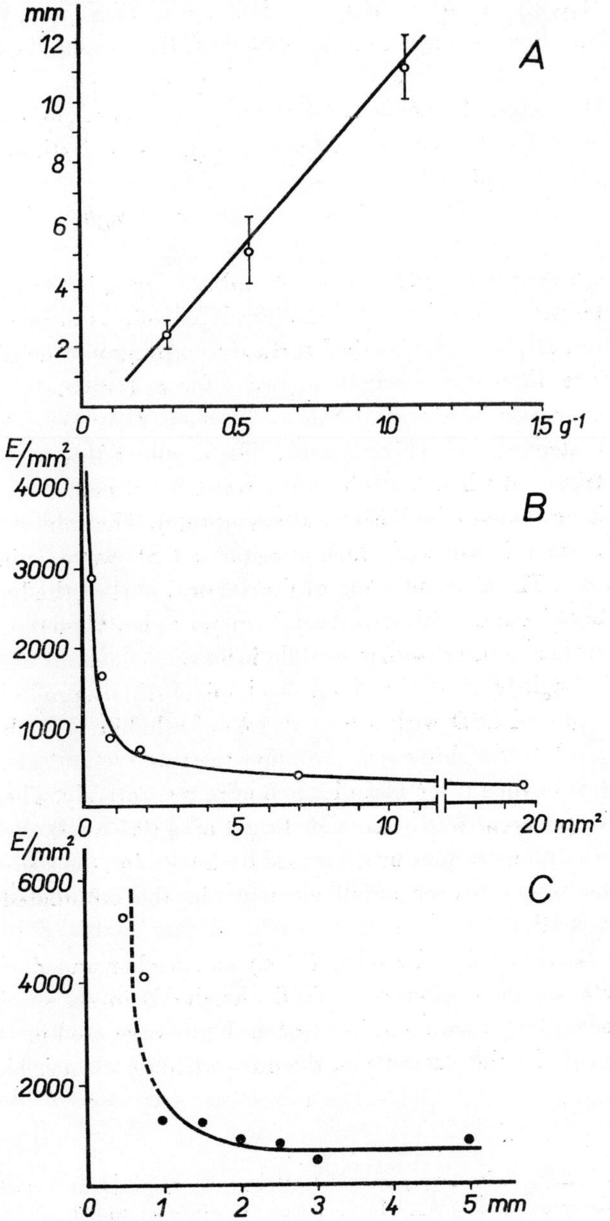

Fig. 2. 1. Some properties of the mechanical stimuli eliciting CSD in rats (Zachar and Zacharová 1963). *(A)* Linear relationship between the threshold height of free fall (ordinate) and the reciprocal mass of the stimulus body (abscissa). Stimulated area, 1.76 mm^2; penetration depth, 1.5 mm. *(B)* Relationship between the stimulated cortical area (abscissa) and threshold density of the kinetic energy (erg mm^{-2}; ordinate). Stimulus mass, 3.76 grams, penetration depth, 1.5 mm. *(C)* Relationship between the penetration depth (abscissa) and threshold density of kinetic energy (erg mm^{-2}; ordinate). Stimulus mass 3.76 grams, stimulated area 1.76 mm^2.

a wave of CSD. Such incidental mechanical initiation of CSD must be carefully avoided in all experiments involving the manipulation of exposed brain. The parameters of mechanical stimuli were systematically studied by Zachar and Zacharová (1961a, b, 1962, 1963). In their basic experiments they elicited CSD in rats by the impact of a falling body on the exposed cortical surface covered by dura. Provided that the mass of the falling body, area of impact, maximum cortical deformation, and time of contact remain constant, the threshold can be expressed by the minimum height of free fall. Experimental manipulation with the above factors proved that the threshold height is directly proportional to the reciprocal value of the mass (Fig. 2.1 A), which indicates that the actual stimulus is the energy E determined by the equation,

$$E = mgh$$

where m is the mass of the stimulus body, g is the gravitation constant, and h is the height of free fall. The above relationship is only valid, however, when the falling rod displaces the cortical surface to a minimum depth of 1.0 to 1.5 mm (Fig. 2.1 C). The threshold energy is minimal for rod diameters 0.5 to 1.0 mm. The threshold expressed as energy per unit of surface (E/mm^2) is a hyperbolic function of the stimulated surface (Fig. 2.1 B). The shape of this curve suggests that SD can only be triggered when a minimum percentage of neural elements in the stimulated region is activated (the horizontal asymptote). The minimum volume of cortex, the maximum activation of which can start a CSD wave, is indicated by the vertical asymptote. The exact plotting of the vertical part of the hyperbola is impossible, however, because rods with a contact diameter of less than 0.5 mm may easily pierce the brain surface and cause irreversible injury.

Slightly suprathreshold mechanical stimuli produced reversible effects and elicited repeated CSD with a high degree of reliability. Zachar and Zacharová (1961a) used the latter technique to examine the relative and absolute refractory periods, which last in the rat for 14 and 2 to 3 min, respectively. The above times apply to 1.75 mm^2 target area. With a smaller target area (0.5 mm^2) the duration of the relative refractory phase cannot be decreased by increasing the stimulus energy (Fig. 2. 2), probably because recovery of all elements in the stimulated region is necessary for CSD initiation.

Zacharová and Zachar (1966) and Zachar and Zacharová (1962) used mechanical stimuli for comparison of SD thresholds in six species of laboratory animals. The same target area and immersion depth were used in all animals and corrections were made for the elasticity of the dura when necessary. The lowest thresholds were found

---

Fig. 2. 2. Refractory phase of CSD in rats examined by repeated mechanical stimuli (Zachar and Zacharová 1961a). *(A)* Incidence of SD with test stimuli of different intensity (t, dots; $t+5$, circles; $t+10$, crosses); t is the value of the threshold stimulus in millimeters of free fall at different times after application of the conditioning stimulus (abscissa). Stimulated cortical area, 1.76 mm^2; stimulus mass, 3.76 grams; penetration depth, 1.5 mm. *(B)* Same as *(A)* but stimulated cortical area 0.44 mm^2. *(C)* Relative refractory period of CSD expressed as the increment of the mechanical stimulus (millimeters above threshold) needed to elicit CSD in 100 % cases (ordinate). Time after conditioning stimulus on the abscissa. Stimulated cortical area, 1.76 mm^2; stimulus mass, 3.76 grams; penetration depth, 1.5 mm.

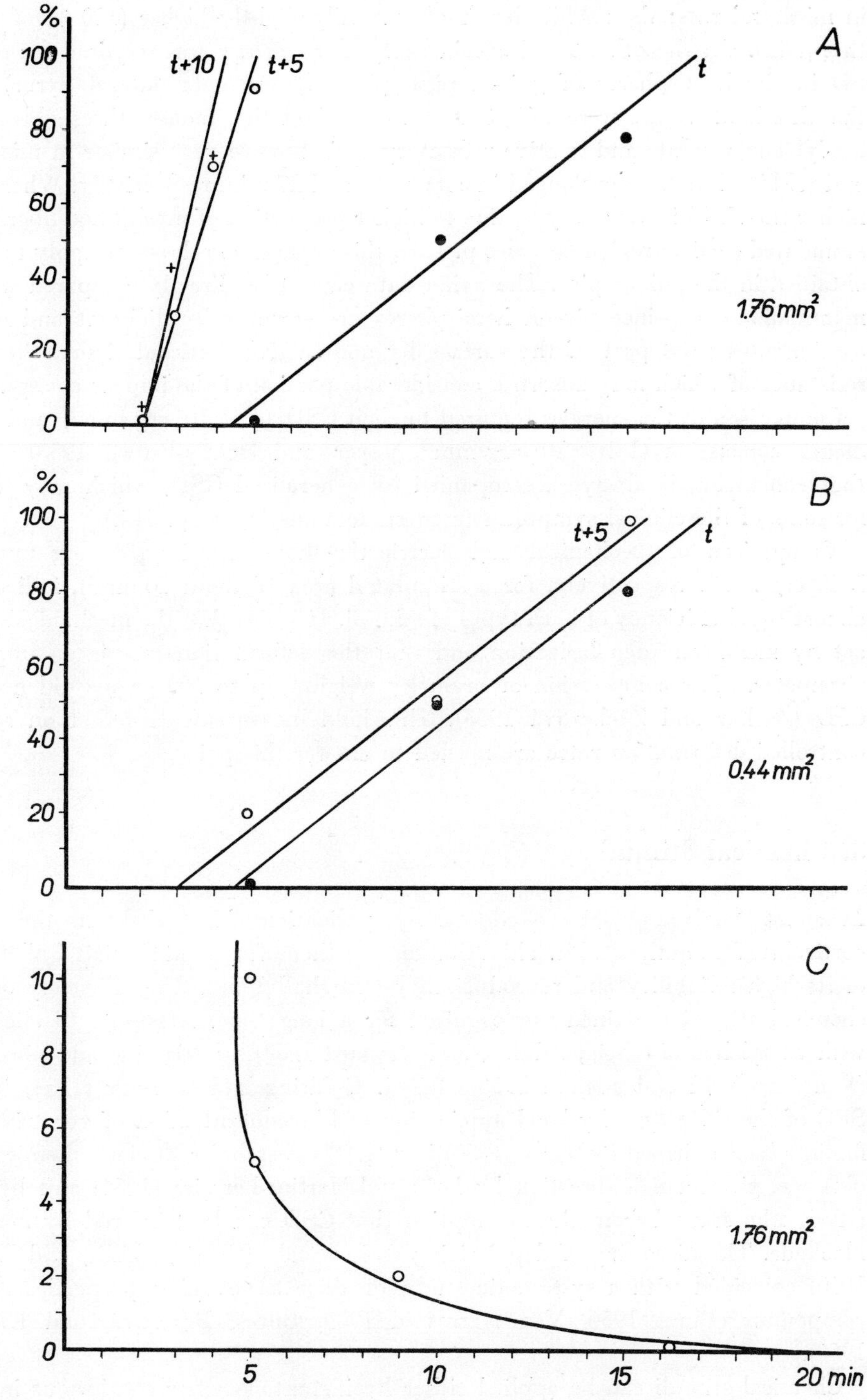
%
100
80
60
40
20
0
t+10
t+5
t
A
1.76 mm²
%
100
80
60
40
20
0
t+5
t
B
0.44 mm²
10
8
6
4
2
0
C
1.76 mm²
5
10
15
20 min

in mice and rats; the rabbit threshold was only slightly higher (120 % of the rat threshold). On the other hand considerably more energy was required for evoking SD in the hemispheres of guinea pigs, pigeons, and cats (lateral gyrus) where the threshold values were 250, 310 and 400 % of the mouse threshold, respectively. The absolute and relative refractory periods were very similar in mice, rats, and rabbits, but were prolonged in cats to 12 and 27 min, respectively. Whereas the higher threshold in cats may be due to higher proportion of myelinated fibers in the stimulated cortical region (see also p. 147), this explanation does not apply to results obtained in the guinea pigs. The avian data cannot be directly compared with the mammalian ones, since pigeon hemispheres are structurally different and covered over a substantial part of the surface by nonreactive corticoid tissue, the elastic resistance of which may absorb a considerable portion of the impact energy.

Comparison of the energies required to elicit CSD (4×10^2 erg mm^{-2}) and experimental concussion (1.2×10^5 erg mm^{-2}, Meyer and Denny-Brown 1955) confirms that concussion is always accompanied by generalized CSD, which may account for some of the clinical symptoms (retrograde amnesia, see p. 315.)

Comparison of mechanical and electric threshold energies (350 erg mm^{-2} and 1000 erg mm^{-2}, respectively, for a stimulated area of about 10 mm^2), indicates an almost equal efficiency of both types of stimuli. It seems that the mechanical stimuli act by membrane depolarization and that the deformation rate is an important parameter. Slow compression of brain by weights up to 100 grams did not elicit CSD (Zachar and Zacharová 1963). Threshold measurements based on solenoid controlled deformation rates are needed to answer this point.

3. Chemical Stimuli

Leão and Morrison (1945) evoked CSD by application of 1 % KCl onto the exposed cortical surface in the rabbit. This stimulus was then often used to elicit CSD because of its high reliability and reproducibility (Marshall 1959). The efficiency of other chemical stimuli remained unrecognized for a long time. Attempts to elicit CSD with acetylcholine (Essig, Adkins, and Barnard 1953), prostigmine and pilocarpine (Van Harreveld and Stamm 1953c) failed. Goldring and O'Leary (1954) induced SPC of the CSD type by local application of low concentration of veratrine. This finding was confirmed by Bureš (1956) in rats. The search for efficient chemical stimulus was given a new direction by Leão and Martins-Ferreira (1954) and by Bureš (1956) who started from the assumption that CSD can be triggered by metabolic blockade. The discovery of depolarizing amino acids (Curtis, Phillis, and Watkins 1960) coincided with a systematic study of the CSD-evoking properties of these compounds (Bureš 1956, Van Harreveld 1959, Bureš, Burešová, and Křivánek 1960).

Chemical stimuli can be applied either by instantaneous or continuous injection

(Curtis 1964). Whereas in the first case the focus simultaneously expands in space and decays in time, in the second case a more or less steady concentration gradient is established. Application of drugs onto the cortical surface combines both above modes, but over short time intervals it rather resembles continuous injection. As the bulk of data has been obtained with this technique, it will be considered first.

The basic parameter of a chemical stimulus is the surface concentration of the applied solution, which plays an important role in determining the depth of the transcortical concentration gradient. On the other hand the effect is independent of the amount of the solution, provided that a certain minimum volume has been exceeded. Application of a filter paper or a cotton pledget soaked with the solution has approximately the same initial effect as flooding the exposed cortical region.

An important variable is the area of contact. Thresholds measured over an area of 15 to 20 mm^2 are increased by 35 % when the contact surface is reduced to 7 mm^2 (Bureš 1962). Although no systematic measurements are available, the threshold seems to increase further with smaller openings, the relationship probably being similar to that found in mechanical stimuli.

In some respects chemical stimuli resemble electrical and mechanical ones, however, they are distinguished by their protracted action. The substance applied onto the cortical surface gradually penetrates into the cerebral tissue. The resulting gradient depends on the surface concentration (which can be assumed constant over a short period), on the diffusion coefficient of the substance, and on the rate of its removal into the blood stream. The steepness of the vertical gradient cannot be easily established, but radial measurements indicate that the subthreshold effects subside rather abruptly over a distance of approximately 1 mm.

Vertical distribution of K^+ after 15 min of subarachnoid perfusion with 40 mM KCl was established by Pape and Katzman (1972a) in the cat anterior sylvian gyrus. The specific activity of the tracer (^{42}K) dropped from 100 % at the surface to 50 % and 10 % at the depth of 1.0 and 2.5 mm, respectively. The gradient was somewhat less steep after 1 hr perfusion (65 % and 25 % at 1.0 and 2.5 mm, respectively). In another paper, Pape and Katzman (1972b) recorded membrane potentials of glia cells at different depths during the first 2 min of perfusion. A cell 10 μ deep reached maximum depolarization after 13 sec, whereas a cell at 380 μ required about 2 min to approximate the new plateau. The calculated extracellular K^+ level after a 2-min perfusion approached 50 % of the surface concentration already at the depth of 400 μ. An analogous method was employed by Gibson and McIlwain (1965), who recorded membrane potentials of incubated cortical slices after addition of 1 μl of 0.1 to 0.5 M KCl to the slice surface. Good agreement was found between the observed course of depolarization and the calculations based on K^+ diffusion from an instantaneous planar surface source to the intracortical point of recording.

A steep concentration profile of K^+ was directly measured with potassium selective microelectrodes in rat cerebral cortex washed for 1 to 2 min with 40 mM KCl (Gerstein and Bureš, unpublished results). Egorov and Kuznetsova (1972) measured the impedance of the cerebral tissue at different depths below the cortical surface, treated with 10 to 25 % KCl. The high impedance zone was about 0.5 mm thick. It was surrounded by a narrow region of slow impedance oscillations, which triggered the individual SD waves.

The rate of removal is proportional to the concentration and can be estimated by measuring the radioactivity decay of a known amount of labeled compound applied onto the cortical surface. For about 5 mg of KCl solution applied onto a 4 mm trephine opening the ^{42}K activity decreased with a biological half time of about 40 min (Burešová 1956). Needless to say, local application of substances must prevent tangential spread of the solution over the cortex. This is simple in rats, where the brain is usually tightly pressed against the edges of the trephine opening, but may be a serious problem in animals with wide epidural and/or subdural spaces (rabbit, cat).

The protracted action accounts for another peculiarity of chemical stimuli, that is, generation of repeated CSD waves by a single application of suprathreshold concentrations of the active agent. Such stimuli establish a focus, the center of which is fully depolarized. Cortical SD waves are generated at the periphery of the focus, where the concentration of the depolarizing substance approaches threshold. After each SD wave, neurons in the threshold zone pass through a sequence of absolute and relative refractoriness and can be depolarized again by the threshold stimulus only when sufficiently recovered. Interwave intervals of 2 to 4 min seen with highly suprathreshold stimuli (25 % KCl) correspond well with the duration of the absolute refractory period established by Zachar and Zacharová (1961a).

With the gradual removal of the drug the depolarized area shrinks and so does the surrounding liminal zone, the diminution of which correlates with the prolongation of the interwave interval. As the liminal zone slowly retreats toward the center of the focus, it contains more and more injured neurons, which do not actively contribute to the CSD process. Therefore, when the concentration gradient does not extend beyond the damaged region, generation of the SPCs stops even when the surface concentration of the drug is still above threshold (Fig. 2.3).

Cutting or removing the dura may cause brain edema in rats and mice (Beránek, Fantiš, and Gutmann 1955). Since application of test solution onto the altered tissue

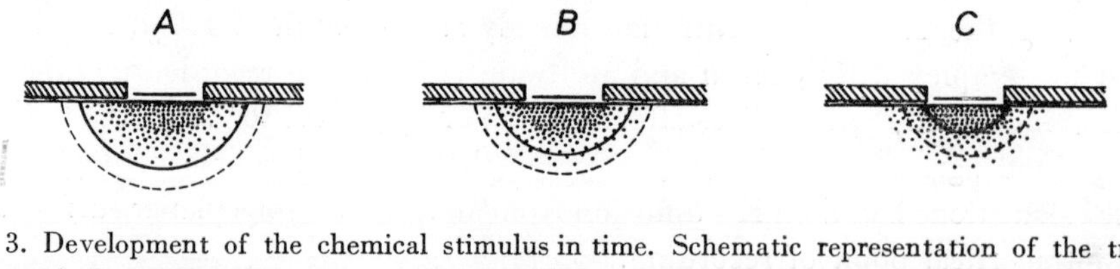

Fig. 2. 3. Development of the chemical stimulus in time. Schematic representation of the trephine opening with the applied filter paper and the underlying cortex. Damage due to the action of hypertonic KCl solution indicated by stippling of decreasing density. Threshold zone (between the full and dashed circular lines) is located at the undamaged periphery of the focus at first *(A)* but gradually retreats into the damaged tissue *(B* and *C)*. For details see text.

will give erroneous results, drugs are usually applied onto the intact dura in rats. In young animals the dura is permeable for most drugs used for CSD initiation. In rats aged 5 to 6 months the thickening dura acts as a diffusion barrier which increases the threshold concentration of epidurally applied substances. Diffusion is limited in a similar way by arachnoid membrane in cats (Pape and Katzman 1972b).

The technique of threshold estimation is important when data obtained in different studies are to be compared. Most reliable is determination of the ED_{50} concentration, that is, of a concentration that elicits SD in 50 % of the cases. The procedure should always go from lower to higher concentrations with an interval of at least 20 to 30 min between applications. It is desirable that the concentrations used form a geometrical sequence covering the whole range from subthreshold to supramaximal stimuli in four to six steps. Probit analysis (Finney 1950) or the moving average method (Weil 1952) was used in the actual calculation of ED_{50} and its standard deviation. In other studies (Van Harreveld 1959) threshold was defined as the lowest concentration that elicits CSD in each hemisphere. Accuracy of this method depends on the width of the step separating the threshold concentration from the preceding subthreshold concentration. With close spacing of concentrations, average thresholds estimated in this way are not significantly different from ED_{50} values. The data obtained with surface application of drugs are summarized in Tables 2.1 and 2.2.

Table 2.1.

Threshold Concentrations of Inorganic Ions

Author	Substance	Animal	Threshold (ED_{50} M)	log $ED_{50} \pm \sigma$log ED_{50}
Bureš (1962)	LiCl	Rat		
Bureš (1956)	NaCl	Rat		
Leão, Morrison (1945)	KCl	Rabbit	0.13	
Bureš, Burešová (1956b)	KCl	Rat	0.08	—1.097±0.024
Van Harreveld (1959)	KCl	Rabbit	0.11±0.01	
Bureš (1962)	RbCl	Rat	0.052	—1.280±0,053
Bureš (1956)	NH_4Cl	Rat	0.124	—0.907±0.023
Bureš (1962)	KBr	Rat	0.133	—0.876±0,063

Inorganic Ions

Potassium chloride is the most important member of the group of inorganic ions. The ED_{50} threshold in rats (Bureš 1956) is lower than the mean threshold reported by Leão and Morrison (1945) and by Van Harreveld (1959) for the rabbit. The difference is probably technical in nature rather than biological. Sodium and lithium chlorides do not elicit SD even as saturated solutions. On the contrary, rubidium chloride is slightly more effective than the potassium salt (Table 2.1). The sequence $Rb^+ > K^+ \gg Na^+$, Li^+ corresponds to the lyotropic series (Diamond and Wright 1969) characterized by decreasing ionic radius and increasing hydrated size.

Ammonium chloride was reported by Benitez, Pscheidt, and Stone (1954) to decrease EEG activity in the area of application, but the phenomenon was not recognized as CSD. Van Harreveld (1959) failed to elicit CSD with 0.1 M NH_4Cl, while 0.2 M solutions evoked seizures in the rabbit cortex. In the rat NH_4Cl elicited SD with high reliability (Bureš 1956).

Examination of the role of anions accompanying the potassium showed that the potassium threshold is raised by two thirds, when Cl^- is substituted by Br^-. On the contrary the threshold is low for the fluoride that evokes CSD with a threshold concentration of 0.01 M, even when potassium is replaced by sodium. The resulting sequence of threshold concentrations resembles the permeability order Br^- (1.6) $>$ Cl^- (1.0) $>$ F^- (0.2) found in the internally perfused squid axon (Tasaki, Singer, and Takenaka 1965) and corresponds to the free solution mobilities of the respective anions. Whereas the bromine—chlorine difference can perhaps be accounted for by membrane—ion interaction, the effect of F^- ions is due to interference with glycolysis (see p. 35).

The CSD threshold of the different inorganic ions can be explained by taking into account their action on the resting membrane potential of cortical neurons. According to Goldman (1943) and Hodgkin (1958) the membrane potential E_m depends on the ion concentrations on both sides of the membrane and on the relative membrane permeabilities P for different ions according to the equation

$$E_m = 58 \log \frac{P_K [K_i] + P_{Na} [Na_i] + P_{Cl} [Cl_e]}{P_K [K_e] + P_{Na} [Na_e] + P_{Cl} [Cl_i]}$$

For the resting membrane the relative values of $P_K : P_{Na} : P_{Cl}$ are approximately 1 : 0.01 : 0.5. Increasing the extracellular concentration of monovalent cations or anions leads to depolarization or hyperpolarization of the membrane, respectively. An increase of the extracellular potassium concentration by two or three times decreases the membrane potential by 18 or 30 mV. Such depolarization affects the membrane properties and the $P_K : P_{Na}$ ratio changes to 1 : 20. As a result of the permeability change sodium moves into cells accompanied by Cl^- and water, while K^+ moves out of the cells (see p. 89). If the $P_{Na} : P_K$ ratio is 1 : 100 in the resting membrane, it is impossible to elicit CSD even by highly hyperosmotic solutions of NaCl and LiCl. On the contrary, the neural membrane seems to be more permeable for Rb^+ than for K^+. Similar arguments apply to the anionic effects. Increasing the chloride concentration in the extracellular fluid increases the resting membrane potential (see p. 51). The difference between KBr and KCl thresholds is perhaps due to a higher membrane permeability for Br^-. On the other hand, the F^- effect can only be explained by its metabolic action. Membrane permeability depends on the presence of Ca^{2+} in the extracellular fluid. Reduction of extracellular calcium probably accounts for SD initiation by local application of powerful chelating agents like EDTA (Harmony, Fernández-Bouzas, Toro, and Szava, 1973).

Metabolic Inhibitors

Starting from the similarity between anoxic depolarization of the cerebral cortex (see p. 72) and CSD, Martins-Ferreira (1954) and Leão and Martins-Ferreira (1954) attempted to elicit local anoxia by applying NaCN solution to the exposed rabbit cortex. Cortical SD could be evoked in this way with threshold concentrations of 0.025 M NaCN. Other inhibitors of glycolysis and respiration — for example, sodium iodo-acetate, sodium fluoride, and sodium azide—were also effective in unspecified higher concentrations and produced a series of depressions occurring in 5 to 10 min intervals. Martins-Ferreira (1954, 1955a) elicited repeated CSD waves with 0.1 M NaF. More quantitative results were obtained by Bureš (1956) and by Bureš, Burešová, and Křivánek (1960). The lowest threshold was observed with 2,4-dinitrophenol and ouabain, the highest with NaF and NaN_3 (Table 2.2). Sedláček (1967a, b) obtained very similar results with NaF, NaCN, and ouabain in newborn guinea pigs and in 21-day old chick embryos.

Metabolic inhibitors evoke CSD by different mechanisms. Whereas NaCN and NaN_3 are poisons of oxidative metabolism, NaF and iodoacetate primarily interfere with glycolytic processes. Decoupling of oxidative metabolism from the synthesis of high-energy phosphates accounts for the effect of 2,4-dinitrophenol. The final

Table 2.2.

Threshold Concentrations of Metabolic Inhibitors

Author	Substance	Animal	Threshold (ED_{50} M)	log $ED_{50} \pm \sigma$log ED_{50}
Leão, Martins-Ferreira (1954)	NaCN	Rabbit	0.025	
Bureš (1956)	NaCN	Rat	0.0015	—2.82±0.09
Leão, Martins-Ferreira (1955)	NaF	Rabbit	0.1	
Bureš (1956)	NaF	Rat	0.01	—1.98±0.09
Bureš (1956)	2,4-Dinitrophenol	Rat	0.0002	—3.68±0.26
Bureš (1956)	NaN_3	Rat	0.025	—1.61±0.08
Bureš (1956)	CH_2ICOOH	Rat	0.009	—2.05±0.02
Bureš (1956)	Strophanthin	Rat	0.0003	—3.56±0.02

result of the above interactions is a breakdown of the sodium pump, the function of which maintains the normal ion distribution across the membrane. Whereas potassium chloride depolarizes the membrane from the outside, metabolic inhibitors do the same from the inside. The final link is not energy metabolism but the metabolic mechanisms of active transport. This is why it is possible to elicit CSD by ouabain, which selectively inhibits the Na^+,K^+-sensitive ATPase without interfering with the glycid and energy metabolism. The ability of ouabain to evoke CSD has been confirmed by Aquino-Cias, Harmony, and Guma (1967). Blockade of the oxidative metabolism by DNP, cyanide or anoxia did not elicit SD in the isolated chicken retina (Van Harreveld and Fifková 1972), probably because this preparation may derive energy for the Na^+ pump from glycolysis. Iodoacetate, glucose-free solutions, and ouabain were effective.

Other CSD-evoking substances can be included in this group only with qualifications. Goldring and O'Leary (1954), Martins-Ferreira (1954, 1955a), and Bureš (1956) elicited CSD with 0.1 to 0.01% veratrine, which potentiates the K^+ effect in excitable tissues. Aconitine has a similar effect (Bureš 1962). Little is known of the mechanism of action of these alkaloids. The possibility of eliciting CSD with $HgCl_2$ (1 to 5 %), demonstrated by Bureš and Koshtoyants (1955), is probably due to blocking of the reactive -SH groups in the neuronal membranes and to the resulting increase of membrane permeability.

Depolarizing Amino Acids

Bureš (1956), Van Harreveld (1959), and Bureš, Burešová, and Křivánek (1960) examined the CSD threshold of a group of acidic amino acids, which were later shown by microelectrophoretic injection techniques to be effective excitants of neurons (Curtis, Phillis, and Watkins 1960, Krnjevič and Phillis 1963, Eccles 1964). The results are summarized in Table 2.3. Although the threshold concentrations were somewhat different with epidural application in rats and cortical application in rabbits, the relative activity of some compounds was quite similar. Thus the D-glutamine threshold was 4.2 times lower than the L-glutamine threshold in rats and D-glutamate was 4.0 times more effective than L-glutamate in rabbits. Curtis and Watkins (1963) found that homocysteic acid is about 5 times and N-methyl-D-aspartic acid about 200 times more efficient than glutamic acid in evoking CSD in the cat cerebral cortex. On the other hand N-methyl-L-aspartic acid was found to be only slightly more active than either the D or L configurations of the glutamic acid. The difference in the activities of the D and L configurations is perhaps due to absence of the D forms in brain, which is not equipped for their metabolic removal. This accounts for the higher extracellular concentration of these substances. Van Harreveld and Fifková (1970, 1971) reported that the transparency increase accompanying retinal SD (see p. 135) can be elicited by superfusion with 0.05 mM homocysteic acid, 0.5 mM

Table 2.3.

Threshold Concentrations of Amino Acids

Author	Substance	Animal	Threshold (ED_{50} M)	log $ED_{50} \pm \sigma \log ED_{50}$
Bureš (1956)	DL-Glutamate	Rat	0.224	
Bureš (1962)	L-Glutamate	Rat (dura removed)	0.034	—1.47±0.13
Van Harreveld (1959)	L-Glutamate	Rabbit	0.015	
Van Harreveld (1959)	D-Glutamate	Rabbit	0.004	
Bureš (1956)	L-Glutamine	Rat	0.077	—1.11±0.05
Van Harreveld (1959)	L-Glutamine	Rabbit	0.080	
Bureš, Burešová, Křivánek (1960)	D-Glutamine	Rat	0.017	—1.77±0.07
Van Harreveld (1959)	L-Aspartate	Rabbit	0.017	
Bureš, Burešová, Křivánek (1970)	L-Aspartate	Rat	0.089	—1.05±0.05
Van Harreveld (1959)	L-Asparagine	Rabbit	0.013	
Bureš, Burešová, Křivánek (1960)	L-Asparagine	Rat	0.055	—1.26±0.07
Van Harreveld (1959)	L-Aminoadipic Acid	Rabbit	0.035	
Curtis, Watkins (1963)	Homocysteic Acid	Cat	30% of glutamate threshold	
Curtis, Watkins (1963)	N-Methyl-D-Aspartic Acid	Cat	0.5% of glutamate threshold	

glutamate, 5.0 mM aspartate, and 5.0 mM glutamine. Whereas the amino acids listed in Table 2.3 elicit CSD at low concentrations, other structurally related compounds (Table 2.4) are inactive or even block CSD initiation (see p. 53). This indicates that the depolarizing effect is not due to the metabolic action of these substances but rather to the fact that the active molecules are accurately keyed to receptor sites on the neuronal membrane. As a consequence the membrane permeability for sodium and other ions increases. Demonstration of movement of sodium chloride and water into the neural elements of the retina, caused by increased concentration of glutamate or glutamine in the medium, actually preceded the electrophysiological analysis (Ames 1956).

Although the above evidence appears to be quite conclusive, it must be pointed out that the depolarizing amino acids do not elicit SD with the same reliability as KCl solution. Curatolo, Marchetti, Salleo, and Brancati (1967) failed to initiate CSD by local treatment of cat cerebral cortex with 2% L-glutamate or 2% L-aspartate. Also DoCarmo and Leão (1972) were unable to trigger SD in rabbits and rats by topical application of glutamate (up to 200 mM), aspartate, and asparagine. These compounds elicited local depolarization attaining 20 to 25 mV in amplitude

Table 2.4.

Comparison of the Chemical Formulas of Amino Acids (Isoglutamine, α - Ketoglutarate, Glycylglutamine, Glutamine, Glutamic Acid, γ - Aminobutyric Acid, Asparagine, Aspartic Acid, β - Alanine, Succinic Acid) that Can or Cannot Elicit CSD (Active Substances in Frames)

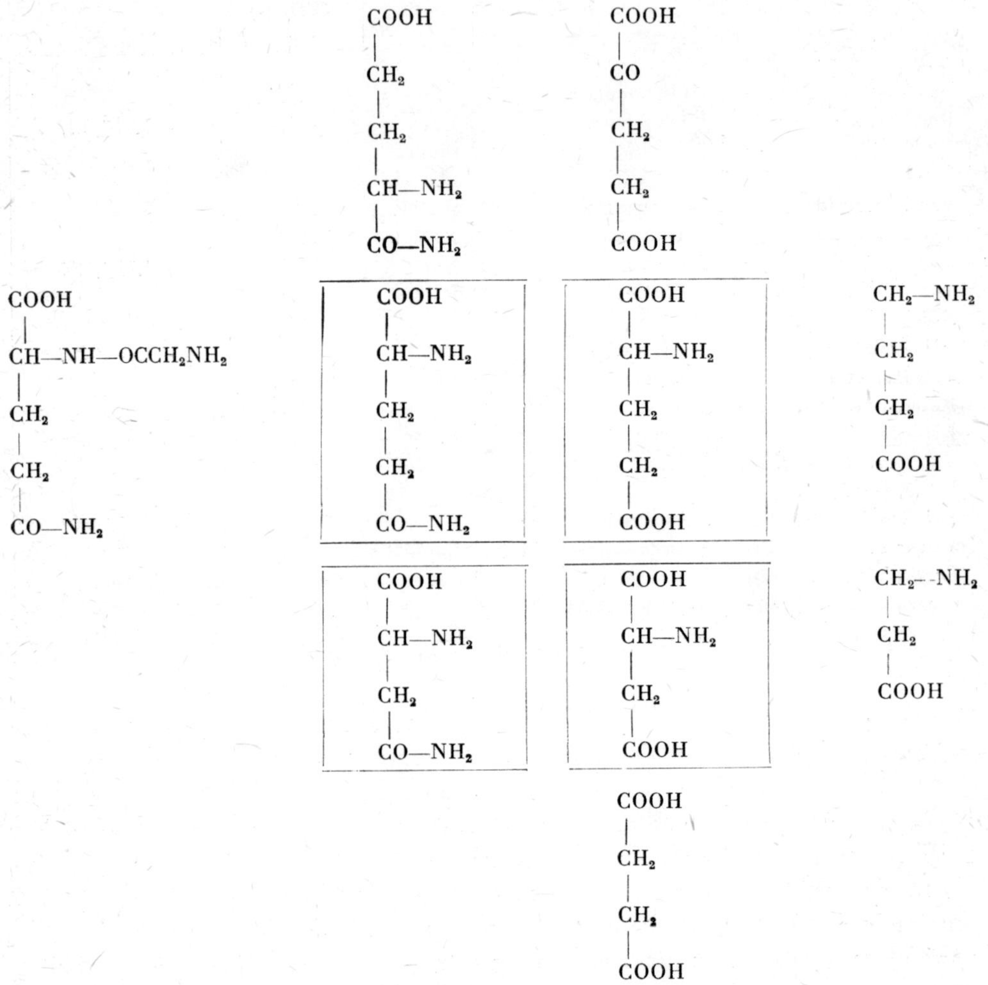

both in cerebral cortex and hippocampus, whereas glutamine evoked delayed depolarization only in hippocampus. The CSD susceptibility of the treated area was so much increased, however, that CSD was often elicited by incidental mechanical stimuli (cardiac and respiratory pulsations of brain).

Whereas ions (group 1) depolarize the membrane by changing the electrolyte equilibrium from the outside, and the inhibitors (group 2) by interfering with active transport from inside the cell, the amino acids (group 3) affect the membrane directly, probably by changing its sievelike properties. Even in groups 2 and 3 potassium probably plays an important role, however, since K^+ released from depolarized neurons and accumulated in the extracellular space may considerably contribute to the overall depolarizing effect.

The above studies used the surface application technique. Less attention was paid to intracerebral injection. Although the theory of instantaneous or continuous point sources was developed and experimentally verified in connection with microelectrophoretic injections of drugs (Curtis 1964), it was usually applied for distances not exceeding 300 microns (Herz, Ziegelgänsberger, and Färber 1969). Threshold measurements of electrophoretically applied potassium ions indicated (Janebová 1971) that CSD can be triggered by 0.6 μg of K^+ injected 1 mm below the cortical surface. Slightly higher threshold values were obtained with pressure injection of KCl (about 1 μg K^+, Matsuura and Bureš 1971). The difference is perhaps due to the facilitatory effects of current applied in the electrophoretic experiments. The absolute thresholds established with the injection technique are by an order of magnitude lower than those determined by surface application (5 mg of 0.6% KCl solution applied onto the cortical surface contain approximately 15 μg K^+), evidently because the active substance is more efficiently distributed through the critical volume of neural tissue. Attempts to use focal injection to determine the size of this critical volume are described in Chapter 7.

Since only minimum amounts of the active substance are injected, the dynamics of the response is different. When the threshold is estimated at various intervals after a conditioning subthreshold injection into the same area, the facilitatory effect decays with a half time of 2 min, which characterizes both the diffusion and removal rates of the substance (Matsuura and Bureš 1971).

4. Local Cooling

Local cooling is similar to the metabolic inhibitors since it may decrease energy metabolism below the critical level. Zacharová and Zachar (1961) are the only authors who have explored the properties of this stimulus in some detail. Cooling was performed with a conical silver thermode, the base of which was formed by a circular silver plate 3 mm in diameter. The cannula was counterbalanced in such a way that it touched the cortex without exerting pressure. Cooling fluid of a given temperature was circulated through the cannula at a rate ensuring constant temperature of the thermode throughout the application period.

Provided the area cooled is constant, the main parameters of the stimulus are probe temperature and duration of cooling. The hyperbolic relationship between the two parameters plotted in Fig. 2.4 shows that approximately 12 °C is the "rheobase". Much lower temperatures are required for eliciting CSD with cold pulses shorter than 5 sec. With repeated CSD waves, threshold decreases (CSD appears at brain temperatures of about 15 °C).

Cooling of the superficial 0.5 mm of cortex below the probe (about 5 mm^3) by 20 °C requires 5 × 20 millical, corresponding to 0.42 joule. Expressed as energy per square millimeter of stimulated cortical surface, the threshold is approximately 400,000 erg mm^{-2}, that is, by three orders of magnitude higher than the electrical and mechanical threshold. This striking difference indicates that cooling affects the whole cell volume, whereas the mechanical and electrical stimuli act more specifically on the sensitive surface structures. Temperatures sufficient to trigger CSD are practically always reached when cooling probes are used for functional elimination of subcortical structures. The possible initiation of CSD under these conditions must be always taken into account.

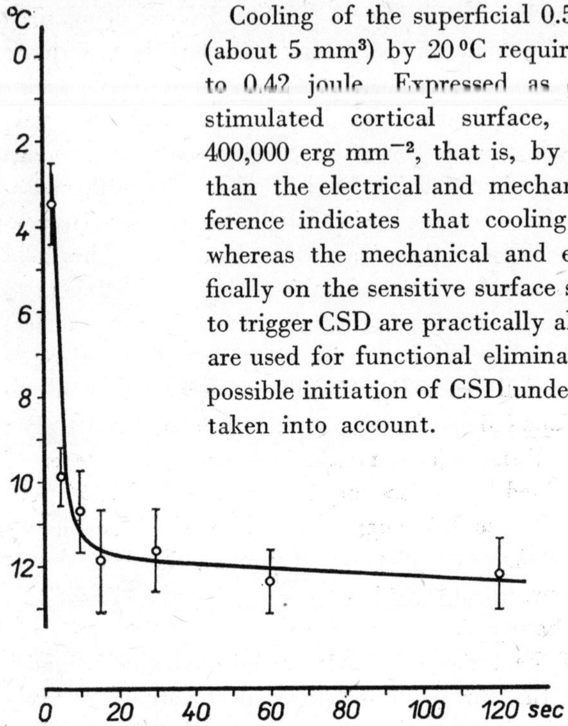

Fig. 2. 4. Relationship between the probe temperature producing CSD in 50% of the cases (ordinate) and duration of the cold impulse (abscissa). Vertical bars denote the confidence limits of the mean values established by probit analysis for p=0.05 (Zacharová and Zachar 1961).

5. Neural Activity

Whereas electrical, mechanical, chemical, and thermic stimuli can elicit CSD reliably and reproducibly, neural activity is a rather poor stimulus. Leão (1944a), Leão and Morrison (1945), and Marshall (1959) could elicit CSD in the opposite hemisphere by stimulating different parts of the corpus callosum in the rabbit. Van Harreveld and Stamm (1953c, 1954b) demonstrated that cortical afterdischarge evoked by faradic stimulation in the rabbit can carry CSD into brain regions considerably remote from the stimulated site. Koroleva and Kuznetsova (1972) reported that application of 10 to 25% KCl on the cerebral cortex of rats may elicit CSD not only from the area treated, but also from a remote KCl focus, the activity of which stopped earlier. Activation of the remote focus, demonstrated by the technique of dynamic diagrams (Koroleva 1970), is probably mediated by the neuronal discharge triggered in deep cortical layers by KCl induced depolarization of cortical surface (Koroleva and Kuznetsova 1971). After subconvulsive dosages of metrazol, CSD can be evoked in the rabbit visual cortex by intense rhythmic visual stimuli (Van Harreveld and Stamm 1955). All these results are isolated observations rather than regular phenomena. Bureš (1962) was not able to elicit CSD in rats by prolonged (20 min) supramaximal stimulation (1 Hz to 3.5 Hz) of the sciatic nerve. Only when the cortical projection area was treated with 5 or 10% metrazol, were evoked responses considerably increased and in 35% cases CSD was evoked after 5.5 min of 3.5 Hz stimulation (Fig. 2.5). The facilitatory effect of metrazol is discussed in Chapter 3. The possibility of inducing retinal SD by a single flash of light under special conditions is described in Chapter 6.

It can be concluded that nerve impulses can elicit CSD only exceptionally, for example, when driven at a high rate by electrical stimulation and enhanced by pharmacologically increased excitability.

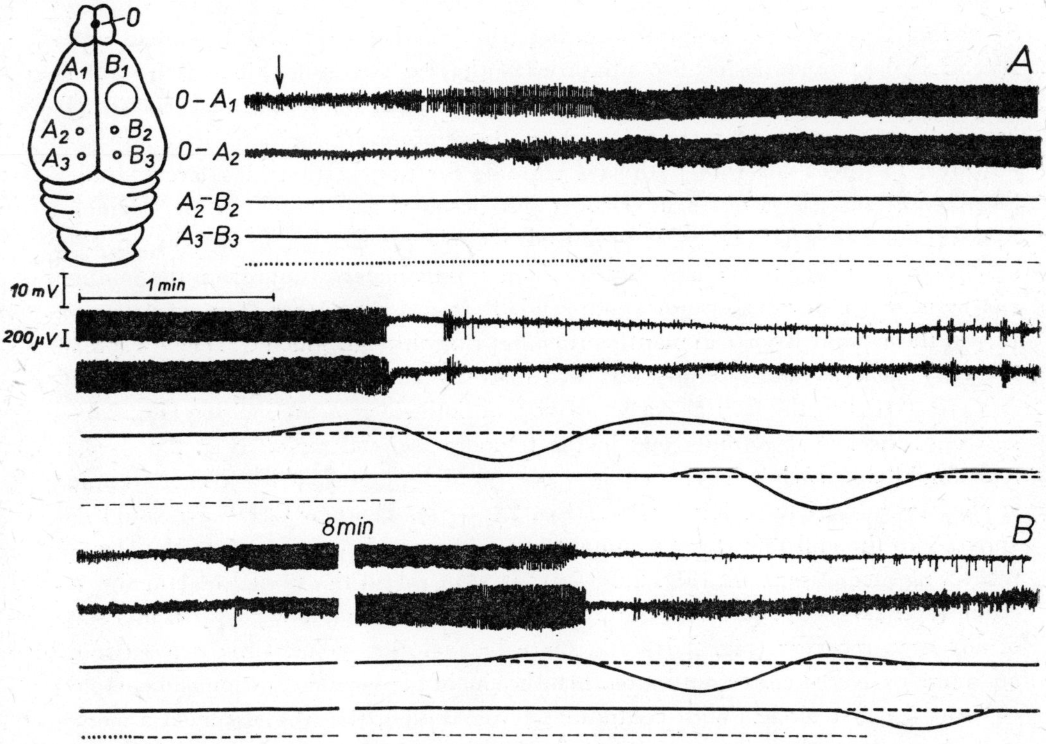

Fig. 2. 5. Cortical SD elicited in the rat by stimulation of right sciatic nerve after application of 10% metrazol onto the left somatosensory cortical area. *(A)* Immediately after metrazol application. *(B)* 30 min after metrazol application. The inset diagram shows the distribution of the electrodes. Arrow denotes the metrazol application; dotted line the sciatic stimulation at 1/sec; dashed line the sciatic stimulation at 3.5/sec. Calibration: 100 µV for EEG; 10 mV for SPC (Bureš 1962).

6. Focal Injury

Although injury may induce CSD, it is extremely difficult to define it as a stimulus and to separate the injury proper from concomitant mechanical stimulation. Cortical SD evoked by insertion of an electrode into the cortex is due to the indentation of surface rather than to damage of neurons along the electrode tract (Marshall 1959). Besides direct cell damage, cutting or stabbing may cause ischemia. The possibility of evoking CSD by occlusion of the terminal artery was reported by Kempinsky (1954). The results are essentially similar to general anoxic effects which are discussed in greater detail in Chapter 4.

7. Entrapped Wave of Spreading Depression

Spreading depression is a selfpropagating reaction that continues to spread until it reaches the boundaries or discontinuities of the reactive tissue. Since each wave is followed by 1 to 2 min of absolute and 5 to 10 min of relative refractoriness, SD cannot turn around and retrace its steps. By appropriate incisions it is possible, however, to direct SD into pathways suitable for propagation in a circle. Under ideal conditions SD is not a final effect but becomes a selfperpetuating stimulus. Shibata and Bureš (1971, 1972) produced a circle preparation in rats by making a 5-mm long parasagittal transcortical incision approximately 4 mm from the midline and between 1 mm rostrally and 4 mm caudally from bregma (Fig. 2.6). The incision turned the expanded cortical mantle into a flat ring through which CSD could spread not only medially and laterally but also rostrally and caudally from the incision. A wave started in the frontal cortex moved on both sides of the incision (Fig. 2.6 — 1,2) until the two wavefronts met in the temporo-occipital region (Fig. 2.6 — 3,4) and annihilated each other. A circle wave could be launched by a new stimulus applied to the parieto-occipital cortex (Fig. 2.6 — 3). The new CSD wave could not spread into the still refractory occipital cortex, but could propagate into the already recovering medial segment (Fig. 2.6 — 4). It went round the frontal end of the incision (Fig. 2.6 — 5) and found the area in which the previous wave expired in a state of advanced recovery (Fig. 2.6 — 6). Once beyond this point, CSD entered more and more recovered cortex until it reached the site of the second injection and completed thus the first circle. With continuing reverberation, the SPC assumed a stereotype shape due to regular movement of CSD along the circular pathway (Fig. 2.7). One cycle lasted 5 to 6 min on the average and the reverberation usually stopped spontaneously after 4 to 8 cycles because of increasing refractoriness or because an interfering "extrasystolic" CSD wave was generated.

Still better results were obtained with CSD reverberation around a circular lesion induced by thermocoagulation of cerebral cortex. Ten cycles could be generated on the average with lesions 4 mm in diameter under normal conditions, but reverberation could be facilitated by systemic application of a pyrrolopyrimidine compound BW-271 (2-methyl 4-benzyl-amino pyrrolo [2,3-d] pyrimidine) (15 mg/kg) to the average number of 40 cycles.

In accordance with the mathematical model proposed by Wiener and Rosenblueth (1946) circulating CSD wave can only be produced in the presence of an obstacle the

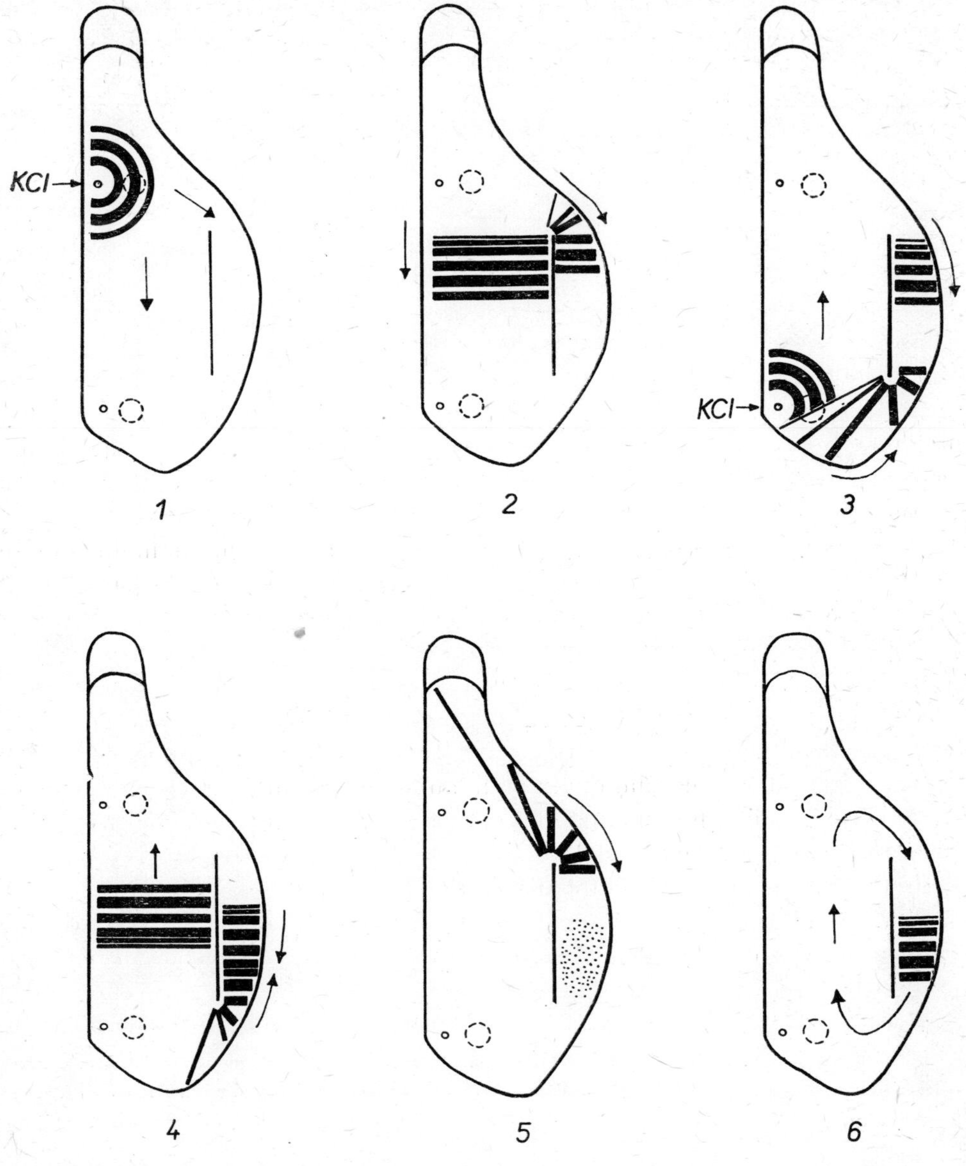

Fig. 2. 6. Diagram illustrating the method of launching the circuit wave of SD in rat cerebral cortex. Position of the negative SPC indicated by heavy black lines. Stippling denotes the region where the first CSD wave expired. For details see text (Shibata and Bureš 1972).

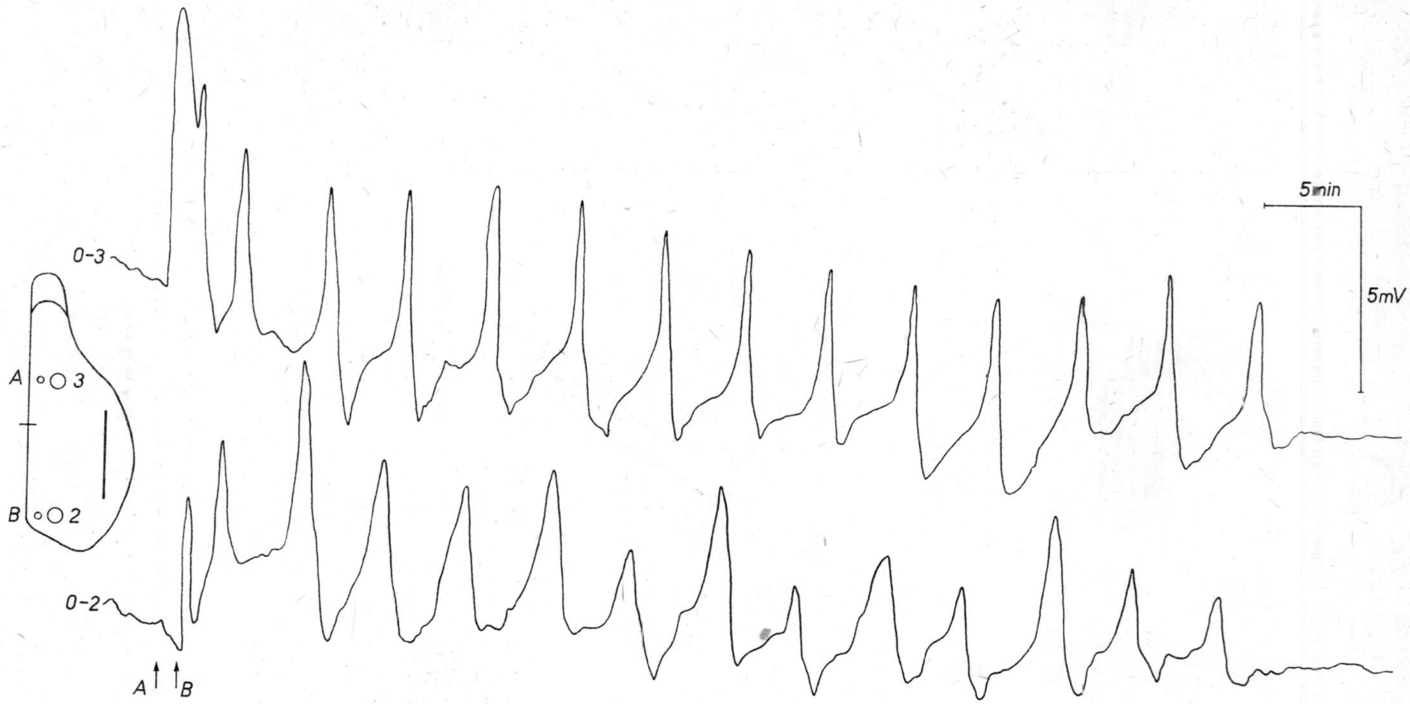

Fig. 2. 7. Entrapped CSD wave in the rat. Position of the recording (2, 3) and stimulating *(A, B)* sites is shown in the inset brain diagram. Comparison of SPC recordings (0—3) and (0—2) indicates clockwise circulation of CSD. Note that the first two SPC waves in lead (0—2) are triggered by the injections *A* and *B* respectively. Alternation of higher and lower SPCs in lead (0—2) indicates gradually developing propagation block in the area of recording (Shibata and Bureš 1972).

circumference of which exceeds the CSD wave-length. The cortical segments between the lesion and the boundary of the cortex must be wide enough to ensure reliable CSD transmission. Satisfactory results were obtained with lesions 3 to 5 mm in diameter surrounded by at least 2 mm of intact cortex. Reverberation cannot be initiated by repeated stimulation of a single point or by simultaneous stimulation of several points, but requires at least 2 stimuli applied to 2 different points and separated by an interval equal to the refractory period plus the conduction time between the two stimulated loci. The second CSD wave must be elicited from a point close to the lesion so that it hits the obstacle end on, not tangentially. In the latter case, two waves travelling around the obstacle in opposite directions would prevent reverberation. The other edge of the incipient circle wave must touch the boundary of the cortex, since otherwise the outer end of the wave, at first limited by refractory tissue, will gradually turn around and follow the first wave. The above conditions are best satisfied by injection into the medial segment, the width of which is approximately equal to the critical diameter (see p. 164). The second stimulus can be considered as affecting the whole wave-rear between two boundaries, which is another prerequisite of stable reverberation theoretically postulated by Selfridge (1948).

The circle wave can be deliberately stopped by an appropriately timed interfering wave or by reversible blockade of a segment of the circular pathway. Also a general increase of refractoriness induced by 1-min asphyxia causes an immediate cessation of CSD reverberation in rats (Shibata and Bureš 1973).

Reverberating SD was also found in the ring shaped preparation of isolated chicken retina (Martins-Ferreira, Albuquerque, and Bureš, unpublished), where the circle wave could be initiated by blocking SD propagation in one direction by anodic polarization. The circular SD wave spread around the ring with a 10 min period for several hours and resembled in many respects the entrapped wave of excitation in the ring preparation of medusa bell (Kinosita 1937, Horridge 1956).

Chapter 3

Blocking and Facilitating Influences

Although SD can be evoked by various chemical and physical stimuli described in the preceding chapters, it represents a highly stereotyped, stimulus-independent reaction. This indicates that different stimuli trigger complex chain reactions, converging on a common link which is at the same time the first link of the autoregenerative process of SD. The nature of the hypothetical reaction can be elucidated by examining procedures that either block or enhance SD initiation. Processes underlying the actual spreading mechanism can also be studied with similar methods.

I. Local Interference with Initiation of Spreading Depression

Local blocking effects can easily be established by determining the threshold concentration of the active agent in the region pretreated with the solution of the antagonist or by finding the minimum concentration of the antagonistic substance that, when added to a suprathreshold concentration of the active agent, prevents SD initiation.

Divalent Cations

The latter technique was used to demonstrate the blocking effect of divalent cations in rat cerebral cortex (Bureš and Burešová 1956b, c). Different amounts of $MgCl_2$, $CaCl_2$, $SrCl_2$, or $BaCl_2$ were dissolved in 2% KCl and the mixture was applied across the intact dura to cortical surface exposed by trephine openings 4 to 5 mm in diameter. A typical experiment is illustrated in Fig. 3.1. Statistical determination of the blocking ratio, R^{2+}/K^+ revealed an inverse relationship between the blocking effect and the atomic weight of the divalent cations (Fig. 3.2), Mg^{2+} being the most and Ba^{2+} the least efficient K^+ antagonist. In another series of experiments $CaCl_2$ was added to 1, 2, 5, or 10% KCl solutions. The relationship between the Ca^{2+}/K^+ blocking ratio and KCl concentration was found to be a logarithmic one (Fig.3.3). Low concentrations of $CaCl_2$ decreased the effect of suprathreshold KCl solutions by reducing the number of slow potential waves generated by a single application of the mixture. This was probably due to the fact that in the cortex different surface concentrations of K^+ and Ca^{2+} generate concentration gradients of different slope and depth. A blocking effect must be achieved at the periphery of the focus where SD develops when the extracellular K^+ concentration exceeds a given threshold. If Ca^{2+} increases the SD threshold of this region, so that an otherwise effective K^+ concentration becomes subthreshold, SD initiation is prevented. Van Harreveld and Fifková (1970, 1971) used 10 mM $MgCl_2$ to prevent appearance of spontaneous SD waves in isolated chicken retina. A 20 mM $MgCl_2$ solution antagonized the effect of 0.2 mM but not of 2.5 mM glutamate.

A similar blocking effect of Mg^{2+} and Ca^{2+} was demonstrated for other SD stimuli (Table 3.1). The blocking concentrations were roughly related to the degree by which the concentration of the active agent exceeded the threshold. A quantitative comparison of results is impossible, however, since the diffusion constants of the various agents in cortical tissue are not known.

Table 3.1.

Blockade of the Chemically Initiated CSD by Divalent Cations (Bureš 1962)

CSD initiated by	n	Blocking Substance	Blocking Concentration	
			$\log ED_{50} \pm \sigma \log ED_{50}$	ED_{50} (M)
KCl 0.268 M	35	$CaCl_2$	—1.036±0.019	0.092
KCl 0.268 M	35	$MgCl_2$	—1.523±0.057	0.030
Strophanthin $4.08 \cdot 10^{-4}$ M	52	$MgCl_2$	—1.509±0.063	0.031
CH_2ICOOH $1.34 \cdot 10^{-2}$ M	35	$MgCl_2$	—0.959±0.037	0.110
2,4-Dinitrophenol $2.72 \cdot 10^{-3}$ M	100	$CaCl_2$	—1.67 ±0.071	0.021

Divalent cations also block the effect of mechanical stimuli (Zachar and Zacharová 1963). The blocking effect increased again in the order Mg, Ca, Sr, Ba. Determining the blocking concentrations of Ca^{2+} for mechanical stimuli of different intensities made it possible to estimate roughly the equivalence between chemical and mechanical stimuli (Fig. 3.3). Calcium chloride also partly antagonized the effect of local cooling (Zacharová and Zachar 1961).

The above results indicate that divalent cations display a universal antagonism against all stimuli capable of eliciting SD. It seems that they interfere with the last link of the converging reaction chains which is essential for the mechanism of SD propagation. The most probable sites of action are cellular membranes that are stabilized (Höber 1945, Shanes 1958, Cerf 1963) by divalent cations. In the giant axons the membrane conductance and permeability is decreased (Cole 1949) and the level of threshold depolarization is increased (Frankenhäuser and Hodgkin 1957).

The relative potency of alkaline earths to block the potassium effect may throw light on the mechanism of antagonistic action. According to Diamond and Wright (1969) the sequence $Ba^{2+} < Sr^{2+} < Ca^{2+} < Mg^{2+}$ (the order of free solution mobilities)

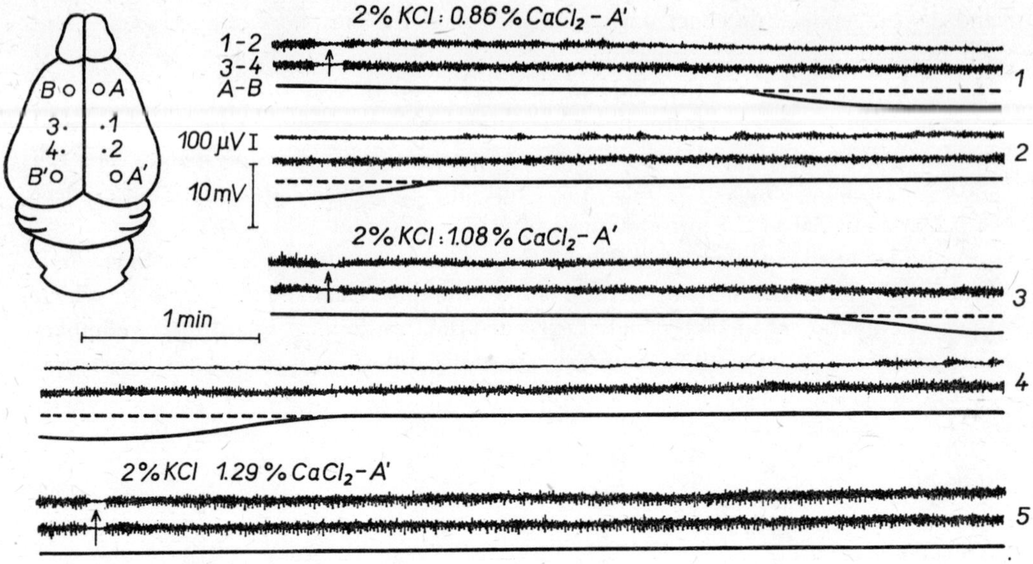

Fig. 3. 1. Blockade of CSD initiation in rats by addition of different concentrations of $CaCl_2$ to the effective 2% KCl solution. (1, 2, 3, 4) Needle electrodes for EEG. *(A, B, A', B')* Trephine openings for SPC recording or for application of the chemical stimuli; CSD was evoked by the first two KCl : $CaCl_2$ mixtures (records 1, 2 and 3, 4) but was blocked with the third one (record 5). Calibration: 100 μV for EEG; 10 mV for SPC (Bureš and Burešová 1956b).

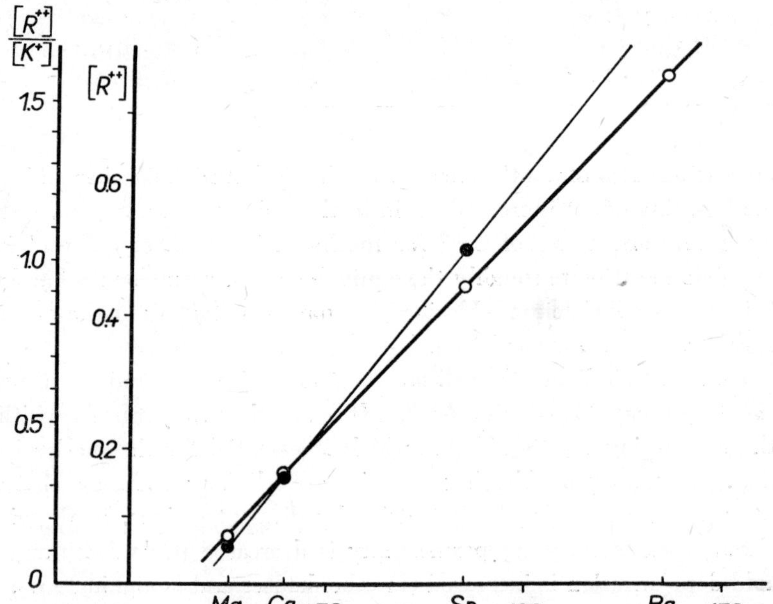

Fig. 3. 2. Relationship between the atomic weight of divalent cations (abscissa)and their blocking effect on CSD initiated by slightly suprathreshold $(t + 2 \text{ mm})$ mechanical stimuli (dots, thin line,

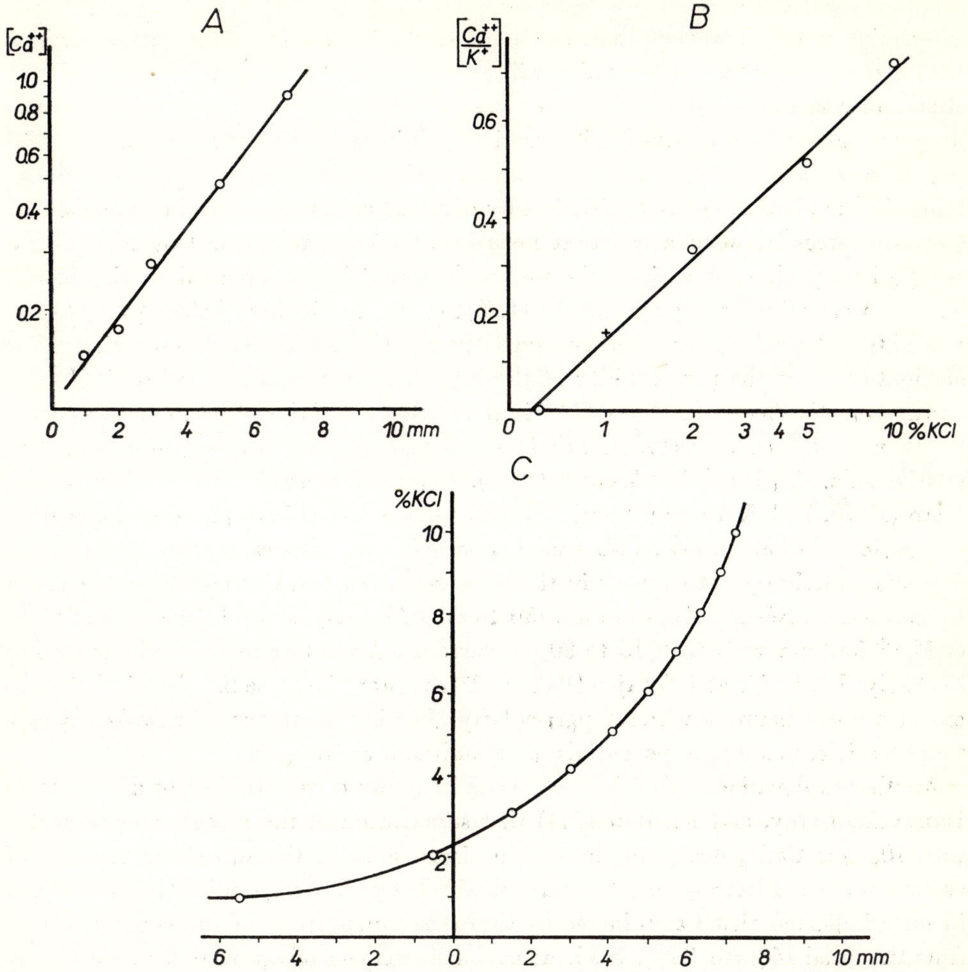

Fig. 3. 3. Relationship between the intensity of mechanical or chemical stimuli and treshold concentration of $CaCl_2$ preventing CSD initiation. *(A)* Mechanical stimulus intensity expressed in millimeters of free fall above threshold on the abscissa. Threshold concentration of the blocking $CaCl_2$ solution (M) on the logarithmic ordinate (Zachar and Zacharová 1963). *(B)* Intensity of the chemical stimulus expressed by concentration (%) of the KCl solution on the logarithmic abscissa. Threshold blocking ratio of molar concentrations $[Ca^{2+}] : [K^+]$ on the ordinate (Bureš and Burešová 1956b). *(C)* Equivalence of mechanical and chemical stimuli at suprathreshold intensities, calculated from the combined relationships *(A)* and *(B)*. Note that $CaCl_2$ concentration blocking the action of 2 % KCl does not signinificantly influence the mechanical threshold stimuli, probably because they affect deep cortical layers not yet reached by Ca^{2+} ions (Zachar and Zacharová 1963).

Zachar and Zacharová 1963) or by 2 % KCl solution (circles, heavy line, Bureš and Burešová 1956b). Ordinates: blocking molar concentrations (ED_{50}) of divalent cations $[R^{2+}]$ for mechanical stimuli or the blocking ratio $[R^{2+}]/[K^+]$ for chemical stimuli (ED_{50}).

occurs in membranes with low negative ionic charges. In this case the ion-to-site interaction is much weaker than the ion-to-water attraction. The smallest cation with highest free energy of hydration will have the smallest affinity for the membrane sites under these conditions. The reverse sequence $Mg^{2+} > Ca^{2+} > Sr^{2+} > Ba^{2+}$ arises at strong sites where ion-to-site interaction dominates over hydration energy. This sequence can also be expressed in membranes with closely spaced sites. It has been found in the blockade of SD initiation by divalent cations and can be explained by coulomb forces between a constant negative charge in the neural membrane and the positively charged cations the radius of which is proportional to the atomic weight. A very similar sequence, Mg^{2+} (1.25) > Ca^{2+} (1.00) > Sr^{2+} (0.50) > Ba^{2+} (0.29), was obtained by Goldner, Cassidy, and Titball (1967) for the capability of alkaline earths to restore the permeability of the intestine after treatment with EDTA.

Antagonistic effects of K^+ and Ca^{2+} in the electrical activity of brain were reported by Bonnet and Bremer (1937), Libet and Gerard (1938), Feldberg and Sherwood (1957), John, Tschirgi, and Wenzel (1959). Recently Krnjević (1965), Somjen and Kato (1968), and Kato and Somjen (1969) reported that iontophoretic application of divalent cations from five-barreled micropipettes depresses the spontaneous or evoked discharges of neurons in the cat cerebral cortex. Cortical neurons excited by continuous release of glutamate (30 to 60 nA) were silenced by 10 sec of Ca^{2+} or Mg^{2+} iontophoresis with 15 to 80 nA currents. According to intracellular studies by Kelly, Krnjević, and Somjen (1969) Ca^{2+} and Mg^{2+} increase the electrical threshold of cortical neurons without particularly affecting spontaneous or evoked synaptic potentials, membrane potentials, or membrane resistance.

Another explanation of the Ca^{2+} effect can be inferred from the recent finding (Van Harreveld, Dafny, and Khattab 1971) that superfusion of the rabbit cerebral cortex with 100 mM $CaCl_2$ decreases the specific impedance of the superficial 0.6 mm of cortical tissue. Electron micrographs obtained by the freeze-substitution method in mice indicated that $CaCl_2$ increased the extracellular space of the cerebral cortex from the usual 14% to 33%. Such enormous increment of extracellular volume may considerably decrease the efficiency of humoral interaction between neurons and even prevent SD initiation.

Sodium Chloride

A weak blocking effect of sodium chloride was demonstrated with solid NaCl added to 1% KCl solution to concentrations of 20 to 40% NaCl (Bureš 1962). No SD was elicited by local application of this mixture onto rat cerebral cortex. The blocking effect was maintained even when during subsequent applications the NaCl: KCl ratio was reduced to 5 : 1, but with a further decrease of NaCl concentration to 1%, the 1% KCl started to evoke SD again. On the other hand, attempts to establish the blocking effect by gradually adding increasing concentrations of NaCl to 1%

KCl failed, probably because the aftereffects of the preceding SD wave facilitated the initiation of the following one. This peculiar hysteresis is illustrated in Fig. 3.4, which shows how the threshold of the antagonistic effect depends on the direction from which it is approached. The exact mechanism of the above effect is obscure but it can be surmised that the blockade is due to the hyperpolarizing action of the increased Cl^- concentration in the extracellular fluid, which is only insufficiently counteracted by the slight depolarizing effect of Na^+ ions (see p. 34). The antagonistic effects of Cl^- ions on SD were also reported by Leão (1961, 1963), who found electrical or mechanical threshold of CSD in the rabbit markedly raised by concentrated NaCl solutions (280 mM) and decreased by the dilute ones (30 to 40 mM). Chloride ions could be substituted by bromide or nitrate, but not by acetate, sulphate, thiocyanate, and thiosulphate. Non-electrolytes (sucrose, glucose, glycerol) had little effect on the CSD threshold even when applied in high concentrations.

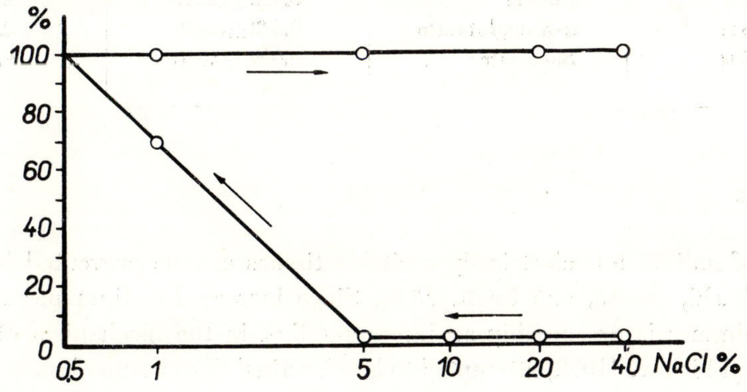

Fig. 3. 4. Blockade of CSD initiation by NaCl added to 1 % KCl. Concentration of the added NaCl solution (weight/volume percent) on the logarithmic abscissa. Percentage of CSD waves evoked by the respective NaCl : KCl mixture on the ordinate. Arrows indicate the sequence in which the NaCl concentration was increased or decreased in the process of threshold estimation (Bureš 1962).

Tricarboxylic Acid Cycle Intermediates

Metabolic reactions of brain slices to increased K^+ concentration (see p. 111) can be prevented by adding citrate, α-ketoglutarate, or succinate (Lippset and Crescitelli 1950, McIlwain 1954) to the medium. When neutral sodium salts of these acids are dissolved in 1% KCl, mixtures containing rather high concentrations of these substrates do not elicit SD (Table 3.2) (Bureš 1956, Bureš 1962), whereas even 40% glucose does not prevent the initiation of SD. The analogy between brain slices and SD was not complete, however. Thus lactic acid blocked SD but did not suppress the potassium-induced metabolic reaction in brain slices. The weak antagonistic effects are probably due to an improved energy balance of the neurons. The blocking effects may be partly obscured by the chelating activity of some of the above substances, which may influence the SD threshold in exactly the opposite way (Harmony 1969).

Table 3.2.

Blockade of CSD Initiation by Adding Substrates of Oxidative Metabolism to the Effective KCl Solution (Bureš 1956)

CSD Initiated by KCl	Metabolic Substrate	Blocking Ratio Substrate/K^+	
		$\log ED_{50} \pm \sigma \log ED_{50}$	ED_{50} (M)
0.134 M	Lactate	0.196 ± 0.041	1.57
0.134 M	Citrate	0.410 ± 0.021	2.57
0.134 M	α-Ketoglutarate	0.473 ± 0.038	2.97
0.134 M	Succinate	0.999 ± 0.018	9.97

Tetrodotoxin

Movement of sodium into electrically excitable tissues can be prevented by tetrodotoxin (Narahashi, Moore, and Scott 1964). Since increased sodium permeability of neural membranes is presumably an important link in the mechanism of SD, Van Harreveld and Fifková (1972) attempted to block retinal SD by superfusing the preparation with 6 μM tetrodotoxin. Subsequent application of 1mM glutamate caused the typical release of labeled glutamate from the preloaded retina (see p. 115), but absence of the transparency change indicated blockade of the intracellular electrolyte transport. Tetrodotoxin did not prevent the development of the transparency change elicited by isotonic KCl, however. These results are in a good agreement with findings in cortical tissue slices (Okamoto and Quastel 1970) where tetrodotoxin prevents the sodium uptake caused by glutamate, but not that induced by potassium chloride. Sugaya, Takato, and Noda (1971) reported that electrical stimulation of a cortical region treated with tetrodotoxin fails to elicit SD but that SD can be evoked from the same area by KCl.

Stimulus-Specific Antagonism

Some SD-evoking stimuli act through specific metabolic mechanisms that can be blocked by appropriate means. Thus Bureš and Koshtoyants (1955) reported that the thiol group poison $HgCl_2$ evokes SD when applied on an exposed cortical surface.

Supply of -SH groups in form of cysteine or glutathione antagonizes the effects of $HgCl_2$. Whereas a filter paper soaked in 5% $HgCl_2$ evoked on the average 5.8± 1.0 SD waves when applied on intact rat cortex, the same stimulus remained ineffective when applied onto an area pretreated for 5 min with 10% glutathione. The action of glutathione was restricted to $HgCl_2$ and did not affect the KCl threshold.

Similarly, the SD-evoking effect of glutamine could be antagonized by glycylglutamine (Bureš, Burešová and Křivánek 1960, Bureš 1962). In the cortex pretreated for 10 min with the latter substance the glutamine SD threshold increased from the normal 0.077M to 0.270M but the KCl threshold remained unchanged. Competitive inhibition was suggested to account for the finding (Van Harreveld and Fifková 1971) that the SD elicited in isolated chicken retina by glutamate can be prevented by pretreatment with pyroglutamate.

The stimulus specificity of the antagonism indicates that the substances used do not affect the final common link of the converging reaction chains, but that they interrupt these chains at some earlier stage — for example, glutathione by supplying reactive SH groups selectively blocked by $HgCl_2$, and glycylglutamine by competitive inhibition of glutamine.

2. Local Facilitation of Initiation of Spreading Depression

The problem of local facilitation can be traced back to the early studies on SD in cats and monkeys. In these animals SD is a rather elusive phenomenon the incidence of which was believed to be increased by exposure of the cerebral cortex to pathological conditions (Marshall 1959). Various possible influences were tested: radical internal dehydration by intravenous injection of concentrated sucrose solution (Marshall 1950); cooling of the mineral oil covering the exposed cortex (Marshall, Essig, and Dubroff 1951); prolonged exposure to air (Marshall and Essig 1951), washing the cortical surface with isotonic sucrose (Essig and Marshall 1950), washing with Tyrode solution with ten times the normal KCl content (Marshall, Essig, and Witkin 1951), or washing with 0.004 to 0.008 M NaF solution (Leão and Martins-Ferreira 1956). The facilitating effect of the above procedures was later confirmed by Van Harreveld and Bogen (1956) in the retrosplenial area of the rabbit, that is, in a region otherwise refractory to SD (see p. 118). Unfortunately some of the facilitating procedures were rather complex and their action is poorly understood. Only cooling and potassium ions are stimuli that would elicit SD at higher intensities. As pointed out by Leão and Martins-Ferreira (1956), any chemical substance that elicits SD by local application, can be used in subthreshold concentrations to facilitate the initiation of SD in the treated area.

Starting with this notion, Zachar and Zacharová (1961b) analyzed the interaction of two subthreshold stimuli quantitatively. They determined the mechanical threshold stimulus in a cortical region before and after treating it with subthreshold concentrations of KCl or 2,4-dinitrophenol. Figure 3.5 shows that even highly subthreshold stimuli, which never elicit SD, start to do so under these conditions. The threshold of the mechanical stimulus decreased 6 min after drug application from the initial 19 gmm to approximately 15 and 11 gmm after 0.3 or 0.6 % KCl, respectively, and to 9.4 gmm after 0.27 to 0.54 mM 2,4-dinitrophenol. No change of the mechanical threshold could be detected 15 min after KCl application, whereas a slight decrease was still observed at the same interval after application of 2,4-dinitrophenol.

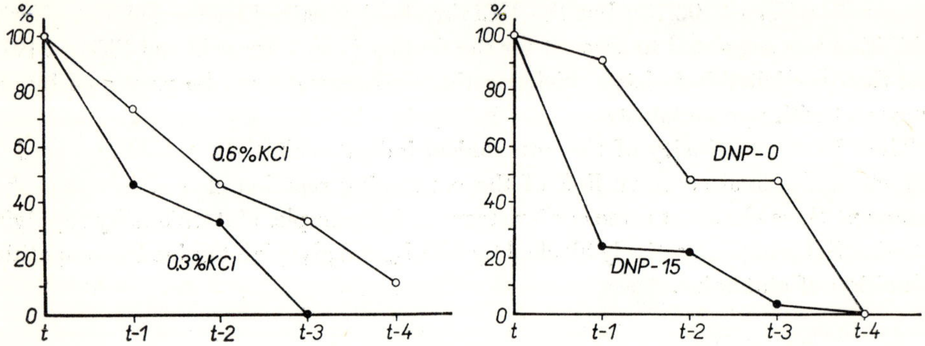

Fig. 3. 5. Dependence of the percentage of occurrence of CSD (ordinate) on the intensity of the subthreshold mechanical stimulus (abscissa) applied to cortical area treated with 0.6 or 0.3 % KCl or with 0.27 to 0.54 mM 2,4-dinitrophenol (DNP - 0). *(t)* threshold value of mechanical stimulus in millimeters of free fall of the stimulus body. Fifteen minutes after removal of the filter paper soaked with DNP the facilitation nearly disappeared (DNP—15) (Zachar and Zacharová 1961a).

Similar results were obtained with local cooling. The threshold of mechanical stimuli applied to a cortical region cooled for 1 min to 15 °C dropped to 60% of the original value and this facilitating effect outlasted the actual cooling for approximately 30 min (Zacharová and Zachar 1961).

In contrast with the above results is the finding that two closely subthreshold mechanical stimuli do not summate when applied in rapid succession. On the contrary a subthreshold conditioning stimulus significantly decreases the effectiveness of a suprathreshold stimulus applied within 1 min to the same region (Fig. 3.6) (Zachar and Zacharová 1961b). It seems that the second stimulus affects the same neural population and since most neural elements are still refractory, it does not release enough of the additional transmitter substance to initiate SD. This refractoriness is a remarkable example of occlusion and may also account for other puzzling findings, for example that trauma (Marshall 1959) or moderate neural activity (Grafstein 1956a) can sometimes prevent SD initiation. The same stimuli may elicit SD when strong enough, or facilitate its initiation by other stimuli with which they overlap in the subliminal fringe.

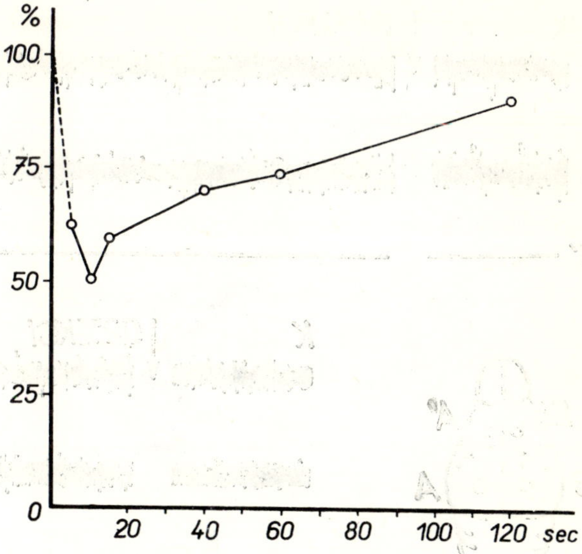

Fig. 3. 6. The time course of relative refractoriness after the subtreshold mechanical pulse (2 mm below threshold). The testing stimulus was 1 mm above threshold. Ordinate: the percentage occurrence of CSD. Abscissa: the interval between the conditioning and testing stimulus (Zachar and Zacharová 1961a).

3. General Influences on Initiation of Spreading Depression

Asphyxia

Besides local influences SD can also be affected by general metabolic conditions, especially those interfering with the energy metabolism of neurons and decreasing their resistance to depolarization. As brain gets more than 95% of its energy from oxidative processes, anoxia was the most obvious procedure to test. According to Leão and Morrison (1945) and Leão (1947) faradic stimulation of cerebral cortex, applied during cerebral circulatory arrest, failed to elicit SD. These results were confirmed by Van Harreveld and Stamm (1953b) who stressed, however, that asphyxiation did not prevent initiation of SD by direct current applied 30 sec after the start of circulatory arrest. Bureš and Burešová (1960a) examined the effect of a brief asphyxia (evoked by 45-sec compression of thorax in rats) on a subthreshold chemical stimulus. A typical experiment in an anesthetized rat is shown in Fig. 3.7. Neither a subthreshold solution of KCl (0.2 %) nor asphyxia and ischemia lasting for 1 min or less (Leão and Morrison 1945, Van Harreveld and Stamm 1953b) elicited SD when applied alone. A 45-sec asphyxia, induced 2 min after application of 0.2 % KCl onto the exposed cortical surface, evoked SD in 80 % of the cases, however (Fig. 3.8). Subthreshold concentrations of other substances and spontaneous subthreshold foci of SD are influenced in the same way.

Similar results were obtained when applying KCl at different intervals after a 45-sec asphyxia. Efficiency of 0.2 % KCl was slightly raised (to 30 %) for 2 min only, efficiency of 0.4 % KCl was clearly increased (80 to 100 %) for slightly less than

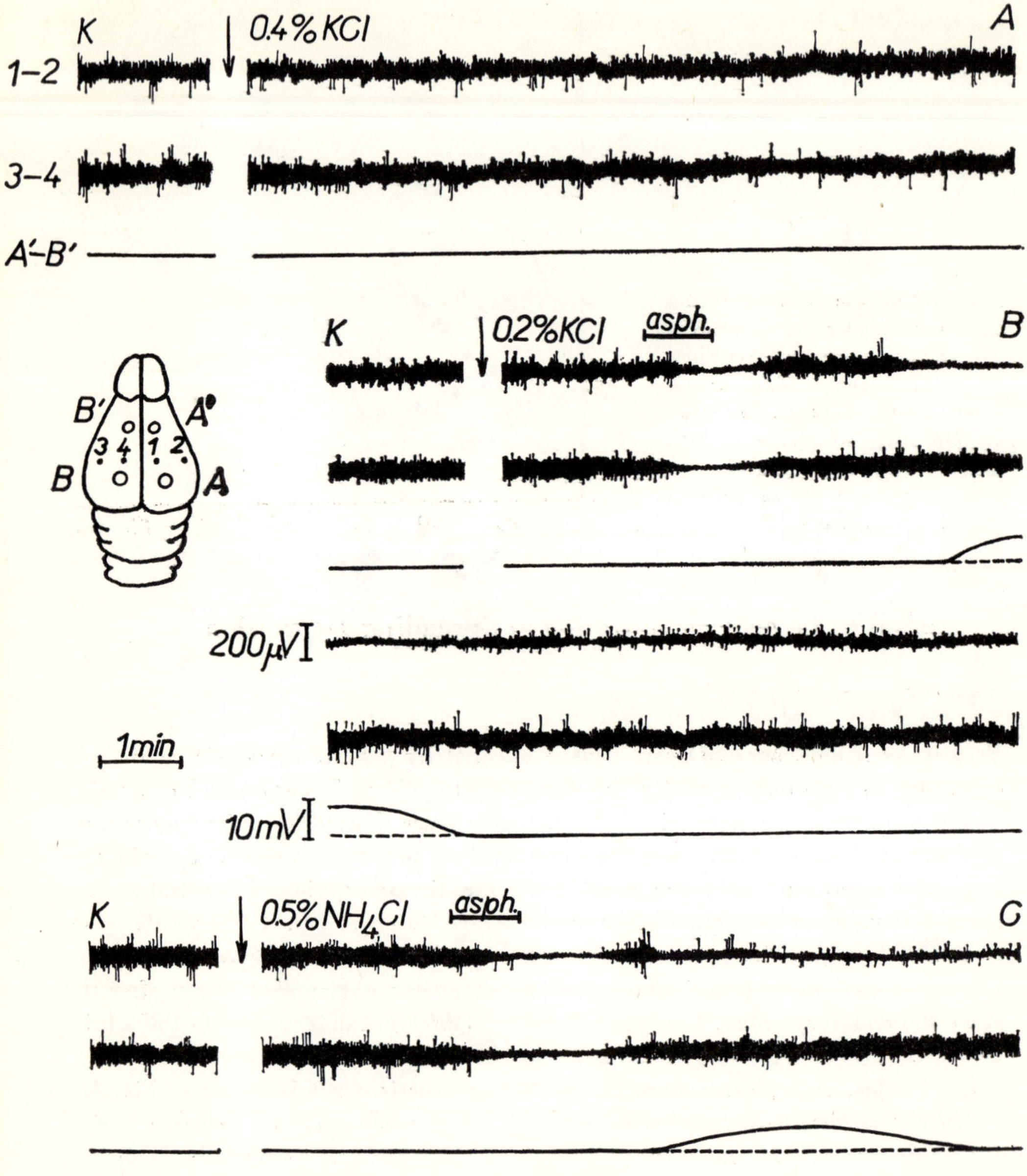

Fig. 3. 7. Activation of subthreshold foci of SD by asphyxia. (1—4) Steel needle electrodes for EEG recording. *(A', B')* Small trephine openings (3 mm in diameter) for application of calomel cell electrodes. *(A, B)* Large trephine openings (5 mm in diameter) for application of drugs. *(K)* Control recording. Arrows denote application of the substance evoking SD. Horizontal bar (*asph*) corresponds to duration of asphyxia. *(A)* 0.4 % KCl did not evoke CSD. *(B)* 0.2 % KCl solution may start CSD when followed by 45- sec asphyxia, which alone is ineffective (see absence of CSD in the other hemisphere). *(C)* Asphyxia can also activate a subthreshold NH_4Cl focus. Calibration: 200 μV for EEG; 10 mV for SPC. Upward deflection indicates negativity of *(A)* (Bureš and Burešová 1960a).

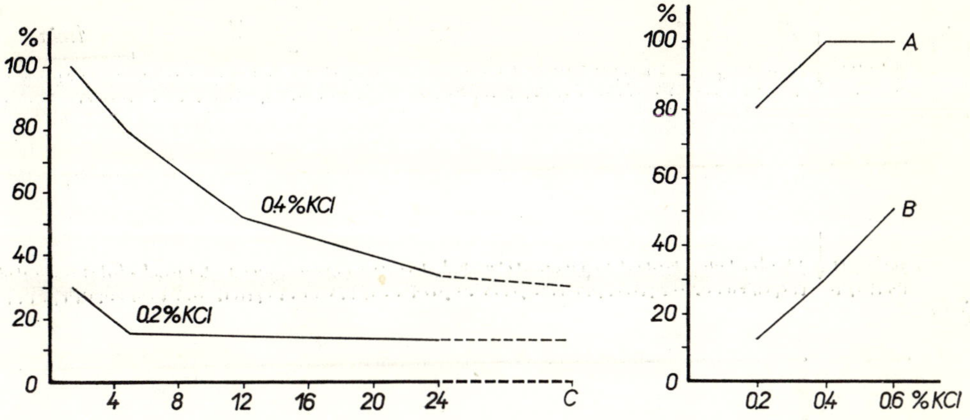

Fig. 3. 8. Changes of CSD susceptibility following 45-sec asphyxia (left) and activation of subthreshold KCl foci *(B)* by 45-sec asphyxia *(A)* (right). Ordinate: percentage of CSD waves evoked by the application of the respective KCl solution (left) or by 45-sec asphyxia (right). Left abscissa: time from 45-sec asphyxia to KCl application in minutes. *(C)* Control level. Right abscissa: KCl concentration used to establish the subthreshold focus.

10 min (Fig. 3.8). Thus both local application of drugs and asphyxia have aftereffects, the respective half times of which seem to be 30 to 45 min and 5 to 10 min, respectively. The mutual interaction of both processes was best demonstrated by experiments in which a subthreshold KCl focus was repeatedly activated by 30-sec asphyxia applied at regular intervals. When this interval was brief (10 to 15 min) the focus decayed very slowly and up to 10 SD waves could be generated in sequence. With longer intervals between asphyxias (20 to 30 min) the focus disappeared much faster. It seems that the decreasing activity of the focus is counteracted by the effect of asphyxia. The minimum interval at which the two processes balance each other is about 10 min under the above conditions.

The cumulative aftereffects of asphyxia could be demonstrated in rats, in which several asphyxias (four to six) were applied within 1 to 2 hours. A 0.6 % KCl solution applied in these animals evokes a train of four to six SD waves instead of the usual single one. Depletion of energy resources and their slow restoration is probably responsible for the above effects.

Hypoglycemia

Resistance to depolarization is also decreased by a reduced supply of glucose, the most important substrate of brain metabolism. Bureš and Burešová (1960a) found in anesthetized rats a considerable decrease of KCl threshold after intravenous injection of insulin (0.1 IU/kg). A typical example is shown in Fig. 3.9. The most

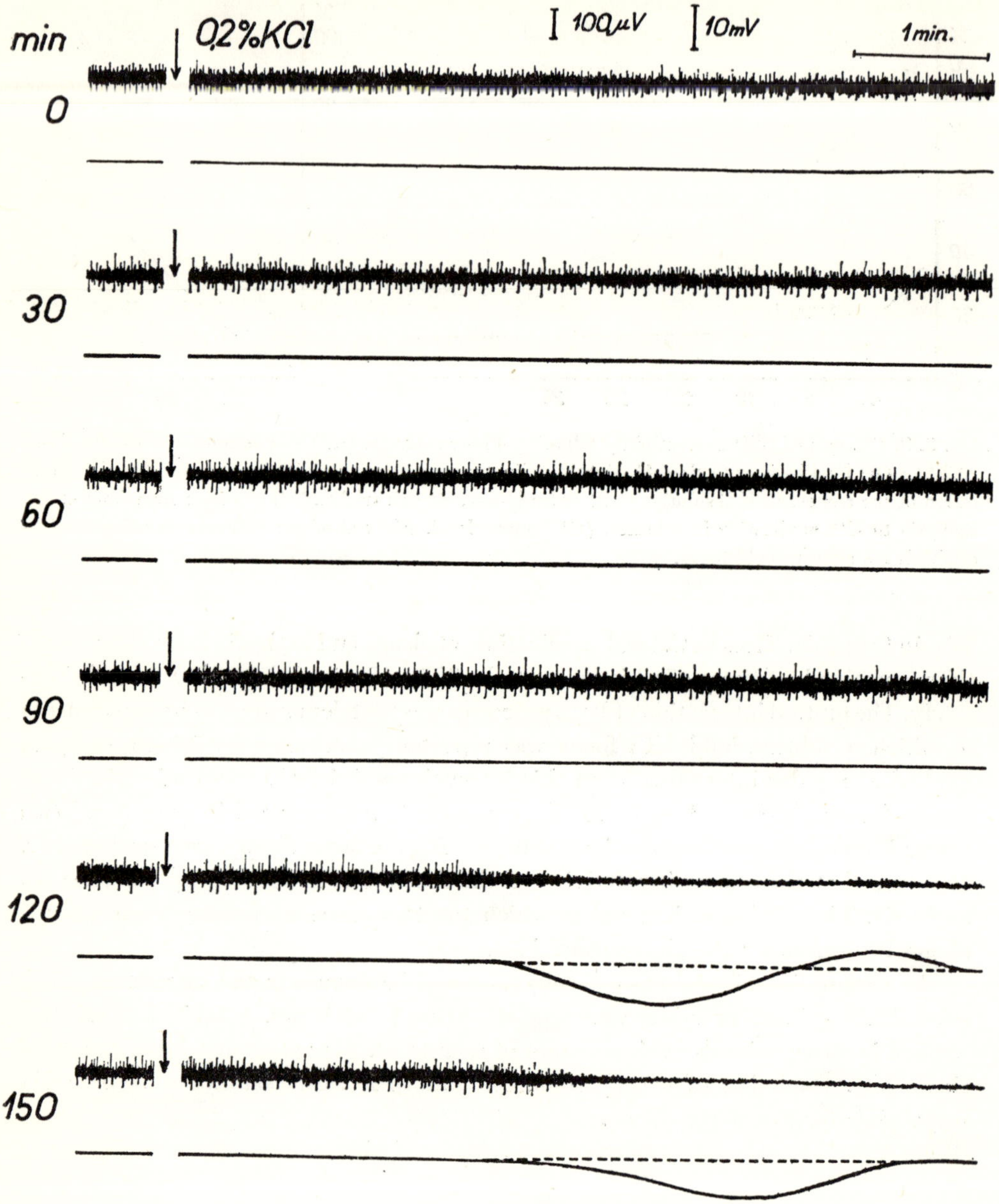

Fig. 3. 9. Effect of insulin (0.1 I. U./kg) on CSD susceptibility. Numbers on the left side indicate time in minutes after insulin injection. The subthreshold 0.2 % KCl started to evoke CSD 2 hours after insulin administration (Bureš and Burešová 1960a).

significant effect was observed 2 hours after insulin injection when the threshold dropped to 0.22 % KCl as compared with 0.54 % KCl in control animals. The insulin effect could only be revealed with repeated applications of subthreshold KCl solutions, however. A single application of a filter paper soaked in 0.2 % KCl was usually ineffective, even when applied during maximal hypoglycemia. The facilitating effect became manifest only in regions in which the increased level of extracellular K^+ had been maintained for some time. In further experiments (Burešová, Bureš, and Křivánek 1960) the dynamics of the facilitating effect was analyzed and compared with the course of the blood sugar curve. As shown in Fig. 3.10, both processes had a similar time course, but the changes of SD threshold were delayed approximately 1 hour. The threshold was maximally decreased in experiments in which the treatment of cerebral cortex with subthreshold KCl solutions coincided with maximum hypoglycemia.

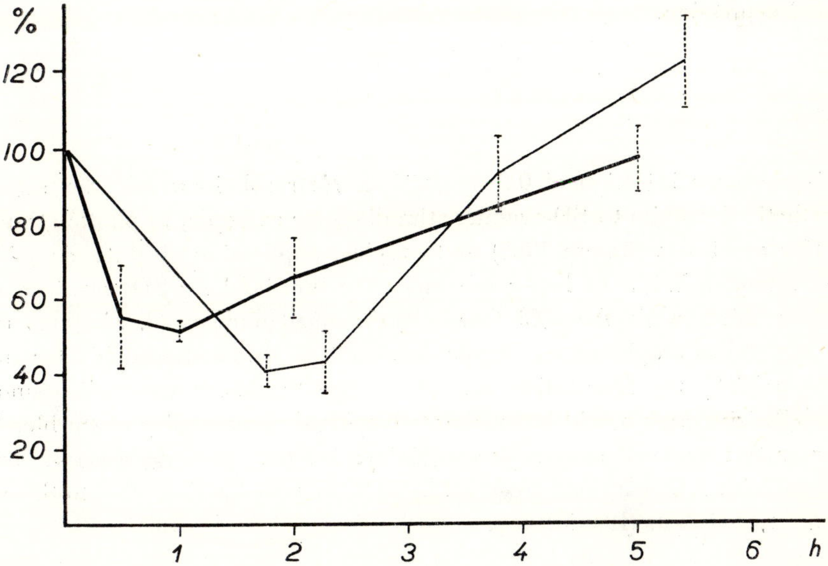

Fig. 3. 10. Changes of blood sugar concentration (heavy line) and threshold concentration of KCl (thin line) at various intervals after insulin administration (0.1 I. U./kg). Abscissa: hours since insulin administration. Ordinate: blood sugar concentration or KCl threshold in percentage of control values. Vertical dotted bars denote standard errors of the mean (Burešová, Bureš, and Křivánek 1960).

Recovery from the insulin effect was considerably retarded when the KCl solution evoked an SD wave. In this case application of the same subthreshold KCl concentrations at 1-hour intervals repeatedly evoked SD waves. It seems that each SD wave facilitated initiation of the following one by slowing down the recovery processes. Of course, the facilitating effect can only be observed in a certain critical interval.

All the above findings indicate that insulin-induced facilitation of SD is not primarily due to hypoglycemia but rather to a slowly developing depletion of substances essential for maintaining the active transport of ions across cellular membranes.

Adrenalectomy

The distribution of electrolytes between extracellular and intracellular compartments is maintained by active transport controlled by hormones of the adrenal cortex. According to Burešová and Poupa (1959) the KCl threshold is reduced 8 to 9 days after adrenalectomy by approximately 30 %. This change can be reversed by deoxycorticosterone but not by cortisone. Besides facilitating SD initiation, the electrolyte shifts induced by adrenalectomy prolong the duration of the SPC and of the EEG depression.

Metrazol

Slow intravenous injection of 0.2 to 0.25 g Metrazol increases the sensitivity of anesthetized rabbits to SD-evoking stimuli — for example, to photic stimulation (Van Harreveld and Stamm 1955) or to topical application of glutamic acid (Van Harreveld 1959). With the latter substance the threshold for SD was decreased to about one third, while the KCl threshold remained unchanged. Since no marked effect of metrazol on glutamate metabolism could be demonstrated (Potter and Van Harreveld 1962) the facilitation cannot be due to slower metabolic removal of this depolarizing amino acid but rather to increased permeability of the blood brain barrier or to increased membrane sensitivity. A slight local decrease of threshold was found with KCl solutions dissolved in 10 % metrazol and applied to the exposed cortical surface in rats (Bureš 1962).

Systemic Application of Depolarizing and Hyperpolarizing Agents

Most narcotics do not interfere with SD initiation even in dosages causing complete cessation of spontaneous EEG activity. This is not true, however, for higher concentrations of ether vapours administered for periods of 45 to 60 min (Van Harreveld and Stamm 1953a). When respiration was maintained artificially, 7% ether vapours increased SD threshold and 10% ether abolished SD completely after 20 min administration. As these levels of ether anesthesia are still reversible and characterized by considerable spontaneous EEG activity, the abolition of SD cannot be ascribed to injury but rather to partial depolarization of neurons. The depolarizing action of ether may perhaps explain the amnesic effect of ether anesthesia described by Pearlman (1966).

Essentially similar results were obtained with sublethal dosage of NaCN (6mg/kg, i. p.) which also causes partial depolarization of cortical neurons. This level of histotoxic anoxia (Bureš 1957b) abolishes spontaneous EEG activity and decreases the demarcation potential of the cerebral cortex to approximately 50%. Even very strong chemical stimuli (10% KCl) failed to elicit SD under these conditions, which resemble in many respects a protracted SD. It is probable that neural effects of many intoxications have a similar mechanism (Goldring, O'Leary, and Lam 1953). Other drugs may elicit repeated CSD waves starting from cortical surface. This was shown to be the case for methionine sulfoximine seizures in the rabbit (Johnson, Goldring, and O'Leary 1965). It seems that even some anesthetics may act in this way (Norton and Jewett 1967, see p. 354). Fifková and Van Harreveld (1970) took advantage of the high permeability of the blood brain barrier in chicken embryos and elicited SD in the striatum by rapid intravenous injection of glutamate (40 mg) in embryos at 18 to 19 days of incubation.

In contrast with the long list of depolarizing agents there are only a few factors inducing clear-cut hyperpolarization of central neurons. The most reliable of these is hypercapnia due to increased CO_2 content in the inspired air. According to Van Harreveld and Stamm (1953c) 7 to 15% CO_2 changed SD in the rabbit cortex into a spreading convulsion without affecting the concomitant SPC. These observations were recently confirmed by Caspers and Simmich (1966). On the contrary, Laget and Neverlée (1962) reported in rats breathing 12% CO_2 a diminution of SPC amplitude approximately proportional to the increase of cortical steady potential. The CO_2 effects were pertinently discussed by Marshall (1965).

4. Local Effects on Propagation of Spreading Depression

The preceding pages were concerned with processes taking place in the area of stimulus application, where stimulus-specific reactions are tightly interlaced with the actual SD mechanism. As both types of phenomena cannot be reliably separated, it is difficult to decide how much the agents affecting SD initiation influence the process of spreading. Spreading of SD far beyond the limits of the stimulus action is the most important sign of SD, the elucidation of which is of prime importance for understanding the mechanism of this phenomenon. One of the obvious approaches to these problems is the analysis of agents affecting velocity, intensity, and extent of SD in regions invaded from a remote area.

Local Facilitation

Subthreshold concentrations of most substances, the local application of which facilitates SD initiation (see p. 53), can also facilitate SD propagation. Thus treatment of the rabbit retrosplenial area with Tyrode solution, the K^+ concentration of which was increased ten times, makes this brain region accessible to SD waves generated in the adjacent neocortex (Van Harreveld and Bogen 1956). Local application of subthreshold concentrations of KCl (Marshall, Essig, and Witkin 1951, Freygang and Landau 1955) or of metabolic inhibitors (Leão and Martins-Ferreira 1956) considerably facilitates spreading of SD in the gyrencephalic brain of cats. Leão and Martins-Ferreira (1961) used either hypotonic NaCl (30 to 40 mM) or isotonic sodium acetate (160 mM) to facilitate SD in cerebellum, superior colliculus and bulbus olfactorius of the rabbit. After 20 to 30 min of treatment SD could be easily and regularly evoked in these regions otherwise partially or completely refractory to SD. Attempts to influence the rate of spreading in a similar way were less convincing. An experiment performed by Bureš (1962) is illustrated in Fig. 3.11. Spreading depres-

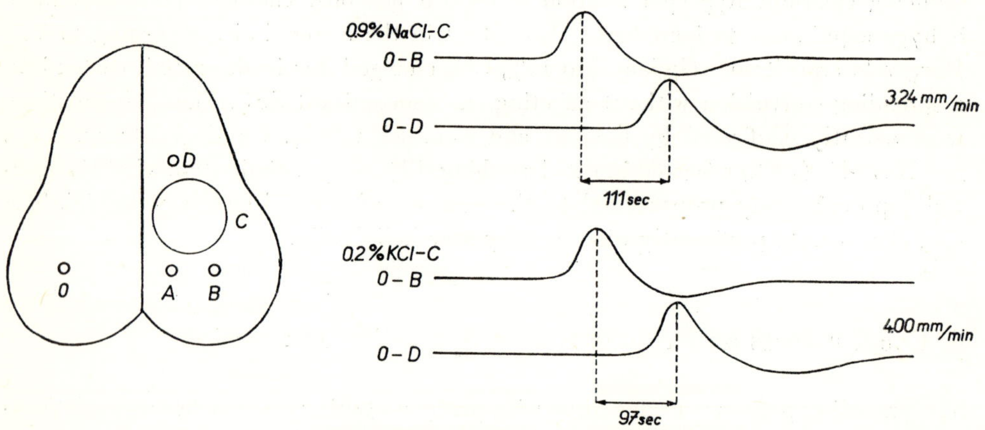

Fig. 3. 11. Faster propagation of CSD through a cortical area pretreated with 0.2 % KCl. The inset diagram shows the distribution of the trephine openings over the rat brain. Cortical SD was evoked from trephine opening *(A)* and SPC recorded from trephine opening *(B)* and *(D)*, after area *(C)* was treated either with 0.9 % NaCl (above) or with 0.2 % KCl (below). Spreading rates across area *(C)* are calculated from the *(AB)* and *(AD)* distances and corresponding delays (Bureš 1962).

sion was elicited from trephine opening A and recorded in two cortical regions B and D to one of which SD penetrated through an area 4 mm in diameter, treated with 0.2% KCl. Comparison of velocities indicates that SD spreads through the K^+-treated region faster than through the normal cortex. The difference is relatively small, however.

Local Blockade

There are only a few ways to prevent reversibly the penetration of SD into a given brain region. According to Leão (1944a) SD stops at a narrow strip of cocaine-treated cortex in the rabbit. Grafstein (1956b) repeated these experiments in the isolated cortical slab of the cat. A 2-mm-wide filter paper applied across the whole width of the slab stopped SD propagation when soaked with 5 % procaine hydrochloride. A 2% solution was ineffective. Leão (1961, 1963) reported slow propagation or blockade of CSD in a cortical region treated with hypertonic (280 mM) NaCl, NaBr or $NaNO_3$. Choline chloride or tetraethylammonium chloride exerted an even more powerful blocking action.

Ochs and Hunt (1960) studied penetration of CSD into a cortical island formed by subpial incisions, disrupting all cortical layers with the exception of the molecular layer. This narrow bridge of cortical tissue, consisting predominantly of dendrites, can mediate effective spread of SD into the island. Treatment of the area of incision with 1% GABA or 0.1% nicotine caused a reversible blockade of the SD passage through the subpial bridge. The same concentrations of GABA or nicotine did not block SD in normal cortex, evidently because blocking concentrations were not attained in deeper cortical layers.

The most powerful blocking action is exerted by divalent cations, especially Ca^{2+} and Mg^{2+} (Bureš and Burešová 1956b, c, Bureš 1960, Burešová and Bureš 1960).

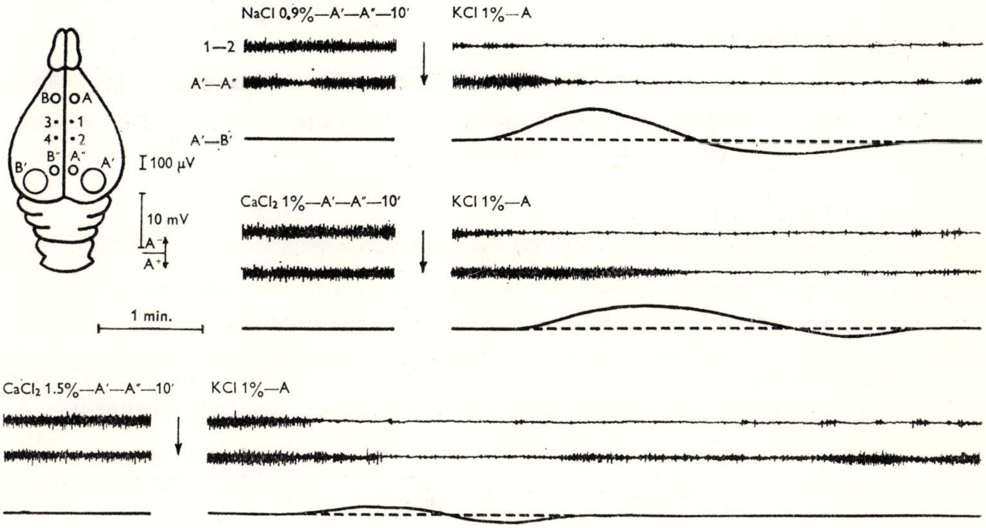

Fig. 3. 12. Block of propagation of CSD into a cortical region protected by different concentrations of $CaCl_2$. (1, 2, 3, 4) Steel needle electrodes for EEG recording. (*A' A" B' B"*) Trephine openings for $CaCl_2$ application. (A, B) Trephine openings for evoking CSD by application of 1% KCl. Calibration: 100 μV for EEG; 10 mV for SPC (Bureš and Burešová 1956c).

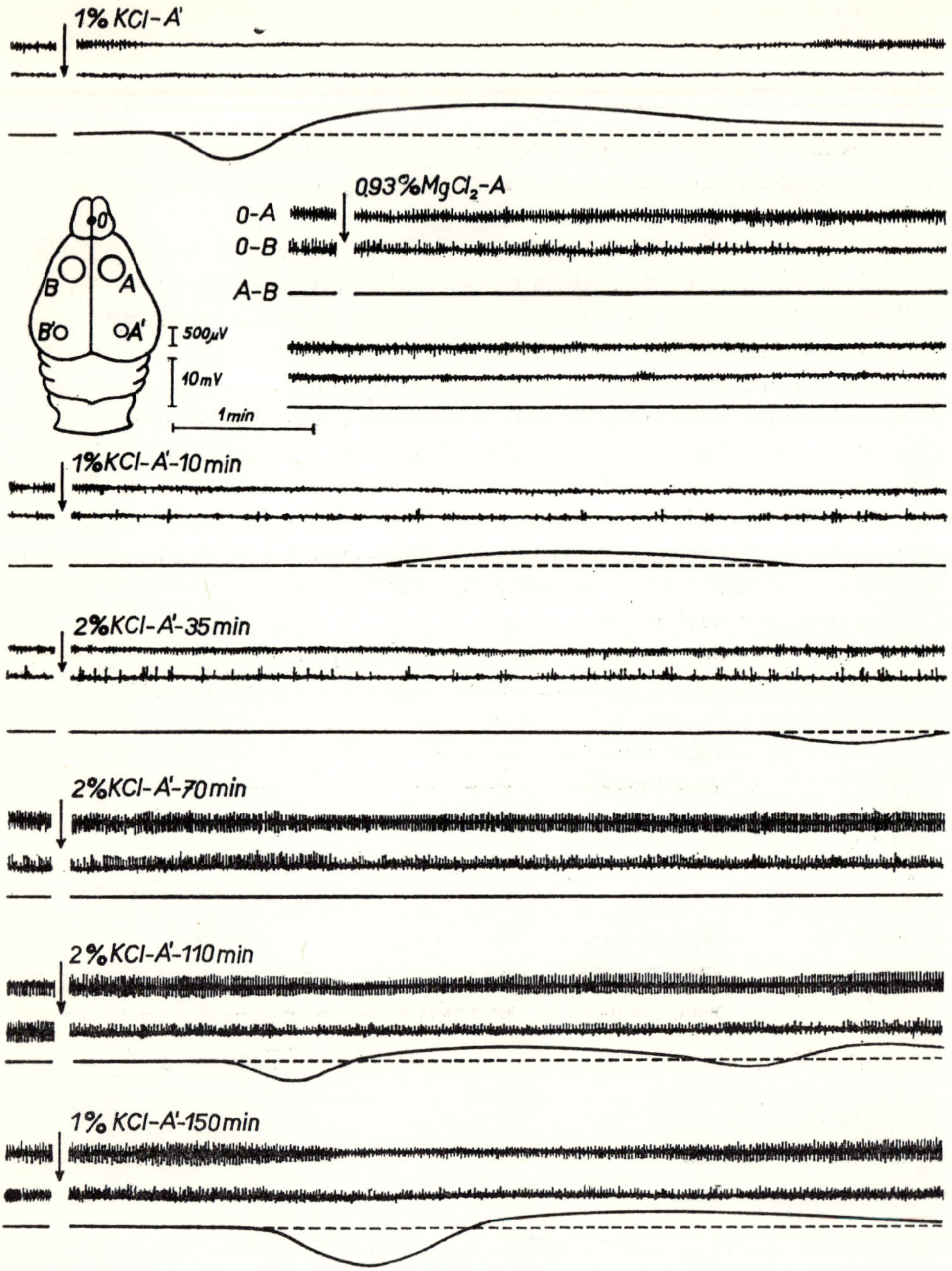

Fig. 3. 13. Protection of somatosensory evoked responses (left sciatic nerve stimulation at 1/2 sec) against the CSD effect by treatment of the cortical projection area with 0.93% $MgCl_2$. *(A, B)* Trephine openings for recording the evoked potentials and the SPC. (A', B') Trephine openings for eliciting CSD by application of 1% KCl or 2% KCl. Calibration: 500 µV for EEG; 10mV for SPC. (First

A typical experiment is illustrated by Fig. 3.12. First, saline was applied to areas *A*', *A*'' in which the SD wave evoked from area *A* was recorded. Then $CaCl_2$ solutions of different concentrations were applied to *A*' and *A*''. Spreading of SD into the treated region was examined 10 min later. When $CaCl_2$ concentration reached 1.5 %, the wave of depression ceased to enter the protected areas. This was indicated by shorter and less marked depression of EEG activity and by decreased amplitude of the negative SPC.

Divalent cations can also protect cortical evoked responses in the treated area. As shown in Fig. 3.13, 0.93% $MgCl_2$ causes an initial reduction of evoked responses in the treated region protected against SD invasion. After 30 to 60 min evoked responses recover and since the protective effect against SD is still pronounced, they remain unaffected by SD waves generated from remote areas. It is only after several hours that the protective effect disappears, the negative waves start to enter area *A*, and the evoked response begins to show the characteristic reduction again.

The average reduction of SPC in the protected areas is shown in Fig. 3.14. By interpolating these values it is possible to estimate the concentrations

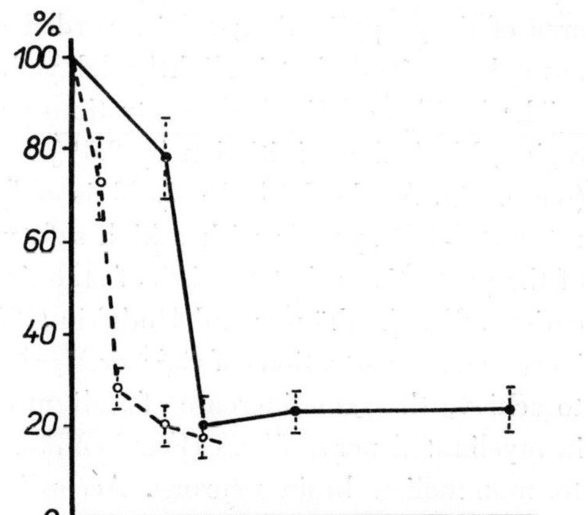

Fig. 3. 14. Blockade of CSD propagation in the rat cortex by divalent cations. (Above) Amplitude of the negative SPC (in percentages of control values) penetrating into a cortical area pretreated for 10 min with different concentrations of $CaCl_2$ (full line) or $MgCl_2$ (dashed line) indicated on the abscissa. (Below) Amplitude of the negative SPC (in percentages of control values) penetrating into a cortical area at different times after the 10-min pretreatment with 0.05 M $MgCl_2$ was terminated. Dotted vertical bars indicate the standard error of the mean values (Bureš 1960).

---

recording) CSD under control conditions. (Second and third recordings, continuous) The effect of $MgCl_2$ alone. (Further recordings) CSD waves evoked at indicated intervals after $MgCl_2$ application (Burešová and Bureš 1960).

of $MgCl_2$ and $CaCl_2$ causing 50% lowering of SPC amplitude as 0.042 and 0.12 M, respectively. Slightly higher concentrations give maximum protection.

A closer analysis of the time course of the protective effect demonstrated gradual penetration of the divalent cations into deep cortical layers. During the first few minutes after $CaCl_2$ or $MgCl_2$ application, well-developed surface positivity indicated SD passage through deep layers (Bureš 1960). The maximum blocking effect was reached 10 min after drug application and then subsided slowly with a half time of 30 to 40 min (Fig. 3.14), probably proportional to the decrease of the drug concentration. The treated region is protected not only from single but also from repeated SD waves produced by 25% KCl. The protective effect is confined to the area of drug application; SPC recorded only 2 mm outside the treated area has a normal amplitude but is slightly delayed.

The $MgCl_2$ and $CaCl_2$ concentrations preventing penetration of SD into the treated region, blocked SD initiation by 2.4% KCl if they were added to this KCl solution (see p. 46). As the KCl threshold is only 0.6% KCl, this finding indicates that in rat cortex SD spreads with a high safety factor through all layers. The mechanism of the protective effect consists of stabilization of the cell membrane by the divalent cations. Frankenhäuser and Hodgkin (1957) have shown in squid axons that with increased concentrations of Ca^{2+} or Mg^{2+} a higher degree of depolarization is required to achieve the same increase of sodium conductance. Similar results were obtained in myelinated nerve fibres (Frankenhäuser and Meves 1958) and recently extended to mammalian brain neurons. According to Krnjević (1965), Somjen and Kato (1968), and Kato and Somjen (1969) microelectrophoretic application of divalent cations depresses discharges of neurons evoked by glutamate or by synaptic influences. The effect seems to be a predominantly postsynaptic one, since intracellular recording reveals an elevation of electrical threshold unaccompanied by any significant changes of spontaneous and evoked PSPs, membrane potential, or membrane resistance (Kelly, Krnjević, and Somjen 1969). Burešová, Shima, Bureš, and Fifková (1963) recorded unit activity in cortical areas treated with 0.1 M $MgCl_2$. This solution did not suppress the firing of deeply located neurons. On the contrary it protected them against the direct effect of SD evoked from a distance. Depression of surface activity in a cortical area treated with 0.1 M $MgSO_4$ was reported by Bindman, Lippold, and Redfearn (1962) while normal potentials persisted at a depth of 1 mm below the surface.

The blocking effect of GABA (see p. 63) is also probably due to the stabilizing effect on the cell membrane (Curtis, Phillis, and Watkins 1959). Unlike divalent cations, GABA does not penetrate in sufficient concentration into the deep cortical layers and cannot therefore cause a complete block of SD in normal cortex. This restriction does no apply to the isolated chicken retina, where SD can be suppressed by GABA or glycine (Van Harreveld and Fifková 1971).

5. General Influences on Propagation of Spreading Depression

Body Temperature

Analysis of temperature dependence of different biological functions may provide important information on the nature of the underlying mechanisms. As electrochemical processes are described by equations in which temperature appears in Kelvin degrees, an increase or decrease of temperature in the biologically permissible limits does not substantially influence concentration, diffusion, or membrane potentials ($Q_{10} \doteq 1.0$). On the other hand, the rate of metabolic processes is strikingly dependent on temperature variation within the same range ($Q_{10} = 3$ to 4). The quantitative relationships between body temperature and different manifestations

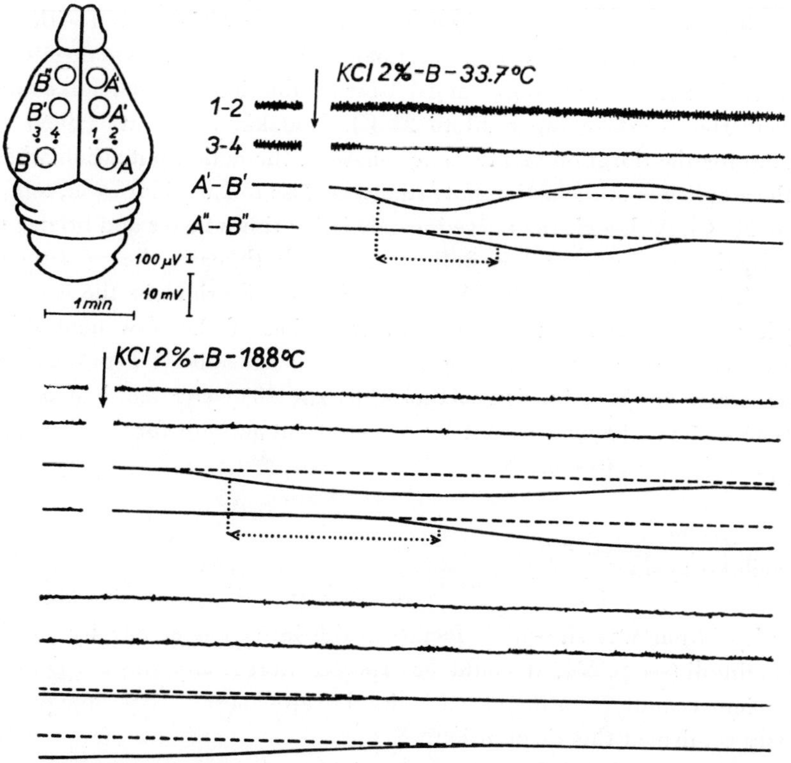

Fig. 3. 15. Influence of reduced body temperature on CSD in rat. (1, 2, 3, 4) Steel needle electrodes for EEG recording. *(A', A", B', B")* Trephine openings for application of wick calomel cell electrodes. Cortical SD was evoked by applying a filter paper soaked with 2% KCl onto the trephine opening *B* (arrow) at colonic temperatures 33.7 (above) or 18.8 °C (below). The dotted horizontal bars indicate the delays with which the SPC records reach 50% of the negative maximum at the proximal and distal electrodes. This delay and the distance *(B', B")* was used for calculating the spreading rate. Calibration: 100 μV for EEG; 10 mV for SPC (Bureš, Burešová, and Zacharová 1957).

of SD were studied by Bureš, Burešová, and Zacharová (1957) in anesthetized rats, the colonic temperatures of which were varied between 42 °C and 17 °C by passing warm or cold water through copper tubing coiled around the animals' bodies. The spreading rate, duration, and amplitude of the negative SPC was established for at least two temperature levels in each rat. A typical experiment is illustrated in Fig. 3.15. With decreasing body temperature the SPC became more prolonged and its conduction slower. On the other hand the amplitude of the slow negative wave remained unchanged, even when body temperature dropped below 20 °C, that is, at a time when the spontaneous EEG was nearly absent and the SPC remained the only manifestation of SD.

Figure 3.16 summarizes the results of the above experiments. The spreading rate and the duration of the negative slow potential (measured at 50% of maximum) changed with a Q_{10} equal to 1.7 and 2.0, respectively, the amplitude of the slow potential with a Q_{10} equal to 1.0. These values agree surprisingly well with analogous Q_{10} data for action potentials in nerve fibers. Chatfield and Lyman (1954) found in nerves of the rat tail a Q_{10} of 2.0 and 1.1 for conduction rate and spike amplitude, respectively (temperature range 13 to 23 °C). Hodgkin and Katz (1949) reported a Q_{10} of 2.0 for the duration of the rising phase of the action potential, whereas the Q_{10} for the amplitude of the action potential was close to 1.0 (giant axon, temperature range 5 to 20 °C). Although the nerve impulse is 10^5 times faster and briefer than the SPC of SD, the similar Q_{10} values indicate that in both cases the amplitude of the electrical change depends on the electrochemical equilibrium in the cellular membrane, whereas the spreading rate and the duration of the slow potential depend on more complex processes regulating membrane permeability. Temperature dependent decrease of the K^+ diffusion coefficient (2.5×10^{-5} cm^2 sec^{-1} at 38 °C, 1.7×10^{-5} cm^2 sec^{-1} at 18 °C) can contribute to but not account for the observed reduction of spreading rate (see p. 162).

Anoxia and Asphyxia

Since asphyxiation was shown to facilitate the initiation of SD by subthreshold chemical stimuli (see p. 55), it could be expected that it also affects SD in a similar way in regions remote from the area of stimulus application. Experimental evidence only partly confirmed this assumption.

Leão and Morrison (1945) showed that 1 min of cerebral circulatory arrest produced after SD had been evoked from the frontal cortex did not stop SD propagation to the occipital cortex. In a later study Leão (1947) investigated the effect of asphyxiation on the slow potential change of SD. A 1-min asphyxiation enhanced and prolonged the negative slow potential in areas that had just been entered by SPC and caused appearance of a second negative wave in regions in which the negative potential started to decline or to change into the positive phase. These results were confirmed

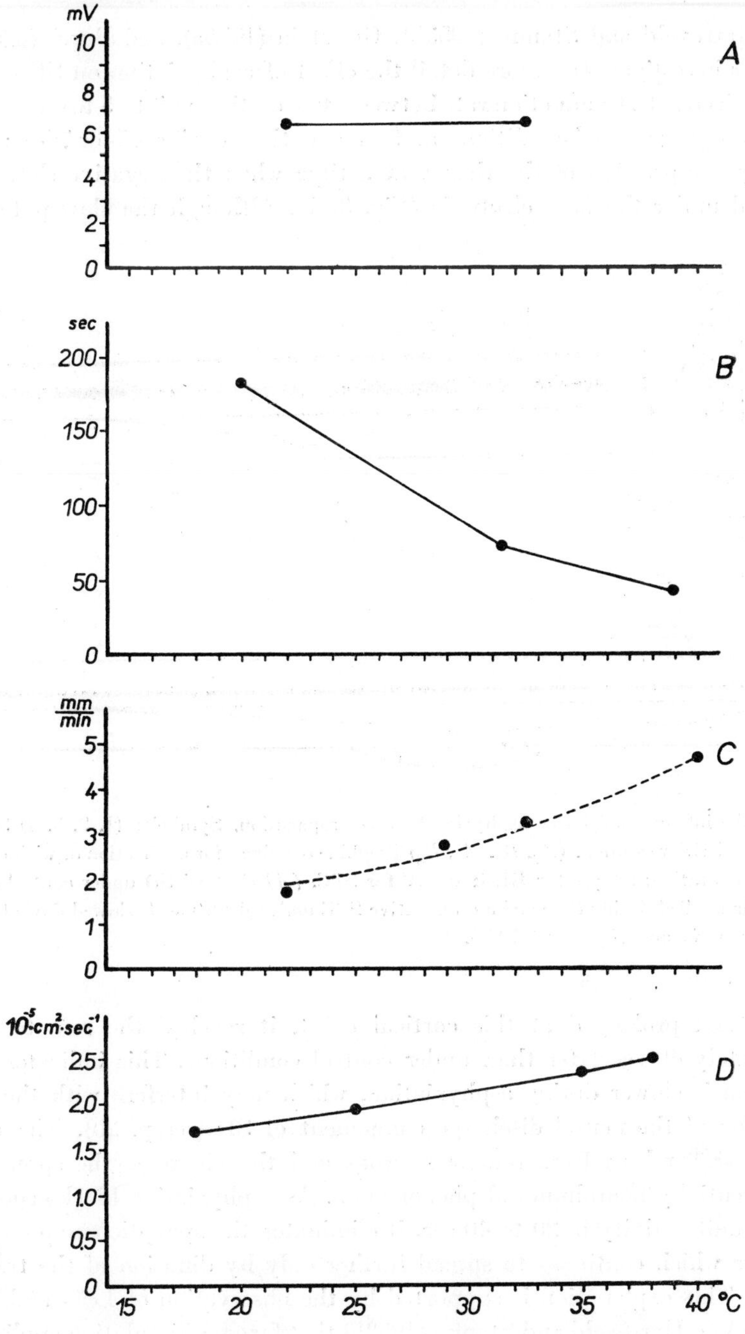

Fig. 3. 16. Dependence of the CSD parameters on body temperature (abscissa). *(A)* SPC amplitude (mV), *(B)* Duration (sec) of the SPC exceeding 50% of maximum negativity. *(C)* Spreading rate (mm/min). Dashed line corresponds to the theoretical curve calculated for $Q_{10} = 1.7$. *(D)* Diffusion coefficient of K^+ in free solutions ($10^5 cm^2 sec^{-1}$).

by Van Harreveld and Stamm (1953b), Grafstein (1956a), and Bureš (1957b). The last author investigated in more detail the effect of asphyxiation on SD conduction in anesthetized rats. Conduction rate between two cortical points 5 to 6 mm apart was established under normal conditions at first and then during 45- or 75-sec asphyxia evoked by compression of the thorax at a time when the negative slow potential culminated under the near electrode (Fig. 3.17). Although the slow potential was

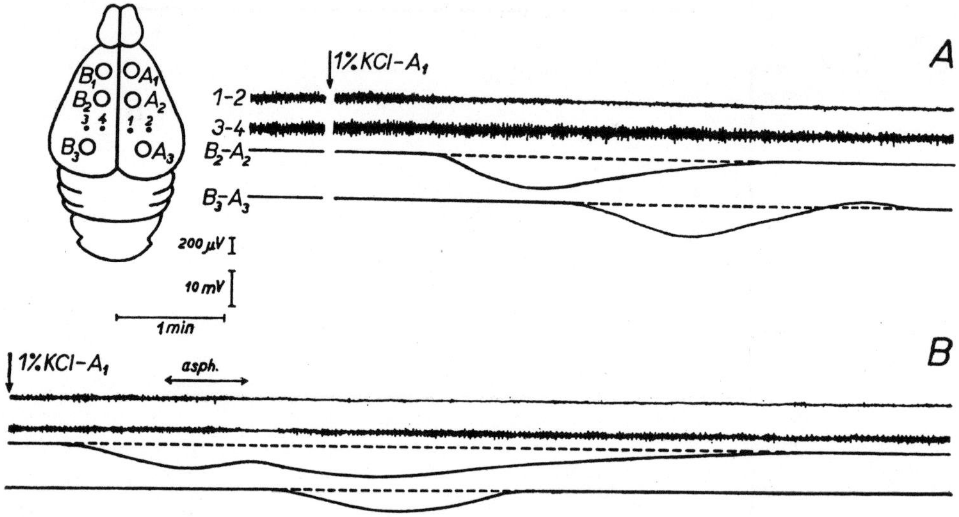

Fig. 3. 17. The influence of 45-sec asphyxia on CSD propagation. Symbols: (1, 2, 3, 4) Steel needle electrodes for EEG recording. (A_2, B_2, A_3, B_3) Trephine openings for application of wick calomel cell electrodes. Calibration: 200 μV for EEG; 10 mV for SPC. *(A)* Cortical SD under control conditions. *(B)* Asphyxia applied during the maximum negative SPC under electrode A_2 slowed down CSD propagation between A_2 and A_3 (Bureš 1957).

enhanced and prolonged at this cortical point, it reached the remote electrode approximately 40 sec later than under control conditions. This indicates that SD propagation is slower during asphyxiation, which may interfere with the synaptic stansmission of the neural discharge component of SD (see p. 20). The discharge may cause K^+ release from remote neurons and thus increase the spreading rate of this essentially neurohumoral phenomenon. As asphyxiation blocks spontaneous EEG and unit activity in 20 to 40 sec, it eliminates the synaptic component of the SD process which continues to spread further only by diffusion of the transmitter substance. This explanation is supported by the observation of Leão and Morrison (1945) and Van Harreveld and Stamm (1953b) that faradic stimulation applied during asphyxiation does not elicit SD. On the other hand, asphyxiation also leads to release of K^+ from neurons and finally to depolarization (see p. 76). With longer duration of asphyxiation the retardation of SD is compensated for by the slower developing facilitation. This may explain why 45- and 75-sec asphyxiation cause the same delay of CSD. Evidence for the possible dissociation of the aerobic and anaerobic components of SD mechanism was also obtained by Leão and Martins-Ferreira (1959) who decsribed in the hippocampal SPC two phases differentially sensitive to ischemia. When the circulation was interrupted at SPC onset, the negativity was halted at a level markedly below the normal one. Upon release of the circulation the negative potential first rose to full amplitude and only then returned to the baseline.

Hypoglycemia

Martins-Ferreira (1954, 1955b) influenced CSD in the rabbit by high dosage of insulin, which decreased the blood sugar level to 20mg per 100 ml. Under these conditions the negative cortical SPC was increased to 30 mV and prolonged to 5 min. Administration of glucose immediately returned the SPC to control values. According to de Mello and da Silva (1960), CSD in the hypoglycemic rabbit is characterized by two phases — a rapid initial negativization which then more slowly increases to maximum. The slow phase is absent during ischemia but develops upon release of the arterial occlusion. Similar two-phase SPCs were also described by Leão and Martins-Ferreira (1959) in the exposed rabbit hippocampus.

Chapter 4
Anoxic Depolarization

Short-lasting anoxia or asphyxia (about 1 min) used in the preceding chapter does not elicit SD, but more prolonged interruption of the oxygen supply (2 to 5 min) evokes in the cerebral cortex a well-defined reaction called by Marshall (1959) "asphyxial (or anoxic) SD". Use of this term is not quite justified by the electrophysiological manifestations of the process, which starts several minutes after EEG activity has completely disappeared and develops simultaneously in many cortical points. Although neither EEG changes nor regular spreading characterize the cortical effects of prolonged anoxia, other signs clearly point toward a close relationship with SD. Since the most obvious of these is a striking negativization of cortical surface, the term "anoxic (ischemic, asphyxial) depolarization" is more commonly used in this context.

1. Asphyxial Slow Potential Change

Anoxic depolarization was first described in the rabbit cerebral cortex by Leão (1947). The finding was soon confirmed in a number of studies (Leão 1951, Goldensohn, Schoenfeld, and Hoefer 1951, Goldring and O'Leary 1951, Van Harreveld and Stamm 1953b, Kempinsky 1954, Grafstein 1956a, Bureš 1957b, Bureš and Burešová 1957, Benešová, Bureš, and Burešová 1957). The absolute amplitude and shape of the negative wave varied according to the conditions of recording; it was usually low and brief when the depolarization also affected the reference region (for example, the ventricle, skull bones over intact cortex). Placement of the indifferent electrode on really inactive tissue is therefore essential, but considerable separation of the active cortical electrode from the remote reference electrode increases the possible contamination of the recorded potential difference by extracortical dipoles. The location of the reference electrode also determines the absolute base-line level of the cortical steady potential which may vary from positive to negative values depending on the amount of injury in the reference region (periostal or intraventricular electrode). Perhaps the most justified absolute values can be obtained by measuring the cortical injury potential. As pointed out by Marshall (1959) the maximum demarcation potential is generated by the potential difference between the fully depolarized somatodendritic membranes of cortical neurons and their intact corticofugal axons. The corresponding membrane potential difference amounts to 60 to 80 mV, but the actual *IR* drop between source and sink depends on the resistivity of the cortex and on the internal resistance of the sources. The proportionality between the average membrane potential measured by intracellular electrodes and the demarcation potential was confirmed by Bureš, Fifková, and Mareš (1964) and by Mareš (1964) (see p. 144).

A typical experiment showing the changes of the demarcation potential after decapitation in an anesthetized rat is shown in Fig. 4.1. The initial potential difference does not change, or may even slightly increase during the first 2 to 3 min, but then rapidly declines to zero. Thermocoagulation of intact cortical surface at this stage of ischemia elicited only a small demarcation potential, indicating that the cortical neurons had already been depolarized (Bureš 1957b).

The depolarization change also depends on the exact mechanism of the interruption of oxygen supply. Bureš and Burešová (1957) pointed out that anoxia evoked by respiration of pure nitrogen is accompanied by a more rapid development of anoxic depolarization than asphyxia elicited by clamping of the trachea. In the latter case accumulation of CO_2 in the blood causes an initial increase of the cortical steady

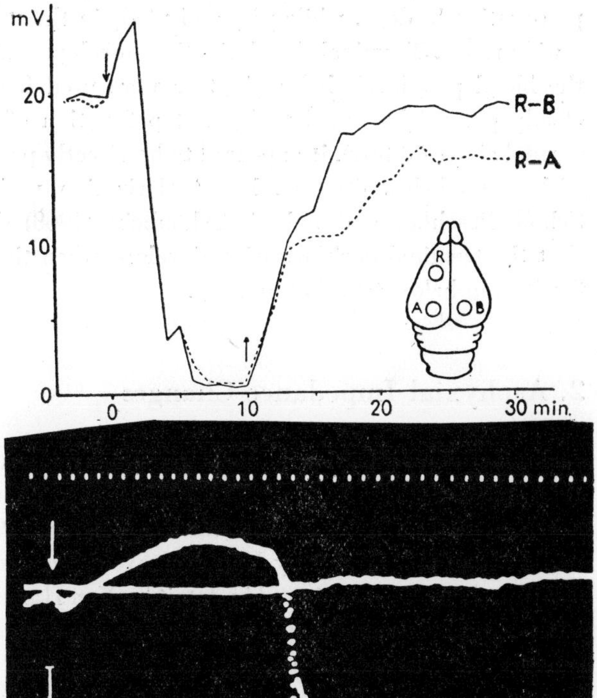

Fig. 4. 1. Terminal anoxic depolarization in the rat cerebral cortex. The inset diagram shows distribution of trephine openings. *R* is a cortical area destroyed by thermocoagulation, *A, B* is the intact cortex. (Above) Changes of the cortical demarcation potential during and after 10 min of reversible ischaemia (between arrows). (Below) Oscillographic recording of the rapid phase of depolarization. Horizontal trace corresponds to the reference potential. Calibration: 10 mV; time mark 10 sec (Bureš, Petráň, and Zachar 1960).

potential, which counteracts to some extent the depolarizing effect of the simultaneously developing pO_2 drop. Brain ischemia caused by circulatory arrest is actually an asphyxia limited to brain that is separated from the oxygen supplies in the rest of the body. The relationship between the cortical steady potential, arterial pO_2, pCO_2, and EEG activity was carefully analyzed by Speckmann and Caspers (1963, 1967) and by Caspers, Schütz, and Speckmann (1963) in curarized rats. According to the results of these authors, asphyxia (stopping artificial respiration) elicits after 5 to 10 sec a low initial negativity (hundreds of microvolts), followed after 10 to 20 sec by an intermediate positivity, which finally changes into extensive terminal depolarization. Whereas the initial negativity corresponds to activation of cortical neurons (arousal triggered from chemoreceptors), the ensuing positivity closely corresponds to the increase of pCO_2 and decrease of pH in the arterial blood. The terminal depolarization starts when cortical pO_2 reaches a critical level independent of pCO_2 and pH, usually at the time when cardiac failure has reduced the cerebral blood flow to zero. The effects of asphyxia on circulation were eliminated in a study by Hirsch, Scholl, Dickmans, Eisolt, Gaehtgens, Mann, and Krankenhagen (1968) in which steady potential of the lateral gyrus was measured in the isolated head preparation in dogs, while pO_2 and pCO_2 in the perfusing blood were changed over a wide range. Terminal depolarization developed with a latency of 1 to 2 min when the blood pO_2 levels below 40 torr were used for perfusion. Whereas the cortical steady potential seemed to be a step function of arterial pO_2 (depolarized below, normal above 40 torr), it appeared to be directly proportional to pCO_2 (depolarization with pCO_2 below 40 torr, hyperpolarization with pCO_2 above 40 torr). Hirsch, Scholl, Paschke, and Schmid-Schönbein (1968) showed with the same technique that the terminal depolarization develops when the perfusion pressure is mantained for 10 min below 60 to 40 mm Hg.

2. Asphyxial Impedance Changes

Asphyxial depolarization is accompanied by marked increase of the impedance of the asphyxiated brain tissue. This impedance change was first demonstrated with a bridge method by Leão and Martins-Ferreira (1953) and confirmed by Freygang and Landau (1955) and by Van Harreveld and Ochs (1956). The technical aspects of the problem were reviewed in detail by Van Harreveld (1966). A typical experiment in the rat is illustrated in Fig. 4.2. After the onset of brain ischemia cortical impedance (mainly its resistive component) rises only slightly for 2 to 3 min. At the time when the anoxic depolarization develops, the impedance suddenly increases by more than 50% during 1 min. After this jump, impedance continues to rise slowly and reaches approximately 400% of the initial level after several hours.

The close correlation between the fast components of asphyxial depolarization and impedance increase indicates that the two phenomena are different manifestations of the same basic process, which was systematically studied by Van Harreveld (1966). The sudden impedance increase is accompanied by an increase of the diameter of apical dendrites (+27 %) and of the perikarya of pyramidal cells (+12 %) indicating a 50% increase of nerve cell volume (Van Harreveld 1957). Electron micrographs of freeze-dried surface layers of cerebral cortex of the mouse showed

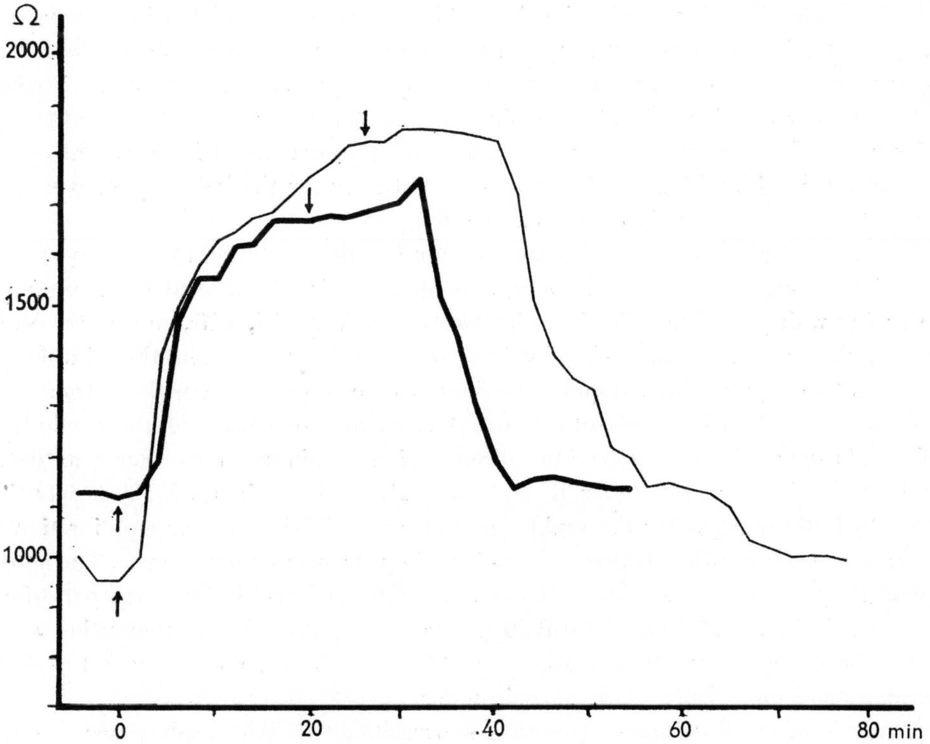

Fig. 4. 2. Changes of cortical impedance during and after transient cortical ischemia in the rat. Heavy line indicates 20-min ischemia, thin line indicates 24-min ischemia, arrows indicate the onset and termination of ischemia. Ordinate: cortical impedance between two silver electrodes (3 mm in diameter, 6 mm intercentral distance, measuring current 10 μA, 1000/sec) applied onto the frontal and occipital cortices of the same hemisphere (Bureš, Petráň, and Zachar 1960).

that the extracellular space is reduced from the usual 20% to approximately 6% during asphyxial depolarization (Van Harreveld and Malhotra 1967). Using the freeze substitution technique, movement of chloride into the apical dendrites was shown to occur during the rapid impedance increase (Van Harreveld and Schadé 1959). Together with the finding that the membrane potential of cortical neurons rapidly decreases at the time of asphyxial depolarization (Collevijn and Van Harreveld 1966), all these results are compatible with the hypothetical mechanism of SD (see Chap. 6).

Blockade of oxidative metabolism arrests the sodium pump and causes slow accumulation of potassium (or of other depolarizing substances) in the extracellular space. When the concentration of the depolarizing agent reaches a critical level, the sodium permeability of the membrane suddenly increases and sodium moves into the cells. Since at this time the sodium influx exceeds the sodium outflux by a considerable amount, electroneutrality of the intracellular compartment can only be maintained by simultaneous influx of chloride ions. The transport of substantial amounts of extracellular ions into cells generates osmotic gradients, the development of which is prevented by movements of water maintaining equal osmolarity of the extracellular and intracellular fluids. The asphyxial impedance increase is due to a net loss of extracellular ions or, in other words, to a relative decrease of the volume of the extracellular fluid, which provides the main pathway for the low-frequency electric currents used in conductivity measurements.

The K^+ release from the asphyxiated cortex was demonstrated by the superfusion technique (Bureš and Křivánek 1960), and recently directly verified by intracortical recording with potassium selective microelectrodes (Vyskočil, Kříž, and Bureš 1972). During the first few minutes of asphyxia K^+ activity slowly rose until the critical level of 11 mEq/l was reached. Rapid potassium release increased then the extracellular potassium level in a few seconds to 75 mM. This change coincided with the rapid phase of anoxic depolarization. Potassium accumulation continued more slowly until the 100 mM level was reached after 10 min asphyxia. The maximum K^+ concentration attained immediately after the rapid phase of depolarization reflects equilibration of potassium concentration between extra- and intracellular compartments. The subsequent slow K^+ increase is probably due to liberation of chemically bound potassium. Even the 100 mM K^+ level was still 20% below the 125 mM K^+ concentration which would be theoretically obtained when all brain potassium (100 mM/kg wet weight) forms an aqueous solution with all brain water.

Analysis of small samples of cortical subarachnoid fluid in asphyxiated foetuses of rhesus monkey revealed a 7-fold increase of K^+ concentration and a significant rise (10%) of the total osmolarity (Bito and Myers 1972). The latter finding was explained by the assumption that chemically bound cations (predominantly K^+) are displaced from the lipidic binding sites by NH_4^+ released by glutamine-glutamate conversion.

Asphyxial depolarization can thus be considered an extreme case of SD evoked simultaneously in wide cortical areas by interference with oxidative transport mechanisms. Since this type of SD proceeds in the complete absence of repolarization processes, the depolarization is more profound and the water and electrolyte shifts are more pronounced. Even the asphyxial depolarization is reversible, however, when oxygen supply is restored in time (see p. 82).

3. Factors Influencing Asphyxial Depolarization

The close relationship between mechanisms of SD and asphyxial depolarization explains why both processes are similarly influenced by different local and general agents. Some factors are specific to asphyxial depolarization, however. The latency of asphyxial depolarization depends on the oxygen reserves available to the brain. Thus according to Speckmann and Caspers (1967) stopping of the respiration pump after prolonged administration of pure oxygen evokes in rats no terminal depolarization until 8 min after cessation of the EEG. De Valois (1966) found that anoxic anoxia (respiration of N_2) induced under conditions of hyperbaric oxygenation (3 ATA) evoked a less-pronounced conductivity decrease in rabbit cerebral cortex than under normal pressure. Since hyperbaric oxygenation did not increase the half time of the conductivity drop caused by stagnant anoxia (de Valois 1966), it seems that significant oxygen reserves cannot be established in the brain but only in the whole body.

After oxidative metabolism has been eliminated, the polarity of neuron membranes is maintained by anaerobic glycolysis. Benešová, Bureš, and Burešová (1957) demonstrated that the half time of terminal depolarization is decreased from the usual 100 sec to 49 sec in hypoglycemic rats (blood sugar level below 50 mg/100 ml) and increased to 126 sec in hyperglycemic rats (blood sugar level over 200 mg/100 ml). Decreased latency of anoxic depolarization in hypoglycemic rats was confirmed by de Mello and da Silva (1960). Local application of 20% glucose solution on the exposed cortical surface also caused a 20-sec delay of anoxic depolarization in the treated region. (Longer delays cannot be expected under these conditions since anoxic depolarization initiated in the adjacent regions spread into the treated area which had a diameter of 5 mm).

At the end of 10-min brain ischemia in rats the levels of glycogen and glucose were decreased by 52 and 75 %, respectively, whereas the lactic acid level was increased to 410% (Fig. 4.3). These data indicate an intensive glycolytic utilization of glucose and glycogen. As demonstrated by the unmeasurably low creatine phosphate level, the glycolytic processes alone cannot maintain the levels of high-energy phosphates that serve as a direct source of energy for metabolic transport mechanisms. A rapid recovery of creatine phosphate started immediately after the circulation had been restored. The normal level was reached in approximately 6 min, whereas cortical repolarization was complete in about 8 min. A close relationship between these two parameters was demonstrated during the whole recovery period (Křivánek, Bureš, and Burešová 1958, 1959).

Asphyxial depolarization is delayed therefore under all conditions slowing the exhaustion of the high-energy compounds. Body temperature was the most obvious variable to be examined in this connection. Bureš and Burešová (1957) found the half time of anoxic depolarization (N_2 anoxia) prolonged from 2.4 min at 36 °C to 4.9 min at 21 °C (colonic temperatures). Benešová, Bureš, and Burešová (1957) found in unanesthetized rats that the half time of asphyxial depolarization (decapitation) increased from 105 sec at 36 °C to 119 sec at 30 °C and to 145 sec at 20 °C. These times were considerably increased by intravenous allobarbital (25 mg/kg) or chlorpromazine (10 mg/kg) administered 2 to 3 hours prior to decapitation. Collewijn and Schadé (1962b, 1964a) found the latency of the rapid impedance rise (cardiac arrest) increased from 3.6 min at 37 °C to 4.9 min at 28 °C in rabbits and

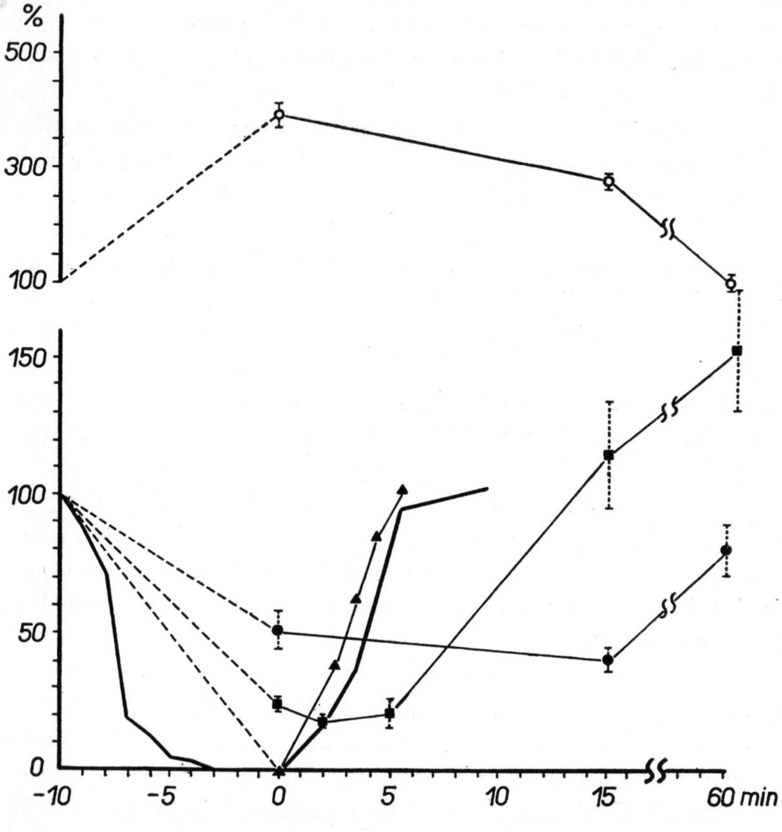

Fig. 4. 3. Relationship between levels of glucose (squares), glycogen (dots), lactic acid (circles), creatine phosphate (triangles), and cortical demarcation potential (heavy line). Abscissa: time before or after termination of 10 min brain ischemia. Ordinate: All values are expressed in percentages of the respective control levels. The vertical dotted bars denote standard errors (Křivánek, Bureš, and Burešová 1959).

from 1.3 to 5.1 min within the same temperature range in the rats. The latency was not further increased by cooling the rabbits to 18 to 20 °C, probably because of a simultaneously developing cardiovascular insufficiency. It must be pointed out, however, that the conductivity measurements differ from the potential recording in an important aspect; whereas hypothermia does not significantly influence the cortical demarcation potential, it decreases cortical conductivity proportionally to the decrease of temperature. Cortical conductivity at 20 °C reaches only 70%

of the conductivity at 37 °C. This is largely due to the temperature effect on the diffusion coefficient of the electrolyte solutions concerned. Histochemical analysis of chloride shifts indicated that circulatory arrest at 20 °C causes similar shifts of ion distribution as in normothermic animals (Collewijn and Schadé 1964b).

The significance of local metabolic reserves for the rate of asphyxial depolarization was demonstrated by Duda, Zachar, and Ruščák (1958) who found faster depolarization in a hemisphere subjected to repeated SD waves prior to asphyxiation. The decreased glycogen content (Křivánek 1958) may be responsible for the reduced resistance to anoxia in this case.

Whereas the above factors influence the latency of terminal depolarization by changing the rate of metabolic exhaustion, it is also possible to affect directly the membrane processes underlying the actual depolarization. Divalent cations, which were shown to block the initiation and propagation of SD (Bureš and Burešová 1956b, c, Bureš 1960) can also be used to delay the onset of anoxic depolarization. Bureš and Burešová (1957) evoked terminal depolarization in rats by intraperitoneal injection of NaCN (7 mg/kg) and followed its development in normal cortex and in cortical regions pretreated for 10 min with different concentrations of $CaCl_2$ or $MgCl_2$. As shown in Fig. 4.4, 0.1 M solutions of both substances increased the de-

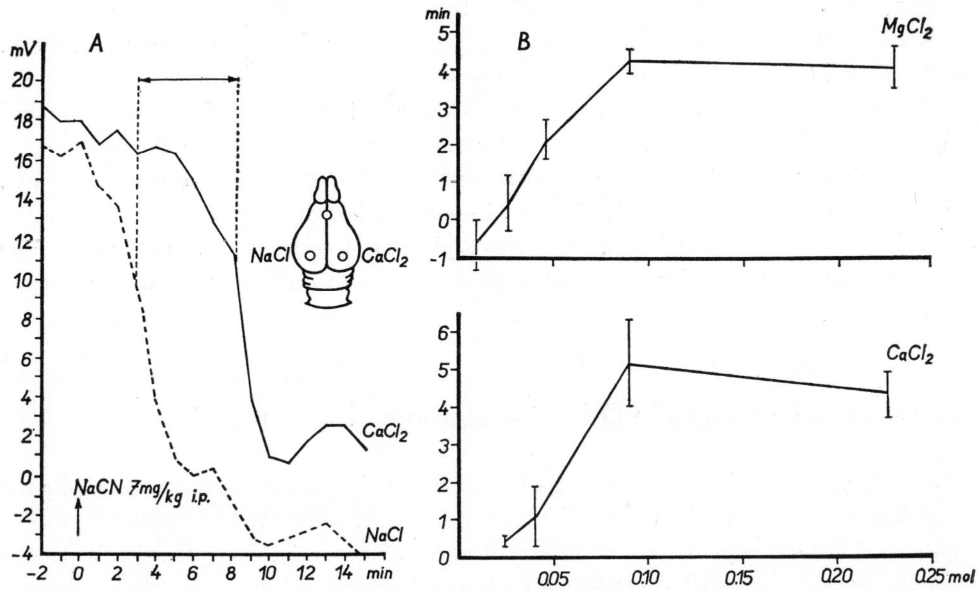

Fig. 4. 4. Delayed onset of terminal anoxic depolarization in cortical areas treated by divalent cations. *(A)* Example of typical experiment in the rat. Inset diagram shows the distribution of electrodes. Ordinate: cortical demarcation potential measured between thermocoagulated area and the intact cortical surface (NaCl) or the pretreated region ($CaCl_2$). Abscissa: time after intraperitoneal injection of NaCN (7 mg/kg). Horizontal arrows indicate the delay with which 50% depolarization was reached in the protected area. *(B)* Average delay (ordinate) of anoxic depolarization (at 50 % of maximum depolarization) in cortical areas treated with different concentrations of $MgCl_2$ or $CaCl_2$ (abscissa) (Bureš and Burešová 1957).

polarization half times by 4 min on the average. $MgCl_2$ seemed to be slightly more efficient than $CaCl_2$. Application of more concentrated solutions did not increase the depolarization delay. Although the relatively small cortical area (5 mm in diameter) treated with divalent cations was surrounded after a few minutes by depolarized cortex, it could maintain its polarity so long because it was protected by magnesium or calcium ions against SD invasion from the adjacent regions.

The effect of divalent cations on the asphyxial impedance change was recently investigated in cats by Adey, Bystrom, Costin, Kado, and Tarby (1969). Both $MgCl_2$ and $CaCl_2$ solutions delayed the onset of the impedance change by several minutes, but the evaluation of this effect was difficult because of the considerable resistivity increase (20 to 30%) caused by $CaCl_2$. The asphyxial impedance increase was delayed by topical application of tetrodotoxin in a similar manner as by $CaCl_2$ (Tarby, Costin, and Adey 1969) and the effect was still more pronounced after combined pretreatment of the cerebral cortex with $CaCl_2$ and tetrodotoxin. The authors suggested that tetrodotoxin delays the asphyxial impedance increase by changing the membrane properties of the nerve cells (blockade of sodium channels) but that calcium changes the properties of extracellular macromolecules (mucopolysaccharides) and reduces the availability of water and electrolytes for transmembrane migration.

A different explanation of the calcium effect was offered by Van Harreveld, Dafny, and Khattab (1971) who found that superfusion of rabbit cerebral cortex with isotonic $CaCl_2$ caused not an increase but a 50 % decrease in impedance of the upper cortical layers (about 0.6 mm deep). Electron micrographs revealed a corresponding increase of extracellular space (from 13.7 % in the untreated to 32.6 % in the treated cortex). The delayed asphyxial depolarization and impedance increase can be partly due to the fact that the potassium released from the asphyxiated neurons diffuses into a larger extracellular volume and reaches the critical concentration later than under normal conditions.

4. Asphyxial Changes in Other Neural and Nonneural Tissues

Fifková, Bureš, Koshtoyants, Křivánek, and Weiss (1961) demonstrated an asphyxial depolarization change in rat cerebellum. After decapitation the cerebellar injury potential (15 mV) decreased with a half time of 2.1 min. Van Harreveld (1961) also found in the cerebellar cortex an asphyxial increase of impedance that was more gradual but otherwise similar to that in the cerebral cortex. Asphyxial water and electrolyte shifts in the cerebellum were demonstrated both by light (Van Harreveld 1961) and electron microscopy (Van Harreveld and Malhotra 1966).

An asphyxial impedance increase was also reported in the rabbit hippocampus (de Valois 1966). With stagnant anoxia conductivity decreased slightly more slowly in the hippocampus than in the neocortex (4.3 and 3.7 min, respectively) but with histotoxic anoxia evoked by CO intoxication, hippocampus was affected earlier than neocortex.

Asphyxial depolarization was observed in the gray matter of the spinal cord by Van Harreveld and Hawes (1946). Unlike in the cortex, it started within 8 to 9 sec after circulatory arrest and culminated after 2 to 2.5 min when it reached values up to 25 mV. This asphyxial depolarization was accompanied by a conductivity decrease that proceeded rapidly at the beginning and slowed down after the first 5 min of asphyxia (Van Harreveld and Biersteker 1964). Microelectrode analysis of the spinal asphyxial potential (Collewijn and Van Harreveld 1966, Biersteker, Collewijn, and Van Harreveld 1966) indicated that it is due to a rapid depolarization of dendrites caused by increased sodium permeability. Depolarization of spinal motoneuron somata proceeds much more slowly, probably as the result of arrest of the sodium pump. What accounts for the differences in asphyxial depolarization of cortical and spinal neurons remains unclear.

Myelinated axons are relatively resistant to anoxia. Ventral root fibers are still excitable 1 hour after circulatory arrest and provide a stable source for the sinks in the dendrites and later also in the somata. The cortical asphyxial potential is thus mainly due to the potential difference between the depolarized somatodendritic membranes and the polarized corticofugal axons. Depolarization of the endings of afferent fibers may contribute to the generation of the asphyxial potential, however. Biersteker, Collewijn, and Van Harreveld (1966) demonstrated that asphyxial potentials in the dorsal roots of cats were caused by depolarization of the intraspinal section of the primary afferent fibers, probably by a mechanism similar to presynaptic inhibition.

Circulatory arrest also increases the impedance of nonneural tissues. Van Harreveld and Biber (1962) examined the conductivity changes in the asphyxiated submaxillary salivary gland, liver, kidney, and skeletal muscle. The highest conductivity decrease was found in the liver (85 to 90% within 30 min). The impedance of kidney was doubled in 10 min, but later it increased slowly, reaching 300% after 2 hours. The conductivity of the salivary gland decreased slowly during the first 10 to 20 min but then the decrease accelerated and 20 to 30% of the initial level was reached after 90 min. The slowest conductivity decrease was found in muscle (20% in the first hour and 30% in the second hour). Histochemical methods demonstrated that the impedance increase is accompanied by a loss of extracellular electrolytes, which either leave the tissue with blood or move into cells. The above conductivity changes are not fast enough to be compared with the rapid asphyxial impedance change in the cerebral cortex. It seems, therefore, that they are due to the arrest of ion pumps rather than to sudden changes of membrane permeability for sodium.

5. Electrical Indication of the Revival Capacity of the Brain

The mammalian neocortex tolerates without permanent damage ischemia lasting for 6 to 10 min (Schneider 1956). This time span can be considerably prolonged by hypothermia and drugs, that is by agents that also delay the onset of anoxic depolarization (Benešová, Bureš, and Burešová 1957). Although irreversible damage appears after the period of so-called revival time (considerably exceeding the half-time of terminal depolarization), the assumption seemed to be justified that the two phenomena are related and that it would be possible to use the cortical steady potential to indicate the probability of successful revival.

Correlation between cortical polarity (defined as the cortical injury potential) and revival expectancy was tested by Bureš, Burešová, Benešová, and Křivánek (1959) in rats cooled with the technique described by Andjus (1951) and Andjus and Smith (1955) to rectal temperatures near 0 °C and subsequently reanimated. Colonic temperature, ECG, EEG, and cortical demarcation potential were recorded. As shown in Fig. 4.5 the spontaneous EEG disappeared between 20 and 15 °C and the heart stopped around 10 °C. Reanimation was started 10 to 30 min after cardiac arrest by slowly warming the trunk and applying artificial respiration. Cardiac action appeared after a few minutes and cortical polarity returned within 20 to 30 min to initial levels. In the experiments in which the cortical polarity decreased to zero during cooling, heart action could sometimes be restored but the cortex remained depolarized. From more than 50 experiments in which colonic temperature was reduced below 5 °C, rats in which reanimation started with a cortical polarity of approximately 5 mV could be successfully reanimated in 70 % of the cases, whereas resuscitation of animals with a fully depolarized cortex was successful in only 15 % of cases.

Interpretation of the above results is confused by the fact that reanimation may fail because of cardiac damage. Incomplete depolarization of the cerebral cortex can nevertheless be considered as a prognostically favorable sign for reanimation in the whole organism. Speckmann and Caspers (1967) arrived at the same conclusion in experiments in rats in which they correlated the time after the onset of the terminal depolarization with the probability of successful reanimation. This probability was 100% during the first 30 sec of depolarization, but decreased to 0% when maximum depolarization was reached (after 180 sec on the average). In this case as well, success of reanimation was determined by cardiovascular factors. Recovery of brain function is possible even after complete depolarization has occurred, provided that oxygen supply to the brain is restored soon enough.

The above was shown in rats by Křivánek, Bureš, and Burešová (1958, 1959) and by Burešová and Bureš (1958) with a technique for transient brain ischemization (Opitz and Thorn 1949). After exposing the trachea a rubber band was passed underneath it and used to compress the neck of the animal until blood was prevented from reaching the brain. Although some blood flow was maintained through the spinal

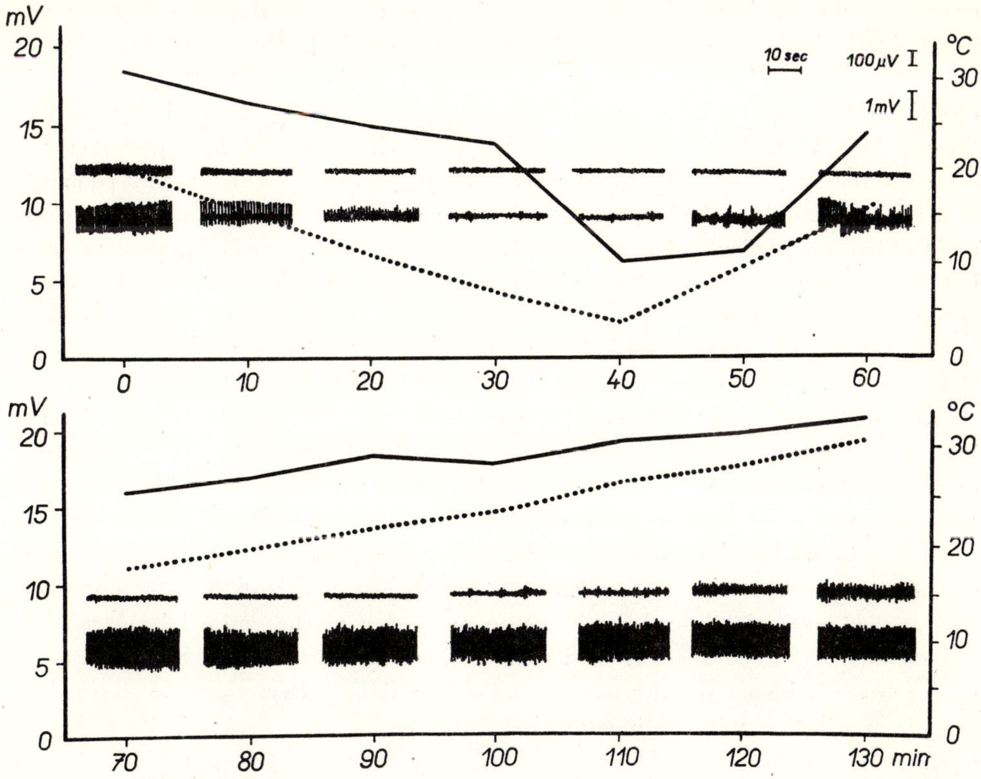

Fig. 4. 5. Cortical demarcation potential (full line), EEG (upper recording), ECG (lower recording), and colonic temperature (dotted line) during cooling of the rat and during subsequent resuscitation. Abscissa: time in minutes. Ordinate: cortical demarcation potential on the left (mV); colonic temperature (°C) on the right. Calibration: 10 sec for the EEG and ECG samples; 100 µV for EEG; 1 mV for ECG. The first phase of cooling (until 20 °C) was omitted. Rewarming and artificial respiration started after 40 min. Note that rapid decrease of cortical polarity followed cardiac arrest and that cortical polarity had recovered long before the EEG appeared (Bureš, Burešová, Benešová, and Křivánek 1959).

and vertebral arteries under these conditions, anoxic depolarization developed with a half time approximately equal to that after decapitation (2.1 and 1.8 min, respectively). From the onset of ischemization artificial respiration was applied through the free trachea, so that cardiac activity remained normal. After different delays the rubber band was released and the return of cortical polarity was observed. Repolarization following 10-min ischemia proceeded with a half time of 4 min and was completed within 6 to 8 min (Fig. 4.3). After a 20-min ischemia, cortical repolarization was slower, reaching after 8 min only 25 % of the initial value (Křivánek, Bureš, and Burešová 1959).

Reversibility of asphyxial depolarization lasting for 30 min was confirmed by Speckmann and Caspers (1966) in rats with ligated carotid arteries breathing low oxygen mixtures. Also Hirsch, Scholl, Dickmans, Eisolt, Mann, and Krankenhagen (1968) found in the isolated dog head that cortical polarity is restored even after 20 to 30 min ischemia, greatly exceeding the revival time of the brain. Their data seem to indicate, however, that the longer the preceding ischemia, the slower the repolarization. In several experiments in which circulation had been restored after 30-min asphyxia the initial level was not attained at all. The authors conclude that it is impossible to find a correlation between cortical polarity and the development of irreversible brain damage. Also Hossman (1971) reported complete repolarization of cat cerebral cortex after ischemia lasting up to 90 min.

Similar considerations prompted Burešová and Bureš (1958) to use cortical impedance as an index of revival capacity since cortical impedance continues to rise even after the depolarization is completed. It can be expected, therefore, that a definite increment of impedance (corresponding to hydration of cells, electrolyte shifts, and hydrolysis of intracellular molecules) indicates irreversible collapse of vital brain functions. Reversible ischemization of rat brain was achieved by the technique described above (see p. 82). Impedance was measured between two Ag-AgCl disc electrodes applied to the cerebral surface (interelectrode distance, 6 mm) using a bridge method and a 500-Hz measuring current. Neck compression was applied until the impedance increase reached a predetermined level ranging from 175 to 300% of the initial value. Cardiovascular functions were maintained during brain ischemization by noradrenaline injections. After release of the rubber band, resuscitation was continued either until spontaneous respiration reappeared or until 90 min had elapsed. A marked decrease of revival probability (defined as recovery of spontaneous breathing within 90 min of resuscitation) was observed in rats in which cortical impedance exceeded 250% of the initial value at the end of ischemization. Irreversible cortical damage occurred, however, even in rats in which the asphyxial impedance rise was less marked and was acutely reversible. This was shown in rats overtrained with an appetitive-aversive conditioned reaction (see p. 234) and subjected to ischemization until impedance increased by 50, 75, or 100 %. Retention of the task was tested for 3 days following ischemization. The results are summarized in Fig. 4.6. Whereas the impedance increase by 50 and 75% was compatible with recovery of conditioned reactions in 70 to 90% of the animals, the 100% group displayed serious impairment of cortical function. That cortical damage is quantitatively related to the amplitude of the impedance change was demonstrated in another group in which cortical impedance was maintained for about 40 min at the 150% level by briefly releasing the neck compression from time to time. In spite of the long duration of this partial ischemia, conditioned reactions recovered in all rats by the second day after asphyxiation. It must be stressed that during partial ischemia of this type the cerebral cortex is permanently depolarized from the third or fourth minute.

Conductivity changes accompanying the recovery of the cerebral cortex from asphyxiation were studied in the rabbit by Van Harreveld and Tachibana (1962).

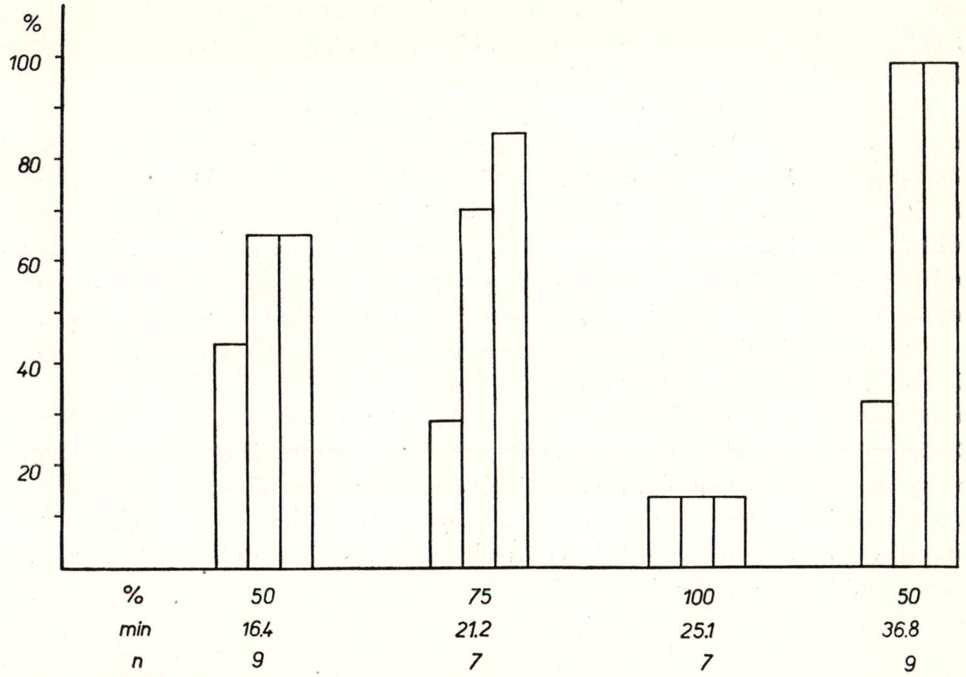

Fig. 4. 6. Relationship between the increment of cortical impedance during brain ischemia and retention of pretrained conditioned reactions during the first 3 days following resuscitation (columns 1, 2, 3). The numbers below the columns indicate the maximum impedance increase (in percentage of control values) during ischemia, the duration of ischemia, and number of animals in the respective groups. Ordinate: percentage of animals in which conditioned reactions reappeared on the first, second, and third day of resuscitation (Burešová and Bureš 1958).

Cerebral asphyxiation was induced by clamping arteries supplying the head and was maintained for 15 to 75 min. Cortical conductivity decreased to 58 and 42% of the initial level after 15- and 75-min asphyxiation, respectively. During 15-min reoxygenation a rapid return of conductivity to normal values was found in most animals asphyxiated for up to 60 min, but little or no recovery was seen in the 75-min group. With restitution of normal cortical conductivity dendritic diameter reverted to preasphyxial values and chloride ions were removed from the cellular elements. The authors point out that acute reestablishment of cortical impedance and ion distribution in brains seriously damaged by 30- to 60-min asphyxiation indicates a marked difference between the mechanisms maintaining normal ionic distribution and the processes necessary for survival of nerve cells. The vulnerability of the latter is perhaps due to damage of enzymatic systems indispensable for normal cell function. The neuron can live until the supply of the inadequately produced enzymes is exhausted and then dies, sometimes hours or days after asphyxia. Ischemization of cat cerebral cortex (Hossman 1971) caused a similar impedance increase (165 % and 243 % after 10 and 60 min, respectively) which was acutely reversible when the circulatory arrest had not lasted more than 90 min.

The results of the above studies indicate that unlike cortical polarity cortical impedance can be used as a sign of impending damage. Acute reanimation failed when the impedance increased to approximately 250% of the initial level during asphyxia. It also seems that incomplete ischemization can be maintained within safe limits when cortical impedance does not increase above 150%. Whether a meaningful correlation exists between a certain level of asphyxial impedance increase and onset of permanent morphological changes has to be established by further experiments.

The interest in the electrical symptoms of brain revival capacity was stimulated in recent years by the clinical need to determine objectively that irreversible brain death had occurred and that resuscitation can be stopped. An EEG silence lasting for 24 hours, which is often taken as a criterion of brain death, is evidently not a safe symptom of irreversible damage. A single impedance measurement would provide more meaningful prognostic information provided that reliable methods for specific impedance estimation were developed which would make it possible to obtain absolute values and to make conclusions from them.

Chapter 5

Chemical Aspects of Spreading Depression

The purpose of the chemical exploration of the brain is to study the interrelationship between functional manifestations of neural activity and the underlying chemical processes, and to describe the mechanism of such correlations. Spreading depression possesses many features that make it particularly suitable for chemical analysis. Spreading depression evoked in one hemisphere does not spread to the contralateral one, which can thus serve as a control. Furthermore, the rate of SD propagation is slow enough to allow chemical analysis under proper experimental conditions.

Several manifestations of SD indicate that chemical changes may play an important role in this remarkable pattern of functional alteration in the cerebral cortex. As has been already mentioned (p. 67) the temperature coefficient (Q_{10}) for spreading rate and duration of SPC was found to be about 2, which fits fairly well with that for chemical reactions ($Q_{10} = 2$ to 4). No temperature dependence was observed for the SPC amplitude. Since the first SD studies it has been known that partial oxygen pressure decreases in the depressed region of the cerebral cortex (Van Harreveld and Stamm 1952, Marshall 1959, Van Harreveld 1954, 1959, Lukyanova and Bureš 1967). Originally this decline of oxygen tension was ascribed to vasoconstriction of the cortical vessels. This assumption seemed to be supported by the observation that in the rabbit cortex initial vasoconstriction took place during SD (Van Harreveld and Ochs 1957, Van Harreveld and Stamm 1952). However, no initial vasoconstriction has been observed in the cat and rat cerebral cortex (Marshall 1959, Van Harreveld and Ochs 1957). The predominant, and in the case of rat and cat, exclusive, vasomotor reaction is vasodilation, as demonstrated in studies using either cooled (Burešová 1957a, Seylaz and Molnar 1966) or heated (Sonnenschein and Walker 1956) thermocouples, histological technique (Van Harreveld and Ochs 1957), determination of hemoglobin content, and isotope technique (Burešová 1957a), as well as measurements of cortical volume (Marshall 1959). Therefore decrease in pO_2 in the cortical area invaded by SD can be explained only by increased O_2 consumption. Apparently changes taking place in the cerebral cortex during SD trigger biochemical processes controlling oxidative metabolism in the tissue required to provide additional production of energy.

More direct evidence for a possible role of some chemical substance(s) in the mechanism of SD propagation has been postulated by Grafstein (1956a). The spreading rate of SD evoked in isolated slabs of the cat's cerebral cortex could be affected by polarization of the tissue. Propagation of SD toward the cathode was found to be faster than in the opposite direction. It was suggested that SD is a neurohumoral reaction transmitted by some positively charged particle, the diffusion of which is influenced by the electric field. Taking into consideration that the wave of negativity is preceded by a short neuronal discharge, Grafstein came to the conclusion that SD represents a combination of both electrical and chemical mechanisms. The potassium ion has been suggested in the role of the SD "transmitter".

Supporting evidence for this potassium hypothesis has been presented by Bureš (1956) who showed that the chemical compounds evoking a typical metabolic reaction in cerebral cortex slices *in vitro* (increased aerobic glycolysis) elicit SD *in vivo*. Substances preventing this reaction *in vitro* also prevented initiation of SD *in vivo* when added to effective KCl solution in the proper concentration (for details see p. 51).

Regardless of the indirect nature of all of this evidence an hypothesis including the following general points seemed to be justified: Potassium ions released from the nerve cells by the action of SD-eliciting agents (mechanical, thermal, chemical, or electrical stimulations) accumulate in the extracellular space and affect the metabolism of cortical cells in a manner similar to that demonstrated in *in vitro* experiments when the K^+ concentration is increased to the appropriate level above the normal extracellular concentration. This is obviously an oversimplification, but perhaps it is sufficiently clear to show the way in which chemical analysis of the problem has been carried out to verify this hypothesis experimentally. Apparently two main problems required solution. First, whether release of potassium ions and their migration actually take place (if so, whether the concentration achieved is sufficient to exert an effect on adjacent cells to ensure the propagation of SD); second, the chemical changes shown *in vitro* in cerebral cortex slices should be experimentally demonstrated *in vivo* in the course of SD. Were these elementary processes shown to occur, various additional questions would arise. (a) Are the presumed ion shifts and chemical changes great enough to be analyzed quantitatively? (b) What is the origin of potassium ions supposedly accumulating in fairly high concentration in the extraneuronal space? (c) Are all these changes reversible and is the rate of recovery sufficient to explain the autoregenerative nature of SD? (d) Are they correlated with the steady potential changes and is such a correlation experimentally demonstrable?

1. Ion and Water Transport and Distribution during Spreading Depression

The most commonly used and simplest methods of determination of ions in tissue are the atomic absorption or flame photometric measurements preceded by digestion of the tissue in a mineral acid. This approach could not be applied in the case of SD elicited by a single KCl application. It was found that no net changes in water, sodium, or potassium contents took place in the whole cortex after 30 or 60 min of repeated SD waves evoked by 25% KCl (Křivánek, unpublished). The possibility remained, however that shifts in ion distribution between cellular and extracellular compartments might occur. Such changes are more difficult to detect. One possible approach is histochemistry, as used by Van Harreveld and Schadé(1959) to demonstrate chloride ion shifts in the course of SD. This method is based on treatment of the frozen tissue with an ethanolic solution of $AgNO_3$, which reacts with chloride ions to form an AgCl precipitate. Subsequent reduction with pyrogallic acid shows a dark silver precipitate in areas corresponding to chloride location. Accumulation of chloride in the apical dendrites during SD has been demonstrated in the rabbit cortex situated laterally to the parasagittal sulcus. The adjacent retrosplenial area, into which SD does not normally propagate (see p. 118), served as a control (Van Harreveld 1958). Together with the previously demonstrated increase in impedance, the shift of chloride ions obviously reflects transport of NaCl into apical dendrites. By this method chloride transport can be visualized only in structures with a radial arrangement of neurones. It is therefore not applicable to the whole cortex or to other structures with a different structural organization. Another disadvantage is the obvious difficulty of making quantitative measurements.

Some attempts have also been made to study histochemically the distribution of potassium ions during ischemization (Collewijn and Schadé 1962a). The method resembles the histochemical technique for chloride detection. It is based on precipitation of K^+ ions by sodium cobalt hexanitrite, which is then transformed into black cobalt sulfide with ammonium sulfide. The known drawbacks of histochemical methods in general, and particularly of those concerned with the determination of soluble substances of small molecular size, seriously limited the use of this method for potassium detection.

A more accurate method, which would allow not only more precise measurements but also a more dynamic approach to electrolyte analysis during SD, was desirable. Two such methods were introduced at the same time independently by Bureš and Křivánek (1958, 1960) and Brinley, Kandel, and Marshall (1960). In Brinley's procedure the cortical surface was loaded topically with a radioactive isotope of potassium. The output of ^{42}K into Ringer's solution washing the rabbit's cortical surface was followed in both depressed and normal cortex. Significantly elevated release of ^{42}K was found in cortex through which the slow potential wave was passing. Each wave was accompanied by a striking increase of ^{42}K output with a maximum up to 400% above baseline. In the second method (Bureš and Křivánek 1960, Křivánek and Bureš 1960) an isotonic solution (usually 0.25 M sucrose) was perfused under low pressure through a small metal or plastic cannula fixed to the edges of a trephine opening 5 mm in diameter in the rat's skull. The solution was allowed to flow at a constant rate through the cannula and after contact with the cerebral cortex was gathered for analysis (Fig. 5.1). Concentration of both sodium and potassium in the outflowing fluid was determined by flame photometry. The results were practically identical with those of Brinley, Kandel, and Marshall (1960). When SD-evoking drugs were added to the washing fluid (mainly 2,4-dinitrophenol), an increased outflow of potassium from the cerebral cortex was indicated by an increase in concentration in the outflow solution. As expected, a similar increase (up to 400%) could be found when the cannula was placed in a region not directly affected by the SD-eliciting agent. Efflux of sodium was also increased, but to a much smaller

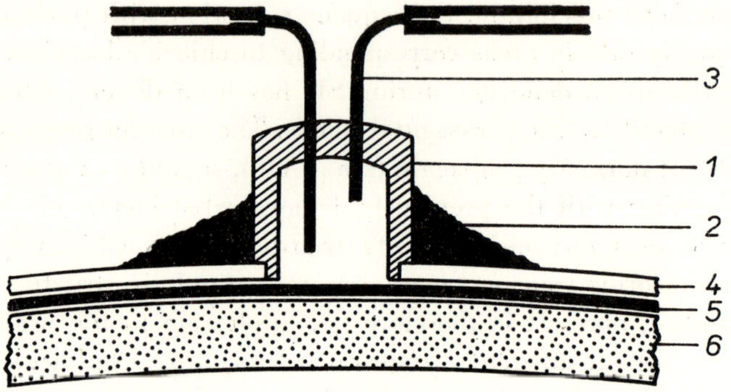

Fig. 5. 1. Diagram of the epidural cannula. (1) the body of the cannula; (2) phosphate cement or acrylic resin; (3) tubes through which the washing fluid flows; (4) cranial bone; (5) dura; (6) cortex (Bureš and Křivánek 1960).

extent. Using a flame photometer with an extremely small jet that allowed measurements of ion concentrations in very small volumes it was possible to take samples of the outflow at relatively short time intervals (2 min as compared with 15 to 20 min in the previous case). This setup made it possible to correlate K^+ output with different phases of the steady potential change passing through the washed cortical region. As in the experiments of Brinley, Kandel, and Marshall (1960) a close correlation between the occurrence of the wave and increased outflow of potassium was found. Moreover a correlation between SPC voltage and the percentage increase of potassium outflow was found in some cases (Křivánek and Bureš 1960) (Fig. 5.2). Analogous ion shifts were also observed during cerebellar SD (Fifková, Bureš, Koshtoyants, Křivánek, and Weiss 1961) and in the striatum of chick embryos (Sedláček 1969). A similar correlation between recovery of the resting potential (2.5 min) and of potassium content (1 min) in isolated cerebral cortex slices following electrical stimulation (10 min) has been demonstrated *in vitro* (Cummins and McIlwain 1961, Hillman, Campbell, and McIlwain 1963).

To employ this method for quantitative estimation of ion shifts in the cerebral cortex the assumption was made that the potassium concentration in the washing fluid is in equilibrium with that in the compartment from which it is freely diffusible. It may be in contact with the "extraneuronal space". A relative increase in potassium concentration in the washing fluid would then correspond to that in this compartment. An elevation of K^+ concentration by a factor of five or six that was found experimentally (Křivánek and Bureš 1960) was presumed to reflect a similar increase in extracellular concentration, that is, from the usual 3 mEq/1 (estimated from the potassium concentration in the cerebrospinal fluid — Van Harreveld 1966) to 15 to 20 mEq/l. This figure is necessarily an underestimation, since the inertia of the superfusion technique and the fact that at any time the negative SPC peak did not occupy more than 50 % of the superfused area, tend to smooth the sharp temporal and spatial gradients. The extracellular K^+ levels reached during SD must probably exceed 30 to 40 mEq/l to account for the observed changes of K^+ efflux. To estimate whether this increase would be sufficient to reach the threshold concentration for eliciting SD, another assumption was made: that the mechanism of potassium action on cortical cells during SD is identical irrespective of whether the K^+ ions were added externally or released endogenously into the extraneuronal space. It would then be possible to compare the estimated threshold concentration of K^+ ions for evoking SD with that reached by extracellular K^+. Correction would have to be made for

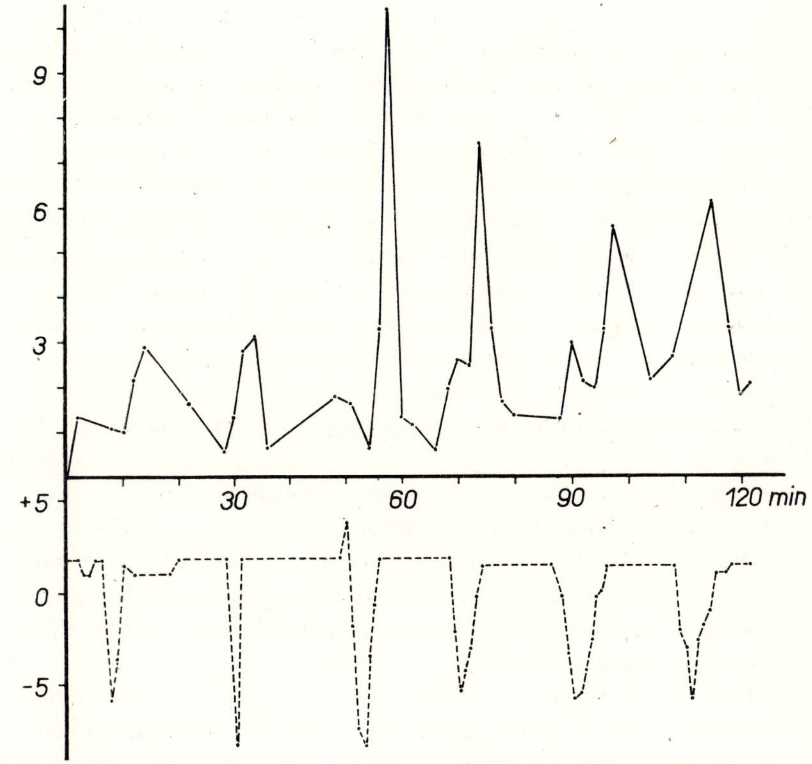

Fig. 5. 2. Time relation between the course of SPCs (below, ordinate in mV) and K^+ release into 0.9 % NaCl (above, ordinate in $\mu M \times 10^2$) (Křivánek and Bureš 1960).

the dilution of externally applied potassium ions that obviously takes place before the latter reach their site of action by diffusion. The threshold concentration of 80mM KCl found with epidural application in rats (see p. 33) is then quite compatible with the extracellular K^+ increase inferred from the superfusion experiments. Similar results were reported by Fertziger and Ranck (1970) who exposed the cat suprasylvian gyrus to ^{42}K and superfused it with 3 to 120 mM solution of unlabeled KCl. The ^{42}K efflux did not change until the KCl content in the perfusate reached 45 to 60 mM. These concentrations triggered SD and caused a stereotyped increase in ^{42}K efflux (about 2.3 times) indicating SD initiation.

One crucial question still remained to be solved. What is the origin of the potassium accumulated in the compartment in contact with the washing fluid? The changes found could be a mere reflection of simultaneous changes in the blood vessel dimension that have been shown to take place during SD. An altered permeability of the blood-brain barrier could be another possibility. The proposed mechanism of SD propagation could be borne out only by proof that the released K^+ is of intracellular origin. To solve this problem, the observations reported by Katzman and Leiderman (1953) were employed. The authors showed that after injecting rats with ^{42}K, isotope equilibrium with intracellular potassium was achieved only after 24 hours. This means that at appropriate time intervals after ^{42}K injection, a higher specific activity of potassium is measured in the extracellular compartment than in the intracellular one. If the potassium released during SD were of intracellular origin, the specific activity of the potassium in the washing fluid would decrease because of "contamination" of the highly labeled extracellular potassium with slightly labeled intracellular cations. If potassium in the washing fluid were of extracellular and/or blood origin, the specific activity of potassium would not change. It was shown that the specific activity of potassium in the washing fluid was significantly decreased in the course of SD, so that the released potassium ions originated in the intracellular space. The conclusion can be drawn that during SD potassium ions released by depolarization of the excitable membranes of cortical cells accumulate in the extracellular space. The concentration achieved is sufficient to depolarize the membranes of adjacent cells.

The above conclusion was confirmed by direct measurement of extracellular potassium activity with the cation selective electrodes. Using gross glass electrodes covered with collodion (sensitive area 3 mm^2) applied to pial surface of the cerebral cortex of monkeys, Meyer, Gotoh, and Tazaki (1961) found that seizure activity and SD are accompanied by accumulation of extracellular K^+, but no quantitative interpretation of these data was attempted.

Vyskočil, Kříž, and Bureš (1972) used the potassium sensitive liquid ion exchanger microelectrodes prepared according to Walker (1971). To prevent distortion of the potassium electrode readings by the steady potential fields arising in the area of recording, the potassium microelectrode was glued to another capillary microelectrode filled with 1 M NaCl, the distance between the parallel tips of the two capillaries being less than 10 μm. The K^+ concentration was estimated from the potential difference between the two capillary electrodes. The SP changes in the area of recording were related to a wick calomel cell electrode placed on the occipital muscles. The potassium electrode introduced into the parietal cortex stabilized after a few minutes at a potential corresponding to 3.0 mM K^+. As the SD wave elicited from the occipital cortex approached the potassium electrode inserted 1 mm below the cortical surface, its potential rose at first slowly and then abruptly (10 mV/sec) to about 60 mV. This potential change corresponded to a K_e^+ increase to 60 mM and was maintained for 20 sec. The potassium potential then started to decline along an S-shaped curve. The slope of the steepest part of the recovery phase was several times lower (3 mV/sec) than the slope of the initial K^+ increase. The SP recording reflected the major features of the potassium potential, but was of lower amplitude (20 mV). During recovery of the SD the SP reached the predepression level when the K_e^+ was still 6 mM above the resting value. This is in good agreement with Goldman's equation from which it follows that the membrane potential is influenced at K_e^+ levels below 6 mM mainly by the Cl^- and Na^+ gradients. The amplitude of the SD potassium potential did not markedly change over the first millimeter. At 1.5 mm depth the maximal K_e^+ shift was less marked (40 mM) and the potassium rise time was prolonged indicating K^+ diffusion from a remote active region into the passive space around the recording electrode. The SD potassium potential disappeared 2 mm below the cortical surface, where the SP changed to low positivity. The above findings were confirmed in cat cerebral cortex by Prince, Lux, and Neher (1973) who found with microelectrodes of the same type that extracellular potassium increased during SD from the resting level of 3.25 mM up to 80 mM.

The duration of SD evoked by a single application of even 25% KCl is limited to about 2 to 3 hours (see p. 224). Since the concentration of topically applied KCl progressively decreases due to diffusion from the site of application, the frequency of the isolated slow potential waves also decreases. For some purposes (see p. 103) it is desirable to keep the SD process at a maximum level for several hours. This can be done by repeated application of KCl at about 40-min intervals, usually for 4 to 5 hours. Relatively prolonged overloading of cerebral cortical tissue with hypertonic KCl solutions could affect ionic and water metabolism to a serious extent. Figure 5.3 summarizes the results of measurements of potassium and water contents in the hemicortices and "subcortices" (cerebrum without cortex and cerebellum) from brains treated either by 25% KCl or by saline. In contrast to a single application of 25% KCl, a net increase of K^+ content was found after 5 hours of repeated KCl application. A relatively fast recovery occurred after KCl application had been discontinued. On the other hand water content, which can be measured more accurately, appeared to recover in two phases. The major fraction (about 70 %) recovers in 24 hours, whereas a residual portion required much more time to reach normal values. During this interval some residual irregularities in distribution that are undetectable by the analytical method used, may also be reversed. Even though a relatively long time is necessary for complete recovery, the electrolyte and water shifts seem to be completely reversible. This concerns only cortical regions outside the area of KCl application that is seriously damaged (Křivánek 1969a).

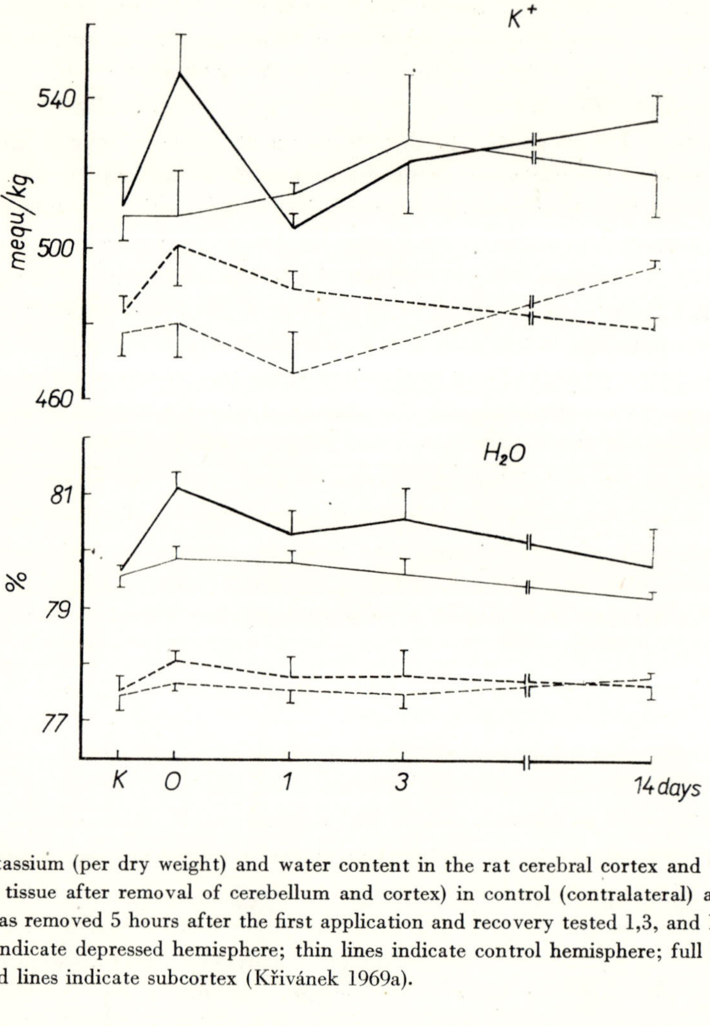

Fig. 5. 3. Potassium (per dry weight) and water content in the rat cerebral cortex and "subcortical" region (brain tissue after removal of cerebellum and cortex) in control (contralateral) and depressed tissue. KCl was removed 5 hours after the first application and recovery tested 1,3, and 14 days later. Heavy lines indicate depressed hemisphere; thin lines indicate control hemisphere; full lines indicate cortex; dashed lines indicate subcortex (Křivánek 1969a).

2. Spreading Cortical Depression and Labile Chemical Compounds in the Brain

In the previous section data were summarized that support the view that potassium ions may play a decisive role in the SD phenomenon. The hypothesis was advanced that the chemical events underlying the SD process are analogous to those obtained in in vitro experiments with cerebral cortex slices exposed to an increased concentration of K^+ in the incubation medium. Ashford and Dixon (1935) and Dickens and Greville (1935) found a stimulating action of potassium ions on respiration and aerobic glycolysis of cortical slices. Later this finding was extended to studies of various aspects of brain metabolism as affected by changes in the electrolyte composition of the medium, in particular potassium and calcium. In spite of the great effort invested in the study of the K^+ effect on the metabolism of glucose, glycogen, ion and water transport, transmitters, lipids, and proteins in cerebral cortex slices, its mechanism has not yet been fully elucidated.

To verify a possible analogy between this effect of potassium *in vitro* and the manifestations of SD *in vivo*, it was necessary to carry out more direct analyses of those chemical systems that respond most clearly to the presence of K^+ *in vitro*, that is, systems engaged in the metabolism of glucose and compounds involved in the storage and transfer of chemical energy. To measure the concentration of these labile substances in the brain it is essential to protect them from the extremely fast decomposition that takes place in the immediate post mortem period. The most common approach is to freeze rapidly the dissected brain or severed head, or sometimes even the whole animal, by immersion into a liquid gas. At low temperatures chemical reactions proceed extremely slowly, so that under appropriate conditions it is possible to recover in the test tube brain constituents in amounts approaching those existing in vivo. To follow changes in glucose metabolism the levels of glycogen, free glucose, and lactic acid were determined in various phases of SD.

The level of glycogen 20 to 30 min after a single application of 2 or 25% KCl decreased by 30% as compared to that in the opposite hemisphere which had been kept relatively intact (Fig. 5.4). The change was large enough and the rate of recovery sufficiently slow for the decrease to be detected in the whole hemisphere (Křivánek 1958). On the other hand changes in the content of free glucose and lactic acid were much smaller and so did not reach the level of statistical significance (Křivánek 1958, 1961).

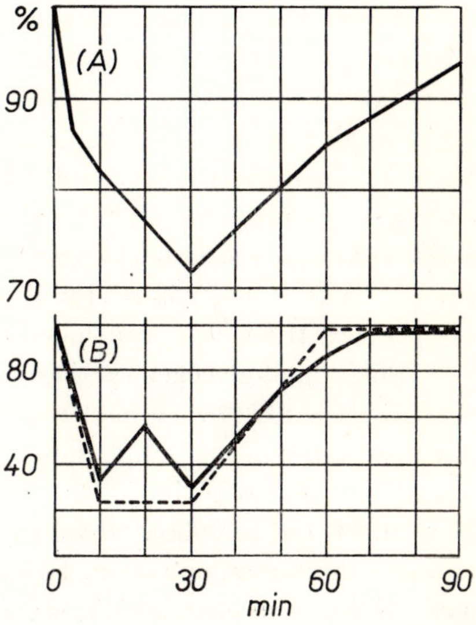

Fig. 5. 4. Temporal correlation between changes in brain glycogen (Křivánek 1958) and the inhibition of conditioned reflexes (Bureš and Burešová 1960b) accompanying CSD evoked by 2 % KCl. *(A)* Glycogen content during SD expressed as percentage of the glycogen content in the control hemisphere. *(B)* Percentage of rats with correct responses in conditioned reflex experiments. Dashed lines indicate alimentary conditioned reflexes; solid lines indicate avoidance reactions.

Since SD elicited in the cortex is limited to cortical tissue (see p. 118), only cerebral cortices were taken for analysis in further experiments. For this purpose cortical slabs were dissected from the frozen brain under continuous cooling with liquid nitrogen. Cooling was maintained until enzymes were inactivated by homogenizing frozen cortical samples in protein precipitating agents such as trichloracetic acid, perchloric acid, or $Ba(OH)_2 + ZnSO_4$. With this technique the SD-elicited decrease of glucose level was fairly high (—30 %), especially when a more specific (chromatographic) method was used for determination. Under similar experimental conditions, the lactic acid content in cortical slabs was found to have increased up to 100 % above the normal level (Křivánek 1961, Ruščák and Duda 1959).

Accumulation of lactate raises the question of possible pH changes during SD. Methodologically this is a rather difficult problem (Marshall 1965) since the potential corresponding to the pH change must be distinguished from the SPC of SD. Rapoport and Marshall (1964) measured the pH of the rabbit cortex during SD elicited by both electrical (tetanic stimulation) and chemical (2% KCl) stimuli. Potential changes were recorded independently with a glass membrane pH electrode and with a pore Ag-AgCl electrode applied onto the cerebral cortex against a reference electrode. From the difference between the two records (pH electrode recorded both SPC and pH) an acidic shift of -0.027 ± 0.005 pH unit was found in the positive phase of SPC after making corrections for possible errors. This finding shows that only very small (0.05) pH changes occur during SD. The previous assumption by Tschirgi, Inanaga, Taylor, Walker, and Sonnenschein (1957), Tschirgi and Taylor (1958) that SPC is accompanied by alcalinization and can be entirely accounted for by a jugular-cortical pH difference formed across the blood-brain barrier appears, therefore, to be erroneous. It seems that the great buffer capacity of the cerebral cortex prevents excessive pH shifts in spite of the rather high accumulation of lactate.

Since vasodilation occurs during SD, a decrease in the glucose level is unlikely to be due to a decrease of the glucose supply. Changes in the content of the compounds mentioned above support the view that glucose consumption is increased to such an extent that supply from the blood stream becomes insufficient to cover demands and a net decline in the glucose level takes place. Moreover mobilization of glycogen reserves takes place as has been shown experimentally by measuring incorporation of ^{14}C from glucose into glycogen during CSD. Specific activity of glycogen in the depressed cortex was higher by 47 % as compared with that in the contralateral, intact cortex. It has been concluded that increased rate of glycogen breakdown rather than inhibition of glycogen synthesis is responsible for the fall of glycogen level during SD (Křivánek 1972b). No matter how small the reserves of glycogen are in the brain (about an order of magnitude lower than in liver or muscle), glycogen can be transformed to glucose-6-phosphate and serve as an additional source of energy (Kerr and Ghantus 1936). Obviously two possible general mechanisms can be activated by the potassium action. First, energy demand is suddenly increased (enhancement of oxygen consumption, see p. 87) and substances that could serve as an energy source are utilized. These compounds are then catabolized at a higher rate. This enhancement of glucose uptake and catabolism could be considered as a consequence of the potassium effect, and corresponds to restoration of the membrane polarity by reestablishment of the asymmetric distribution of ions across the neuronal membrane. The process is obviously an energy-dependent one. The theoretical possibility remains, however, that the increase of glycolysis, in spite of elevated oxygen consumption, is an expression of some kind of reversal of the Pasteur effect induced by potassium action. Under normal conditions an increased consumption of oxygen is followed by a decresed rate of glycolysis (smaller amount of lactic acid formed). Potassium-induced uncoupling of oxidation from the synthesis of macroergic phosphates decreases the efficiency of the energy-producing processes. In this case the potassium ions would be engaged in the chemical changes of SD more directly than in the first one.

In this connection it was important to know whether SD is accompanied by any changes in the level of energy-rich phosphates. An attempt was made to measure levels of creatine phosphate (CrP), adenosinetriphosphate (ATP), and inorganic phosphate during SD. Estimation of CrP in the whole hemisphere revealed only a slight decrease during SD elicited by mechanical or chemical stimuli (Zachar and Ruščák 1958). Thanks to the relatively low rate of SPC propagation through the cortex, it is possible to freeze the particular area of the cortex in which the SPC undergoes a definite phase of development. To demonstrate experimentally a possible correlation of the labile phosphate level with the development of SD, propagation of a single SPC was monitored electrophysiologically. At various phases of de- or repolarization, the corresponding cortical region was frozen in liquid nitrogen. It was shown that in the region in which the amplitude of negativity reached its maximum, the CrP level was decreased by more than 40 % (Křivánek 1961). This change is fairly high if we consider the fact that in the slab of the cortex taken for analysis the degree of depolarization varies and certainly is not maximal at the time of fixation. The maximum of the slow potential wave is limited to a narrow band that is not large enough to allow chemical analysis by the method used. As soon as polarity of the cortex started to recover, CrP was found to be at its normal level. Inorganic phosphate content increased by an amount that is stoichiometrically related to the CrP decline. In spite of a very rapid change in CrP no changes in ATP were seen in the depolarized regions of the cerebral cortex (Fig. 5.5). It is generally accepted that CrP can serve *in vivo* as an "energy buffer" reversibly offering its phosphate to the ADP and thus maintaining the level of ATP even when consumption suddenly rises. Short-lasting increases of ATP utilization are covered by CrP, the level of which drops transiently. A similar effect (rapid drop of CrP) can be achieved in cerebral cortex slices *in vitro* by raising the potassium concentration in the medium (Heald 1954, Sugawara and Wada 1957) or by electrical stimulation (Heald 1954). There is a close correlation between the recovery of polarity in depressed tissue and the CrP level. In the cortical region invaded by the negative slow potential (Fig. 5. 6) the CrP level is decreased by about

40%, but as soon as the maximum negativity passes there is a rapid recovery to the normal value. It seems that complete recovery of CrP even precedes that of the slow potential (Křivánek 1961). A similar observation was made during recovery of cortical polarity from the terminal depolarization evoked by brain ischemia (see p. 77).

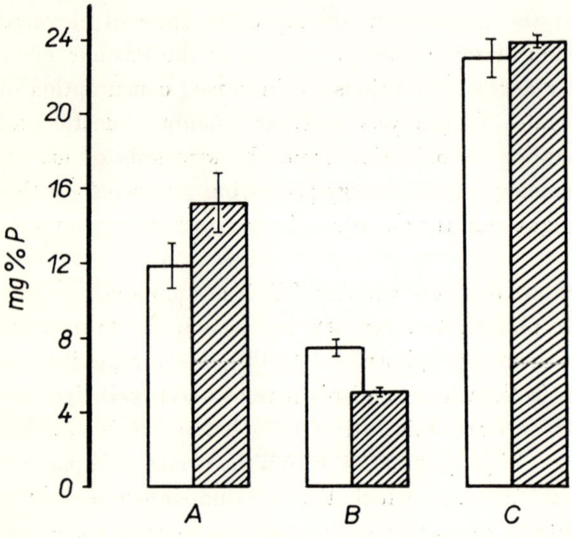

Fig. 5. 5. Inorganic phosphate *(A)*, creatine phosphate *(B)*, and ATP *(C)* in the cerebral cortex at the moment of passage of the maximum negativity of the slow potential wave (shaded columns) and in control cortex (white columns) (Křivánek 1961).

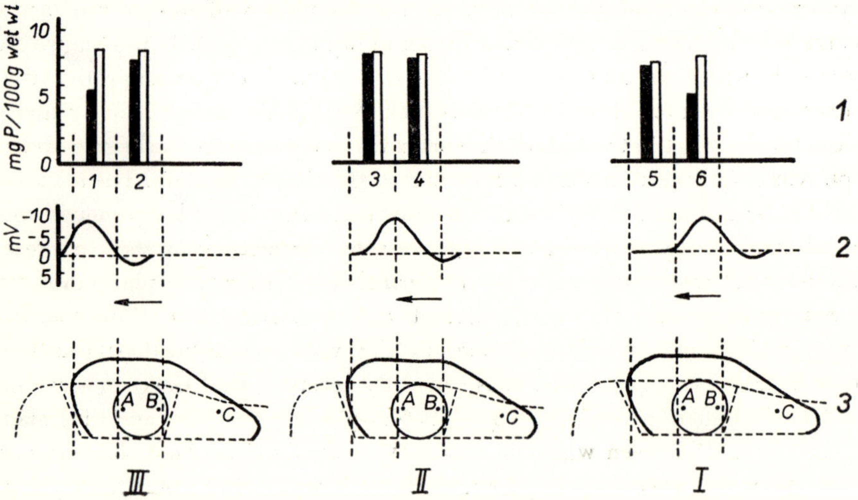

Fig. 5. 6. Changes in creatine phosphate level in the cerebral cortex of rats corresponding to the various phases of the negative wave of SD shown in (2). Black columns represent experimental values and white columns the corresponding control values from the contralateral hemicortex. Differences obtained in (1) and (6) are statistically significant for $P < 0.01$. (3) Diagrammatic representation of the positions of the electrodes *(A,B)* in relation to the point of application of KCl *(C)* (Křivánek 1961).

A close correlation between recovery rates of both resting potential and CrP was also demonstrated *in vitro* after electrical stimulation of cerebral cortex slices (Hillman, Campbell, and McIlwain 1963). Once the relatively rapid changes in the levels of the labile compounds had been demonstrated an attempt was made to answer the question of whether the recovery rate of the slow potential change correlates with the recovery rate of the chemical changes occurring during SD. The aim of this study was to analyze the chemical basis of the refractory period of SD, that is, the time interval between two successive waves of the slow potential. For this purpose only one SPC wave was elicited with 1% KCl. The development of SD was checked electrophysiologically. At various time intervals (minutes) after recovery of cortical polarity, the brain was frozen in liquid nitrogen, and glucose, lactic acid, and glycogen were determined in the cortical slabs. The polarity was considered as completely recovered when the curve of the slow negative potential crossed the baseline. From that point it takes approximately 5 min before another wave can be initiated from the same area of cerebral cortex by the same stimulus (see p. 28). Obviously repolarization alone is not a sufficient indicator of recovery. As shown in Fig. 5.7, five min after restoration of cortical polarity neither glucose nor lactate content have reached normal value. There is fairly good correlation of glucose and lactic acid recovery with the recovery of EEG amplitude. The 10-min period into which recovery of all the above parameters fits well (except the glycogen level which returns after long delay) corresponds to the relative refractory period of SD. Summation of the glucose and lactic acid changes should appear with short interwave intervals when waves of the slow potential develop in tissue in which residual changes induced by the preceding SD wave are still present. (An equal efficiency of each SD wave must be assumed). However, lactate and glucose were shown to be affected to the same degree irrespective of SD duration (Křivánek 1961). The possibility remains that the origin of the electrophysiological and biochemical parameters is not exactly the same. Steady potential differences are recorded in the uppermost layers of the cortex, whereas the EEG might reflect electrical events located in more remote structures. The location of the chemical compounds analyzed is obviously not only in the upper portion of the cortex. Hence only some shifts in phase of differentially located events might take place.

Lack of cumulative biochemical effects of single slow potential waves has been demonstrated also in studies of the SD effect on levels of both glycogen (see p. 95) and protein synthesis (p. 107). Neither different KCl concentrations nor prolongation of their action for hours by repeated application of 25% KCl made the effects more pronounced. As this is obviously a general phenomenon it was tempting to speculate that the SD effect is confined only to some compartment(s) or specialized structures of cortical tissue, the rest of it being relatively intact. Apical dendrites might be such structures. They represent a large membrane that could be primarily involved in responses to ionic changes in their environment. This assumption is supported by the finding that chloride ions and water shifts caused by SD are mainly localized in the apical dendrites of the cerebral cortex (Van Harreveld 1958, see p. 118). Also Ochs and Hunt (1960) came to the conclusion that apical dendrites play a major role in the propagation of SD. Quantitative histochemical studies of the distribution of glycolytic and oxidative enzymes throughout the cortical layers led Lowry, Roberts, Leiner, Wu, Farr, and Albers (1954) to the assumption that regions rich in dendrites are particularly active and that "brain metabolism is quantitatively the metabolism of dendrites".

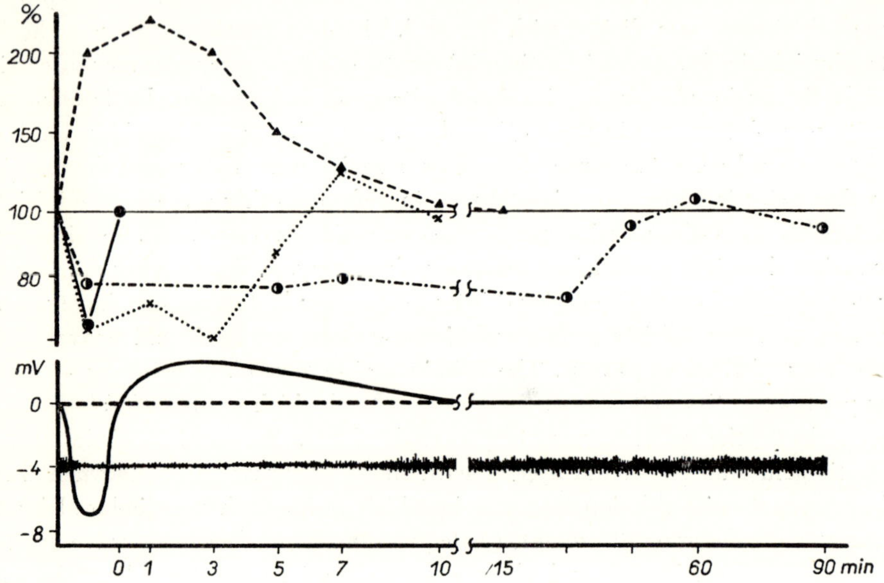

Fig. 5. 7. Percent change in lactic acid (▲ —— ▲), phosphocreatine (● — ●), glycogen (◑ — . — ◑), and glucose (× . . . . . ×) accompanying changes in dc potential (▬▬▬) and EEG activity. Abscissa: time after complete repolarization (Křivánek 1962).

3. Amino Acids and Spreading Depression

Since the metabolism of amino acids is closely bound with that of carbohydrates and since some amino acids are thought to play an important role in brain function (GABA, glutamic acid), possible involvement of amino acids in the mechanism of SD was studied.

Some amino acids are potent SD-eliciting agents, glutamate, glutamine, and aspartate being particularly active (see p. 36). No changes in their content in the cerebral cortex 30 or 60 min after topical application of 23 or 25% KCl could be found. The same was true for alanine, aspartate, and GABA (Ruščák 1964, Křivánek 1960). It was demonstrated in cerebral cortex slices *in vitro* that incorporation of ^{14}C from uniformly labeled glucose into glutamic acid and GABA increased after concentration of K^+ ions in the medium had been elevated to 100 mM (Rybová 1959, Kini and Quastel 1959). Using intraperitoneally administered ^{14}C-labeled glucose and evoking SD by 25% KCl, specific activities of glutamate, glutamine, aspartate, alanine, and GABA were determined and related to the total activity of the soluble fraction (trichloracetic acid extracts) to determine the relative specific activity. Only a slight increase of relative specific activity of GABA and alanine was observed (Fig. 5.8) (Křivánek 1972b). No changes in the ammonia level were found (Křivánek 1960).

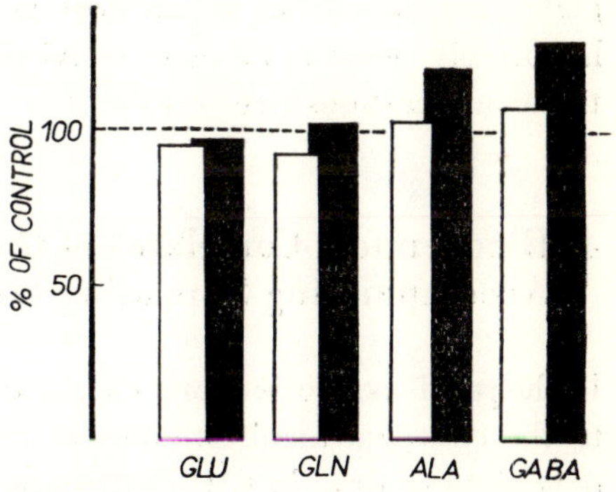

Fig. 5. 8. Levels of some free aminoacids (white columns) and specific activities of their ^{14}C (from ^{14}C-glucose) as related to the total radioactivity of the soluble fraction (black columns). Duration of SD 1 hour. GLU — glutamic acid; GLN — glutamine; ALA — alanine; GABA — gamma-aminobutyric acid.

While SD alone does not exert any appreciable effect on brain amino acids, a different picture was obtained with SD elicited in the oligemic brain after ligature of both carotids. Electrical and biochemical characteristics are qualitatively the same as in the case of conventional SD, only more pronounced. The slow potential wave recovers more slowly and the decrease of creatine phosphate level is even detectable in the whole hemisphere (Duda, Ruščák, and Zachar 1958, Ruščák and Duda 1959). The decline of free glucose and glycogen levels as well as enhancement of the lactic acid content has been found. Moreover, citrate content was slightly decreased while pyruvate and oxoglutarate remained unchanged (Ruščák and Ruščáková 1971). Altered levels of some amino acids are the main feature distinguishing this kind of SD. After 30 min SD elicited in the cerebral cortex of rats by 3M KCl leads to a decrease in amino nitrogen, glutamate, glutamine, and aspartate, whereas alanine as well as gamma-aminobutyric acid levels were found to be increased (Ruščák 1961, 1962b). Not only KCl but even salts not normally evoking SD (LiCl, NaCl, $CaCl_2$) were shown to cause an increase of alanine and gamma-aminobutyrate when applied topically in a 3M concentration on the cortical surface of rats with carotid ligature (Ruščák 1962a).

In rabbits (Van Harreveld 1959) but not in rats (Bureš, Burešová, and Křivánek 1960) glutamate has been reported to evoke SD at a lower threshold concentration than KCl. Using the technique of cortical superfusion (Bureš and Křivánek, 1960), Van Harreveld and Kooiman (1965) demonstrated an enhanced release of ninhydrin-positive material from the cerebral cortex during SD. When SD was evoked in vitro in the isolated retina that had previously been loaded with radioactive glutamate, increased output of ^{14}C glutamate and to lesser extent ^{14}C aspartate were observed (Van Harreveld and Fifková 1969, 1970). On the basis of these experiments Van Harreveld advanced the hypothesis that glutamate rather than potassium is responsible for the membrane changes occurring during SD. After being released into the extracellular space, glutamate increases the permeability of the cellular membranes to sodium, which is the first step in the action of all agents evoking SD. No definite experimental data have yet been furnished to prove the glutamate hypothesis which does not deny the role of potassium. The potassium hypothesis seems to be more convincingly supported by experiments and quantitative considerations (see p. 155).

4. Biochemical Correlates of the Functional Changes Accompanying Spreading Depression

In the previous two sections chemical changes were described that are closely related to the electrical manifestations of SD. Some of them, for example the outflux of potassium or drop in CrP content, were shown to coincide with the development of the negative slow potential. As pointed out in Chapters 1 and 9 (see p. 218) SD is accompanied by a serious impairment of the basic functions of the cerebral cortex. Evoked responses are suppressed and unit activity is inhibited. Conditioned reflexes disappear and learning ability is abolished. It seems therefore that generation and transmission of electric impulses are severely impaired. Possible changes in the enzymatic systems which are supposed to play an important role in chemical synaptic transmission have been studied under conditions of SD.

Of interest was the question of the role of the cortical cholinergic systems in the functional changes accompanying SD. The failure to find a significant correlation between changes in functional activity of the brain and acetylcholinesterase (AChE) activity may often be due to the fact that chemical analysis was performed in large samples of tissue in which modification of functional activity was not uniform and the corresponding effect on the AChE activity was rather small. A method has been developed therefore for colorimetric estimation of AChE activity in very small samples of the brain tissue (1 mg wet weight) in which the change of functional activity and the corresponding response of AChE was expected to be maximally developed (Křivánek 1972a). The samples for analysis were cut with an injection needle from 1 mm thick frozen coronal brain sections dissected in a stereotaxic apparatus from the frozen head of the rat. Portions of the motor cortex obtained in this way were homogenized and 10-μl aliquots were then subjected to the procedure for determination of AChE activity based on Hestrin's method (1949).

Since it has been shown that barbiturate anesthesia does not interfere with SD and because most of the previous experiments have been carried out in anesthetized rats, the same experimental setup was used in the case of AChE measurements. A single application of 25% KCl on the surface of one hemisphere did not induce statistically significant changes in AChE activity although some tendency to rise above the normal levels as compared with the contralateral cortex and expressed per unit of protein content appeared after 30, 60, and 120 min of SD. However, prolonged treatment of the rat cerebral cortex by repeated application of 25% KCl (PCSD see p. 93) onto the cortical surface resulted in a significant increase of AChE activity. After 4 hours of SD a 16% increase in AChE activity was found. In spite of this relatively high activity increase the return to normal was rapid. Less than 2 hours appeared to be sufficient for recovery from 4 hours of KCl action (Fig. 5.9).

Since the tissue samples had the same volume, enzymatic activity could be expressed per volume; and thus progressive decrease of AChE with longer intervals after SD initiation was found. The decrease of protein content, to which the AChE activity was related was much more marked than the decrease of AChE activity; that is, the ratio of AChE to protein increased (Křivánek 1972a). The experiment performed in unanesthetized rats showed that protein content after 5 hours of SD was only 90 % of normal (Křivánek 1969a) (see p. 107). The difference in the protein level changes as induced by prolonged KCl action in the two experimental series mentioned is obviously caused by prolonged anesthesia in the former one. It is difficult to maintain the same depth of narcosis for a long time without additional administration of anesthetic (barbiturate in this case). Very often some hypoxic symptoms could be observed. Nevertheless this experiment demonstrates a relatively high stability of AChE. When total protein content decreases, the decline of AChE activity is much slower. So far it is difffcult to determine the basis of this stability. It is possible that only a small portion of cortical synapses is cholinergic in nature. On the other hand the stability may indicate that the functional changes induced by SD are inadequate to influence the AChE activity.

The adrenergic system, especially in the brain stem, has also been subjected to chemical analysis during SD. In 1966 Donoso and Stefano measured the noradrenaline content in hypothalamus, mesencephalon, cortex, and pons-medulla in rats, while SD was evoked by topical application of 20% KCl on both cortices. Ten minutes of SD caused a 30% decrease in the noradrenaline level in the hypothalamus and a 48% increase in the mesencephalon. No changes in cortex and pons were found. In a more recent study a method for the estimation of noradrenaline turnover was used (Schanberg, Schildkraut, and Kopin 1967) to study the SD effect on the metabolism of this transmitter. After intracisternal injection, the tritiated noradrenaline (pulse labeling) rapidly penetrated into the surounding tissue and was metabolized. The rate of disappearance from the brain tissue is an expression of the metabolic rate. Two hours after injecting tritiated noradrenaline, SD was elicited by topical application of 25% KCl onto one hemisphere while the opposite one served as a control. One hour later the animals were killed. In the brain stem (cerebrum devoid of cerebral cortex, subcortical white matter, and cerebellum) the specific

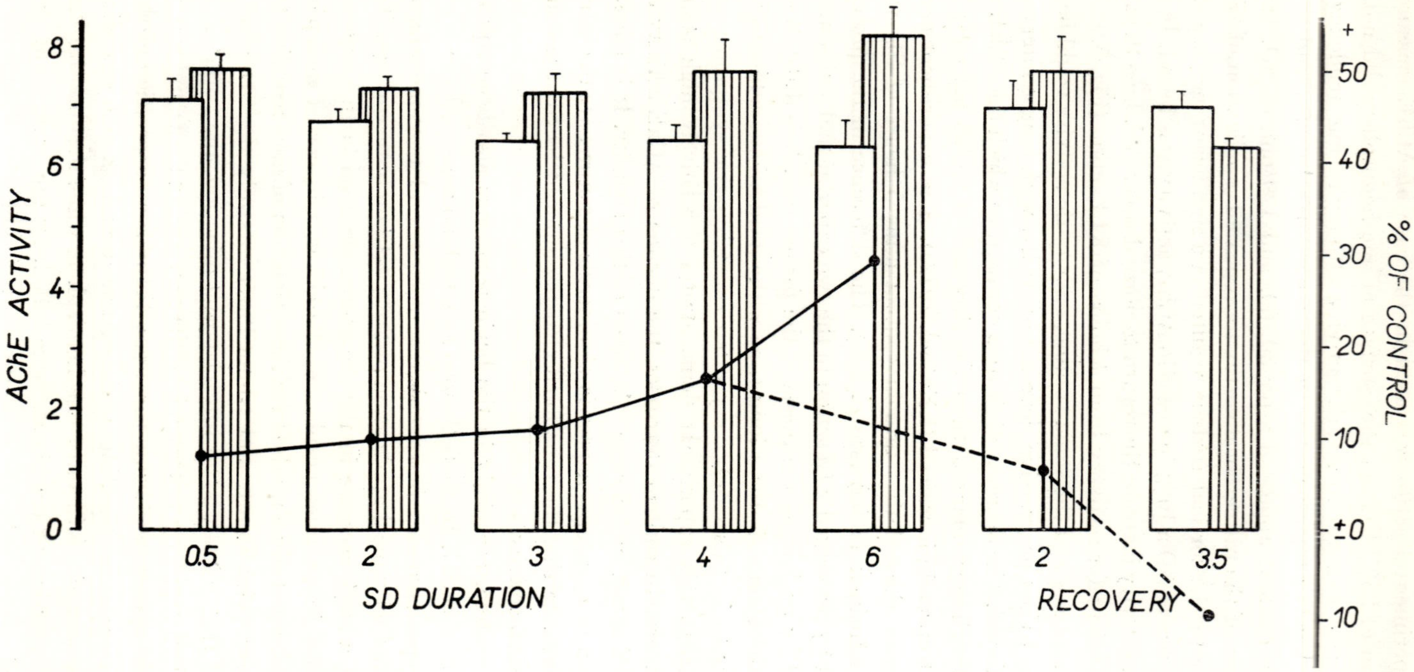

Fig. 5. 9. Acetylcholinesterase activity (as related to the protein content) in the rat motor cortex in the course of the prolonged CSD (2—6 hours), and during recovery (2 and 3.5 hours after removal of 25 % KCl.) White columns are controls; shaded columns are PCSD; solid line is percent of controls during PCSD; dashed line is percent of controls during recovery.

activity of noradrenaline as well as that of normetadrenaline was determined. In the brain stem ipsilateral to the depressed cortex the specific activity of both [^{3}H] noradrenaline and [^{3}H] normetadrenaline was decreased by 32 and 17%, respectively. Increased turnover of the transmitter seems to accompany cortical SD. In the opposite brain stem (contralateral to the depressed cortex) the specific activity of noradrenaline was significantly higher (+33 %) indicating decreased turnover as compared to controls (both hemispheres treated by a single application of NaCl) (Shanberg, Schildkraut, Křivánek, and Kopin 1968). Cortical SD has been recently shown to accelerate the α-methyl-p-tyrosine-induced disappearance of dopamine and to increase homovanillic acid content (dopamine level unchanged) in cerebrum. Therefore, dopamine turnover appears to be enhanced (Keller, Bartholini, Pieri, and Pletscher 1972).

The mechanism by which SD may affect the metabolism of noradrenaline in the areas studied is unclear. It might reflect some functional alterations in brain-stem structures, the electrophysiological, morphological, and behavioral aspects of which are described in Chapter 8. For example, Keller, Bartholini, Pieri, and Pletscher (1972) speculate that disinhibition of the nigro-striatal dopaminergic pathway could be the reason of increased dopamine turnover.

5. Protein Metabolism in the Course of Spreading Depression

Since Hydén's (1959) formulation of his hypothesis of the chemical basis of memory, a possible role of protein and RNA metabolism in brain function and particularly in memory trace formation and storage has been repeatedly studied in a number of laboratories. A study of possible changes in protein metabolism accompanying the learning process can take advantage of the SD technique which makes it possible to compare data from the trained and untrained cortex in the same animal. However, it was necessary to determine the possible effect of SD on protein metabolism in the cerebral cortex.

There were no apparent changes in the total protein content of the cerebral cortex after a single epidural application of 25% KCl. This, however, does not mean that there are no changes in conformation of protein structure. According to Martins-Ferreira and de Oliveira-Castro (1966) SD elicited in the isolated retina *in vitro* is accompanied by changes of light scattering,spreading from the focus in all directions over the retinal surface. This optical change may be an expression of structural rearrangement of the retinal macromolecules caused by SD.

The most studied aspect of protein metabolism is the synthesis of protein during various functional states or during learning. According to the theory mentioned above, memory storage is due to the formation of specific protein that ensures the specificity of response to appropriate stimuli. The incorporation rate of radioactive amino acids into proteins of the brain tissue was used as a measure of the rate of protein synthesis.

When SD was elicited by a single application of KCl, protein radioactivity in the depressed cerebral cortex was considerably decreased (Ruščák 1964, Křivánek 1968, 1970, Bennett and Edelman 1969). Incorporation of ^{32}P into protein and nucleic acid fractions was also diminished (Křivánek 1959). The decrease of the incorporation rate is maximal 1 hour after KCl application when the specific radioactivity of total protein in the depressed cortex is lower by 40% than that in the control (contralateral) cortex. Recovery started between the first and second hour, and after 2 hours the radioactivity of proteins from the depressed cortex reached 80% of the control values. Four to five hours were required for complete recovery.

When maximum SD was maintained for 5 hours by repeated application of KCl and radioactive leucine was injected again 60 min before killing the animal (Křivánek 1969b) incorporation of the labeled amino acid was inhibited in the same way as after a single KCl application. Prolonged action of KCl would obviously not result in accumulation of effects of a single KCl application. Even 8 hours of repeated application of KCl gave the same 30 to 40% inhibition. The absence of a greater effect of the longer-lasting SD may be due to partial recovery of the incorporation rate between the single SD waves. Accordingly, a series of SD waves passing successively over the cortex have no cumulative effects but result in a steady state.

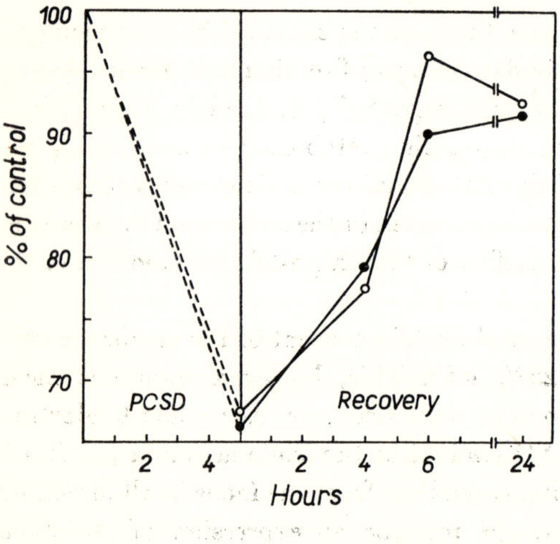

Fig. 5. 10. Specific activity of cerebral cortex protein (cpm/mg protein) expressed as percentage of control values, 1 hour after subcutaneous injection of DL-[1-^{14}C] leucine; 25% KCl was repeatedly applied for 5 hours. The animals were killed at the time interval indicated after KCl had been removed from the cerebral cortex surface. (○ — ○) focal area samples; (● — ●) extrafocal area samples (Křivánek 1969a).

The changes in the protein synthesis found during prolonged SD do not cause any permanent damage, since recovery of incorporation of [^{14}C] leucine can be shown (Fig. 5. 10). Control levels of incorporation were reached in the depressed cortex 6 hours after KCl had been removed from the cortical surface. The degree of inhibition and recovery as well as the time course of both processes appeared to be identical in the cortical region directly treated with KCl and in the cortex unaffected by the externally applied KCl. Therefore inhibition of protein synthesis resulting from the action of externally added KCl does not differ from the effect of SD evoked by a single KCl application. However, prolonged inhibition can cause a small but consistent decrease in the total protein content of the cerebral cortex by about 10 %. This may be partly due to increased hydration, which could account for at most 40 % of the change. Recalculation of protein per dry weight or DNA still showed a statistically significant decrease of about 6 %.

After the main facts on the specific activity of the protein had been established, several other problems remained to be solved: (a) What changes are there in the leucine pool? (b) Would it be possible to demonstrate some specificity of this reaction to potassium, that is, are there any subcellular structures or even some individual proteins the synthesis of which would be specifically sensitive to the increased concentration of potassium ions? (c) Is the inhibition of protein synthesis due to the specific effect of K^+ on some critical link in a complex chain of biochemical reactions leading from individual amino acids to the formation of complex polypeptide macromolecules?

To ascertain whether the lower specific activity of protein during SD was attributable to decreased specific activity of leucine in the free pool or to a slower rate of incorporation into protein, specific activity of the leucine was determined. After 20-min SD, the specific activity of leucine was not decreased, rather it was higher than that of the control samples by about 45 % (Křivánek 1970). The same trend was seen in the specific activity of the whole TCA extract (Bennett and Edelman 1969) and in the specific activity of the total free pool amino acids (the radioactivity of the acid-soluble extract related to the total amino acid content as determined by ninhydrin) for an SD of the same duration (Křivánek 1970). This finding, together with the fact that the levels of the free pool amino acids in the cerebral cortex were not affected by SD (Ruščák 1964), justified the use of specific activity of the total free pool amino acid as an indication of the changes in specific activity of the free pool leucine at various time intervals after initiation of SD. The data indicated that the lower specific activity of proteins in the depressed cerebral cortex was not the result of decreased specific activity of leucine in the free pool. The specific activity of the latter was increased during the whole period studied (10 to 120 min after SD initiation) (Křivánek 1970).

Distribution of the SD inhibitory effect on the protein labeling among the crude subcellular fractions (mitochondrial, microsomal, cell sap) was also studied. Thirty to 40 % inhibition has been found to be evenly distributed (Křivánek 1970). Fig. 5.11 demonstrates the results. To see whether proteins of some mitochondrial subfractions, namely nerve endings particles and pure mitochondria, could reveal a differential susceptibility to the SD action, a double labeling study was undertaken to ensure identical conditions during particles preparation. Practically the same isotope ratios were found, demonstrating again a uniform distribution of the inhibition of the protein labeling through the fractions studied — two nerve endings particles fractions and pure mitochondria (Gaete Avaria and Křivánek 1973).

A possible effect of SD on the composition of the transcallosally transported proteins into synaptosomes has been studied by Bao and Ochs (1972). Proteins had been labeled by topical application of [^{3}H] leucine to the parieto-occipital cortex of anaesthetized rabbits. The decrease of labeling varied but some implications of the morphological aspects of SD have been considered by these authors.

To see whether the inhibitory effect on protein synthesis in vivo would persist under in vitro conditions and also to test whether the entire protein synthetic activity

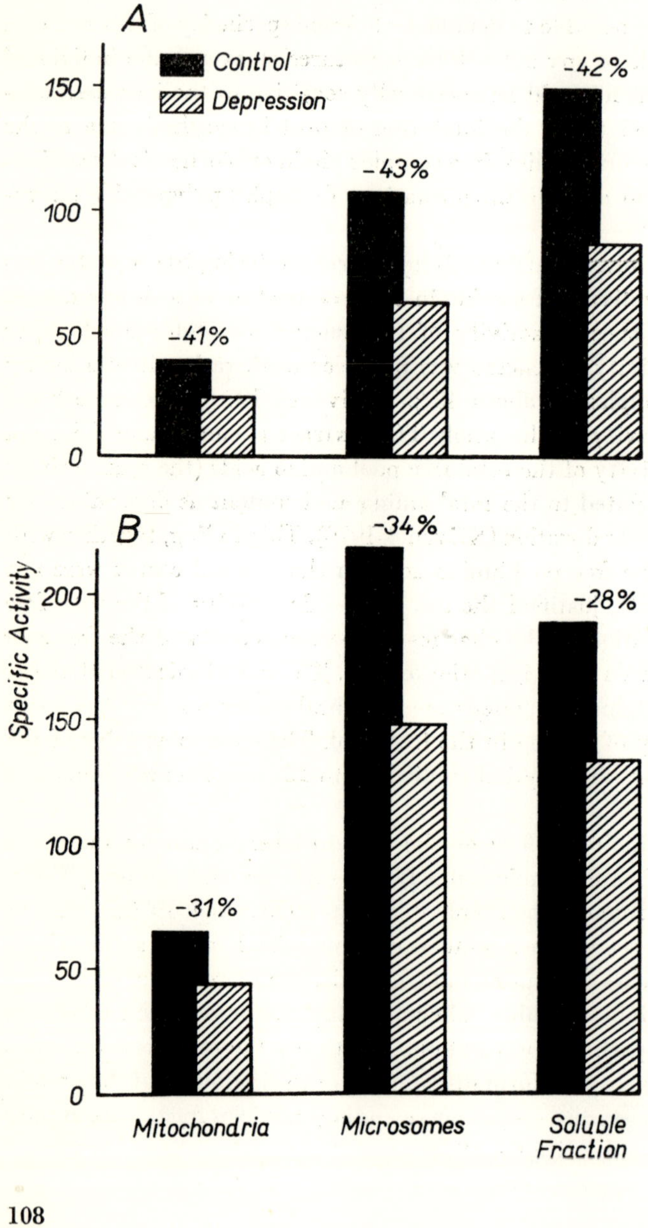

Fig. 5. 11. Effect of CSD (duration 1 hour) on incorporation of DL-[1-^{14}C] leucine into the proteins of the crude mitochondrial, microsomal, and soluble subcellular fractions of rat cerebral cortex. Rats were killed 1 hour after subcutaneous injection of the labeled leucine. *(A)* Data obtained from one group of four animals. Preparation of the purified mitochondrial fraction was according to the procedure of Roodyn, Reis, and Work (1961). *(B)* Data obtained from two groups of four animals. Preparation of the crude mitochondrial fraction was carried out by conventional method (without purification). Ordinate: specific activity in cpm/mg protein. (Křivánek 1970).

of the cerebral cortex had been affected, a cell-free system containing mitochondria microsomes, and supernatant was prepared and augmented with factors essential for its optimum operation.

The cell-free system from the cerebral cortex, which had been treated 60 min with 25% KCl *in vivo*, did not differ from that prepared from the control cortex in its capability to incorporate ^{14}C leucine added *in vitro*.

The failure to find any difference between the in vitro incorporation rates of the in vivo depressed and control cortices could be because the tissue was damaged by preparation to such an extent that a "depressed" brain was studied in both cases. Another possibility remained, however, namely, that shortage of some factor(s) engaged in protein synthesis occurs *in vivo*, but after transfer of the tissue into the medium supplied with an excess of all the essential components, the depressed tissue rapidly becomes "normal". The assumption was made that sensitivity to the depletion would be much more pronounced in the system prepared from the depressed cortex. After decrease of the Mg^{2+} concentration to 20% of its optimum or after complete removal of Mg^{2+} from the incubation medium, the same inhibition of the incorporation rate was found in both normal and depressed homogenate. Identical percentage inhibition of both systems was also found in the medium completely devoid of guanosinetriphosphate (GTP) (Fig. 5.12). Different results, however, were obtained after depletion of oxidizable substrate. Inhibition of labeled leucine incorporation was

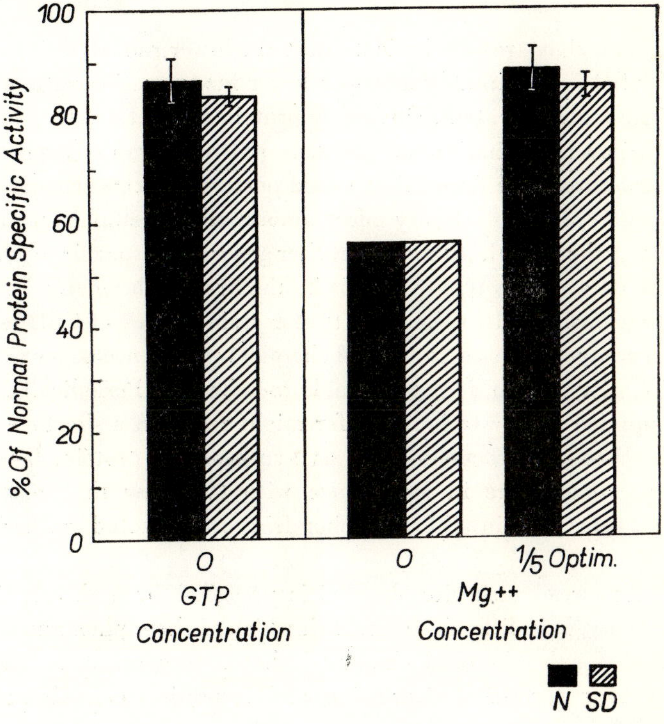

Fig. 5. 12. Protein synthesis of cell-free preparations *in vitro* from the cerebral cortex previously treated with 25 % KCl for 1 hour *in vivo* (shaded columns) as compared with normal preparations from the contralateral cortex (black columns). Media were depleted of some essential factors (Křivánek 1969b).

more apparent in the homogenate from the depressed cortex when no substrate was added to the medium. With progressively increasing substrate concentrations in the medium there was increasing recovery of protein synthetic activity in the homogenates from the potassium-treated cortex. Hence response to the depletion of the oxidizable substrate is the only one in which both types of homogenates differ from each other (Křivánek 1969b) (Fig. 5.13).

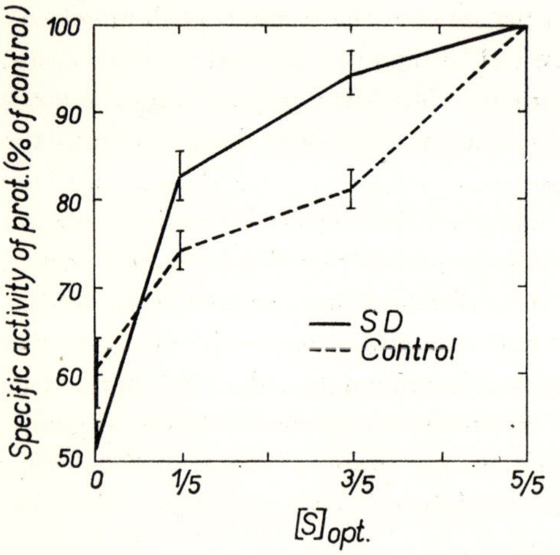

Fig. 5. 13. Effect of substrate concentration on the protein synthetic activity of the homogenates prepared from normal and from the cortices of the mature rats treated with potassium *in vivo*. Percentage of control on the ordinate is referred to the value obtained in the complete medium. Incubation period was 25 min (Křivánek 1969b).

The above results indicate that the lower radioactivity of cortical proteins caused by SD is presumably due to a lower incorporation rate of the precursor amino acid into cortical protein. Obviously protein synthetic activity of the brain was inhibited. However, no individual proteins or their groups localized in various subcellular structures were found that would possess an extra sensitivity to SD. The even distribution of the inhibitory effect among all subcellular fractions in adult animals supports the view that there is a rather general nonspecific mechanism by which SD exerts its effect on protein synthesis in the brain. The many lines of evidence mentioned previously lead to the view that certain phases of CSD activate processes involved in generation of an additional chemical energy necessary for the restoration of normal ion distribution across excitable membranes. Periodically repeated switching of the supplied energy to ion transfer might result in a shortage for other energy requiring biochemical processes such as synthesis of protein. The results of the *in vitro* experiments are in accordance with the view that reactions involving oxidation of substrate in the mitochondria are affected rather than protein synthesis per se.

As already mentioned, SPC is preceded by a shortlasting discharge of neuronal activity. It is difficult to establish which of these phenomena is predominantly responsible for the chemical changes hitherto demonstrated. The possibility of separately evoking spreading depression and spreading convulsion by electrical stimulation of the rabbit cerebral cortex has been claimed by Shirane (1961). Decreased level of glucose and elevated content of lactate was found during spreading convulsion whereas SD was accompanied by an increase of glucose and a fall of lactate.

After the basic chemical aspects of SD have been described, it is necessary to answer the question as to what mechanisms are responsible for the chemical changes accompanying SD.

All the experiments hitherto mentioned have furnished supporting evidence for the suggestion that chemical changes caused by SD in the cerebral cortex *in vivo* are closely related to changes elicited in the brain cortex slices *in vitro* by increasing the potassium ion concentration in the medium above 20 mM. This assumption makes it possible to include in the discussion data from in vitro experiments concerned with the potassium effect.

A great number of papers have been published dealing with the mechanism of K^+ action on metabolism since the first reports by Ashford and Dixon (1935) and Dickens and Greville (1935). Various aspects of the problem were studied but no definite solution has yet been found. Increased oxygen consumption and lactate production (enhancement of aerobic glycolysis), augmented glucose utilization, and a decrease in creatine phosphate and very often also in ATP content have been consistently demonstrated and may be considered as firmly established. It is not clear, however, whether this shift reflects stimulation of cerebral metabolism or some specific impairment of glucose metabolism (reversal of the Pasteur effect). Under normal conditions increased respiration should be accompanied by decreased glycolysis. This so-called "Pasteur effect" seems to be reversed in the potassium-treated brain. Two approaches were used to study changes in energy metabolism as revealed by potassium action. First, those chemical processes were studied that are known to require chemical energy in the form of ATP and CrP (endergonic reactions), followed by more direct processes, in which turnover rates of ATP and CrP were measured. If some kind of general stimulation of metabolism occurred, the rate of endergonic reactions as well as turnover of ATP and CrP would be increased and vice versa. The first approach was to follow the synthesis of glycogen and incorporation of radioactive precursors into the macromolecules of lipids or proteins. Increasing potassium concentration above 50 mM results in inhibition of glycogen synthesis (Kleinzeller and Rybová 1957) *in vitro* as well as *in vivo* (see p. 96). Incorporation of radioactive amino acids ([^{35}S]-methionin, Folbergerová 1961; [^{14}C] glycin, Bassi and Bernelli-Zazzera 1960, Mase, Takahashi, and Ogata 1962) has been shown to be diminished *in vitro* as well as *in vivo* under similar conditions. On the other hand another endergonic process seems to be stimulated when potassium content is augmented in the medium. Incorporation of ^{32}P into phosphoproteins (Tsukada, Takagaki, and Hirano 1958) as well as into phospholipids (Yoshida and Quastel 1962) was reported to be stimulated by potassium *in vitro*. The earlier experiments by Findlay, Magee, and Rossiter (1954) showing an inhibitory effect of potassium on the last two processes are irrelevant since analyses were performed at the end of

4 hours of incubation when reversal of the potassium effect had taken place (Tsukada, Takagaki, and Hirano 1958, Hertz and Clausen 1963).

No definite conclusion has been drawn as far as turnover rates of CrP and adenine nucleotides are concerned. Diminished turnover of "nucleotide labile P", inorganic phosphate, and creatine phosphate was reported by Fonyo, Kovách, Makláy, Leszkowsky, and Meszáros (1958), whereas Tsukada, Takagaki, and Hirano (1958) and Brossard and Quastel (1963) presented the opposite results, that is, stimulation of ^{32}P incorporation into "acid-soluble P" and "7-min nucleotide phosphate". The SD was demonstrated to be accompanied by an increase of CrP turnover. Although short incubation times were used in all three papers cited, they differ in composition of medium and in tonicity as well. It is therefore difficult to make any proper conclusion from these data in spite of the fact that this problem is a crucial one.

The increased oxygen consumption and glycolysis acceleration as a consequence of increased potassium concentration are usually ascribed to the increased level of phosphate acceptors such as ADP and/or AMP as a result of augmented cleavage of CrP and ATP. These are known to stimulate both oxidative and glycolytic pathways of glucose metabolism. Oxidative utilization of pyruvate seems to be accelerated. Potassium-stimulated respiration could be demonstrated with glucose, fructose, pyruvate, and lactate as substrates, but not in the presence of any of the following dicarboxylic acids: succinate, oxoglutarate, fumarate, or malate. Malonate inhibition of respiration is also much more pronounced in the case of stimulated respiration, that is, in the presence of the substrates mentioned above (Ito 1960). Accordingly pyruvate oxidation through tricarboxylic acid cycle would be accelerated. As far as glycolysis is concerned, even less is known about the mechanism of its stimulation in the cerebral cortex by potassium ions. Only recently two papers have been published dealing with changes in glycolytic intermediates in brain slices of the guinea pig (Rollestone and Newsholme 1967, Takagaki 1968). Unfortunately different media were used and also the absolute values of the levels of the critical intermediates (fructosediphosphate, triosophosphate, pyruvate) achieved by added potassium cannot be compared. However, from the concentration ratios of the single intermediates it appeared that in the presence of potassium, glycolysis is affected at the sites previously suggested (Lowry and Passonneau 1964), that is, fructosediphosphate and pyruvate-kinase. To what extent the shifts in levels of these substances are caused exclusively by changes in ADP and/or AMP levels is not clear. A possible additional direct stimulation effect of potassium on pyruvate kinase was suggested (Lipsett and Crescitelli 1950, Takagaki 1968) but not experimentally proved. Intracellular concentrations of neither iP nor ADP and AMP were measured in the Takagaki paper after iP addition to the medium. Therefore an additional effect of high potassium concentration on glycolysis does not seem to prove a specific action. Also confusing is the finding by Rollestone and Newsholme (1967) that a decrease not an increase of ADP and only a slight increase of AMP occurred with high potassium.

The chemical exploration of the phenomenon discussed is hindered by the fact that it is probably confined to only some compartment(s) as suggested earlier (see p. 99). Accurate measurements of the intracellular concentration of the chemical substances is a fairly difficult problem while determination of the compartment most involved in the particular response is almost impossible. This is especially true for brain tissue, the cellular inhomogeneity of which is considerable. No definite proof has been furnished as yet on the extent to which glial cells could participate in the cerebral cortical response to the action of potassium. Van Harreveld and Stamm (1953b) have shown that *in vivo* glial elements alone are not sufficient to ensure SD propagation. Cerebral cortex damaged by transient ischemia did not react with SD to common eliciting agents when the reduction in the number of neurons was excessive. Also SD would not pass through a narrow band of the cortex that had previously suffered local injury resulting in a disappearance of neurons and an increase in glia (Van Harreveld, Terres, and Dernburg 1956). On the other hand respiration of the neurons isolated by manual dissection (Hydén 1959) was shown to be insensitive to a high potassium medium, whereas that of surrounding isolated glial cells ("oligodendroglia") was increased (Hertz 1966). However, this kind of preparation suffers from the serious drawback that dissected neurons are completely devoid of their processes. Clearcut evidence as to the extent to which different kinds of brain cells are affected by potassium ions remains to be presented.

Very little is known about the connection of the chemical events associated with SD with the electrical correlates. Spreading depression *in vivo* and stimulation of glucose metabolism *in vitro* can be elicited by a variety of agents like NH_4^+, Rb^+, a decrease in Ca^{2+} (or the use of EDTA), and by some amino acids (p. 36) as well as by electrical stimulation. Depolarization will result in all these cases as demonstrated *in vivo* by both a shift in the polarity of the cerebral cortex surface and by direct measurements of the resting potential of cortical cells (Collewijn and Van Harreveld 1966, Brožek 1966). *In vitro* the resting potential of cerebral cortex slices has been shown to decline in the presence of potassium ion concentrations comparable with those that could accumulate in vivo during SD (Hillman and McIlwain 1961) and during electrical stimulation (Hillman, Campbell, and McIlwain 1963). Conceivably these agents act by altering the permeability of the excitable membranes in the cerebral cortex. As in peripheral nerves, the presence of sodium ions is essential to evoke the potassium effect in brain preparations. Increased permeability to sodium ions is suggested as being a first step in the action of potassium and related agents (Van Harreveld 1966). Consequently, potassium is released and can elicit depolarization of membranes. Potassium flux rates seem to be enhanced, which might be a result of increased transport rather than increased permeability (Hertz 1968). Sodium fluxes are claimed to be unaffected by potassium ions in the medium of cerebral cortex slices (Hertz 1966). Increased potassium fluxes were also shown by Cummins and McIlwain (1961) in isolated cerebral cortex slices during and immediately after electrical stimulation.

The mechanism by which potassium exerts its effect on the membrane is unclear;

Na, K-activated ATPase, which is located in the membranes and seems to be responsible for a variety of transport phenomena, has been shown to be stimulated by the agents increasing brain respiration mentioned above, and is inhibited by the factors abolishing stimulated respiration such as ouabain (Wollenberger 1947). Transport ATPase might therefore be the site of potassium action. Stimulation of its activity would lead to the increased rate of ATP cleavage, which would stimulate glycolysis and respiration, as mentioned above.

Accordingly, transport ATPase can be considered as a crucial point at which the ion transport couples electrical and biochemical phenomena.

It seems, therefore, that the presence of high concentrations of potassium or of related compounds evoking SD *in vivo* leads to rearrangement of the ions across the excitable membrane by changing the permeability to these ions. This will cause depolarization. Increased uptake of potassium and extrusion of sodium against their concentration gradients require energy, which is generated by stimulation of glucose metabolism by enhancement of ADP or other phosphate acceptors. The metabolism of compounds involved in ion transport is also increased (some phospholipids, phosphoproteins), whereas that of the others not directly related to transport phenomena is inhibited (incorporation of amino acids into proteins) due to a shortage of energy-rich substances. Involvement of cyclic adenosine 3',5' - monophosphate should also be considered since Sattin and Rall (1967) and Shimizu, Creveling, and Daly (1970) have demonstrated that potassium ions and some other depolarizing agents cause an accumulation of cyclic AMP in incubated slices of cerebral cortex.

Chapter 6

Morphological and Developmental Aspects of Spreading Depression

Spreading depression was discovered in the cerebral cortex of the rabbit (Leão 1944a) and mammalian neocortex was used, therefore, in most experiments concerned with the further analysis of this phenomenon. According to Marshall (1959) SD has been observed in the cerebral cortex of the mouse, rat, guinea pig, rabbit, porcupine, marmoset, sloth, cat, and macaque monkey. The squirrel monkey (Rebert 1970) and the Australian phalanger *Trichosurus vulpecula* (Megirian and Bureš, unpublished) have recently been added to this list. The lissencephalic cortex of lower mammals seems to offer particularly suitable conditions for SD. The reaction becomes less reliable und reproducible in higher mammals, for example in cat, monkey, and sheep (Eidelberg, Kolmodin and Meyerson 1965).

1. Cortical Spreading Depression

The uniform structure of the mammalian neocortex led to the assumption that the fundamental properties of SD (rate of spreading, SPC) depend on laminar structures. Research concentrated first on establishing the cortical layers specifically engaged in SD propagation. Leão and Morrison (1945) reported that acute thermocoagulation or transection of the superficial cortical layers blocked SD. Grafstein (1956b) failed to block SD propagation in an isolated cortical slab by thermocoagulation of three upper cortical layers performed 2 weeks before the actual experiment. Destruction of layers IV to VI also failed to block SD, and radial cuts interfered with SD propagation only when extending from the surface to the middle of layer VI or from the base of the cortex to layer I. Whereas these findings indicated equal participation of all cortical layers in the mechanism of spreading, with only shallow subpial cuts Ochs and Hunt (1960) found a transient SD block which became permanent when the transection reached down through layer IV of the rabbbit cortex. Cuts from the subcortical white matter upward did not block the SD when at least the uppermost molecular layer was spared.

In contrast with the above data Sloan and Jasper (1950) claimed that SD can overcome a complete transcortical cut in cats, provided the gap between the wound edges is less than 1.5 mm wide and filled with tissue fluid. Later efforts to repeat this finding which resembled the caffeine spike experiments of Libet and Gerard

(1941), failed. In the experiments by Ochs (1958), SD did not pass across cuts made through the cortex. In a careful study Van Harreveld, Terres, and Dernburg (1956) examined SD propagation across a transcortical section made 3 weeks to 3 months before the experiment. Although the glial scar was often less than 0.1 mm wide, it invariably stopped SD propagation. The small slow potential recorded beyond the scar approached by the SD wave, was evidently due to physical spread of current. The authors concluded that the SD transmission across the cut observed by Sloan and Jasper (1950) was perhaps facilitated by the acute injury potential and release of intracellular material.

The significance of the upper cortical layers for SD was demonstrated by Leão's (1951) experiments in which SPC was recorded from different depths of rabbit cortex with capillary electrodes. The negativity developed in the superficial layers first and then spread into the deep ones, the vertical and tangential spreading rates being approximately equal. Similar results were obtained in the cat by Grafstein (1956b) and in the rat by Monakhov, Fifková, and Bureš (1962a). Ichijo and Ochs (1970) estimated the rate of radial descent of SD into the lower layers of cat cortex by measuring the latency between depression of the direct cortical response and depression of the antidromically activated pyramidal tract cells. The latency-depth relation indicated a spreading rate of 0.75 mm/min between 1 and 2 mm and a rate twice as fast in the upper layers of cerebral cortex. It seems that superficial cortical layers not only have the maximum area of reactive membranes per unit volume of tissue, but also that the horizontal branches of the apical dendrites overlap most extensively in the first and second layers and carry thus the depolarization wave further forward than in the deeper layers (Fig. 6.1). This suggestion was supported by the electron microscopic findings of Van Harreveld and Khattab (1967); they examined with the freeze substitution technique the surface (20 μ) of the mouse cortex invaded by SD and found loss of extracellular space and swollen cellular structures, most probably parts of the closely interdigitating system of apical dendrites. These results convincingly prove that the electrolyte and water shifts accompanying SD depolarization take place even in the uppermost layers of the cortex, but other evidence indicates that similar changes also occur deeper below the surface. During

---

Fig. 6. 1. Vertical distribution of SPC in the cerebral cortex of the rat. (Above) Example of a typical experiment; SPC is recorded with an array of electrodes introduced into various cortical layers as indicated in the inset diagram (left). The recording shows two slow potential waves initiated by a single application of KCl (center). First part of the same record with the time scale magnified three times is shown on the right in order to illustrate the method of delay estimation. Calibration: 3 min, 10 mV. (Below left) Average amplitude of the slow negative potential (ordinate). Abscissa: cortical layers 1—6. Abbreviations: cc, corpus callosum; *S*, nucleus caudatus. (Below right) The relative delay (ordinate) with which SPC attains 50 % of the negative maximum in deep cortical layers (abscissa) as compared with the superficial layers. The dotted vertical bars indicate the standard errors of the mean values (Monakhov, Fifková, and Bureš 1962a).

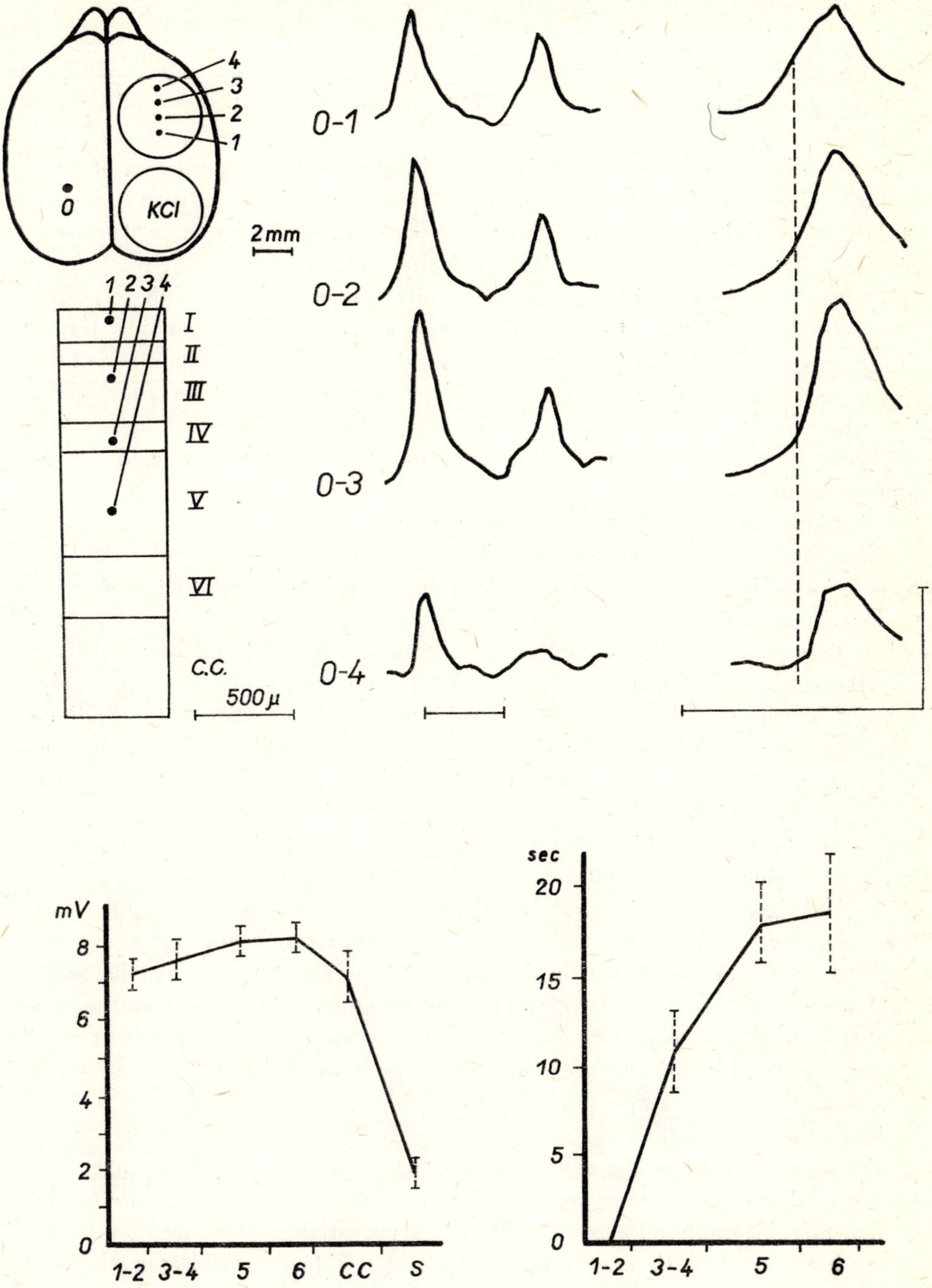
4
3
2
1
O
KCl
2 mm
1 2 3 4
I
II
III
IV
V
VI
C.C.
500 µ
0-1
0-2
0-3
0-4
mV
8
6
4
2
0
1-2
3-4
5
6
CC
S
sec
20
15
10
5
0
1-2
3-4
5
6

SD, Van Harreveld (1958) found a 17% increase in diameter of apical dendrites just below the boundary between molecular and granular layers in the rabbit cortex. With a histochemical freeze substitution method, SD was found to be accompanied by chloride shifts into apical dendrites in layers I to III. During cortical SD in rats Fifková and Křivánek (1965) found an 11% increase in the diameter of perikarya in deeper cortical layers.

On the other hand SD does not always penetrate into the deeper layers of the cat cortex. Ichijo and Ochs (1970) observed full depression of the direct cortical response at the surface, while the pyramidal tract cell responses in the depth remained preserved. Similar results were obtained by Muñoz-Martínez (1970). Anomalous concomitants of cortical SD as increased activity in deep cortical layers (Rosenblueth and García-Ramos 1966) and augmentation of the I waves elicited in the pyramidal tract by direct cortical stimulation (Muñoz-Martínez 1968) are probably also due to failure of downward propagation. Lower density of dendrites in deeper layers may decrease the safety factor of SD and in combination with hyperpolarizing agents (CO_2) may generate radial SD gradients, thus accounting for the modification of the basic process to spreading convulsions.

Conditions for SD initiation and propagation are similar over the whole cortical surface. Significant regional differences were only observed in the medial and lateral boundaries of the neocortex, that is in the retrosplenial and entorhinal regions. Leão (1944a) found in the rabbit that cortical SD does not spread across the parasagittal sulcus that separates the retrosplenial area from the parietal and occipital cortex. Van Harreveld and Bogen (1956) observed SD propagation into this region only in 1 out of 36 rabbits and Van Harreveld and Schadé (1959) confirmed this finding by the elegant demonstration of the sharp boundary of intracellular chlorine transport under the parasagittal sulcus during SD. Since SD seems to be stopped by sulci in gyrencephalic brains, a similar explanation was originally suggested in this case. More important are morphological differences, however, since the retrosplenial area is a part of cingular cortex (Rose and Woolsey 1948), most of which is situated on the medial surface of the hemisphere. Although no sulcus separates cingular cortex from neocortex in the rat, Fifková (1964a) found with an array of capillary electrodes a considerable decrease of SPC in the superficial layer and a corresponding shift of the maximum negativity to deep layers of the agranular segment of the retrosplenial area (Fig. 6.2). The penetration of SPC into the more medially located granular segment occurred in 35% of the cases with a prolonged refractory period (30 min). No slow potential waves were found in the adjoining subiculum forming the transition to hippocampus. The findings are schematically represented in Fig. 6.3. Similar results were obtained in the entorhinal area which forms the occipital part of the pyriform lobe joining the neocortex at the rhinal fissure, and in the more medially located presubiculum and subiculum. The slow potential propagating from the neocortex is preceded in these structures by a negative prepotential appearing in 70 to 80% of the cases and attaining over approximately 1 min an average amplitude

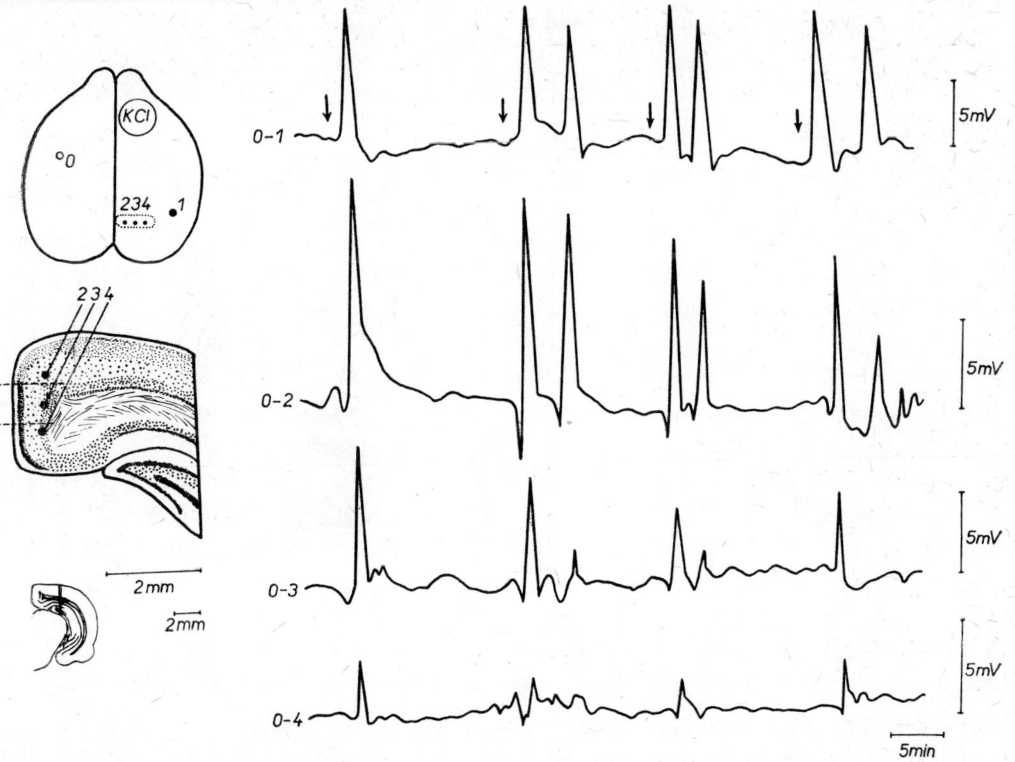

Fig. 6. 2. Multiple electrode recording of SPC accompanying CSD penetration into the retrosplenial cortex. The inset diagram illustrates location of the recording capillary electrodes and of the area of KCl application. (0—1) Control recording from cortical surface. (0—2) Layer V of area retrosplenialis agranularis (segment I); (0—3) layer VI of area retrosplenialis granularis (segment II); (0—4) layer VI of area retrosplenialis granularis (segment III). Arrows indicate application of 2 % KCl to frontal cortex. Calibration: 5 mV and 5 min (Fifková 1964a).

of 2.5 mV. The prepotential can be easily distinguished from the following SPC which is steeper and several times higher in amplitude. It is probably an expression of nonhomogeneity of the reactive tissue; a higher SD threshold in the entorhinal cortex stops SD propagation until diffusion from neocortex raises the extracellular potassium concentration to the new threshold level. The threshold is never reached in 40% of the cases. Further conduction is also unreliable, so that the percentage of the cortical SD waves penetrating into presubiculum and subiculum drops to 39 and 33%, respectively. The adjoining hippocampus is never entered by neocortical SD waves. Besides this lateromedial gradient of SD decrement from neocortex to hippocampus, there is also a rostrocaudal one; the anterior parts of entorhinal cortex seem to offer better conditions for SD development than the posterior ones. All these results are summarized in Fig. 6.3.

The reason for the higher threshold or absence of SD in the retrosplenial and entorhina lcortex must be sought in the overall reduction of the membrane area per unit volume of tissue in regions where the density of perikarya is increased while the density of dendrites is diminished.

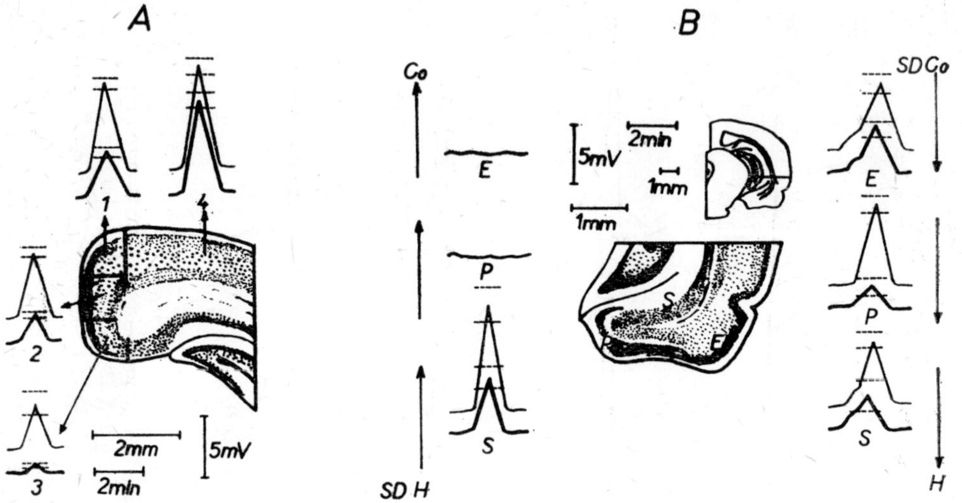

Fig. 6. 3. Spreading depression in the neocortical-hippocampal border region in the rat. *(A)* Comparison of mean SPC amplitudes in neocortex (4) and in different sectors of area retrosplenialis (1, 2, 3). Heavy line indicates mean amplitude of all reactions. Thin line indicates mean amplitude of positive reactions only. The dotted horizontal bars indicate $\pm$ 1 SEM level. *(B)* Mean SPC amplitude in the temporal border regions during cortical *(Co)* or hippocampal *(H)* SD. The direction of arrows indicates from which structure the SD was evoked. Abbreviations: *S*, subiculum; *P*, presubiculum; *E*, area entorhinalis; *Co*, neocortex; *H*, hippocampus (Fifková 1964a).

2. Cerebellar Spreading Depression

Whereas Leão and Martins-Ferreira (1961) and Van Harreveld (1961) were not able to elicit SD in the cerebellum of the rabbit, Rhoton, Goldring, and O'Leary (1960) described a slow potential change resembling cortical SD in cat cerebellum. Fifková, Bureš, Koshtoyants, Křivánek, and Weiss (1961) succeeded in eliciting SD in rat cerebellum both by surface application of 1% KCl and by intracortical microinjection of 25% KCl. The SPCs reached 5 to 6 mV in amplitude and lasted for 70 to 80 sec. They could be recorded with both surface and deep electrodes within the same gyrus. The spreading rate was 2.7 mm/min. No decrement was seen over a distance of 3 mm but atypical slow potential waves (two negative peaks or high initial positivity) were more frequent than in the cortex. Spreading across sulci and from vermis to hemispheres and vice versa was observed only exceptionally. Cortical SD could be reliably elicited in the rabbit vermis pretreated for 20 to 30 min with hypotonic NaCl (30 to 40 mM) or isotonic sodium acetate (160 mM) (Leão and Martins-Ferreira 1961).

3. Hippocampal Spreading Depression

The possibility of eliciting SD in the exposed rabbit hippocampus was first reported by Leão and Martins-Ferreira (1958). The reaction could be evoked in the same way and had approximately the same properties as the neocortical SD. The hippocampal SPC had sometimes two components, a rapid initial phase followed by a slower negativity which could be suppressed by arterial occlusion (Leão and Martins-Ferreira 1959) or by increase of extracellular potassium concentration (Leão and Martins-Ferreira 1965). Bureš, Burešová, and Weiss (1960) demonstrated SD in the exposed dorsal hippocampus of rats and, using microinjection of solid KCl and capillary electrodes, also in the intact hippocampus of rats and cats.

The regular arrangement of cellular and dendritic layers in the hippocampus seemed to offer exceptionally favorable conditions for establishing the role of different portions of the neuron in the SPC generation. Monakhov, Fifková, and Bureš (1962b) used multiple capillary electrodes to study the potential field of SD in dorsal hippocampus with KCl microinjection into the posterior hippocampus. A typical experiment is illustrated by Fig. 6.4 and all data are summarized in Fig. 6.5. The average potential field was characterized by negativity extending over all hippocampal layers with maxima (12 to 13 mV) in the H_1, H_2 and H_4, H_5 pyramids. Slightly lower negativity was recorded from both the upper and lower elements of fascia dentata, probably because they have a less-developed dendritic tree. A rapid decrement of the SPC was observed in the extrahippocampal structures, both above and below the hippocampus. Similarly, as in the neocortex no positive deflections were found in the hippocampus during SD, probably because the source corresponding to the prominent sink is distributed over the rather long efferent hippocampal axons.

Propagation of SD to different parts of hippocampus was studied in detail by Fifková (1964a). After KCl microinjection into the rostral part of dorsal hippocampus, SD spread without decrement into dorsal and posterior hippocampus (Fig. 6.6). Nearly 80% of the SD waves reached the ventral hippocampus and 55% of the SD waves entered the subiculum. Transition to presubiculum and entorhinal cortex was never observed, however (Fig. 6.3). In all hippocampal regions the negative SPC was consistently higher in the layers formed by hippocampal pyramids than in those consisting of granular cells of fascia dentata.

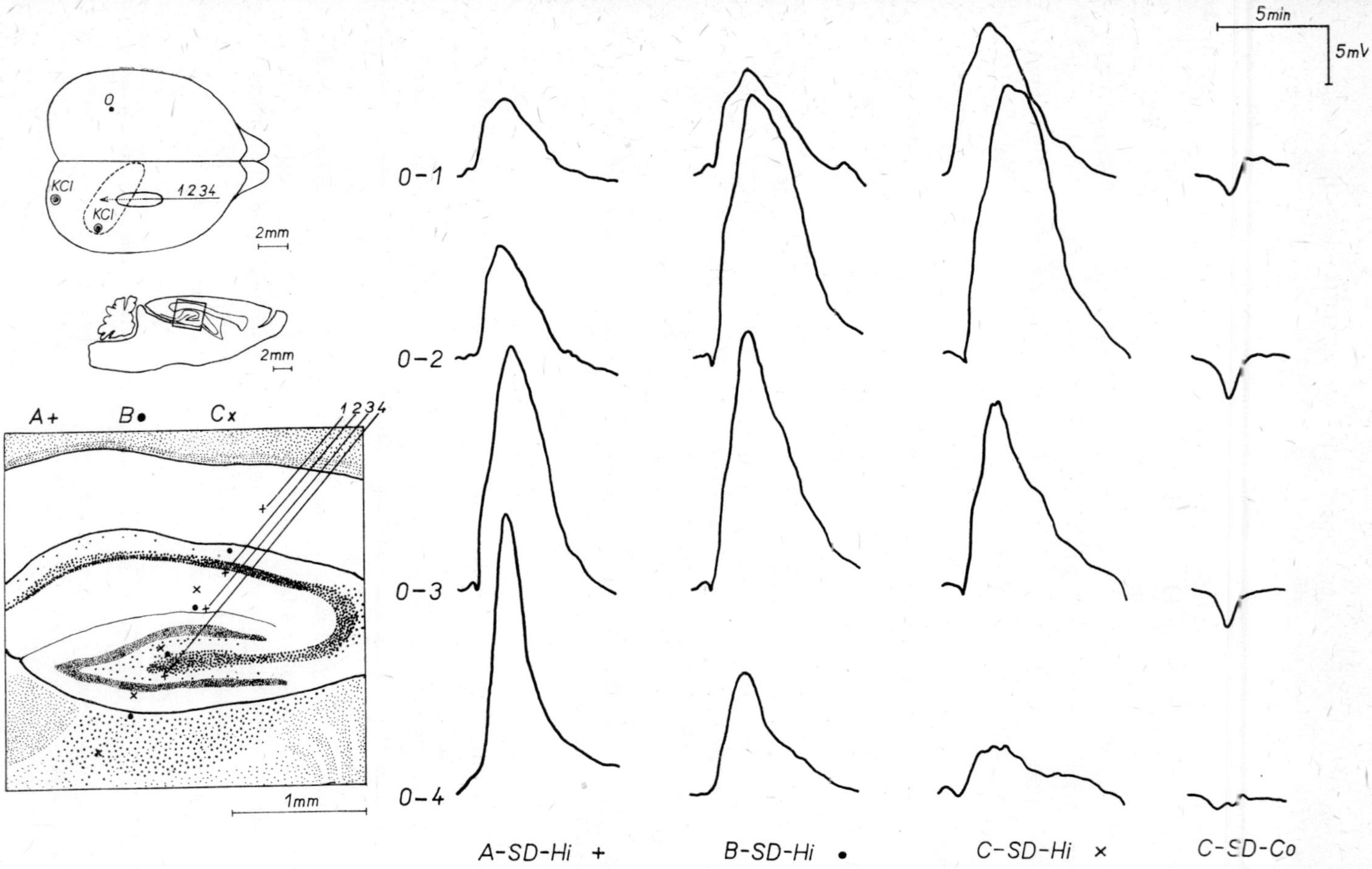

Fig. 6. 4. Slow potential waves of hippocampal SD recorded with an array of four capillary electrodes (1, 2, 3, 4) gradually inserted to three different depths *(A, B, C)*. Electrode location indicated in the inset diagrams, the lowest of which represents a parasagittal brain section in the electrode plane. The last column of the SPC recordings corresponds to a cortical SD recorded with the hippocampal electrodes in position *C* (Monakhov, Fifková, and Bureš 1962b).

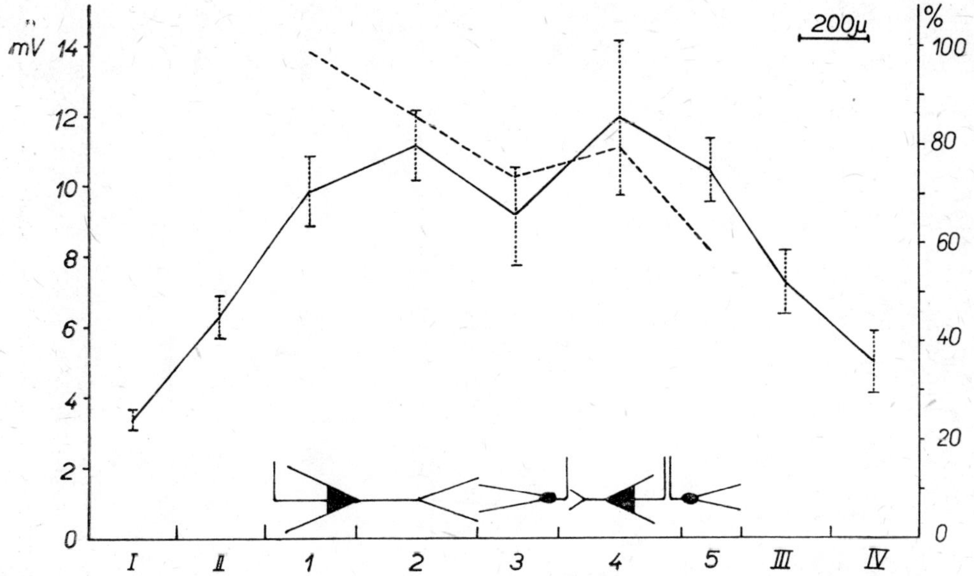

Fig. 6. 5. Steady potential field of hippocampal SD at the height of the negative SPC. Dashed line indicates single electrode data. Full line indicates multiple electrode data. Dotted vertical bars indicate standard errors of the mean. Ordinate: maximum SPC amplitude in millivolts. Abscissa: depth of electrode insertion into the dorsal hippocampus. (I, II, III, IV) Extrahippocampal structures (cortex, thalamus). (1) Alveus, basal dendrites, and cell bodies of H_1 and H_2 pyramids; (2) apical dendrites; (3) molecular and granular layers of fascia dentata; (4) H_4 and H_5 pyramids; (5) lower fascia dentata elements (Monakhov, Fifková, and Bureš 1962b).

4. Caudate Spreading Depression

Spreading depression in the mammalian corpus striatum was first described by Leão and Martins-Ferreira (1958). A detailed analysis of caudate SD in rat, rabbit, and cat was carried out by Fifková and Bureš (1964). Microinjection of 25% KCl into various parts of the corpus striatum evoked SPC, the amplitude (11 to 14 mV), duration (around 60 sec at 50% of maximum negativity), and spreading rate (2.6 to 3.3 mm/min) of which were approximately the same in all three species. Trachtenberg, Hull, and Buchwald (1970) recently examined SD in the caudate nucleus of cats using capillary microelectrodes for SPC recording. Negative slow potentials ranging up to 50 mV propagated at a rate of 2.6 mm/min but did not reach cerebral cortex, claustrum, or contralateral caudate. In the rabbit, whose caudate and putamen are separated by fibers of capsula interna, the delay between slow potential waves recorded from the two structures indicated that SD does not take the shortest pathway between them, rather it circumvents the internal capsule rostrally (Fifková 1966 b). In the rat, caudate and putamen form a complex that is uniformly swept by

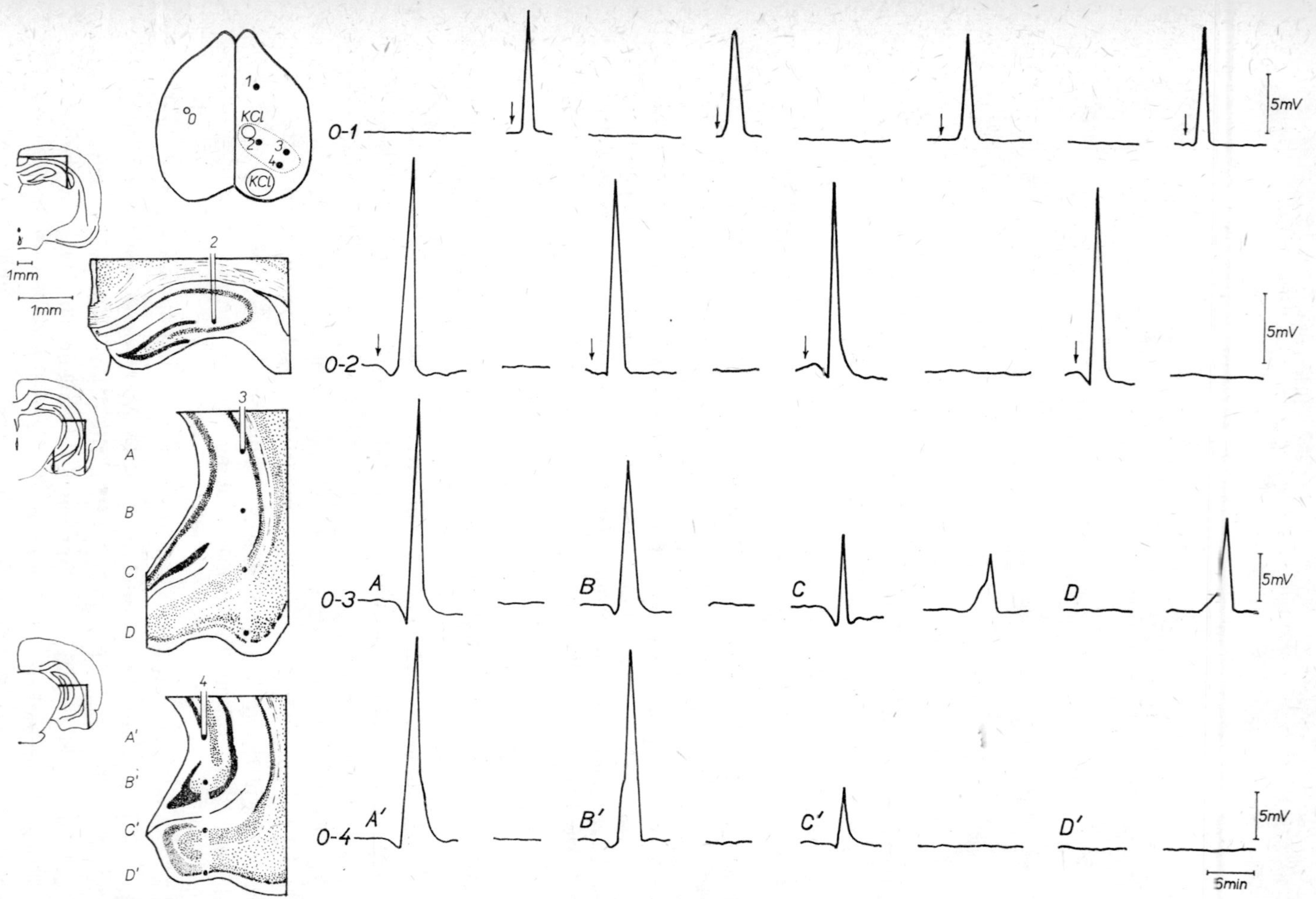

Fig. 6. 6. Propagation of cortical and hippocampal SD into subiculum and entorhinal cortex in the rat. Electrode location indicated in the inset diagram and coronal brain sections. The SPC recordings are from the following locations: (0—1) frontal cortex; (0—2) superior hippocampus; (0—3A) apical dendrites of H_2 pyramids in posterior hippocampus; (0—3B) apical dendrites of H_1 pyramids in the inferior hippocampus; (0—3C) subiculum inferius; (0—3D) area entorhinalis; (0—4A') fascia dentata posterior; (0—4B') H_5 pyramids of the inferior hippocampus; (0—4C') subiculum inferius; (0—4D)' area entorhinalis. In each position of electrodes 3 and 4 one SD wave was evoked from hippocampus and one from occipital cortex (see arrows in hippocampal or cortical recordings) (Fifková 1964a).

SD. The SPC does not enter septal nuclei, the globus pallidus, and the compact part of capsula interna, but it is not completely isolated from the structures in the pyriform lobe. The wave of caudate SD penetrated to lateral nucleus of the amygdala and from there to the neocortex in about 40% of the cases. Similarly, neocortical SD was accompanied in 60% of the cases by SD in the caudate (Fig. 6.7).

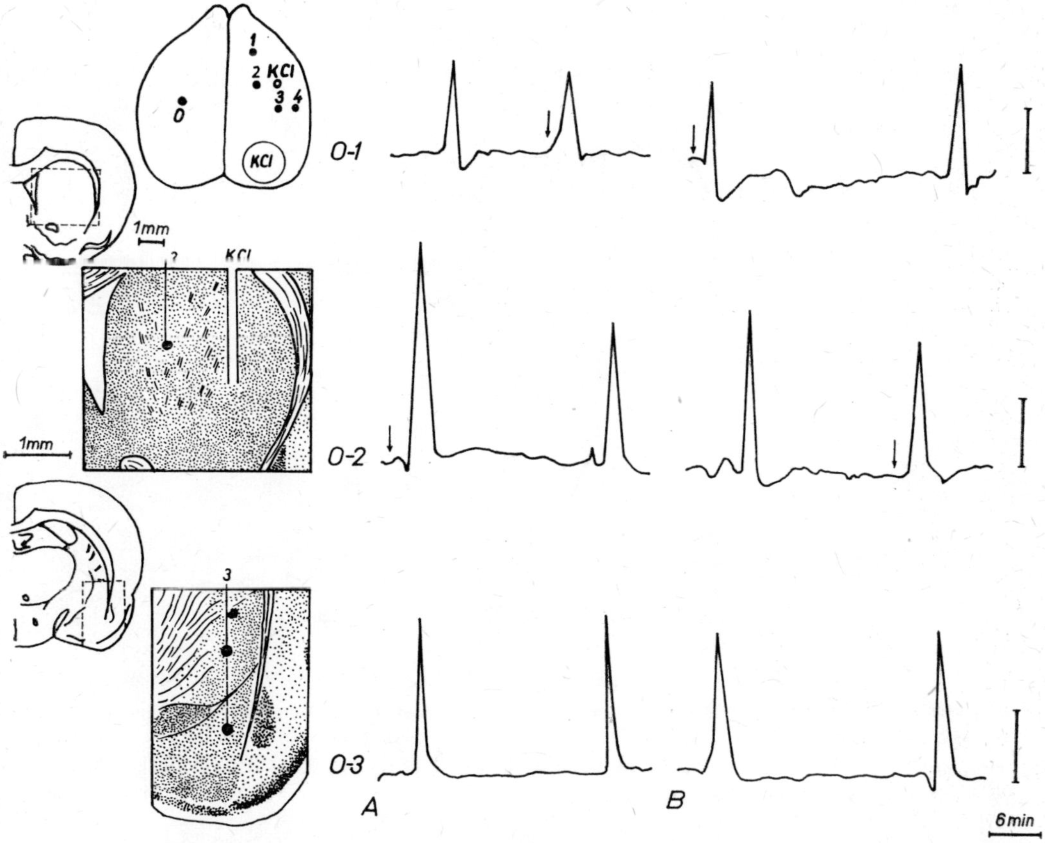

Fig. 6. 7. Propagation of striatal SD to neocortex and of neocortical SD to caudate through the lateral nucleus of amygdala. Location of electrodes indicated in the inset diagram. (0—1) Neocortex; (0—2) caudate; (0—3*A*) putamen—nucleus caudatus complex; (0—3*B*) lateral nucleus of amygdala. Calibration: 5 mV, 6 min (Fifková and Syka 1964).

The pathways involved must be rather long since the delay between cortical and caudatal SPCs was 326 sec (Fifková and Bureš 1964, Fifková and Syka 1964) although the shortest distance between the two recorded points was only 5 mm. Evidently SD cannot use this short route because it cannot cross the thick layer of callosal fibers separating the neocortex from the dorsal and lateral surface of the caudate nucleus (Fig. 6.8). The pathway corresponding most closely to the experimentally established value passes through the claustrum and amygdala. This assumption was confirmed by SPC recording. Cortical SD enters the pyriform cortex, the claustrum, and the amygdala complex with a slight delay, accounting for the frequent occurrence of the negative prepotential (1.5 to 2.5 mV, 1 min duration, see also p. 118). The negative SPC was high in the claustrum and in the lateral nucleus of the amygdala (over 10 mV). These structures were entered by all cortical SD waves,

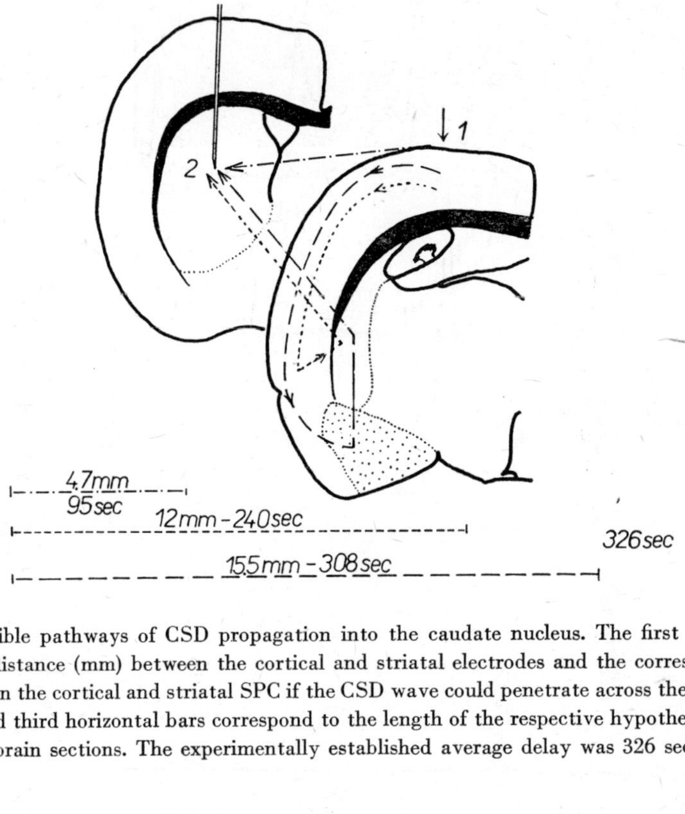

Fig. 6. 8. Possible pathways of CSD propagation into the caudate nucleus. The first horizontal bar indicates the distance (mm) between the cortical and striatal electrodes and the corresponding delay (95 sec) between the cortical and striatal SPC if the CSD wave could penetrate across the callosal fibers. The second and third horizontal bars correspond to the length of the respective hypothetical pathways shown in the brain sections. The experimentally established average delay was 326 sec (Fifková and Syka 1964).

initiated after a prolonged quiet interval (approximately 30 min, Fig. 6.9). Fibers separating the lateral nucleus of the amygdala from the putamen complex form a more important barrier, which was overcome by only 60% of the cortical SD waves. Propagation of SD from caudate to amygdala was also observed in only 38% of the cases, but all SD waves appearing in the amygdala reached the neocortex (42%).

Corticostriatal transmission is characterized by a long refractory period. Whereas repetitive waves of cortical SD are regularly transmitted to the claustrum, only every second wave appears in the lateral nucleus of the amygdala and still fewer reach the caudate nucleus. Figure 6.10 compares the recovery cycle of SD waves spreading between neocortex and caudate and entering from the neocortex into different

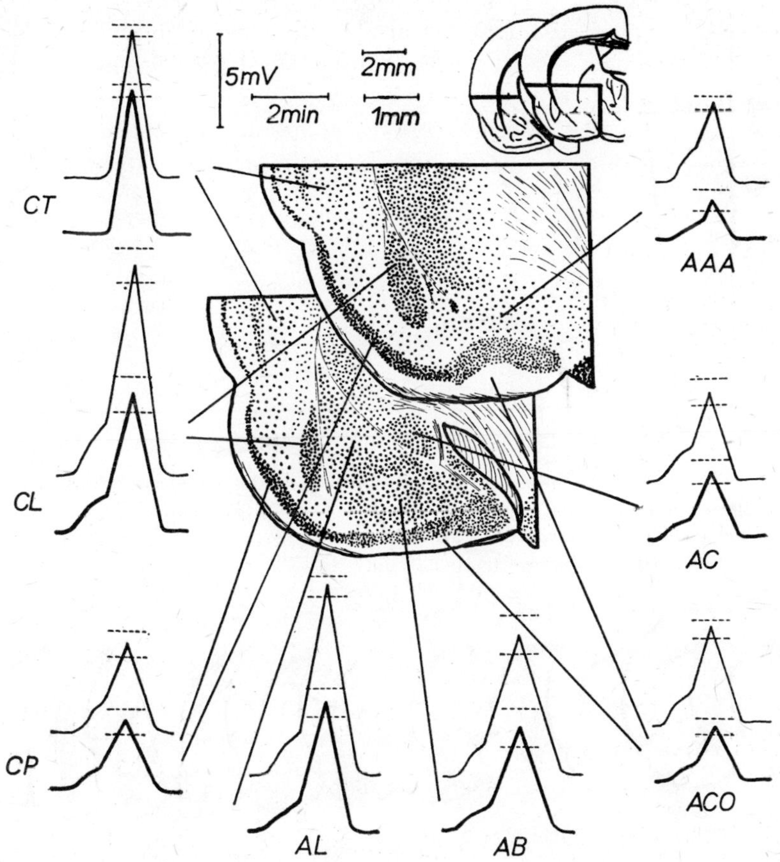

Fig. 6. 9. Average amplitude of SPC propagated into the pyriform lobe from the neocortex. Heavy line indicates all reactions; thin line indicates positive reactions only; dotted horizontal lines indicate ±1 SEM. Symbols: *CT*, temporal cortex; *CL*, claustrum; *CP*, pyriform cortex; *AAA*, anterior amygdalar area; *ACO*, cortical nucleus of amygdala; *AB*, basal nucleus of amygdala; *AL*, lateral nucleus of amygdala; *AC*, central nucleus of amygdala (Fifková 1964a).

structures of the pyriform lobe. Duration of the refractory period is inversely proportional to the safety factor of spreading. Structures with a short refractory period (neocortex, hippocampus, caudate nucleus) are able to generate a new SD wave long before all elements have recovered from depolarization. In the pyriform lobe and the striato-amygdalar boundary SD seems to require full recovery of most elements.

Corticostriatal transmission of SD could be interrupted (Fig. 6.11) by a horizontal transcortical cut parallel with the rhinal fissure and extending between coronal planes — 1.5 and + 3.5 (stereotaxic atlas of Fifková and Maršala 1967) or by a stereotaxic lesion destroying the amygdala and the caudal part of the claustrum (Fifková and

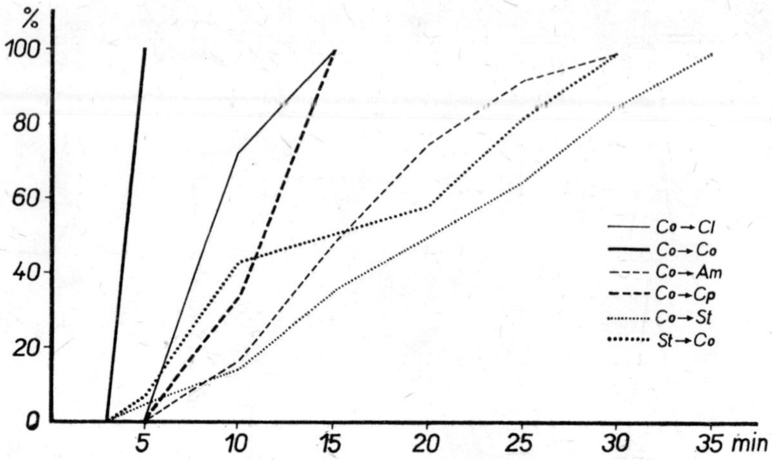

Fig. 6. 10. Recovery cycle of SD penetrating from neocortex into different structures of the pyriform lobe and into the caudate nucleus or from caudate nucleus to neocortex. Percentage of positive reactions (ordinate) to the testing SD wave evoked at various intervals (abscissa) after the conditioning SD wave. Symbols: *Cl*, claustrum; *Co*, neocortex; *Am*, amygdala; *Cp*, pyriform cortex; *St*, corpus striatum.

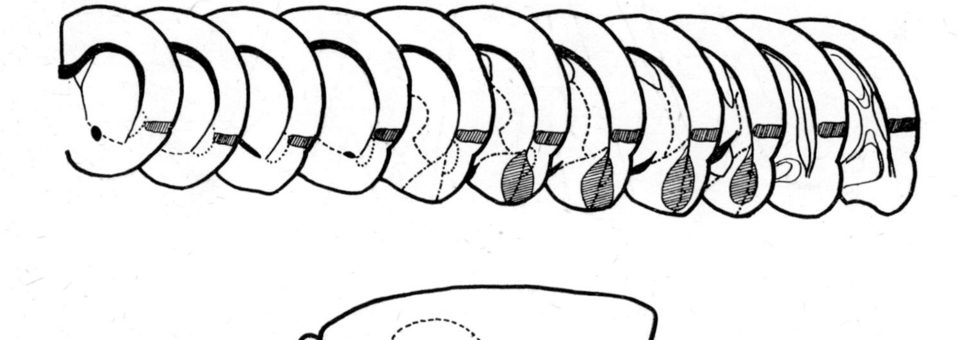

Fig. 6. 11. Schematic illustration of the extent of lesions preventing SD propagation between neocortex and caudate nucleus in rats. (Above) Frontal sections. (Below) Projection of the relevant structures and lesions onto the lateral surface of the hemisphere. Dashed line indicates corpus striatum; dotted line indicates claustrum; dash—dot line indicates amygdala. The arrow indicates the region of assumed corticostriatal transition. Extent of CSD indicated by shading, incomplete SD in the pyriform lobe by dashed shading (Fifková and Syka 1964).

Syka 1964). In a few experiments in which SD transition was not blocked by the lesion it was possible to determine the volume of the remaining tissue bridge mediating SD propagation. The minimum cross-section of such bridge was about 1 mm^2.

The possibility of eliciting SD in the caudate nucleus disproved the assumption that laminar structure is an essential prerequisite for the accompanying SPC. Although devoid of obvious lamination, caudate and putamen form a meshwork of closely interdigitating neural processes, the density of which is evidently the only decisive factor. The source for the current sink is probably again in the efferent myelinated axons. In regions where fibers of the capsula interna pass through corpus striatum, the amplitude of SPC is reduced but the SD propagation is not blocked when enough gray matter surrounds the bundles of myelinated fibers (see also p. 148).

The greater dimensions of the amygdala and septum in the rabbit made it possible to examine the SD susceptibility of these structures adjacent to caudate (Fifková 1966b). With KCl injection into the amygdala, SPC propagated without decrement to all structures of the pyriform lobe, including the pyriform cortex and entorhinal area. The SPC amplitudes ranged from 5 to 10 mV and the velocity was about 2.5 mm/min. Only increased refractoriness at the distal electrode indicated that the structure is not quite homogeneous. Septal SD waves could also be generated by KCl injection into the septum, but their propagation was decremental, the SPC amplitude being significantly higher at the near electrode than at the distal one. Perhaps the autoregenerative mechanism of SD is impaired by the rapid escape of potassium ions into the lateral ventricle that forms the lateral boundary of the narrow strip of septal nuclei.

5. Thalamic Spreading Depression

Since cortex, hippocampus, and caudate are structures characterized by contiguity of grey matter over distance of many millimeters, Fifková's (1964b, 1966a) discovery of SD in the nonhomogeneous system of thalamic nuclei in rats came as a surprise. Using microinjection of 25% KCl into different thalamic nuclei and multiple capillary electrodes for SPC recording, she found in all parts of thalamus negative slow potentials averaging 6 to 9 mV in amplitude and about 1 min in duration. A typical example is given in Fig. 6.12. With KCl injection into the ventrolateral nuclei all SD waves entered the ipsilateral midline and medial nuclei and 75% of them crossed into the contralateral thalamus. Decremental spreading was also found in the rostrocaudal direction; SD waves generated from the ventrolateral and midline nuclei reached ipsilateral posterior nuclei in only 50 to 60% of the cases. Since the midline nuclei mediate the passage of SD from one side to the other, the two gradients combine in such a way that after unilateral KCl injection into the ventrolateral nuclei, only 35 to 40% of the SD waves reach the contralateral posterior nuclei (Fig. 6.13). The average spreading rate was 2.4 mm/min. The 50 and 100% recovery

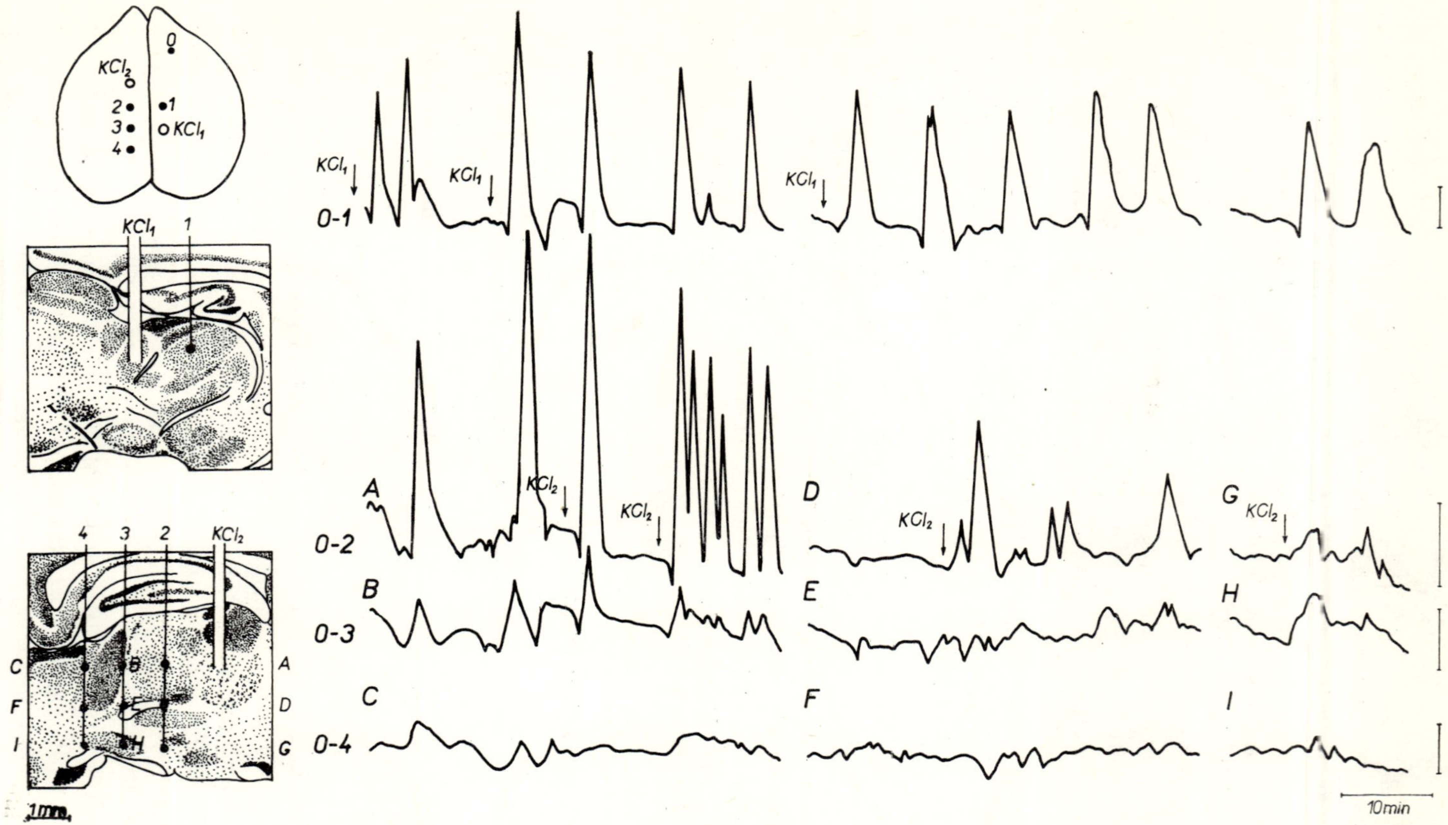

Fig. 6. 12. Thalamic SD in the rat. Location of the injecting cannulae (KCl_1, KCl_2) and of the capillary electrodes is shown in the inset diagram and parasagittal brain sections: (0—1) nucleus mediodorsalis; (0—2*A*) nucleus ventralis pars dorsomedialis; (0—2*D*) zona incerta; (0—2*G*) area hypothalamica lateralis; (0—3*B*) nucleus posterior thalami; (0—3*E*) zona incerta; (0—3*H*) substantia nigra; (0—4*C*) area pretectalis; (0—4*F*) formatio reticularis; (0—4*I*) substantia nigra. The arrows indicate KCl injection either into the right posterior thalamus (KCl_1) or into the left anterior thalamus (KCl_2). Calibration: 3 min, 5 mV (Fifková 1966c).

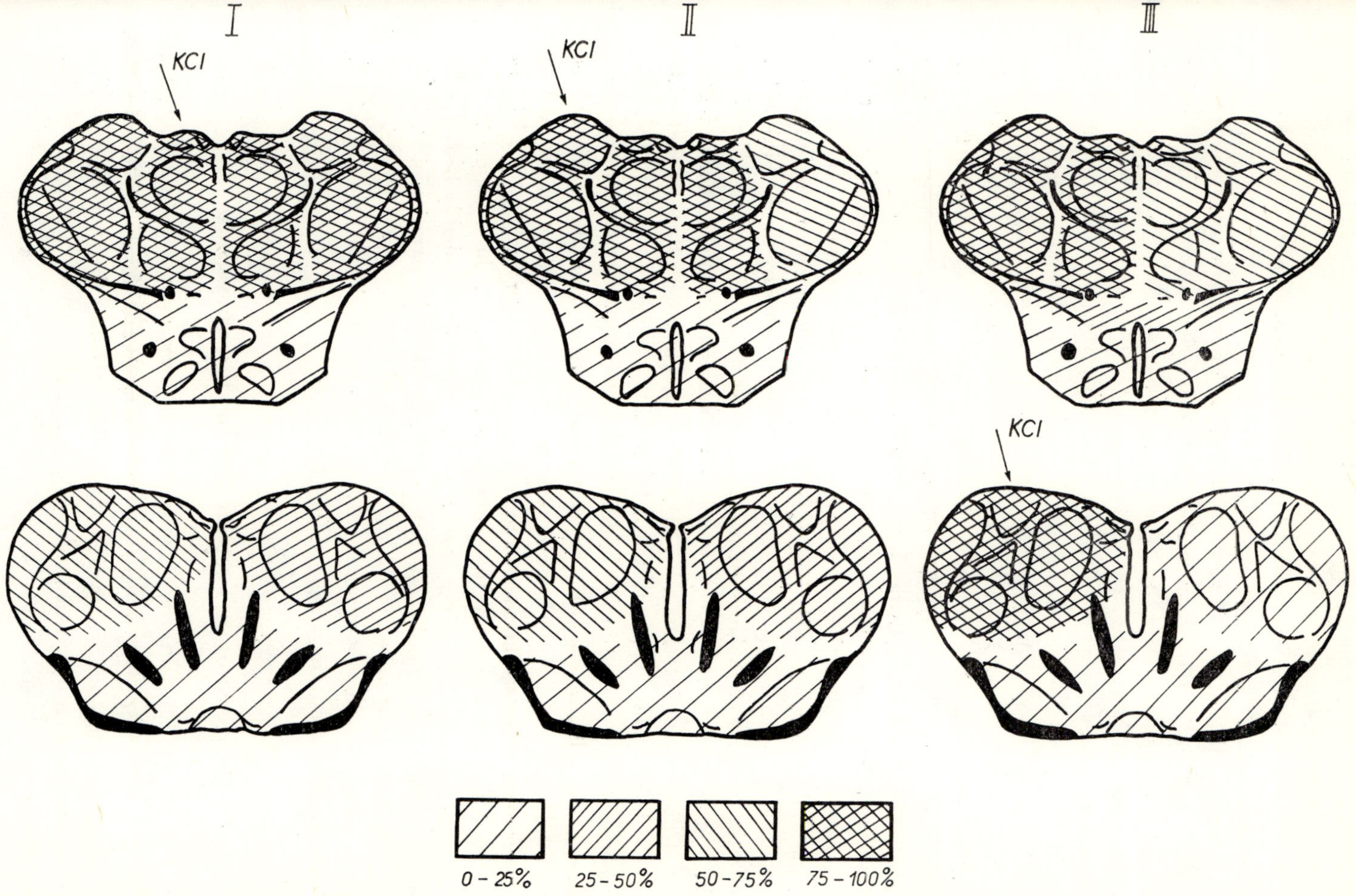

Fig. 6. 13. Incidence of SD waves in different parts of thalamus after KCl injection into medial nuclei (I), ventral nuclei (II), and posterior nuclei (III). Coronal sections through the anterior (above) and posterior (below) groups of thalamic nuclei (Fifková 1966c).

times were 4.0 and 7.5 min in the ipsilateral thalamus, 5 and 10 min in the central thalamus, and 6.5 and 10 min in the contralateral thalamus.

Since the thalamus is fully surrounded by other structures, knowledge of the exact boundaries of thalamic SD is essential. Although the posterior thalamic nuclei are in direct contact with the rostral mesencephalon, thalamic SD reached neither the mesencephalic and bulbar reticular formation nor the inferior colliculus. The superior colliculus was entered by 40% of the SD waves evoked from the posterior thalamus but not from other thalamic sites. The thalamus is separated from the hypothalamus by the zona incerta into which low SPCs penetrated only when KCl was injected into the posterior thalamus. No spread of thalamic SD into hypothalamic structures was observed, however (Fig. 6.13). Similarly, thalamic SD did not propagate into the corpus striatum, separated by the compact capsula interna from the thalamic complex. The hippocampus, enveloping the dorsal, posterior, and also part of the basal surfaces of the thalamus, is often affected by KCl leaking backward along the injection cannula. Even in the hemisphere contralateral to injection 30% of thalamic SD waves invaded the hippocampus, however. This might have occurred either by direct propagation between the two contiguous structures (separated only by the microscopic thalamohippocampal cleft) or as a consequence of seizure activity that is often induced in the thalamus and contralateral hippocampus by the KCl injection.

Some of the features of thalamic SD in rats are specific to this species. The fibers of laminae medullares form so narrow a barrier between the small nuclei of grey matter that they do not interfere with SD propagation although they do somewhat reduce the velocity. This explanation was borne out by experiments with thalamic SD in rabbits (Fifková 1966b) in which individual nuclei appeared to be more isolated than in rats, evidently because of the larger amount of myelinated fibers. The highest SPC amplitude was found in the ventrolateral group (5 to 7 mV), but on the average it was lower than in rats. The most complete spread to other thalamic nuclei was obtained with KCl injections into the ventrolateral group, but the decrements were higher than in rats. The SD never crossed to the other side probably because the midline nuclei proved to be fully resistant to SD. The mutual separation of thalamic nuclei is still more pronounced in the cat in which SD in the ventral anterior and ventral lateral nucleus does not spread to other nuclei (Buchwald and Hull 1967, Trachtenberg, Hull, and Buchwald 1970).

6. Spreading Depression in Tectum and in Olfactory Bulb

Leão and Martins-Ferreira (1961) were able to elicit SD in the superior colliculus of the rabbit only when the exposed structure was pretreated for 20 to 30 min with sodium acetate. Occasional penetration of thalamic SD into the superior colliculus in rats has already been mentioned (see above). Fifková (1966b) used KCl injection into the superior colliculus to elicit SD in this structure in the rabbit and the rat.

Whereas in the rat 8 mV SPCs were registered from all parts of the superior colliculus, the SPC was lower in the rabbit (6 mV). It was found only in the stratum griseum superficiale and medium but not in the stratum griseum profundum which contains too many myelinated fibers. No spreading toward the inferior colliculus or tegmentum was observed.

Ookawa and Bureš (1969) attempted to elicit SD in the optic lobes of the chicken. In most cases microinjection of KCl evoked only local negative potentials, rapidly decreasing with distance. A few SPC changes of the SD type were also recorded but their occurrence probably indicated an abnormal increase of SD susceptibility due to anoxia or injury.

Fully developed SD was observed in the rabbit olfactory bulb treated with isotonic sodium acetate (Leão and Martins-Ferreira 1961, 1963, Leão 1963). The predominant component of SPC was a surface positive wave lasting 40 to 60 sec and attaining 10 mV in amplitude. The reverse polarity is probably due to the fact that the outer surface of the olfactory bulb consists of axons of the receptor cells of the olfactory epithelium. The surface positive SPC could be changed to surface negative when the K^+ concentration in the Ringer was increased to 20 to 40 mEq/l. The same elevation of K^+ did not change the SPC polarity in the olfactory bulb treated with acetate. Sometimes the positive SPC of the first SD wave was followed by negative SPC of the second wave affected by increased extracellular potassium concentration. Surface negative potentials in the olfactory bulb were also evoked by ischemia or by substitution of chloride by thiocyanate.

7. Striatal Spreading Depression in Birds and Reptiles

The possibility of evoking SD in the hemispheres of the pigeon was briefly mentioned in Leão's (1944a) classical paper. Bureš, Fifková, and Maršala (1960) evoked SD in pigeons by application of a KCl solution (in filter papers) onto the exposed cerebral surface and correlated its amplitude and propagation with anatomical structure. The signs of SD, especially the SPC, in pigeons were similar to those in mammals and could be recorded both from the thin layer of the primitive cortex and from the surface of the hyperstriatum. With capillary electrodes it was possible to demonstrate SPC propagation to a depth of 5 mm below the surface. In a later study (Shima, Fifková, and Bureš 1963) this radial spread was examined in detail using multiple capillary electrodes (Fig. 6.14). Spreading depression elicited by KCl microinjection into the hyperstriatum spread throughout the hyperstriatum accessorium and/or ventrale. Only 60 to 70% of hyperstriatal SD waves penetrated across the lamina hyperstriatica into the neostriatum. The more compact lamina medullaris externa completely prevented propagation of neostriatal SD to the paleostriatum (Fig. 6.15). The average SPC amplitude in the hyperstriatum and neostriatum was between 13 to 15 mV, duration of the negative slow potential (at 50% of maximum amplitude) was 35 sec, and the spreading rate within the same structure was approximately 3 mm/min. The spreading rate was slower (2 mm/min) and the refractory period much longer for the propagation between hyperstriatum and neostriatum.

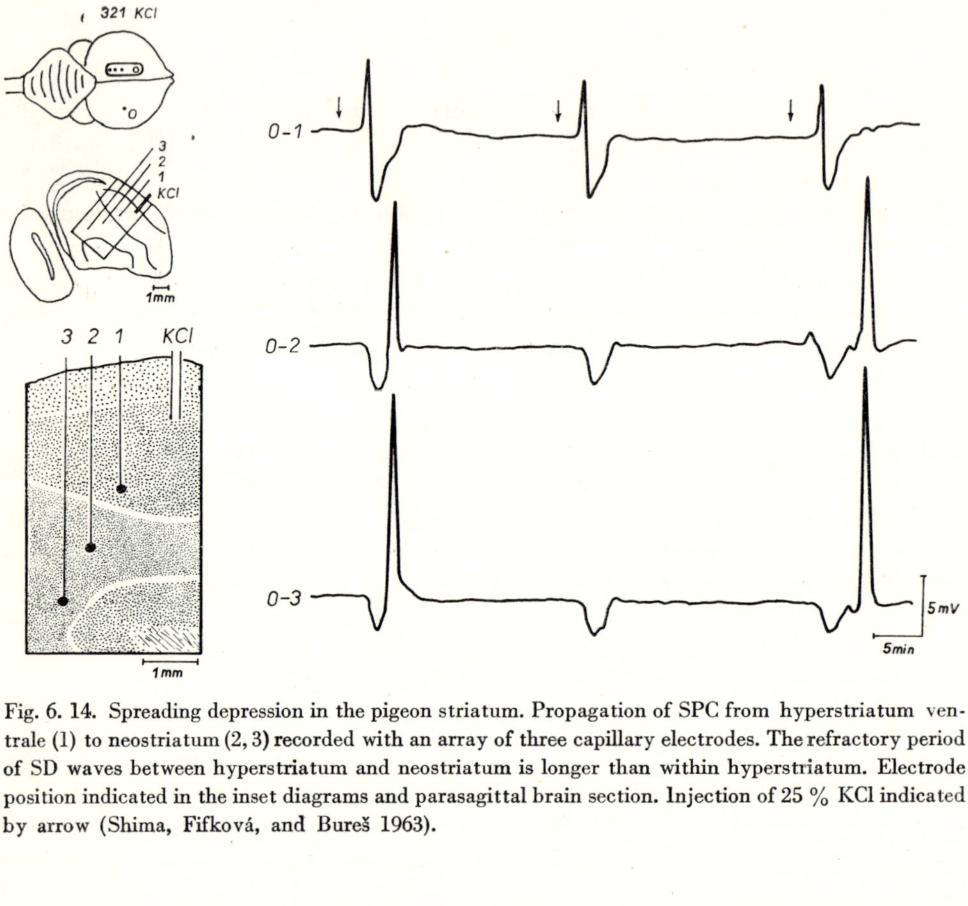

Fig. 6. 14. Spreading depression in the pigeon striatum. Propagation of SPC from hyperstriatum ventrale (1) to neostriatum (2, 3) recorded with an array of three capillary electrodes. The refractory period of SD waves between hyperstriatum and neostriatum is longer than within hyperstriatum. Electrode position indicated in the inset diagrams and parasagittal brain section. Injection of 25 % KCl indicated by arrow (Shima, Fifková, and Bureš 1963).

The EEG changes accompanying striatal SD in the chicken were described by Ookawa and Gotoh (1964) who used surface recording electrodes. Ookawa and Bureš (1969) recorded SPC from the depth of the chicken striatum and obtained essentially similar results as in pigeons. Fully developed SD waves in the hyperstriatum and neostriatum failed to enter ectostriatum and paleostriatum primitivum and appeared irregularly and with reduced amplitude in the border region between these structures.

Martins-Ferreira and Leão (1958) reported the SD process in the cortex and striatum of the alligator, the telencephalon of which resembles in many respects that of birds. The differentiation of prosencephalon is more primitive in the turtle, forming the transition stage between fish and mammals. Tolkunov and Fifková (1964) found in the caudate nucleus and putamen of turtles slow potential waves (6 mV, duration 62 sec) spreading with a velocity of 2 mm/min. Atypical SPCs with rapid onset and a slow decline or with high initial positivity were quite frequent. In a few experiments SD was demonstrated also in the telencephalon of fish (Bureš and Ivanus, unpublished).

Although most data on SD in birds and reptiles are based on SPC recordings, the other manifestations of the process are probably the same as in mammals. Cessation of unit activity in the depressed striatum of pigeons was reported by Burešová, Shima, Bureš, and Fifková (1963) and increase of impedance by Esquibel (1956). Hogberg (1968) used local KCl application to achieve functional ablation of cortex in the painted turtle.

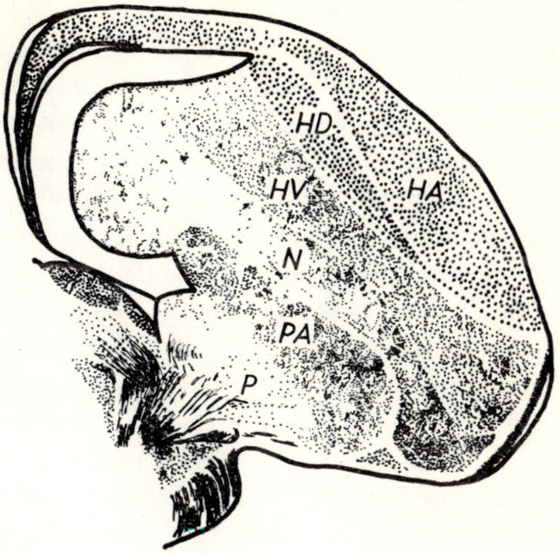

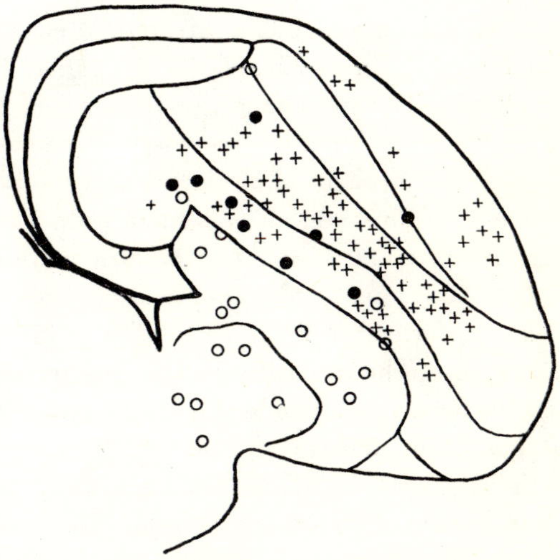

Fig. 6. 15. Schematic representation of the cytoarchitectonic fields and of the incidence of SD on the parasagittal section of pigeon brain about 2.5 mm lateral to the midline. Crosses are points at which SPCs were recorded constantly. Circles are points that SPC failed to enter. Dots are points that showed at least one SPC but not constantly, although SPC simultaneously appeared at other points. Symbols: *HA*, hyperstriatum accessorium; *HD*, hyperstriatum dorsale; *HV*, hyperstriatum ventrale; *N*, neostriatum; *PA*, paleostriatum augmentatum; *P*, paleostriatum primitivum (Shima, Fifková, and Bureš 1963).

8. Spreading Depression in the Retina

Since SD was always associated with the central nervous system, Gouras' (1958) finding of an SD-type of reaction in the excised toad retina was rather unexpected. In the isolated posterior hemispheric segment of the eye local stimulation of exposed retina by mechanical, electrical, or chemical stimuli elicited a local change of color, a grayish spot, spreading with a velocity of 1 mm/min concentrically in all directions. The wave front appeared as an intense brown line sharply separating the normal retina from the affected part. The center of the grayish spot gradually faded into a normal color, some 2 to 3 mm behind the advancing perimeter. The optical changes were accompanied by electrophysiological ones: a sudden negativity of the anterior retinal surface reaching 1 to 2 mV in amplitude and slowly subsiding over 3 to 6 min; a brief (5 to 10 sec) but intense (200 to 300/sec) discharge of unit activity followed by profound depression lasting for 3 to 5 min (similar unit activity changes were reported earlier by Barlow 1953). The local electroretinogram evoked by focal illumination disappeared at the same time. All these manifestations clearly suggest an identity of the retinal process with SD in the brain, especially when taking into account that the slow spreading rate is due to a low ambient temperature (20 °C) and the low SPC voltage to shunting of the electrodes applied to the exposed retinal surface.

Martins-Ferreira (1962) and Martins-Ferreira and Oliveira Castro (1964, 1965, 1966) extended Gouras' observations by experiments in the retina of the toad, chicken and pigeon. Using intraretinal electrodes they found SPCs of up to 25 mV and 1 to 1.5 min in duration accompanied by an increase in impedance lasting for 1 to 2 min. The spreading rate approached 3 mm/min. When the K^+ concentration in the Ringer solution was increased four times, SD could be elicited in the toad retina not only by mechanical or electrical stimuli but also by abrupt changes (increase or decrease) of illumination of a small retinal area (0.3 mm in diameter) (Martins-Ferreira 1962). Using a microphotometric method, Martins-Ferreira and Oliveira Castro (1964, 1966) quantified the optical changes accompanying the retinal SD. Measurements performed in fields 15 to 45 μ in diameter revealed the polyphasic nature of the process. The intensity of light scattered by a given retinal region was first decreased for a few seconds (Fig. 6.16, phase *a*), then abruptly increased to the peak of phase *b* which slowly subsided to the minimum *c*, 1.5 to 3 min after the beginning of the sequence. Light scattering gradually increased again and reached peak *d*, 2 to 5 min later. The base line was restored only after 15 to 30 min. The maximum change of the light scattering (difference *b*—*c*) was about 35% of the base line level. The

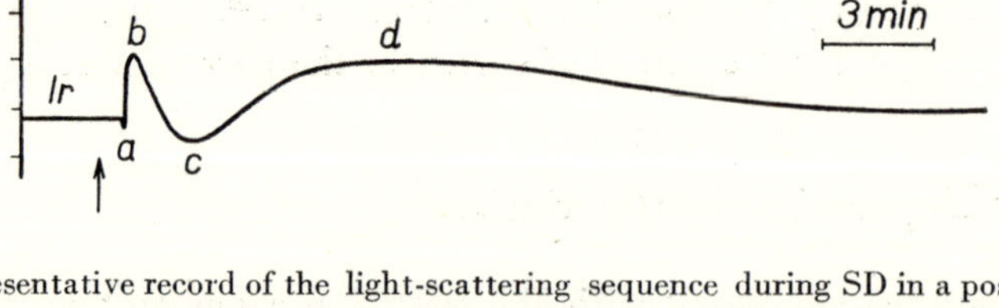

Fig. 6. 16. Representative record of the light-scattering sequence during SD in a posterior hemisphere retinal preparation maintained in the standard Ringer solution. *Ir* is the intensity of light scattering within the retina in the absence of SD. The ordinate is divided into arbitrary units. Arrow indicates time of stimulation (Martins-Ferreira and Oliveira Castro 1966).

optical changes were most pronounced in the inner plexiform layer which consists of a dense network of neuronal and glial processes

A new sequence could be generated before phase *d* was over. In this case phases *a* and *c* of the new sequence were enhanced. Light scattering was similarly increased by hyperosmolar solutions. Hypoosmolar solutions decreased the baseline light scattering and increased the peaks *b* and *d* of the sequence. Phase *d* was fully eliminated by procaine hydrochloride (0.9 mM), by a three-fold increase of K^+ in the Ringer solution and by increasing the ambient temperature. Sodium iodoacetate (0.4 mM) considerably prolonged phases *b*, *c*, and *d*. Van Harreveld and Fifková (1970, 1971b) found that SD elicited by superfusion of isolated retina with KCl or glutamate solutions was accompanied by an increase in light transmission of up to 20 % and lasting for 6 to 8 min.

Whereas phase *d*, which is most sensitive to drugs and temperature, seems to be related to metabolic recovery, phase *b* is directly associated with the slow potential and impedance rise (Martins-Ferreira and Oliveira Castro 1965). Since light scattering depends on hydration of the tissue, the changes induced by SD in the retina are probably analogous to the water or electrolyte shifts observed in the cerebral cortex.

This assumption was supported by further studies (Oliveira Castro and Martins-Ferreira 1968, 1970) demonstrating with ingenious optic methods that SD is accompanied by changes of retinal volume. The SD cycle started with a 30-sec decrease of thickness by maximally 1.5 μ. In the ensuing phase retinal width increased and the change reached a maximum of 4 μ approximately 3 min after SD onset and then slowly subsided. Deformation of retinal surface also indicated volume changes corresponding to the SD wavefront.

Hanawa, Kuge, and Matsumura (1967a, b, 1968) studied retinal SD with a different technique. Dissected bullfrog retina was mounted between two acrylic plates with a 2 mm central hole, so that each side could be bathed with solutions of different composition. The investigators found that a change of transretinal potential resembling SD is most reliably elicited with a Cl^- free Ringer on the vitreous side and 15mM Cl^- on the receptor side (Cl^- substituted by SO_4^{2-}). Under these conditions the receptor side was 0.3 mV positive against the vitreous side. During SD, which could be elicited not only by electric current (vitreous cathode, 0.25 mA) or by mechanical stimulation but also by a single flash, receptor surface developed during approximately 5 sec a 2 to 10 mV negativity followed after 1 to 2 min by a lower but prolonged positivity. The SPC amplitude was independent of the intensity of the suprathreshold stimuli, but was considerably influenced by the recovery cycle of SD which was completed only after 30 min. The electroretinogram was depressed for the duration of SPC, the *b* wave being affected more and longer than the small *a* wave. Unlike Martins-Ferreira and Oliveira Castro (1965) the Japanese team found a small decrease of transretinal impedance during SD. The apparent contradiction was resolved by Martins-Ferreira and Oliveira Castro (1969) who found using transcortical impedance measurement, that the impedance change is markedly dependent on chloride concentration. In normal Ringer, SD was accompanied by an impedance increase of 5 to 12% lasting for 2 to 4 min. After substitution of sodium chloride by sodium sulphate or sucrose the SD impedance change decreased or was even reversed (impedance decrease by 1 to 2% lasting for 15 to 60 sec).

In a later study Hanawa, Kuge, and Matsumura (1968) found that increasing potassium concentration at the receptor surface to 20 mM reduced the retinal SPC to 50%, whereas the same K^+ concentration was ineffective when applied from the vitreous side. The authors suggested that the glial elements of retina, the so-called Müller cells, may be essential for the mechanism of spreading. Processes of these cells extending through all retinal layers envelop the neural and receptor elements and form the inner and outer limiting membranes. Partial depolarization of these cells, but not of their end-feet forming the inner limiting membrane, may account for the negative SPC and for intraretinal release of potassium. The positive shift of SPC is partly due to potassium diffusion from the intercellular space to the bathing solutions.

The role of Müller cells in the mechanism of the retinal SD is not proved but the limiting membranes may also act in a simpler way by reducing the escape of potassium released from neural elements in to the surrounding medium. This may explain why SD can be elicited in a narrow strip of retina, whereas in the brain it cannot pass through the much thicker grey matter layers surrounded by inactive tissue (subiculum, see p. 149). More important is a high density of somatodendritic and glial membranes in the retina, especially in the inner plexiform layer. Remarkably regular branching patterns of dendrites of amacrine cells, described by Oliveira Castro (1966) in the retina of chicken embryo may further enhance the horizontal interaction.

9. Spreading Depression in Tissue Culture.

Walker and Hild (1972) demonstrated recently a phenomenon similar to spreading depression in cultures of rat brain tissue. The explants were grown on cover slips above a hole 100 to 350μ in diameter through which impedance, steady potential and neural activity were recorded by two electrodes applied to the upper and lower pools of the cultivating medium separated by the horizontal glass partition. Current pulses exceeding the density of 10^{-8} Aμ^{-2} for a duration of 0.05 to 5.0 msec produced depression of spontaneous activity lasting for 2 to 20 min and accompanied by a dc shift (2 to 10 mV) and impedance increase (+20 %). Increase of K^+ concentration from the normal 5.2 mM to 8.2 or 12.8 mM in the upper pool diminished or suppressed the neuronal activity. Higher concentrations (50 mM KCl) were required to produce the impedance increase and the slow potential change (upper pool negative). The latter reactions were observed also in cultures from corpus callosum which are free of neurones and display no neuronal activity.

Although the electrical changes recorded in tissue cultures resemble those accompanying SD in the intact brain, it must be pointed out, that spreading has not yet been demonstrated. When depression was produced by mechanical stimulation at some distance from the recording site, the activity change was immediate. Further experiments are required to demonstrate that the interaction of neuronal and neuroglial elements in tissue cultures is strong enough to provide for a propagated autoregenerative process. The potential significance of tissue culture experiments for establishing the role of glia (see p. 145) and for determining the critical density of cellular elements, volume of extracellular space, and dimensions of the reactive tissue, is obvious.

10. Spreading Depression in Invertebrates

The size of the central nervous system of most invertebrates is too small to allow a meaningful study of the problem. Cephalopods with their relatively large and compact brains are, therefore, the only invertebrates in which SD was convincingly demonstrated. Schadé and Collewijn (1962, 1964) found in the retina of cephalopods *(Loligo vulg., Sepia off., Octopus vulg.)* a negative potential (3 to 4 mV) lasting for 4 to 5 min which could be evoked by electrical or chemical (KCl, glutamate) stimuli applied to the anterior retinal surface. The SPC spread with a velocity of 1.9 to 2.7 mm/min and was accompanied by cessation of unit activity, suppression of evoked responses, and by an increase of impedance. Shifts of electrolytes between the retinal elements and the supporting cells (analogous to Müller cells) in the outer segment of the retina were established by histochemistry. The similarity of retinal SD in vertebrates and cephalopods is still more significant when the morphogenetic differences between the two structures are taken into account (the inverted versus everted retina). Functional factors are evidently more important than purely anatomical considerations. The axons of the receptor elements leave the eyeball through small holes in the sclera and form optic or retinal nerves, connecting retina with the optic lobe which is a functional equivalent of the deep retinal layers and optic tectum of lower vertebrates. Retinal SD did not spread through the retinal nerves to the optic lobe, although spreading impedance increase resembling SD could be elicited in the latter structure by direct electrical stimulation. Evoked visual responses in the optic lobe were severely depressed and spontaneous activity of most optic lobe units was markedly reduced during retinal SD (Schadé and Collewijn 1964).

Whereas SD in cephalopods has all the typical signs of the process, it is less probable that SD can be induced by KCl microinjection into different ganglia of the insect nervous system. Rounds (1967, 1968) employed the heading of SD for experiments, in which bursts of ventilatory movements were elicited by injecting 2.5 or 5.0 μl of 25% KCl near the supraesophageal or metathoracic ganglia in the cockroach, but no electrophysiological evidence indicated spreading. As the observed effects were obviously due to local depolarization caused by the injected K^+ ions, "KCl depression" seems to be a more justified term than "spreading depression" in this case.

There is no doubt, however, that such local KCl depolarization can be successfully employed to eliminate portions of the insect nervous system and to study its functional organization.

11. Ontogenetic Development and Susceptibility to Spreading Depression

The development of the brain offers a unique opportunity to correlate morphological and biochemical data with the appearance of various functions. This approach, the merits of which were reviewed in several recent symposia (Kellaway and Petersen 1964, Jílek and Trojan 1968), was also used for analyzing the mechanism of SD.

Bureš (1957a) attempted to elicit cortical SD in rats aged 10, 15, and 20 days and compared the results with those obtained in adult animals. Although no SD could be elicited in 10-day old animals even with a 10% KCl solution, most rats in the 15-day old group reacted with SD in a manner essentially similar to that in adult rats. These findings were confirmed by Fifková (1964c) who covered the period from 10 to 21 days with six equally spaced groups (Fig. 6.17). She found the first SD

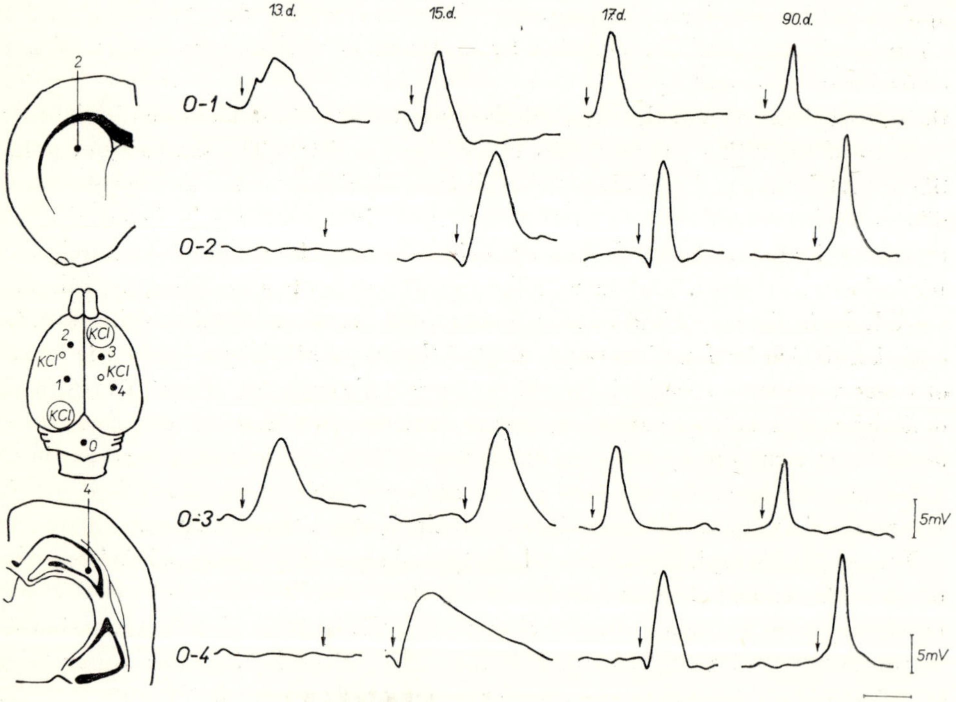

Fig. 6. 17. Development of cortical (0—1 and 0—3), striatal (0—2), and hippocampal (0—4) SD in rats aged 13, 15, 17, and 90 days. Location of electrodes is shown in the inset diagrams and brain sections. Arrows denote application of 25 % KCl to the respective structure (Fifková 1964c).

waves in 40% of 12 to 13-day old rats, but the SPC amplitude was low and the duration of negativity extremely long (5 mV and 300 sec as compared with 11 mV and 85 sec in the 20 to 21-day old group). Fifková (1964c) also determined the SD onset in caudate and hippocampus and found it slightly delayed (by approximately 2 days) in comparison with cortex (Fig. 6.18). Again the first SD waves were low and slow, with occurrence of transitional reactions, characterized by rapid depolarization and prolonged repolarization. Within 4 to 6 days SD assumed the adult type also in these structures (Fig. 6.17). The incidence of cortical SD after the twelfth day of postnatal life in rats was reported also by Tuge, Kanayama, and Chang (1960) and by Deza and Eidelberg (1967)

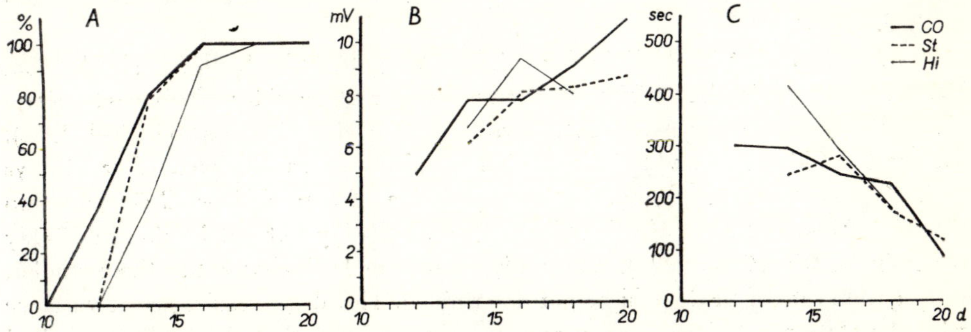

Fig. 6. 18. Development of cortical (heavy line), caudate (dashed line), and hippocampal (thin line) SD in rats. *(A)* Incidence of SD in percentages. *(B)* Amplitude of the negative SPC. *(C)* Duration of the negative SPC (above 50 % of maximum amplitude). Abscissa: age in days (Fifková 1964c).

Schadé (1959) was unable to elicit SD in rabbits aged less than 24 days. The spreading rate of 3 to 4 mm/min and SPC amplitude (7 to 9 mV) were normal but spreading convulsion instead of SD was often found between 24 and 30 days. Néverlée and Laget (1963, 1965) found decremental propagation of SD elicited from the frontal pole of the immature rabbit hemisphere. Local depolarization of the SD type could be generated from the eleventh postnatal day. The SPC reached the somatomotor cortex at 15 to 18 days and the parietal cortex in 19 to 21-day old rabbits. The entire cortex was traversed by SD only at the age of 24 to 25 days. These authors also confirmed Schadé's (1959) observation on the gradual change from spreading convulsion to SD between days 25 to 40. The decremental SD propagation in immature cortex is not a simple function of distance between the stimulus and recording sites, but rather an expression of a maturation gradient. With parietal KCl application SD propagated to the frontal cortex 4 to 8 days earlier than to a similarly remote point in the occipital cortex (Néverlée and Laget 1966, Néverlée 1966). Chemical stimuli (KCl solutions) started to elicit SD much earlier (11 days) than faradic stimulation (20 days). Contralateral SD could be evoked by faradic stimulation only after 35 days of age (Néverlée and Laget 1967).

Unlike rats and rabbits, guinea pigs are born with a more or less mature brain. Bureš (1957a) found in this species an adult type of SD on the first day of postnatal life. This result was confirmed by Sedláček (1967a) and extended to the prenatal period. Slow negative potentials of an SD character could be elicited approximately 1 week before birth, that is in 57-day old embryos. Eidelberg, Kolmodin, and Meyerson (1965) failed to elicit SD in fetal sheep by local application of 1 M KCl onto the exposed cortex, although local depolarization was well developed at the gestational age of 60 days. Terminal depolarization of the SD type develops during brain maturation at the same time when SD appears after KCl application. It could be evoked in guinea-pig embryos (Sedláček and Macek 1966a) by ligature of the umbilical cord just before term, whereas 5 to 10 days earlier the depolarization was slow and gradual.

Development of striatal SD in the chicken was studied by Sedláček (1964, 1966, 1967b). Local application of 25% KCl reduced the EEG activity of adjacent striatal electrodes more in embryos aged 21 days than in 20-day old ones (Sedláček 1964). The first KCl-induced reduction of EEG amplitude was observed after 18 days of incubation (Sedláček 1966). Local application of 3 M KCl or G-strophanthin (3×10^{-4}M) evoked SPC of SD type in 19- and 21-day but not in 15- and 17-day old embryos (Sedláček 1967b). Since only a single dc lead was used in these studies, propagation rate of SPC could be not determined. The above results are at variance with the statement (Tuge, Kanayama, and Chang 1960) that SD could be elicited in the chicken only 6 days after hatching. Sedláček's data were confirmed by Fifková and Van Harreveld (1970), who were able to elicit SD in the striatum of chicken embryos by local application of 25% KCl starting from the sixteenth day of incubation. High permeability of the blood-brain barrier towards glutamate persisting up to the hatching made it possible to elicit SD also by intravenous injection of this substance.

In most of the above experiments SD seems to appear at a definite stage of brain development. Since spontaneous EEG activity appears before SD, that is, between 7 and 15 days of postnatal development in rats (Crain 1952, Schadé 1957, Deza and Eidelberg 1967) and between 8 and 18 days in the rabbit (Schadé 1959), an attempt was made to establish the relationships between SD onset and the level of cortical steady potential (Bureš 1957a) or the membrane potential of cortical cells (Bureš, Fifková, and Mareš 1964). The cortical steady potential, defined as the potential difference between a cortical region destroyed by thermocoagulation and normal cortical surface in the contralateral hemisphere, was found to increase from 2.6 mV at 5 days to 14 mV at 20 days and to 19 mV in 90-day old rats (Fig. 6.19). The highest absolute increment was found between days 10 and 15. Sedláček and Macek (1966a) followed the development of cortical demarcation potential in guinea-pig embryos during the last third of the prenatal period (40 to 65 days of gestation) and found an increase from 3.7 to 7.0 mV over this time span (Fig. 6.19). In full-term embryos removed from the uterus, ligature of the umbilical cord initiated breathing and caused a rapid increase of the demarcation potential to 11 mV, a value comparable to the 14 mV level found in newborn animals (Bureš 1957a, Sedláček and Macek 1965). Demarcation potentials were also studied in the chicken striatum (Sedláček 1966) during the last 9 days of incubation (Fig. 6.19). The steepest increase was observed during the last days before and immediately after hatching. The development of the striatal demarcation potential was nearly the same when the reference electrode was placed on the undamaged surface of the other hemisphere, cerebellum, or optic lobe. Sedláček (1967b) and Sedláček and Macek (1966b) also provided information on the increase of impedance of chick hemispheres during ontogenesis. Their data on high-frequency (10 to 40 MHz) impedance are difficult to interpret but the more conventional 400 and 1000-Hz measurements indicated a considerable increase of impedance corresponding to shrinkage of the extracellular volume during the last 6 days of incubation.

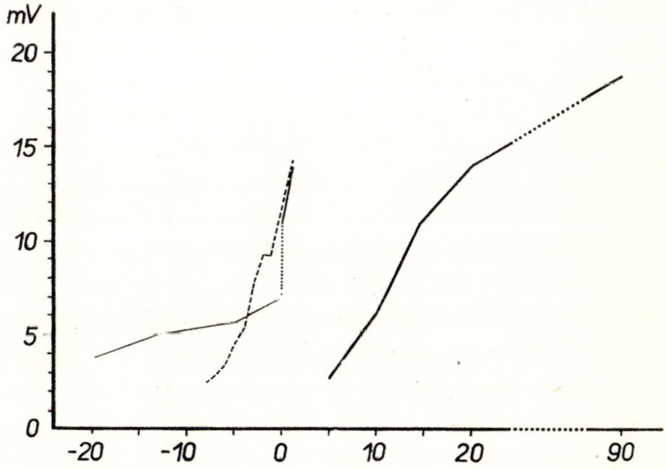

Fig. 6. 19. Development of the demarcation potential in the cerebral hemispheres of rats (heavy line) (Bureš 1957a), guinea pigs (thin line) (Sedláček and Macek 1966a), and chickens (dashed line) (Sedláček 1966) before or after birth. Abscissa: days before (negative values) or after (positive values) birth.

It must be pointed out that the demarcation potential is generated by a potential drop between intact axons leaving the injured area containing depolarized somato-dendritic membranes of the same neurons. The absolute value of the demarcation potential E_d which is proportional to the membrane potential of the axons E_m is reduced by the short-circuiting factor according to the equation,

$$E_d = E_m \frac{R_e}{R_i + R_e}$$

where R_i is the internal resistance and R_e is the resistance of the extracellular fluid. Thus an increase of E_d during development can be due not only to an increase of E_m but also to a relative increase of R_e and/or decrease of R_i. The demarcation potential is reduced a few minutes after death (see p. 72) not because of the depolarization of axons which are rather resistant to anoxia but because the somatodendritic membranes are depolarized in the intact brain where the reference electrode is located. On the contrary, the initial value of the demarcation potential depends on the conditions in the injured region and is little affected by changing the location of the reference electrode.

Bureš, Fifková, and Mareš (1964), Mareš (1964) and Deza and Eidelberg (1967) attempted to find a relationship between the cortical demarcation potential and the average membrane potential of cortical neurons established by the sampling technique (Li and McIlwain 1957). A capillary ultramicroelectrode filled with 3 M KCl was gradually inserted into the cortex, hippocampus, or caudate and all sudden potential jumps corresponding to impalement of cellular elements were measured. The distributions were extremely skewed, the mode class shifting from 0 to 10 mV at 10 to 15 days to 10 to 20 mV after 20 days. The increase of the average membrane potential correlated fairly well with the rise of the demarcation potential (Fig. 6.20).

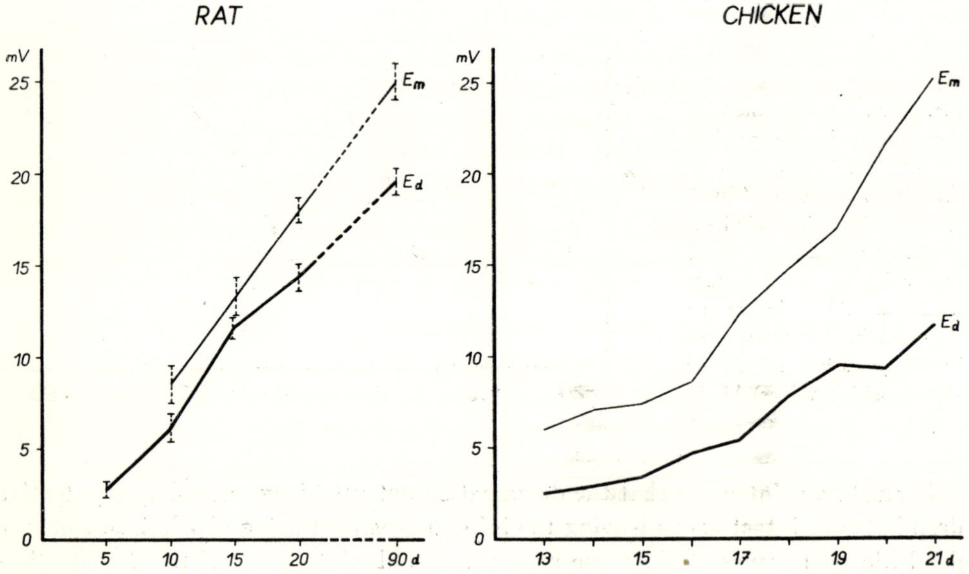

Fig. 6. 20. Development of the average membrane potential of cortical or striatal cells (E_m) and of the cortical or striatal demarcation potential (E_d) in rats or chicken embryos. Abscissa: postnatal or embryonic age in days. Ordinate: potential in millivolts (Mareš 1964, Sedláček 1966, Sedláček and Macek 1968).

Similar results were also obtained with the same technique in chick embryos (Sedláček and Macek 1968). Unfortunately the sampling technique of membrane potential measurements does not discriminate between neurons and glia cells and between perikarya and neural processes. Impalement of the small elements produces an immediate decrease of membrane potential, the value of which remains far below the real one. Taking these qualifications into account, the microelectrode measurements show only a relative increase of membrane potential, which may also reflect such factors as increased size of cellular elements and decreased fragility of membranes.

Whereas cortical demarcation potential is logically related to the membrane potential of cortical neurons, other measurements of the so called cortical steady potential against reference electrodes placed on bone, skin, or exposed sciatic nerve are less well substantiated. Surprisingly, even such measurements performed at different stages of brain maturation showed a gradual positivization of cerebral cortex in rats (Bureš 1957a, sciatic nerve reference; Deza and Eidelberg 1967, bone reference) and in fetal sheep (Eidelberg, Kolmodin, and Meyerson 1965, bone reference). It is not quite clear which dipoles are responsible for generating the steady potential difference under these conditions.

Although SD seems to appear only after the demarcation potential has exceeded 50 % of adult value, this does not necessarily indicate a causal relationship, since other important variables are changing at the same time. Whereas cell division is finished shortly after birth in rat and rabbit brains, the first 18 days of postnatal life are characterized by growth and ramification of cell processes. The packing density of cell bodies (expressed as cell-gray coefficient) decreases because of the growth of axons between days 6 to 12 and of dendrites between days 12 to 18 (Eayrs and Goodhead 1959). Toward the end of the second postnatal week the cellular and extracellular spaces also approach their adult dimensions (Vernadakis and Woodbury 1965), evidently because of a greater efficiency of the metabolic pump (Flexner 1952) indicated by increased oxygen consumption.

At the age when SD appears, neurons are still far from being mature. Dendritic growth continues in rats up to 30 days and myelinization of cortex only starts in the third week. Nevertheless the appearance of SD marks an important point in development when interaction between individual elements and environment becomes strong enough to generate a qualitatively new reaction.

12. The Role of Glia in the Mechanism of Spreading Depression

So far we have tacitly assumed that SD is due to changes taking place in neurons. Advances in microphysiology and microchemistry have stimulated in the last decade interest in the glial elements (Hydén and Egyházi 1963, Kuffler 1967) and led to hypothetical claims that they may account for some features of the SD process (Galambos 1961, Hertz 1965). Although it is impossible to disprove such suggestions completely, the experimental evidence indicates at least that glia alone cannot maintain the process. This was demonstrated by Van Harreveld and Stamm (1954a) in rabbits which were exposed 3 days before the SD experiment to reversible ischemization of the prosencephalon. Usually 35 to 40-min ischemia caused disappearance of EEG activity and heavy neuronal damage. Whereas the loss of nerve cells was nearly complete, neuroglia did not seem seriously affected. These findings could not be considered as a disproof of the participation of glia in SD propagation, however, since it is conceivable that neural manifestations of SD disappear in neuronless cortex while propagation of the glial reaction continues in an unobservable way. To examine this possibility Hull and Van Harreveld (1964) limited the ischemization to an oblong strip of parietal cortex separating the frontal and occipital lobes of the rabbit hemisphere by a 5 mm wide zone, completely free of neurons. Although normal SD could be elicited in front or back of the damaged strip, SPC propagation across the asphyxiated region was interrupted. The blockade occurred even when the asphyxiation only caused a marked decrease in neuron density. Together with the finding that SD does not spread across narrow glial scars (Van Harreveld, Terres, and Dernburg 1956, see also p. 116) available results do not support the hypothesis that SD is essentially a glial process and that the characteristic symptoms are induced by glia-neuronal interaction.

Hertz (1965) suggested that glial cells may take up the potassium ions released from one neuron during SD and transport them to the outer surface of another neuron. This proposal was critically discussed by Wendell-Smith and Blunt (1965) who pointed out that the intercellular spaces provide a sufficiently effective diffusion pathway for movement of ions and that it is unnecessary, therefore, to postulate active participation of neuroglia in the mechanism of SD.

On the other hand, there are good reasons to believe that glia is affected by the SD process and that it may even contribute to some of its properties. Thus the biochemical changes accompanying SD (depletion of glycogen and high-energy phosphates, accumulation of lactic acid) probably occur both in glial and neural elements. Anoxic depolarization of rabbit and rat cerebellar cortex (Van Harreveld 1961) is accompanied by transport of chlorine and water not only into dendrites of Purkyně cells but also into Bergmann fibers, glial elements which run from the cell body in the layer of Purkyně cells upward to form the glial limiting membrane at the cerebellar surface. The diameter of these fibers increased more than the diameter of apical dendrites under comparable conditions (73 and 27 %, respectively). This finding, which was also confirmed by electron microscopy (Van Harreveld and Malhotra 1966) contrasts with Schadé's (1964) claim that in cortical regions invaded by SD, swelling of apical dendrites is accompanied by a decrease in the size of cell bodies of the astrocytes while the oligodendroglia was unaffected. Asphyxia or SD were never accompanied by swelling of nonmyelinated axons (Van Harreveld and Malhotra 1967, Van Harreveld and Steiner 1970). Axons were also unaffected by electrophoretic injection of glutamate (Van Harreveld and Fifková 1971a) which induced gross swelling of dendrites and presynaptic terminals as well as of perinuclear and perivascular glia. It seems that different cellular components of brain, and perhaps even different portions of neurons and glial cells, compete for available chloride ions and water.

Kuffler (1967) has recently reviewed experimental evidence indicating that, unlike neurons, glial cells are linked together by low-impedance connections. Since the glial cell membrane behaves as a perfect K^+ electrode, it is considerably depolarized even by a small increase in extracellular K^+ concentration induced by intense neural activity. A focal depolarization of a group of glial cells causes a potential difference between them and their remote electrically coupled neighbors. Current flow generated in this way may contribute to the cortical demarcation potential or to the SPC accompanying SD, but its relative significance cannot be assessed with reasonable precision at present. As pointed out by Castelucci and Goldring (1970) no potential reversal can be recorded in closed fields generated in this way, since the remote reference electrode "sees" the potential of the spherical source region of the glial syncytium completely enveloping the central sink. A similar mechanism may account for the lack of deep positivity during SD.

13. General Comments on the Morphological Aspects of Spreading Depression

Although some of the above results are controversial, most data point towards several simple conclusions.

(a) High density of neural elements is an indispensable condition for SD initiation and propagation. Whereas the role of dendrites is well proved, participation of unmyelinated axons is still unclear. Glial elements seem to be only passively involved. Cytoarchitecture is of little significance when the surface of neural membranes per unit volume of tissue remains high.

(b) The SD susceptibility is indirectly proportional to the amount of extracellular space and of myelin in a unit volume of tissue. Especially in bundles of myelinated fibers, myelin sheaths reduce the density of neural membranes far beyond the threshold value. Different degrees of dilution of gray matter by myelinated fibers seem to determine the SD susceptibility of various brain structures (absence of SD in reticular formation, presence in corpus striatum) (Fig. 6.21). An increased proportion of myelinated fibers in the neocortex of higher mammals may account for the decreasing SD susceptibility in the cat and monkey.

(c) Thus far SD has only been demonstrated in certain minimum amounts of reactive tissue. In addition to the technical difficulties associated with evoking and recording SD in small volumes of brain, the limiting factor might be the escape of the transmitter substance into adjacent inactive areas. The absolute minimum width of nerve tissue compatible with SD propagation depends of course on the previous

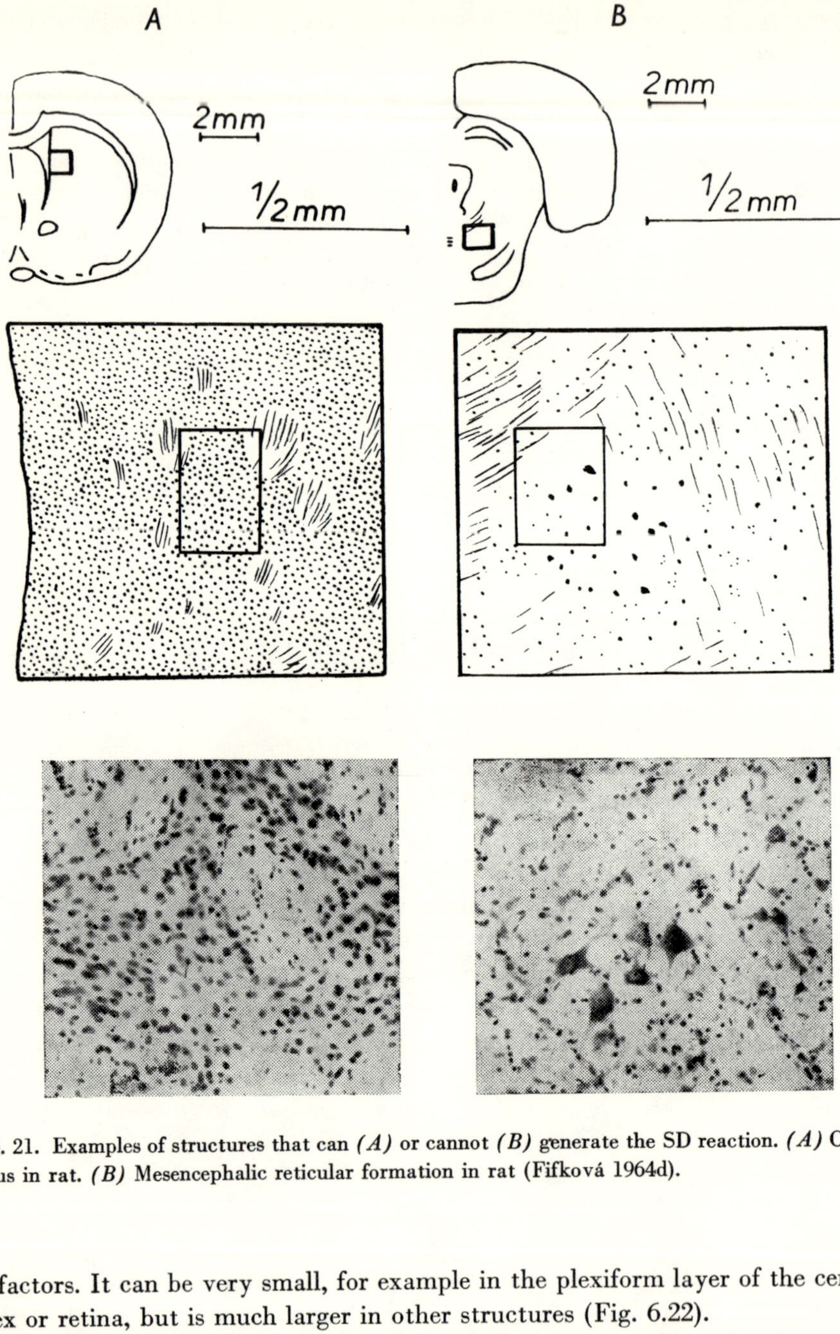

Fig. 6. 21. Examples of structures that can *(A)* or cannot *(B)* generate the SD reaction. *(A)* Caudate nucleus in rat. *(B)* Mesencephalic reticular formation in rat (Fifková 1964d).

two factors. It can be very small, for example in the plexiform layer of the cerebral cortex or retina, but is much larger in other structures (Fig. 6.22).

(d) Any inhomogeneity in the SD susceptibility of brain tissue (a white-matter barrier, transition from a region with low SD threshold to an area with high SD threshold) manifests itself by slowing of the spreading rate, appearance of prepoten-

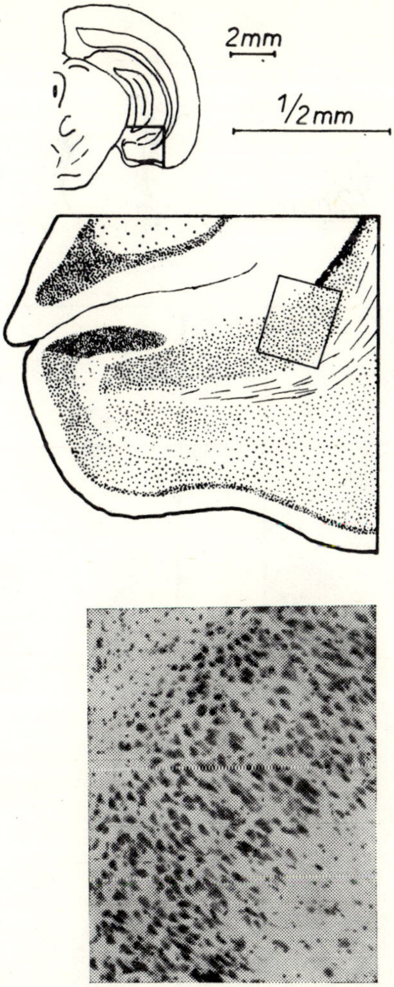

Fig. 6. 22. Example of a narrow continuous cellular strip surrounded by nonreactive tissue that does not support SD propagation in the subiculum hippocampi in rats (Fifková 1964d).

tials, and prolonged refractoriness. Decreased probability of transmission may eventually lead to complete blockade of SD propagation (Fig. 6.23).

Most of the above conclusions are based on electrophysiological recording of SPC. Since the very fact of introducing the recording electrodes into the subcortical structures may change their SD susceptibility (Marshall 1959), it was desiderable to check the crucial results using nonelectrical criteria of SD recognition. Křivánek and Fifková (1965) took advantage of the fact that each SD wave leaves behind a trail of increased lactic acid (100 % increase persisting for 3 to 4 min) that can be

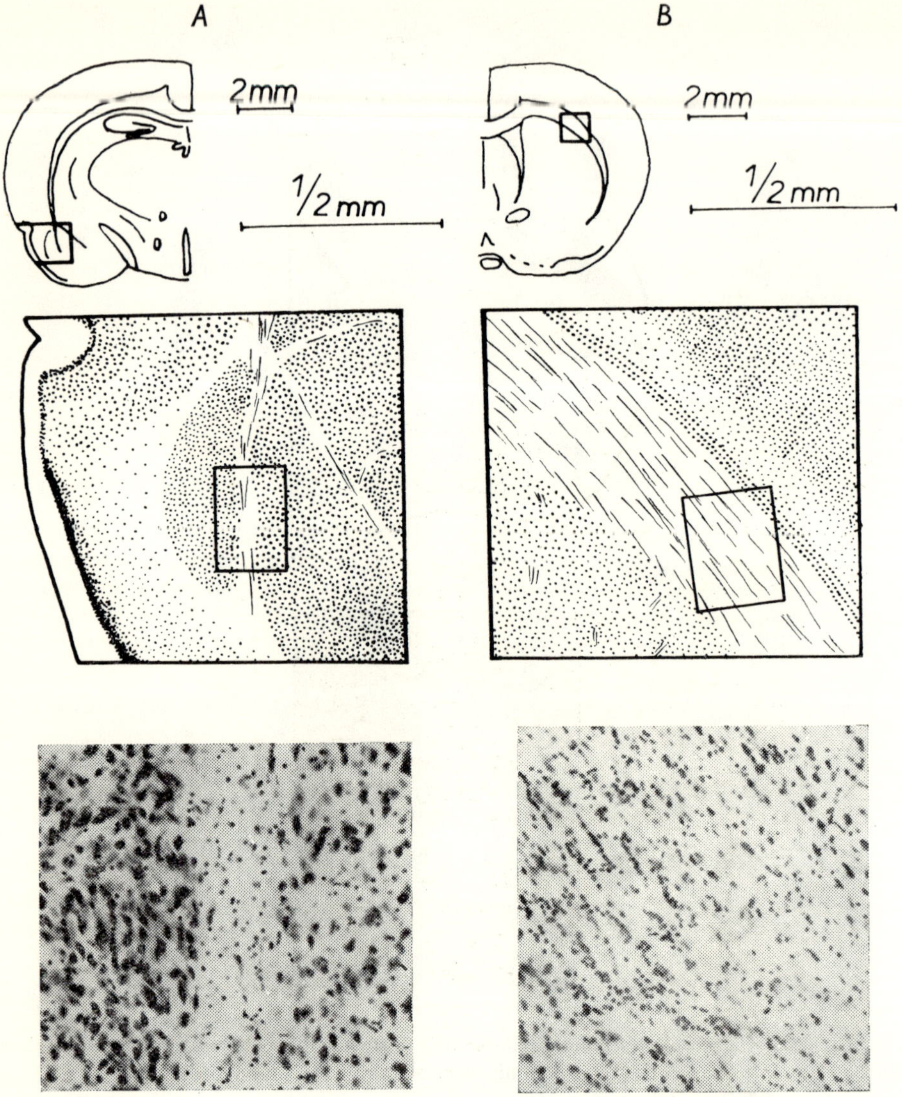

Fig. 6. 23. Examples of white-matter barriers that can *(A)* or cannot *(B)* be crossed by SD waves in rats. *(A)* Capsula interna between claustrum (left) and the lateral nucleus of amygdala (right). *(B)* Corpus callosum between neocortex (top right) and caudate nucleus (bottom left) (Fifková 1964d).

detected by ultramicroanalytic methods in submilligram quantities of tissue. Propagation into amygdala, caudate, retrosplenial and entorhinal cortex was determined for SD waves generated from parietal cortex in rats. At different intervals after KCl application, when the SPC had presumably passed through the examined region, the animal was killed by immersion into liquid nitrogen. The stereotaxic method was adapted to cut from the deeply frozen brain with an electrical saw coronal slices approximately 1 mm thick. Samples of about 0.4 mm^2 surface were cut from the slab with a sharp injection needle and analyzed for lactic acid. Precise location of the areas removed for analysis was verified by histological examination of the rest of the slice (Fig. 6.24).

Using this technique, penetration of cortical SD into the pyriform lobe structures and to retrosplenial area was confirmed. The relative incidence of positive reactions established with SPC recording and microchemical analysis was nearly the same

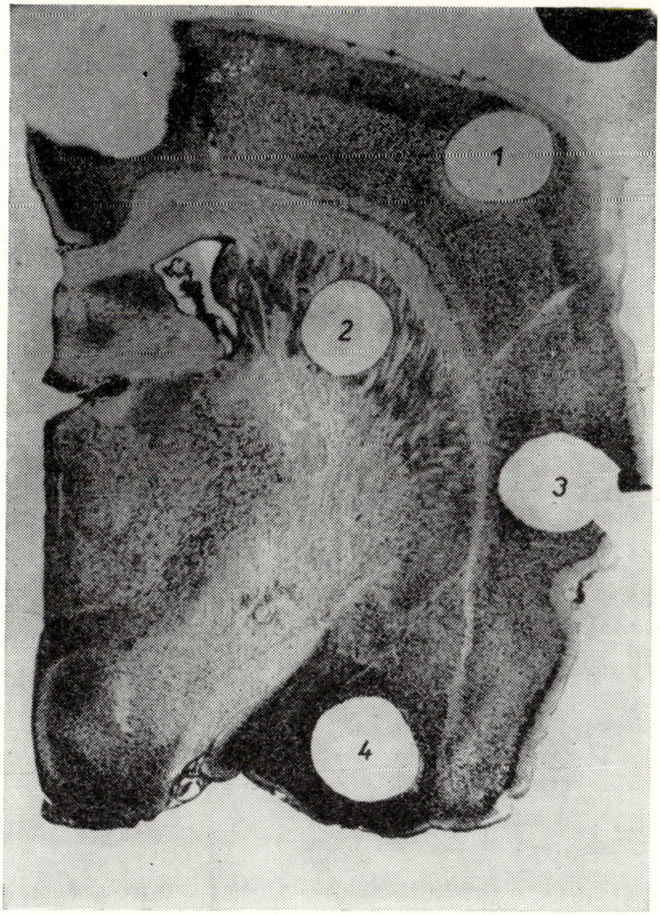

Fig. 6. 24. Location of samples removed for lactic acid determination from a coronal brain section. Areas: (1) parietal cortex; (2) temporal cortex; (3) amygdala (lateral and basal nuclei); (4) caudate (Křivánek and Fifková 1965).

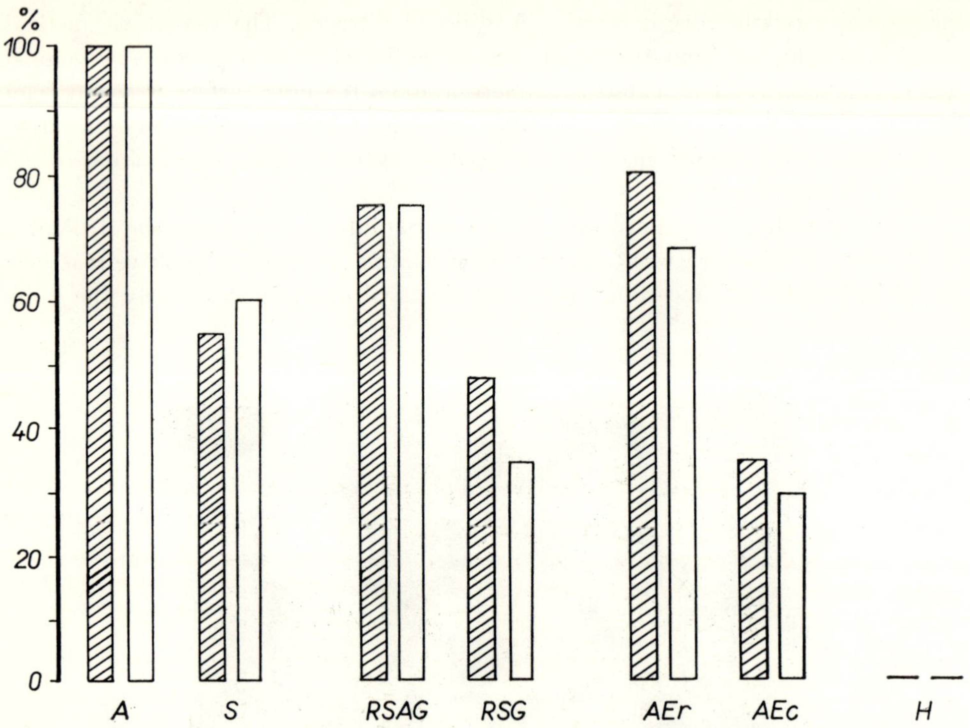

Fig. 6. 25. Percentage of CSD waves entering amygdala *(A)*, corpus striatum *(S)*, area retrosplenialis agranularis *(RSAG)*, area retrosplenialis granularis *(RSG)*, rostral entorhinal area *(AEr)*, caudal entorhinal area *(AEc)*, and hippocampus *(H)* according to electrophysiological (SPC incidence indicated by shaded columns) or biochemical (increased lactate level indicated by white columns) criteria (Křivánek and Fifková 1965).

(Fig. 6.25). It can be concluded, therefore, that insertion of recording electrodes does not significantly change the SD susceptibility of various structures, which is correctly reflected by SPC recording.

Chapter 7

Mechanism of Spreading Depression

At different stages of the history of SD research hypothetical mechanisms have been suggested to account for the available experimental evidence.

1. Vascular Mechanisms

The critical role of the vascular system in the mechanism of propagation was postulated by Leão (1944b) and by Leão and Morrison (1945). According to the first vague hypothesis, cortical vessels release a transmitter substance acting on pial nerve fibers. Marshall's observations (Marshall 1950, Marshall and Essig 1951, Marshall, Essig, and Dubroff 1951) that pathological conditions of the pia-arachnoid membrane facilitate SD in cats and monkeys also provided indirect support for the above assumption. The pia-arachnoid explanation became untenable, however, when it was shown that subpial transcortical cuts, leaving the pial circulation intact, block SD movement (Grafstein 1956b, Ochs 1958, Van Harreveld, Terres, and Dernburg 1956).

Although marked dilation of pial vessels was seen during SD (Leão 1944b), decreased O_2 concentration was found in blood samples taken from the sagittal sinus (Leão and Morrison 1945). Vasoconstriction of intracortical vessels was also indicated by displacement of the cortical surface and by decreased pO_2 in the depressed region (Van Harreveld and Stamm 1952). It was proposed that the electrophysiological signs of SD are due to a wave of vasoconstriction mediated by vasomotor fibers (Roitbak 1955). This explanation contrasted with the finding, however, that high-amplitude SPCs of SD type appear only after more than 2 min of anoxia (Leão 1947, Van Harreveld and Ochs 1956, Bureš and Burešová 1957). Vasodilation rather than vasoconstriction was demonstrated in other studies using heated (Freygang, Landau, and Marshall 1954, Sonnenschein and Walker 1956) or cooled (Burešová 1957a) thermocouples, histological technique (Van Harreveld and Ochs 1957), estimation of hemoglobin content (Burešová 1957a), and measurement of cortical volume (Marshall 1959). Under these conditions the decrease of pO_2 confirmed by Marshall (1959) and Lukyanova and Bureš (1967) cannot be due to a decreased supply but to an increased demand of oxygen. The changes of blood flow must therefore be considered a concomitant rather than the cause of SD.

2. Electric Fields

The electric-field hypothesis, advanced by Sloan and Jasper (1950), was based on the finding that SD can propagate across transcortical cuts. According to this hypothesis the negative slow potential generates current flow causing depolarization of adjacent regions. Most later attempts to demonstrate SD transmission across transcortical cuts failed, however (Ochs 1958, Van Harreveld, Terres, and Dernburg 1956, Grafstein 1956b). The electric-field hypothesis is incompatible with the fact that the extracellular current flow induced by the voltage drop between depressed and undepressed regions is considerably lower than the current density required to trigger an SD wave.

3. Humoral Transmission

Whereas the above hypotheses are of historical interest only, the neurohumoral hypothesis proposed by Burns and Grafstein (1953) has considerable experimental support and its several slightly different versions became widely accepted. According to this hypothesis SD is a chain reaction consisting of a series of causally linked events. Local stimulation evokes depolarization of neurons and release of potassium ions (or of some other transmitter substance) into the extracellular space. When the extracellular potassium concentration reaches a level sufficient to depolarize adjacent neurons, additional potassium is released and the process becomes self-maintained.

4. Potassium Hypothesis

Most electrophysiological signs of SD pointed directly or indirectly towards depolarization of neural elements. Evidence for the accumulation of the depolarizing transmitter substance in the extracellular space during SD was obtained by Bureš and Křivánek (1958), Křivánek and Bureš (1960), Bureš, Burešová, and Křivánek (1960) and Brinley, Kandel, and Marshall (1960) with the superfusion technique (see p. 89). The efflux of K^+ from the depressed region increased four to five times above the control level, evidently because the extracellular potassium concentration increased in a similar way, that is to at least 15 to 20 mEq/l. This figure probably is an underestimation, however, since the inertia and limited spatial resolution of the method tend to smooth out sharp peaks. If the membrane potential during SD corresponds to the equilibrium potential for potassium, the extracellular K^+ can be calculated from the membrane potential values reached during the peak depolarization of SD. Assuming an intracellular K^+ level of 150 mM (Van Harreveld 1966), an average depolarization of 75 % (Brožek 1966, Collewijn and Van Harreveld 1966) corresponds to an increase of the extracellular K^+ level to 60 to 70 mEq/l.

Similar figures can be derived from the finding that bundles of myelinated fibers passing through the gray matter invaded by SD develop a conduction block (Bureš, Hartman, and Lukyanova 1967, Bureš and Fifková 1968), which starts only with extracellular concentrations exceeding 30 mEq/l (Orkand, Nicholls, and Kuffler 1966).

The increase in extracellular K^+ level during SD must be compared with the K^+ concentration required to elicit SD. For KCl solution applied onto the exposed cortical surface covered by dura, the threshold was found to be around 80 mEq/l (Bureš and Burešová 1956b). This seems to be a considerable overestimation, however, since the gradient across the meninges and the escape of KCl into pial capillaries reduce the KCl concentration in the upper cortical layers to a fraction of the surface concentration. With intracortical administration the threshold amount of injected KCl was 2 to $4 \cdot 10^{-8}$ gEq K^+, that is, 20 to 40 times less than the threshold amount required with surface application. Assuming equal distribution around the point of the injection, the overall potassium concentration would be raised to 20 to 40 mEq/l in a 1 μl volume of tissue. It follows from such considerations that during SD extracellular K^+ reaches or exceeds a level sufficient to elicit the response.

5. Glutamic Acid Hypothesis

As another candidate for SD transmitter, Van Harreveld (1959) suggested glutamic acid which is present in relatively high concentration (10 mM/kg tissue) in the brain and can elicit SD in slightly lower concentration than KCl. There was no evidence, however, that glutamic acid is released into the extracellular space during SD. Superfusion of the cerebral surface in rats (Bureš and Křivánek 1962) did not reveal the expected increase of glutamate outflux. With the same technique Van Harreveld and Kooiman (1965) found in the rabbit that the excess ninhydrin-positive material released into the washing fluid during SD mainly stems from blood in pial vessels.

More recently Van Harreveld and Fifková (1970) reported, however, that release of labeled glutamate from the isolated chicken retina preloaded with ^{14}C glutamate is markedly enhanced when diffuse SD is evoked by superfusion with unlabeled glutamate, KCl, or by electrical stimulation. It was not clear, however, whether the glutamate concentration (0.2 mM) attained during retinal SD was high enough to cause SD. Subsequent experiments showed that the correlation between glutamate release and SD presence (indicated by the change of retinal transparency, see p. 137) was not perfect (Van Harreveld and Fifková 1971b, 1972). Thus $MgCl_2$ and GABA suppressed the retinal SD without decreasing the efflux of glutamate. On the other hand, retinal SD elicited by ouabain, EDTA, glutamine, and DL-homocysteic acid was not accompanied by increased liberation of glutamate. Tetrodotoxin blocked the transparency change elicited by glutamate and ouabain, but not that elicited by KCl. These dissociations indicate that glutamate release may be an important, but not indispensable link of the SD mechanism. The tetrodotoxin experiments suggest that potassium induced electrolyte shifts are independent on glutamate release and can proceed inspite of the blockade of the glutamate sensitive sodium transport. Unlike potassium, glutamate does not depolarize the myelinated axons and cannot account, therefore, for the conduction block caused by SD in the fibers penetrating through the depressed gray matter (Bureš and Fifková, 1968, see p. 208). Whereas the experimental evidence completes the case for the transmitter role of potassium, the postulated glutamate role has yet to be demonstrated. Although the potassium and glutamate hypotheses are not mutually exclusive, an experiment by Grafstein (1956a) indicates that the transmitter is a positively rather than a negatively charged particle. When a tangential polarization gradient was established in the isolated cortical slab, SD moved faster from positive to negative pole than vice versa. For all these reasons, we shall use the potassium hypothesis in the further considerations. It must be pointed out, however, that the general mathematical analysis of the mechanism of SD is independent of the nature of the transmitter and therefore also applies to glutamate.

6. Concomitant Phenomena

Although the increment of K^+ concentration in the extracellular fluid is crucial for the mechanism of spreading, it is only a link of a complex chain of metabolical and physiological events. At first the increasing potassium level causes a net inward K^+ flux. When depolarization reaches the critical level, the membrane permeability to sodium suddenly increases and action potentials are generated. Net inward movement of sodium is followed by net outward movement of potassium. As more sodium enters than potassium leaves the cells, Na^+ is accompanied by Cl^-, the accumulation of which in cortical dendrites has been histochemically demonstrated by Van Harreveld and Schadé (1959). The net movement of NaCl into cells induces shifts of water, resulting in an increase of intracellular volume (Van Harreveld 1958) and in a corresponding reduction of extracellular space, thus causing a marked increase in impedance (Van Harreveld and Ochs 1957). Hydrolysis of intracellular components, for example of high-energy phosphates (Křivánek 1958), may also increase the intracellular osmolarity and thus contribute to swelling of neurons.

All of these changes continue until the increasing extracellular K^+ concentration depolarizes the membrane to a level at which action potentials cease to be generated. At this point the potassium efflux starts to decrease and influx to increase until the net potassium movement is reversed. As active transport removes sodium ions from the intracellular compartment, potassium returns to the cells until the normal ionic equilibrium is again obtained. Excess extracellular potassium is also removed by blood flow.

7. A Mathematical Model of Spreading Depression

A. L. Hodgkin (personal communications 1959, 1970, see also Grafstein, 1963) proposed a theoretical model of SD based on mathematical methods introduced by A. F. Huxley (unpublished). It is assumed that at each cortical point the rate at which K^+ enters or leaves the cells is a cubic function of the excess K^+ concentration in the extracellular space and can be expressed by the equation,

$$f(y) = \frac{y\,(y_0-y)\,(y_a-y)}{Ty_a^2} \qquad (7.1)$$

where y is the excess extracellular K^+ concentration, y_0 is the threshold of K^+ excess, y_a is the maximum of K^+ excess, and T is the time constant of the process. As follows from Eq. (7.1) and the corresponding Fig. 7.1 there is no net movement of K^+

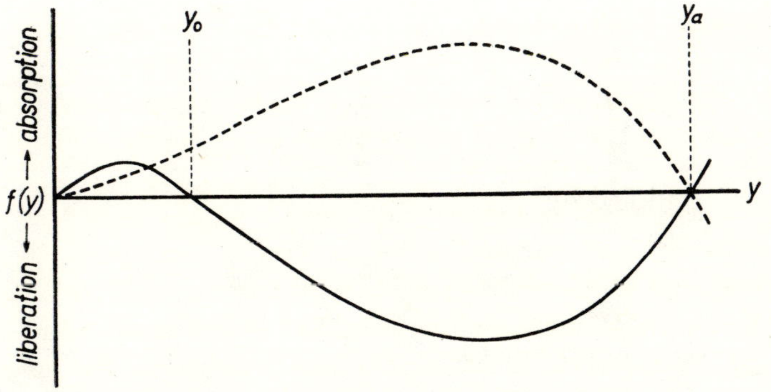

Fig. 7. 1. Potassium movement across the neuronal membrane as a function of extracellular potassium concentration. Full line indicates curve for increasing extracellular potassium. Dashed line indicates curve for decreasing extracellular potassium (CSD recovery).

across the membrane under resting conditions ($y = 0$), when the threshold is reached ($y = y_0$) and when the K^+ concentration is maximum ($y = y_a$). Net K^+ absorption occurs with $y < y_0$, whereas K^+ is released from cells when $y_0 < y < y_a$. The diffusion of K^+ ions is described by Fick's law,

$$D\,\frac{\partial^2 y}{\partial x^2} = \frac{\partial y}{\partial t} \qquad (7.2)$$

where D is the diffusion coefficient of K^+ ion in the extracellular space, x is the distance in the direction of the diffusion gradient, and t is time. Taking into account K^+

movements across the cellular membranes, the diffusion processes underlying SD can be expressed by the equation,

$$D \frac{\partial^2 y}{\partial x^2} = \frac{\partial y}{\partial t} + f(y) \tag{7.3}$$

For a wave propagating at a constant velocity u, Eq. (7.3) changes into

$$\frac{D\,\mathrm{d}^2 y}{u^2 \mathrm{d}t^2} = \frac{\mathrm{d}y}{\mathrm{d}t} + f(y) \tag{7.4}$$

When substituting

$$z = \frac{\mathrm{d}y}{\mathrm{d}t} \tag{7.5}$$

we obtain

$$\frac{\mathrm{d}^2 y}{\mathrm{d}t^2} = \frac{\mathrm{d}}{\mathrm{d}t}(z) = \frac{\mathrm{d}z}{\mathrm{d}t} = \frac{\mathrm{d}z\,\mathrm{d}y}{\mathrm{d}y\,\mathrm{d}t} = \frac{\mathrm{d}z}{\mathrm{d}y} z \tag{7.6}$$

and Eq. (7.4) becomes

$$\frac{D}{u^2} z \frac{\mathrm{d}z}{\mathrm{d}y} = z + \frac{y(y_0 - y)\ (y_a - y)}{T y_a^2} \tag{7.7}$$

This equation is satisfied by

$$\frac{\mathrm{d}y}{\mathrm{d}t} = z = by(y_a - y) \tag{7.8}$$

as can be checked by substituting Eq. (7.8) into Eq. (7.7):

$$\frac{D}{u^2} by\,(y_a - y)\,(by_a - 2by) = by(y_a - y) + \frac{y(y_0 - y)\,(y_a - y)}{T y_a^2} \tag{7.9}$$

and after dividing by $y(y_a - y)$

$$\frac{D}{u^2} b^2\,(y_a - 2y) = b + \frac{y_0 - y}{T y_a^2} \tag{7.10}$$

or

$$y \left(\frac{1}{T y_a^2} - 2 \frac{D b^2}{u^2} \right) + \frac{D b^2}{u^2} y_a - b - \frac{y_0}{T y_a^2} = 0 \tag{7.11}$$

Should this linear combination be equal to zero for all possible y, then the coefficients of y and of the constant term must be equal to zero,

$$\frac{D b^2}{u^2} y_a - b - \frac{y_0}{T y_a^2} = 0 \tag{7.12}$$

$$\frac{1}{Ty_a^2} - 2\,\frac{Db^2}{u^2} = 0 \tag{7.13}$$

Solving Eq. (7.13) for b we obtain

$$b = \pm\,\frac{u}{y_a\sqrt{2DT}} \tag{7.14}$$

By eliminating u from Eqs. (7.12) and (7.13) b can also be expressed in a different form,

$$b = \frac{y_a}{2Ty_a^2} - \frac{y_0}{Ty_a^2} = \frac{y_a - 2y_0}{2Ty_a^2} \tag{7.15}$$

Eq. (7.13) can be written in the form

$$u = \pm y_a b\,\sqrt{2TD} \tag{7.16}$$

and substituting for b from Eq. (7.15) leads to

$$u = \pm\,\frac{y_a - 2y_0}{y_a}\sqrt{\frac{D}{2T}} \tag{7.17}$$

As follows from Eq. (7.17) the conduction velocity u depends on the diffusion coefficient D, on the time constant T with which the extracellular potassium concentration reaches the y_a level, and on the relative values of y_0 and y_a. As pointed out by Hodgkin (personal communication), Eq. (7.15) defines the conditions for obtaining a wave starting at $y = 0$ and ending at y_a. If $y_0 > y_a/2$, b is negative and so is dy/dt, indicating that only a wave of decreasing y can be propagated (that is, for $y = y_a$ at $t = -\infty$ to $y = 0$ at $t = +\infty$). Only if $y_0 < y_a/2$, is b positive and a wave of increasing y (that is, from $y = 0$ at $t = -\infty$ to $y = y_a$ at $t = +\infty$) can be generated.

These two cases can also be distinguished by comparing the areas A and B (Fig. 7.2) obtained by integrating Eq. (7.1) so that

$$A = \int_0^{y_0} f(y)dy \quad \text{and} \quad B = \int_{y_0}^{y_a} f(y)dy$$

A wave of increasing y can be obtained if and only if area B is larger than area A. The proof of this proposition was given by Noble and Hall (1963) for the analogous case of a wave of depolarization or repolarization spreading along a fiber.

The experimental evidence bears out the above suggestion. According to the intracellular recording by Collewijn and Van Harreveld (1966) y_0 is about one fifth to

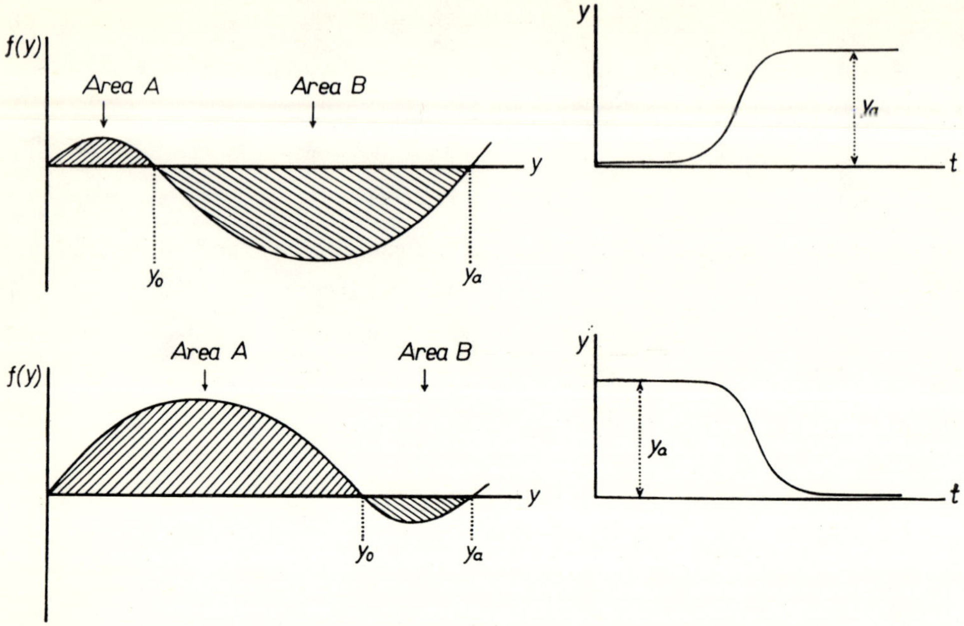

Fig. 7.2. Different time course of the extracellular potassium concentration for $y_o < y_a/2$ (above) and $y_o > y_a/2$ (below).

one fourth of y_a, the two values being close to the figures originally suggested by Hodgkin, that is 30 and 150 mEq/l, respectively. Also the values D and T can be estimated from the slope of the depolarization wave given by Eq. (7.8). By integrating Eq. (7.8) we obtain

$$\int \frac{dy}{y(y_a - y)} = \int b\ dt + C \tag{7.18}$$

Since

$$\int \frac{dy}{y(y_a - y)} = \frac{1}{y_a} \int \left[\frac{1}{y} + \frac{1}{y_a - y} \right] dy = \frac{1}{y_a} \log \left| \frac{y}{y_a - y} \right| \tag{7.19}$$

solution of (7.18) is

$$\frac{1}{y_a} \log \left| \frac{y}{y_a - y} \right| = bt + C \tag{7.20}$$

or

$$\frac{y}{y_a - y} = k \exp(y_a bt) \tag{7.21}$$

If t is defined at $y = y_a/2$ then $k = 1$ and Eq. (7.21) leads to

$$y = \frac{y_a \exp(y_a bt)}{1 + \exp(y_a bt)} \tag{7.22}$$

which can be also written as

$$y = y_a \frac{\exp(0.5\, y_a bt)}{\exp(-0.5\, y_a bt) + \exp(0.5\, y_a bt)} \tag{7.23}$$

or

$$y = \frac{y_a}{2} \frac{\exp(0.5\, y_a \mathrm{bt}) + \exp(0.5\, y_a bt) - \exp(-0.5\, y_a bt) + \exp(-0.5\, y_a bt)}{\exp(-0.5\, y_a bt) + \exp(0.5\, y_a bt)} \tag{7.24}$$

Since

$$\frac{\exp(0.5\, y_a bt) - \exp(-0.5\, y_a bt)}{\exp(0.5\, y_a bt) + \exp(-0.5\, y_a bt)} = \tanh \frac{y_a bt}{2} \tag{7.25}$$

Eq. (7.24) can be written in the form,

$$y = 0.5 y_a\ (1 + \tanh 0.5\, y_a bt) \tag{7.26}$$

and after substituting for b from Eq. (7.14)

$$y = \frac{y_a}{2} (1 + \tanh \frac{ut}{\sqrt{8DT}}) \tag{7.27}$$

According to intracellular recording (Collewijn and Van Harreveld 1966) the maximum depolarization rate is 7 mV/sec and the depolarization is practically completed in approximately 10 sec. These findings are compatible with the value suggested by Hodgkin (Fig. 7.3)

$$\frac{\sqrt{8DT}}{u} \doteq 4 \text{ sec} \tag{7.28}$$

After substituting the experimentally established values in the Eqs. (7.17) and (7.28)

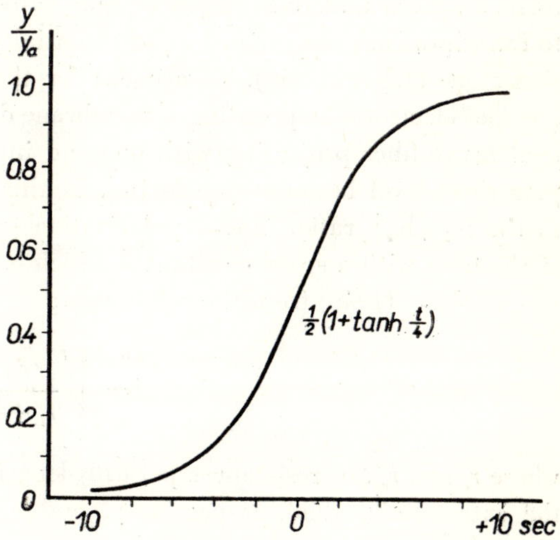

Fig. 7. 3. Increase of the extracellular K^+ concentration as a function of time.

$$u = \frac{150-60}{150}\sqrt{\frac{D}{2T}}$$

and

$$u = \frac{\sqrt{8DT}}{4} = \sqrt{\frac{DT}{2}}$$

we obtain $T = 0.6$ sec. For $u = 3$ mm/min ($=5 \cdot 10^{-3}$ cm/sec)

$$\sqrt{D} = 5 \cdot 10^{-3} \cdot \frac{5}{3} \cdot \sqrt{\frac{6}{5}}$$

$$D = 8.3 \cdot 10^{-5} \text{ cm}^2/\text{sec}$$

This value of D is considerably higher than the diffusion coefficient of K^+ in free solutions ($2.5 \cdot 10^{-5}$ cm²/sec at 38 °C) evidently because depolarization spreads along each neuron by electrotonic mechanisms or by impulse conduction, and between neurons not only by diffusion but also by synaptic transmission. Elimination of the latter component by anoxia (Bureš 1957b) reduces the spreading rate to 2 mm/ /min, which corresponds to $D = 3.6 \cdot 10^{-5}$ cm²/sec, that is, to a value indicating the prime importance of diffusion under these concitions.

8. Electrotonic Spread

Grafstein (1963) used the analysis proposed by Hodgkin for much lower K^+ excess ($y_0 = 2.3$ and $y_a = 9.5$ mEq/l) which in the light of recent evidence (p. 93) seems to be a serious underestimation of real values. As the ratio $y_0 : y_a$ remained one to four, however, she arrived at an essentially similar spreading rate based on diffusion alone (1.5 mm/min). To account for the real velocity of SD, Grafstein (1963) assumes electrotonic spreading of membrane depolarization along neurons. A hypothetical nerve fiber projecting with one end into the region with a high extracellular potassium level becomes depolarized in this region to the potential corresponding to the K_i^+/K_e^+ ratio. The depolarization spreads electrotonically along the length of the fiber with a space constant λ which may be calculated according to Hodgkin and Rushton (1946) from the relationship

$$\lambda = \sqrt{\frac{r_m}{r_i + r_e}} \tag{7.29}$$

where r_i and r_e are resistances per unit length (ohm cm^{-1}) of the axoplasm and of the extracellular fluid, respectively, and r_m is the resistance multiplied by unit length of the membrane (ohm cm). Assuming that the specific transverse resistance of nerve membrane R_m is 800 ohm cm² (Eccles 1957) and that the radius a of the fiber is 0.5 μ, r_m can be calculated from the equation

$$r_m = \frac{R_m}{2\pi a} = \frac{800 \text{ ohm cm}^2}{2\pi 5 \cdot 10^{-5} \text{ cm}} = 2.5 \cdot 10^6 \text{ ohm cm} \tag{7.30}$$

According to Eccles (1953) the specific resistance of axoplasm (R_i) is about twice that of the extracellular fluid (R_e) which amounts to 50 ohm cm (Van Harreveld and Schadé 1960). With the above values r_i can be calculated by inserting into Eq. (7.31)

$$r_i = \frac{R_i}{\pi a^2} = \frac{100 \text{ ohm cm}}{\pi 25 \cdot 10^{-10} \text{cm}^2} \doteq 1.27 \cdot 10^{10} \text{ ohm cm}^{-1} \tag{7.31}$$

Since r_e is much smaller than r_i, it can be ignored in Eq. (7.29) which thus simplifies to

$$\lambda = \sqrt{\frac{r_m}{r_i}} = \sqrt{2 \cdot 10^{-4} \text{ cm}^2} \doteq 1.4 \cdot 10^{-2} \text{ cm} = 140\,\mu \tag{7.32}$$

Assuming further that the membrane capacitance C_m is 6 μF cm⁻² (Eccles 1957), it is possible to calculate the time constant of the membrane from the equation

$$\tau = C_m \cdot R_m = 6\mu F \text{ cm}^{-2} \cdot 800 \text{ ohm cm}^2 = 48 \cdot 10^{-4} \text{ sec} \tag{7.33}$$

This indicates that at a distance of 1λ from the depolarized region of the axon electrotonic depolarization reaches half its final vlaue within 5 msec and the full amplitude within 15 to 20 msec. This rapid electrotonic spread induces changes in potassium movement across the membrane, which can be derived from the flux form of the Nernst equation (Hodgkin and Keynes 1955)

$$\log \frac{\text{flux}_{in}}{\text{flux}_{out}} = -\frac{\Delta E}{60} \tag{7.34}$$

where ΔE is the depolarization in millivots. For resting membrane $\Delta E = 0$ and $\text{flux}_{in} = \text{flux}_{out}$. Depolarization of 10 to 30 mV increases the K^+ outflux approximately 1.5 to 3.0 times. Grafstein (1963) assumed that in 1 sec this increased outflux of K^+ raises extracellular potassium to the level causing firing in adjacent nerve fibers. Spreading depression will thus propagate at a rate of one space constant per second, that is 140μ/sec or 8.4mm/min. The extracellular K^+ concentration probably attains the threshold level more slowly, however, since the electrotonically depolarized dendrites entering an inactive region cannot constitute more than 50 % of the neuropile and the released K^+ is thus distributed into a relatively larger extracellular volume. A spreading rate of one space constant per 2 sec therefore seems to be more reasonable (spreading rate 4.2 mm/min). This velocity can be further increased by impulse conduction along the activated fibers and across the intervening synapses.

9. Critical Mass

All the above considerations do not take into account an important variable: the relative density of active and passive elements in the particular brain structure. In passive elements the K^+ flux only depends on the membrane potential and intracellular and extracellular K^+ concentrations. A tissue composed of such elements would not generate a self-maintained reaction. Glial cells and some dendrites may belong to this category. Thus Van Harreveld and Stamm (1954a) found that SD cannot be evoked in cerebral cortex in which 30-to 70-min asphyxiation damaged most neurons without affecting glial cells. In active elements threshold depolarization changes the membrane permeability for sodium, the influx of which with the consecutive potassium outflux is the decisive event in the mechanism of spreading.

Density of the active elements and corresponding level of interaction determine the safety factor of spreading and the minimum volume of depolarized tissue required to trigger the self-maintained reaction. Depolarization of a single neuron cannot start SD since it only causes a negligible increase of extracellular K^+ in the volume of tissue corresponding to the extent of its dendritic and axonal branching. Unfortunately it is very difficult to stimulate a certain percentage of neurons in a given area without affecting the other elements. Zachar and Zacharová (1963) approached this problem by using mechanical stimuli applied to different volumes of cortex. With the stimulated area 1.5 mm in diameter the threshold was 7.2 gmm/mm^2. The relative refractory phase lasted for 15 min when examined with threshold stimulus but could be maximally shortened to 5 min when the testing stimulus was increased 2.5 times. The difference between threshold stimulus and maximum stimulus corresponds to the ratio of the neurons activated by the threshold stimulus to the total neuronal population of the stimulated area. When the diameter of the stimulated area was reduced to 0.75 mm, the threshold stimulus was increased to 16.3 gmm/mm^2. The duration of the relative refractory period remained unchanged but it could not be shortened even by increasing the stimulus 3.6 times. In this case the threshold stimulus is equal to the maximal one, which indicates that practically all active elements in the stimulated area had to be activated in order to trigger SD (Fig. 7.4) The authors estimated the minimum necessary area as 0.5 mm^2 and taking into account the thickness of cortex, the minimum volume as 1.0 mm^3.

A similar estimate was obtained by Janebová (1971) and by Matsuura and Bureš (1971) with a different technique. By iontophoretic application of K^+ ions or by pressure injection of concentrated KCl solution 1 mm below cortical surface, the threshold was found to be approximately 2 to $4 \cdot 10^{-8}$ gEq K^+. Assuming an instantaneous point source of K^+, diffusion in the homogeneous medium would increase the

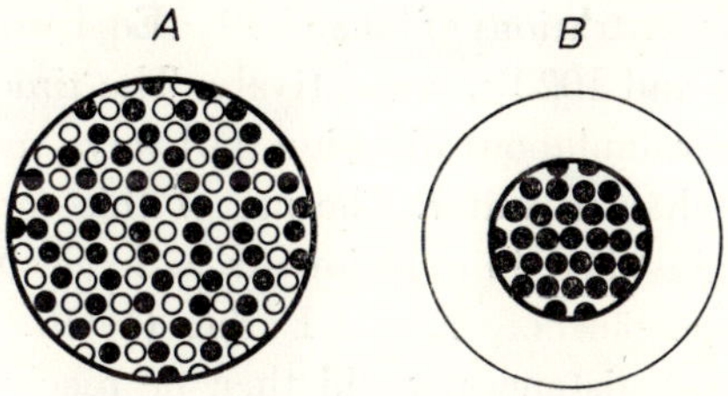

Fig. 7. 4. Schematic illustration explaining why mechanical stimuli applied onto a large trephine opening have a lower threshold and shorter relative refractory period than stimuli applied onto a small trephine opening. Circles are neurons unaffected by the threshold stimulus; dots are neurons depolarized by the threshold stimulus (Zachar and Zacharová 1963).

extracellular K^+ concentration at different distances from the point of application according to the equation (Curtis 1964),

$$C = \frac{10^3 Q \exp\left[\dfrac{-d^2}{4Dt\, 10^8}\right]}{8(\pi Dt)^{1.5}} \tag{7.35}$$

where D is the diffusion coeficient (cm^2/sec) of potassium and C the K^+ concentration (gEq/l) at the distance d (μ) from the point of application of a quantity Q (gEq) of potassium after an interval t (sec) following injection. In every point adjacent to the injection site the potassium concentration increases, reaches maximum, and then decays. The maximal concentration C_{max} is reached after time t (sec) which depends only on the distance d (μ) and on the diffusion coefficient D (cm^2/sec) according to the equation,

$$T = \frac{d^2}{6D\, 10^8} \tag{7.36}$$

After substituting T into Eq. (7.35) we obtain

$$C_{max} = \frac{10^3 Q \exp(-1.5)}{8\,(\pi DT)^{1.5}} \tag{7.37}$$

For the experimentally established single-injection threshold $Q_1 = 3.4 \cdot 10^{-8}$ mol K^+, C_{max} attains 30 mEq/l and 10 mEq/l after 13 and 27 sec at distances 445 and 641 μ, respectively. Assuming the K^+threshold to be within this range, the minimum volume of tissue required for triggering SD would be approximately 0.5 mm^3. The real volume is larger, however, because the injected KCl is distributed mainly to the extracellular space forming about 25 % of the total tissue volume (Van Harreveld 1966). This is the same as if the K^+dosage is increased four times, that is to $13.6 \cdot 10^{-8}$ gEq. In water the maximal concentrations of 30 and 10 mEq/1 would then be reached after 33.2 and 69.0 sec at 705 and 1020 μ, respectively. The time necessary to reach C_{max} is longer, however, since roundabout diffusion pathways make D_K in brain approximately 2.5 times lower than in water. The use of this correction factor for longer distances was recently justified in experiments with electrophoretic application of glutamate by Herz, Ziegelgänsberger, and Färber (1969). The maximal concentrations at the above critical distances would then be reached after 83 and 172 sec, respectively. The real radii of the critical isoconcentration surfaces are probably larger, because potassium ions released from the depolarized neurons add to the injected amount and the area of depolarization is also enlarged by electrotonic spread and impulse conduction. Recording electrode placed 1 to 3 mm from the point of subthreshold KCl injection detected local SPC that attained 16 % of maximal CSD negativity at the 1500 μ distance. Depolarization of this magnitude corresponds to a twofold increase of extracellular potassium. With two simultaneously applied microinjections, 59 % of the single injection threshold Q_1 had to be applied to each point to elicit CSD when the distance was 1 mm. For interfocal distances 2, 3, and 4mm, the double-injection threshold $Q_{1,2}$ was 65, 74, and 97 % of Q_1, respectively. The spatial sumation effect was still significant at 3 mm but undetectable at 4 mm tip separation.

Whereas the spatial summation of two subthreshold foci is complicated by the geometry of interaction, temporal summation is easier to interpret because the K^+ ions are applied to a single point. The threshold amount of KCl required to trigger CSD at different intervals (30 to 480 sec) after injection of 0.8 Q_1, expotentially increased with time from 28.2 % Q_1 at 30 sec to 88.9 % Q_1 at 480 sec with the slope 16.8 % Q_1 for a twofold increase of the interinjection interval. From the time course of the temporal summation it is possible to establish the time t_c during which the critical concentration C_c is reached at the critical distance d_c from the injection. As follows from the experimental data and the computed regression line, 90.5 sec after injection of $0.8Q_1$ it is necessary to apply $0.5Q_1$ in order to trigger SD. Since with $0.5Q_1$ the concentrations are decreased to 50 % at all distances, triggering SD under the above conditions indicates that the concentration reached at the critical distance d_c after an interval t_c following the injection of $0.5Q_1$ is equal to the concentration persisting at this distance (t_c + 90.5) sec after injection of $0.8Q_1$. After substituting into Eq. (7.35) we obtain

$$\frac{10^3\, 0.5\, Q_1 \exp\,[-d_c^2/(4Dt_c\, 10^8)]}{8(\pi D t_c)^{1.5}} = \frac{10^3\, 0.8\, Q_1 \exp\,\{d_c^2\;[4D(t_c + 90.5)\, 10^8]\}}{8(\pi D)^{1.5}\,.\,(t_c + 90.5)^{1.5}} \tag{7.38}$$

Since it can be surmised that d_c corresponds to the maximum concentration that can be attained at this distance by the second injection, we can substitute for it from Eq. (7.36). Equation (7.38) then becomes

$$\frac{10^3\, 0.5\, Q_1 \exp\left[(-t_c 6D\, 10^8)/(4Dt_c 10^8)\right]}{8(\pi D t_c)^{1.5}} = \frac{10^3\, 0.8\, Q_1 \exp\left\{\dfrac{(-t_c 6D 10^8)}{4\, D(t_c + 90.5)10^8}\right\}}{8(\pi) D^{1.5}\, (t_c + 90.5)^{1.5}} \tag{7.39}$$

and after simplifying

$$\frac{0.5 \exp(-1.5)}{t_c^{1.5}} = \frac{0.8 \exp \dfrac{-6t_c}{4(t_c + 90.5)}}{(t_c + 90.5)^{1.5}} \tag{7.40}$$

Equation (7.40) is satisfied by $t_c = 61$ sec which is independent of Q_1 and D. This value of t_c corresponds in aqueous solutions at 37 °C to $d_c = 957\ \mu$ for $Q_1 = 3.4 \cdot 10^{-8}$ mol and $C_c = 2.93$ mEq/l. As pointed out by Krnjević and Mitchell (1960) diffusion of a substance in a multicompartment system involves tortuous pathways. When the boundaries of the extracellular space are considered as spherical, longer distances have to be multiplied by $\pi/2$ and the diffusion coefficient has to be decreased by $(\pi/2)^2$, that is approximately 2.5 times. For $D_K = 1.0 \cdot 10^{-5}$ cm²/sec, d_c decreases to 605 μ and C_c increases to 11.6 mEq/l. The real concentration would be about four times higher, however, since K^+ diffuses into the extracellular space forming approximately 25 % of the total cortical volume. The resulting K^+ concentration of 45 mEq/l is probably higher than the actual threshold, the discrepancy being due to an underestimation of D_K which is equal to $1.0 \cdot 10^{-5}$ cm²/sec only when close to the injection site. When the critical distance is approached more and more K^+ ions are released from neurons, the K^+ diffusion proceeds over shorter distances, and is further enhanced by electrotonic spread and impulse conduction. Because of the combined action of all these factors, D_K increases and may even exceed the value typical for aqueous solution. The critical distance and concentration should thus be sought between 600 and 950 μ and between 12 and 45 mEq/l.

10. Recovery Process

Whereas the attempts to describe quantitatively the processes leading to SD initiation were reasonably successful, the mechanisms underlying the repolarization phase of SPC are less clear. After the net K^+ release has stopped, excess K^+ is removed from the extracellular space by diffusion to inactive tissue, by equilibration with the blood stream, and by active transport into the neurons (Brinley 1963). Simple diffusion from a 2 mm wide layer of cortex would reduce K^+ concentration to 10 % of the initial level only over 6 to 7 min, which is too slow to account for the observed repolarization rates. Removal by circulation is more adequate, since with the flow rate of 0.023 ml $sec^{-1}gram^{-1}$ cortical tissue (Kety 1960) the excess potassium in a 20 % extracellular volume can be reduced to 10 % within 20 sec assuming high permeability of capillary endothelium to K^+ and instantaneous equilibration between extracellular space and blood. With both mechanisms the depressed tissue would lose for each SD wave a definite amount of K^+ (10 to 15 %) but the predicted loss could never be demonstrated with analytical methods (Křivánek and Bureš 1960, Křivánek 1969a). This makes active transport the most probable mechanism of potassium removal. The power of active transport was convincingly demonstrated in cortical tissue slices the neurons of which can be depolarized by electrical stimulation (Hillman and McIlwain 1961). During stimulation the slice loses a measurable amount of potassium (Cummins and McIlwain 1961) which is regained within 1 min after the stimulation is discontinued. Since the membrane potential is restored with the same rate and since the process is associated with increased utilization of energy, it can be considered as an *in vitro* analogy of SD.

Part II

Spreading Depression as a Research Method

Chapter 8

Spreading Depresion as a Tool for Studying the Functional Organization of the Brain

1. Inhibitory Neuronography

Although morphology remans the major source of information on brain organization, modern neuroanatomy cannot develop without using physiological and biochemical methods to characterize the functional significance of anatomically established connections. Such methods are indispensable for tracing multisynaptic pathways, for determining the excitatory and inhibitory nature of nervous connections, and for estimating the degree of convergence in nonspecific systems. The neuronographic technique introduced by Dusser de Barrenne and McCulloch (1936a, b) is a classical example of the application of electrophysiological methods for mapping projection areas and intercentral connections. Local electrical stimulation or local application of strychnine causes a simultaneous discharge of neurons, which is conducted along fiber tracts arising in the stimulated area and can be detected as an appropriately delayed synchronous electric potential even in remote regions. Whereas electrical neuronography reveals both the orthodromic and antidromic connections between the point of stimulation and the point of recording, strychnine does not act on fibers but exclusively on synapses, and initiates only orthodromic conduction from the stimulated region (Frankenhaeuser 1951). The strychnine or electrical neuronography mainly detects phasic intercentral influences; it does not provide information on mutual interaction of nerve centers under resting conditions and/or their tonic interrelationships.

The functional organization of the brain can also be studied by reversing the principles of excitatory neuronography. Activity of a given nerve center is affected by impulses arriving from different sources. Acute elimination of an important afferent influence induces changes of activity in the partly deafferented region that may reveal the inhibitory or excitatory character of the inactivated input, as well as its relative significance. Participation of the eliminated structure in electrophysiological phenomena based on complex interaction can be established in a similar way. Because of the drawbacks of surgical ablation (irreversibility, shock, edema, interference with circulation, retrograde degeneration, glial scars) functional ablation techniques are being used for the above purpose to an ever-increasing extent. An ideal functional ablation technique should be fully reversible; its effects must be uniform and limited to the ablated structure; it must be accompanied by clear-cut electrophysiological signs indicating its extent and duration. Whereas local application of drugs (Brücke, Petsche, Pillat, and Deisenhammer 1959, Magni, Moruzzi, Rossi, and Zanchetti 1959) or local cooling (Dondey, Albe-Fessard, and Le Beau 1962, Fuster and Alexander 1970) have been used for inactivation of restricted areas, transitory elimination of larger cortical and subcortical structures can be achieved by SD. Changes of activity occurring in areas not directly entered by SD can be considered a consequence of the functional elimination, if they coincide with the primary depression. Inhibitory neuronography using SD for achieving functional ablation (Burešová, Bureš, Weiss, and Fifková 1961, Bureš and Burešová 1968b) critically depends on the changes in the depressed region which are described in detail in Chap. 1. The most important feature of SD is the deep depolarization of neural membranes lasting for about 1 min and causing a complete block of neural activity. The depolarization block is preceded by a short-lasting burst of impulse activity (2 to 5 sec) and followed by slow gradual recovery, completed only after 5 to 10 min. The wavelength of the excitatory phase is 100—250 μ, of the depolarization block approximately 3 mm and of the ensuing partial block more than 15 mm. Since the volume of the excited zone is 20 to 50 times smaller than the volume of the depressed tissue, excitatory influences accompanying the onset of SD are overshadowed by depression which becomes the most prominent feature, especially of the later phase of SD development. Nevertheless the possible effects of the excitation phase of SD must always be taken into account when interpreting results obtained with this technique.

Another important prerequisite of neuronographic application of SD is precise knowledge of the extent of the depressed area. The reader should refer to Chap. 6 for the anatomical boundaries of SD in the neocortex, hippocampus, thalamus and caudate nucleus of rats, as well as in the striatum of birds, that is, in the structures used so far in inhibitory neuronography studies.

2. The Effect of Functional Decortication on the Electrical Activity of the Subcortical Centers

Cortical SD in rats sweeps over the entire dorsal surface of the hemisphere but enters only with a decrement the cingular, enthorhinal, and pyriform cortex (Fifková 1964a). Since the total rostrocaudal extent of cortex does not exceed 15 mm, the whole cortical mantle can be covered by a single wavelength of SD elicited from the parietal cortex. Although the functional ablation is predominantly limited to the neocortex, it must be taken into account that 50 % of SD waves may spread through the amygdalar region to the caudate nucleus (Fifková and Syka 1964).

Spontaneous and Evoked EEG Activity

Remote effects of functional decortication in rats have been systematically studied by Weiss (1961a) and Weiss and Fifková (1960, 1961a, b, c). The results are summarized in Fig. 8.1. In unanesthetized, curarized animals, unilateral CSD was accompanied by a decrease of spontaneous EEG in the thalamus and hypothalamus, more pronounced ipsilaterally. On the other hand reticular and hippocampal activity remained essentially unchanged. The hippocampal theta activity which could be evoked by sensory (Weiss and Fifková 1960) or reticular stimulation (Rüdiger, Weiss, and Fifková 1962) and by administration of physostigmine (Bohdanecký, Weiss, and Fifková 1963), was unaffected.

In rats under barbiturate or chloralose anesthesia CSD also decreases the EEG activity in the above two structures (Weiss and Bohdanecký 1963). Somatosensory, auditory, and visual evoked potentials in the specific nuclei of the afferent pathways

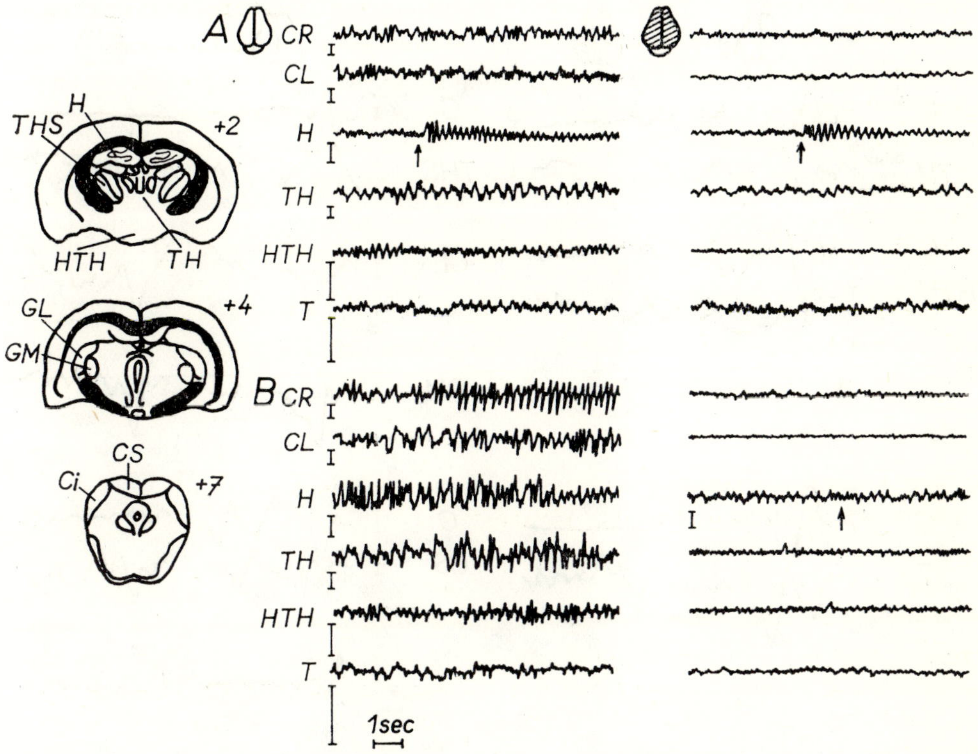

Fig. 8. 1. EEG activity of subcortical structures in unanesthetized curarized rats *(A)* and in rats anesthetized with Dial *(B)* before (left) and during (right) bilateral CSD. Symbols: *CR, CL*, right and left cortex, respectively; *H*, hippocampus; *TH*, thalamus; *HTH*, hypothalamus; *T*, tegmentum. Note that the theta rhythm evoked in the hippocampus by sensory stimulus (arrow) remains preserved also during CSD (Weiss 1960).

at the thalamic (ventral nucleus, medial geniculate body, lateral geniculate body) and mesencephalic levels (inferior colliculus, superior colliculus) were unaffected by CSD (Weiss and Fifková 1961a,b). On the contrary, long latency responses to sensory stimuli recorded in the nonspecific thalamic nuclei, in the hypothalamus, or in the mesencephalic reticular formation were severely depressed (Fig. 8.2). Also cerebellar responses to monocular visual stimuli were considerably reduced by CSD contralateral to the stimulated eye (Roper and Bourassa 1972). It should be pointed out, however, that detection of minute changes of evoked potentials, and particularly of spontaneous activity, is difficult without using sophisticated methods of analysis. The negative results have to be accepted with caution.

The effect of CSD on EEG activity in the thalamic nuclei was also studied in the rabbit (Winocur, Trufant, King, and O'Leary 1950) and in the cat (Sloan and Jasper 1950). Alterations of activity in different thalamic nuclei closely followed penetration of SD into functionally connected cortical regions.

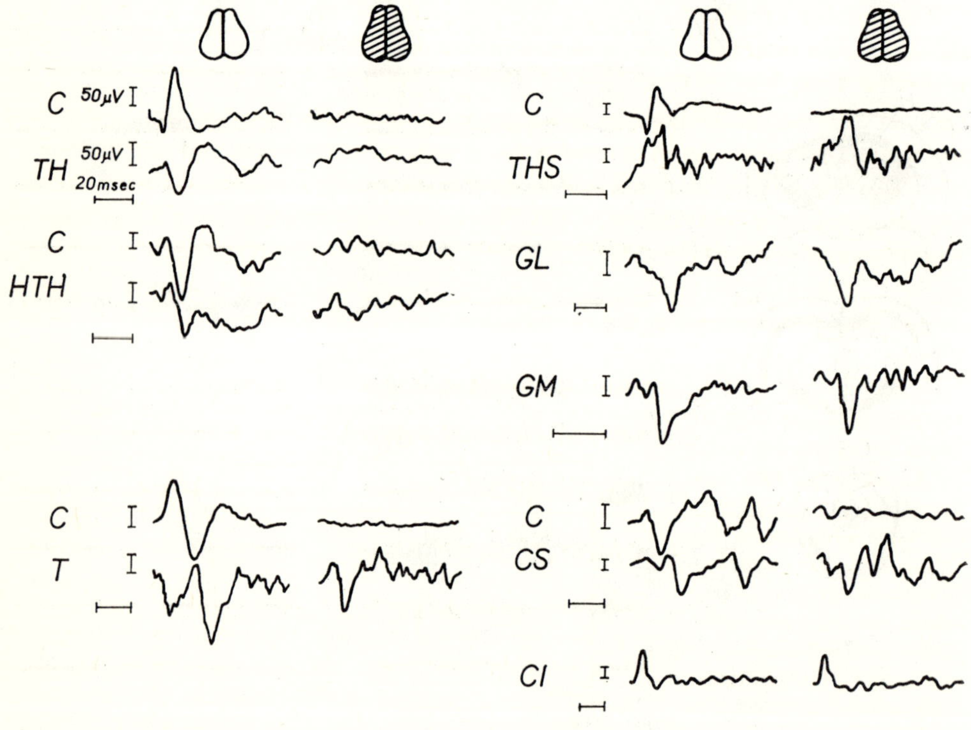

Fig. 8. 2. The effect of bilateral CSD on the evoked responses in nonspecific (left) and specific (right) subcortical structures in curarized unanesthetized rats. Symbols: *C*, cortical projection area corresponding to the stimulus applied; *CS*, superior colliculus; *CI*, inferior colliculus; *GL*, lateral geniculate body; *GM*, medial geniculate body; *THS*, specific thalamic nuclei (ventrobasal complex). Stimuli: *TH, HTH, T, THS*, electrical stimulation of the contralateral sciatic nerve; *GL, CS*, intense flash; *GM, CI*, clicks. See Fig. 8. 1 for schematic brain sections (Weiss 1960).

Unit Activity

The consequences of functional decortication can be demonstrated in a more quantitative way when recording unit activity in remotely affected areas. Changes of spontaneous firing caused by CSD in more than 500 cortical, thalamic, caudate, hypothalamic, hippocampal and reticular neurons were studied in curarized, unanesthetized rats. A whole series of reports (Bureš, Burešová, and Fifková 1961, Bureš, Burešová, Fifková, Olds, Olds, and Travis 1961, Burešová, Bureš, and Fifková 1962, Burešová, Bureš, Fifková, Vinogradova, and Weiss 1962, Rüdiger, Burešová, and Fifková 1962, Burešová, Shima, Bureš, and Fifková 1963, Tolkunov, Burešová, Bureš, Kuznetsova, and Fifková 1965) employed the same technique: unit activity was recorded with capillary microelectrodes (3 M KCl, tip diameter 1 μ) or with stainless steel microelectrodes (tip 2 to 4 μ). The only units used were well isolated, exceeded the peak-to-peak noise by a factor of at least three, and maintained relatively stable spontaneous activity over the 5-to 10-min period preceding CSD initiation.

The number of spikes exceeding the preset threshold amplitude was counted at 0.5 or 1.0 min intervals with an electronic counter. The CSD was monitored by SPC recording from the cortical surface. Only changes of firing rate coinciding with cortical CSD and exceeding the mean predepression rate by more than 3 standard deviations were considered as reactions. A typical experiment and the method of its evaluation is illustrated in Fig. 8.3 showing excitatory reactions of a reticular unit to ipsilateral and contralateral CSD. The inhibitory reaction in a hypothalamic neuron caused by ipsilateral CSD is shown in Fig. 8.4. The results are summarized in Fig. 8.5, showing the relative incidence of units, the activity of which was increased, decreased, or unchanged in the investigated neural populations.

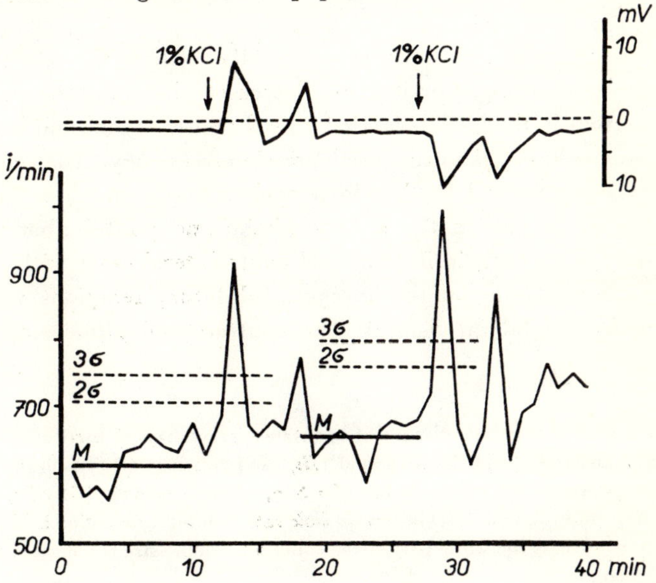

Fig. 8.3. Repeated short increase of reticular unit activity accompanying both ipsilateral and contralateral CSD. (Above) Steady potential, negativity of the left hemisphere downwards. (Below) Firing rate of the unit (spikes/min). Arrows indicate application of 1 % KCl. *M* is the average firing rate during the 10-min predepression interval. The 2 σ and 3 σ levels are indicated by dashed horizontal lines. Abscissa: time in minutes (Bureš, Burešová, Fifková, Olds, Olds, and Travis 1961).

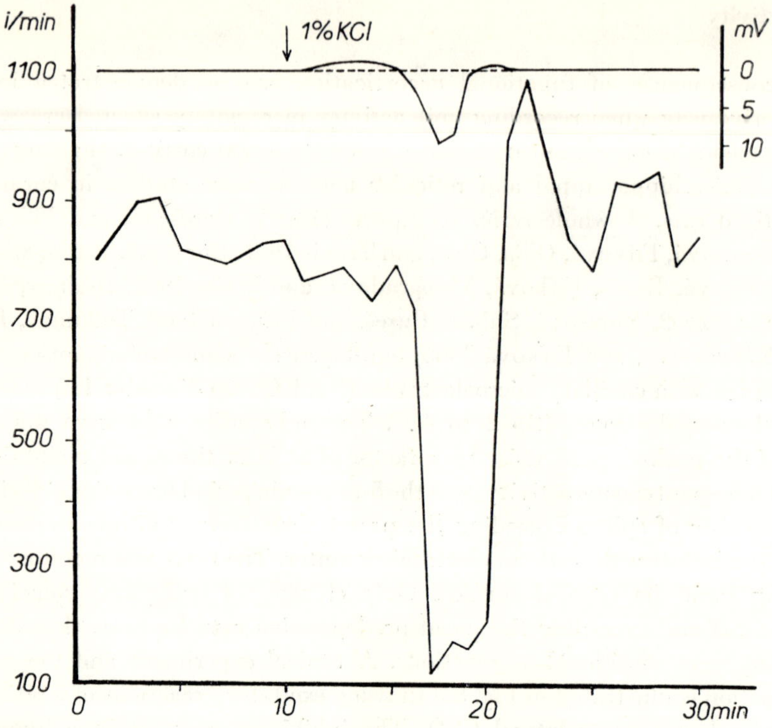

Fig. 8. 4. Decrease of firing rate in a hypothalamic unit during ipsilateral CSD. Description as in Fig. 8. 3. (Bureš, Burešová, Fifková, Olds, Olds, and Travis 1961).

Changes of unit activity essentially confirm the results obtained with macroelectrode recording. Cortical SD decreased the spontaneous activity of 80 to 90% of neurons in the ipsilateral thalamus, hypothalamus, and caudate nucleus for 5 to 6 min to or below 20% of the predepression frequency. The same regions were less affected by contralateral CSD, which evokes fewer and less marked inhibitory reactions. Most neurones in the mesencephalic and pontobulbar reticular formation (60%) reacted to both ipsilateral and contralateral CSD with an activity increase lasting for 2 to 3 min on the average. Inhibitory reactions were less frequent and more prolonged (about 5 min). The contralateral hippocampus resembled the reticular

---

Fig. 8. 5. Survey of changes of spontaneous activity of cortical (*Co*), thalamic (*Th*), caudate (*Cd*), hypothalamic (*Hy*), hippocampal (*Hi*), and reticular (*RF*) neurons caused in rats by contralateral or ipsilateral *SD* in the cortex (*Co SD*), caudate nucleus (*Cd SD*), or thalamus (*Th SD*). *CoSDCI*, effects of ipsilateral CSD in *cerveau isolé* rats. Inhibitory reaction is black, excitatory reaction is shaded; no reaction is the white part of the columns. Sample size is indicated by *n* values (Bureš and Burešová 1968b).

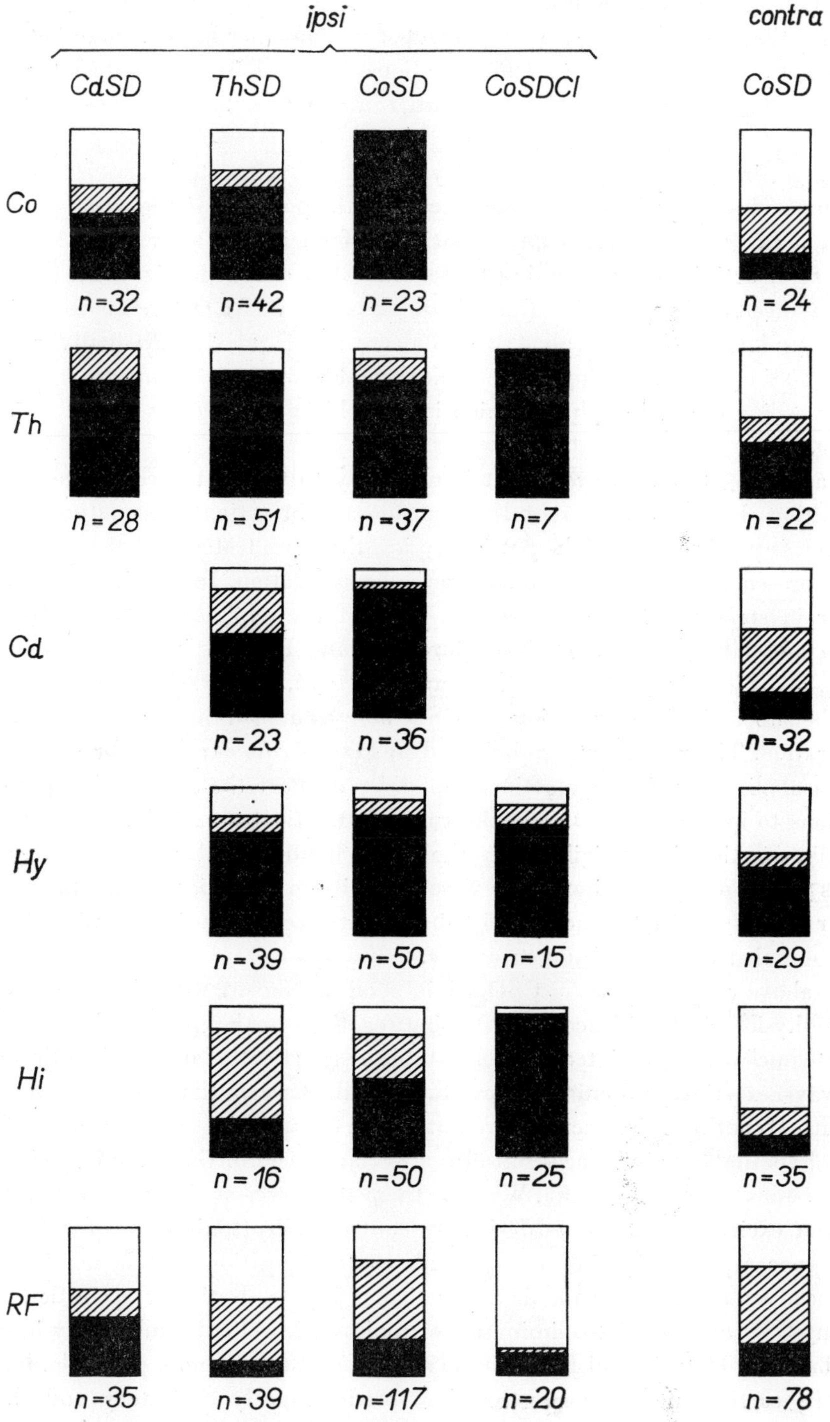
ipsi
contra
CdSD
ThSD
CoSD
CoSDCl
CoSD
Co
n=32
n=42
n=23
n=24
Th
n=28
n=51
n=37
n=7
n=22
Cd
n=23
n=36
n=32
Hy
n=39
n=50
n=15
n=29
Hi
n=16
n=50
n=25
n=35
RF
n=35
n=39
n=117
n=20
n=78

formation in terms of the relative incidence of excitatory and inhibitory reactions, whereas the ipsilateral hippocampus reacted in a manner intermediate between the reticular and thalamic types. Unit reactions recorded in the contralateral cortex during unilateral CSD were also distributed in a manner typical for reticular formation.

Changes in spontaneous unit activity in the ventral posterior nucleus of the cat thalamus, observed while CSD penetrated into the posterior sigmoid and pericruciate cortex (Waller and Feldman 1967) consisted of an initial activation phase (slight increase of activity corresponding to general EEG desynchronization), followed by a pronounced excitation phase (large increase of firing rate lasting for 10 to 150 sec), and a prolonged inactive phase (deep decrease of activity gradually recovering over a 5-min period). Cooling of the critical cortical area caused inactivation without the preceding excitation phase, which is probably generated by the initial SD discharge.

In analysing the above results it is necessary to take into account not only the connections between the cerebral cortex and the investigated structures, but also between any pair of them. The possibility was therefore tested that the unit reactions at the prosencephalic level are due to reticular activation. In a series of experiments the brain stem was transected at the level of the superior colliculus (Burešová, Bureš, and Fifková 1962, Rüdiger, Burešová, and Fifková 1962, Bureš, Burešová, Weiss, and Fifková 1963, Burešová, Bureš, Fifková, Vinogradova, and Weiss 1962) and the subcortical unit reactions to CSD were examined in the cerveau isolé preparation. The results are summarized in Fig. 8.5. As expected, brain stem transection abolished reticular reactions but did not affect thalamic and hypothalamic reactions to ipsilateral CSD. This indicates that reticular participation in the diencephalic reaction is negligible. On the other hand reticular activation probably affects the hippocampus since there were no excitatory reactions in the hippocampus of cerveau isolé rats, and the distribution of reactions to ipsilateral CSD closely resembled that of diencephalic structures.

The above remote effects of CSD are in good agreement with the anatomical and electrophysiological evidence. The striking reactions in the ipsilateral thalamus and caudate nucleus are mediated via well-established corticothalamic and corticocaudate pathways, exerting predominantly excitatory influences on the thalamic and caudate neurons. Hypothalamic reactions are not only a consequence of elimination of direct corticohypothalamic influences but also a tertiary effect of the secondary changes in the thalamus and basal ganglia. Whereas these structures are interconnected through powerful excitatory pathways decisively controlled by tonic corticofugal activity, the hippocampus maintains a more independent position and is nearly equally influenced by corticodiencephalic and reticular inputs. Reticular excitation accompanying CSD can be due to elimination of tonic corticoreticular inhibitory influences postulated by Hugelin and Bonvallet (1957 a, b). It seems more probable, however, that the corticoreticular connections are predominantly excitatory and that the reticular neurons are activated by the corticofugal discharge accompanying CSD onset. The reticular reaction is maintained as long as CSD moves across the critical part of cortex and its duration is prolonged by the slowly decaying reticular afterdischarge. This explanation is supported by the finding that the reticular excitation coincides with CSD invasion into the motor cortex and precedes by approximately 2 min the development of inhibitory reactions in the hypothalamus (Bureš, Burešová, Fifková, Olds, Olds, and Travis 1961). According to Buser, Richard, and Lescop (1969) reversible cryogenic blockade of somatic area I and of motor cortex decreases responses of midbrain reticular units to cutaneous stimuli. Prolonged cortical depression induced by repeated CSD waves decreases the average firing rate of reticular neurons to about 40% (Bureš and Burešová 1964). Waller and Feldman (1967) explained in the same manner the excitation phase preceding inactivation of thalamic neurons during CSD in cats. Because reticular activity is maintained by autorhythmicity and modulated by different inputs, it is little influenced by elimination of a single input, but reacts with clearcut excitation to the discharge appearing at any of the inputs.

In the intact brain, reticular excitation is projected to higher centers where it increases the firing rate of most cells. The changes of unit activity observed during unilateral CSD in the contralateral neocortex, caudate nucleus, and hippocampus (Fig. 8.5) are probably such tertiary effect. In drowsy animals, CSD elicited in one hemisphere is accompanied by EEG desynchronization in the contralateral neocortex, but the arousal reaction cannot be elicited in *cerveau isolé* rats (Weiss 1961b). Also the burst of theta activity accompanying each SD wave (Brožek, unpublished results) is probably a sign of reticular activation. In the ipsilateral hemisphere reticular activation is opposed by the elimination of cortical facilitation, which clearly predominates at the diencephalic level. This assumption was confirmed by Waller and Feldman (1967) who found that thalamic reactions to reticular stimulation disappeared during CSD.

Excitability Changes

Modification of EEG activity and unit activity is accompanied by corresponding excitability changes. Cortical SD in rats increases the threshold for elicitation of recruiting responses in the ipsilateral thalamus (Bureš, Burešová, Weiss, and Fifková 1963) without much affecting the recruiting response evoked from the contralateral thalamic nuclei. The threshold for caudate spindles is also increased by ipsilateral (Fig. 8.6) but not by contralateral CSD (Tolkunov, Burešová, Bureš, Kuznetsova, and Fifková 1965). Rüdiger, Weiss, and Fifková (1962) demonstrated in curarized rats an increased threshold for eliciting the hippocampal theta rhythm by electrical stimulation of the tegmentum. Cortical SD in the hemisphere ipsilateral or contralateral to the side of reticular stimulation increased the threshold to 124 or 117 %, respectively, and bilateral CSD to 168%. Rüdiger and Bureš (1962) found that unilateral CSD increases the threshold of the escape response evoked by electrical stimulation of the tegmentum to 120 %. Decreased excitability of hypothalamic drive centers during CSD results in a decrease in the self-stimulation rate (Rudiger and Fifková 1963) and in an increase in the interference threshold (Rüdiger 1962) (see also p. 305).

The remote changes in spontaneous activity and excitability induced by CSD affect in a particularly striking manner the electrographic signs of sleep. As shown by Weiss, Roldan, Bohdanecký, and Fifková (1964) the slow high voltage activity

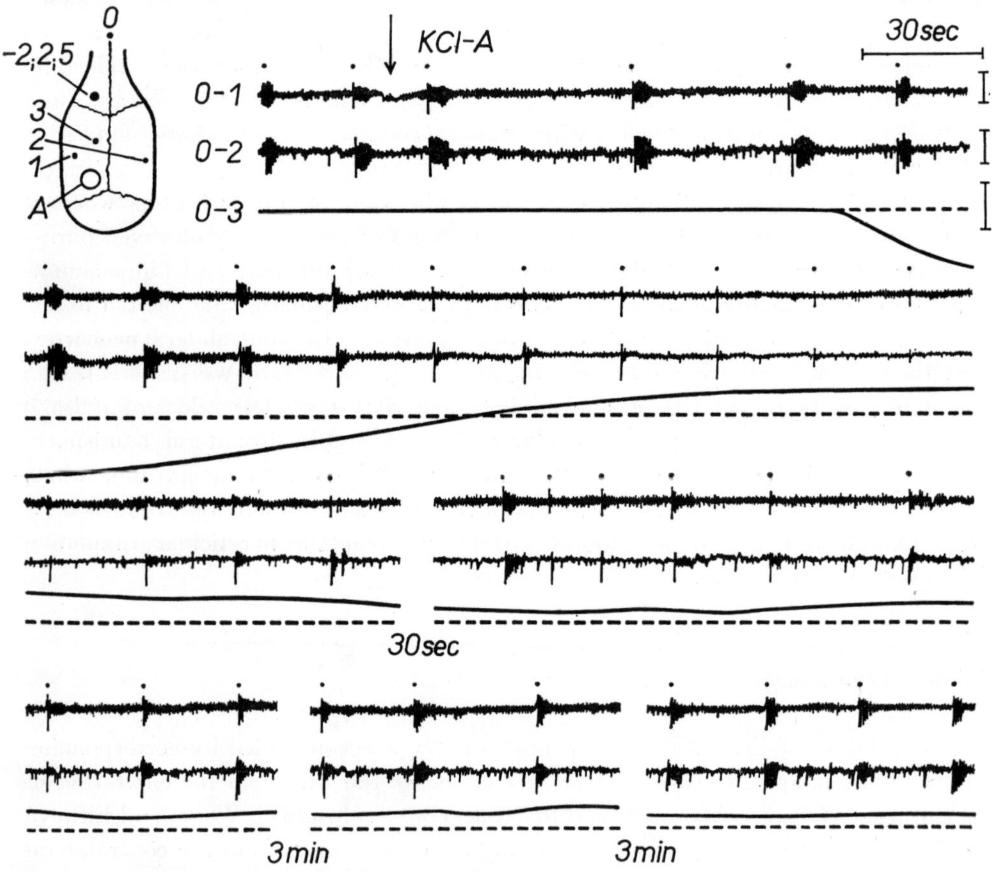

Fig. 8. 6. Effect of CSD on synchronized spindles evoked by stimulation of the ipsilateral caudate nucleus. Symbols: 1, 2, Cortical electrodes for EEG recording; 3, cortical electrode for SPC recording; 0, reference electrode; (—2; 2; 5), stimulating electrode in the head of the caudate nucleus. Arrow denotes application of KCl to cortical area *(A)*. Caudate shocks indicated by dots. Calibration: 500 μV for EEG, 10 mV for SPC. Negativity of the cortical surface is down ward (Tolkunov, Burešová, Bureš, Kuznetsova, and Fifková 1965).

typically present in the mesencephalic tegmentum during the telencephalic phase of sleep (Jouvet 1962) disappears during bilateral CSD. The hippocampal theta activity characteristic for the rhombencephalic (paradoxical) phase of sleep is nearly absent during functional decortication. Although they appear to be behaviorally asleep, functionally decorticated rats do not display any of the usual electrophysiological manifestations of sleep, which may be considered another example of the well known dissociation between EEG and behavior (Bradley and Elkes 1957). Unilateral CSD did not suppress the sleep cycle but considerably prolonged the duration of phase 1 (slow sleep) from 10 min in normal rats to nearly 23 min in functionally hemidecorticated animals. The spontaneous arousal reaction preceding phase 1 was also prolonged (from 1 to 2 min) whereas phase 2 (paradoxical sleep) was shortened from 2.5 min to slightly more than 1 min.

The rather simple scheme of corticosubcortical relationships based on inhibitory neuronography does not always agree with the experimental evidence obtained with other techniques. Reticular responses to sensory stimuli were found to be diminished during elimination of the respective cortical projection areas by local cooling (Borenstein and Buser 1960, Durinian and Rabin 1963, Rabin 1965). These results are in good agreement with the finding that in unanesthetized rats unilateral CSD decreases the arousing effect of contralateral trigeminal stimulation (Weiss and Bureš 1959, see also p. 256, Fig. 10.3). Corticocaudate influences were demonstrated with a similar technique in cats. Encabo and Buser (1964) and La Grutta, Abbadessa, Avelone, and Commare (1966) reported a decrease in auditory evoked potentials in the caudate nucleus after application of isotonic KCl onto the auditory cortex. Giammanco and Paderni (1967) found that potassium blockade of the somatosensory cortex affected in the same manner caudate responses to sciatic nerve stimulation. Spontaneous activity of the head and body of the caudate nucleus (Paderni and Giammanco 1967, 1968) was decreased from 80 to 150 μV to 30 to 60 μV during KCl-induced depression of the ECoG in the frontal cortex (sigmoid gyri) but was unaffected by occipital depression (lateral gyrus). Functional blockade of cortical projection areas also decreases the amplitude of sensory evoked potentials in nonspecific thalamic nuclei (Rabin 1964, Buser, Bruner, and Sindberg 1963) but according to the latter authors it does not affect evoked responses in the specific thalamic relays. Meschersky and Gustson (1964) and Gustson (1963) described reduction of visual evoked responses in the lateral geniculate body during CSD in the rabbit. Santibañez and Espinoza (1968) reported a striking reduction of hypothalamic evoked potentials to sensory stimuli during SD induced in cat cerebral cortex by mechanical stimulation. Whereas all the above findings support the notion of predominant cortical facilitation of subcortical centers, Narikashvili (1963) reported an increase of evoked responses in specific thalamic nuclei during postparoxysmal cortical depression in cats. An increase of auditory and visual evoked responses in the ventral medial nucleus of the thalamus during cortical cooling was observed by Massion and Meulders (1961).

The discrepancies in the above findings are due not only to the different functional ablation techniques used, but also to the difficult interpretation of gross EEG potentials. Without microelectrode recording it is often impossible to decide whether the observed reduction of the evoked potentials is due to inhibition or occlusion. Thus the decrease of long latency reticular responses to sensory stimuli during CSD (Weiss and Fifková 1961b) could be due to occlusion brought about by excitation of 60% of reticular units (Bureš, Burešová, and Fifková 1961). Microelectrode recording of reticular unit reactions to single-shock stimulation of the sciatic nerve or to auditory stimuli revealed, however, that during suppression of cortical evoked potentials, sensory reactions are decreased in 60% of reticular units, the spontaneous activity of which remained unchanged (Bureš and Burešová 1964). The decrease of reticular responses (Fig. 8.7) seems to be due to elimination of corticoreticular feedback and to reduction of reticular excitability following the brief initial excitation. An increased threshold of the tegmental escape reaction during repeated CSD waves in one hemisphere was also found by Rüdiger and Bureš (1962).

Units in the ventral posterior nucleus of the cat thalamus (Waller and Feldman 1967) continued to respond to lemniscal stimulation throughout the inactivation phase caused by cortical SD, but at the same time they ceased to react to reticular stimulation. This important observation indicates that CSD may modify evoked potentials even in the specific relay nuclei when the sensory stimuli cause marked activation of their reticular inputs. It is understandable that the tonic unit reactions to prolonged sensory stimuli are affected by these mechanisms more than the phasic responses to the brief stimuli used to modify the EEG activity (Fig. 8.7). The tonic reactions offer better opportunity for full development of feedback mechanisms involving different levels of the sensory pathways as well as various nonspecific structures. This assertion is illustrated by the different effects of CSD on the EEG and unit responses in the ipsilateral inferior colliculus. Whereas macroelectrode recording revealed no changes of evoked potentials to clicks (Weiss and Fifková 1961a, Fifková and Bureš 1966), reactions to prolonged auditory stimuli (0.2 to 2.0 sec) decreased during functional decortication in 50% and remained unchanged in only 37% of collicular neurons (Burešová, Marusyeva, Bureš, and Fifková 1964).

Cortical SD was also employed to differentiate between local and remote sources of EEG activity. Schwartzbaum, Kreinick, and Mello (1972) found that the 7 Hz EEG activity accompanying reinforcing licking behavior in rats is not diminished during ipsilateral CSD. This observation suggests an extracortical origin of the observed rhythms. Bureš, Burešová, Weiss, and Fifková (1963) failed to suppress the monopolarly recorded recruiting responses in rat cerebral cortex by CSD which blocked recruiting in bipolar recordings. Such result indicates differential contribution of extracortical generators to the monopolar and bipolar records.

In other studies CSD was applied to test the independent existence of the so called "mirror focus" which develops in a cortical area symmetrical to the primary epileptic focus established by local application of drugs or by other means. The dependent mirror focus is suppressed by CSD ipsilateral to the primary focus. Activity of the

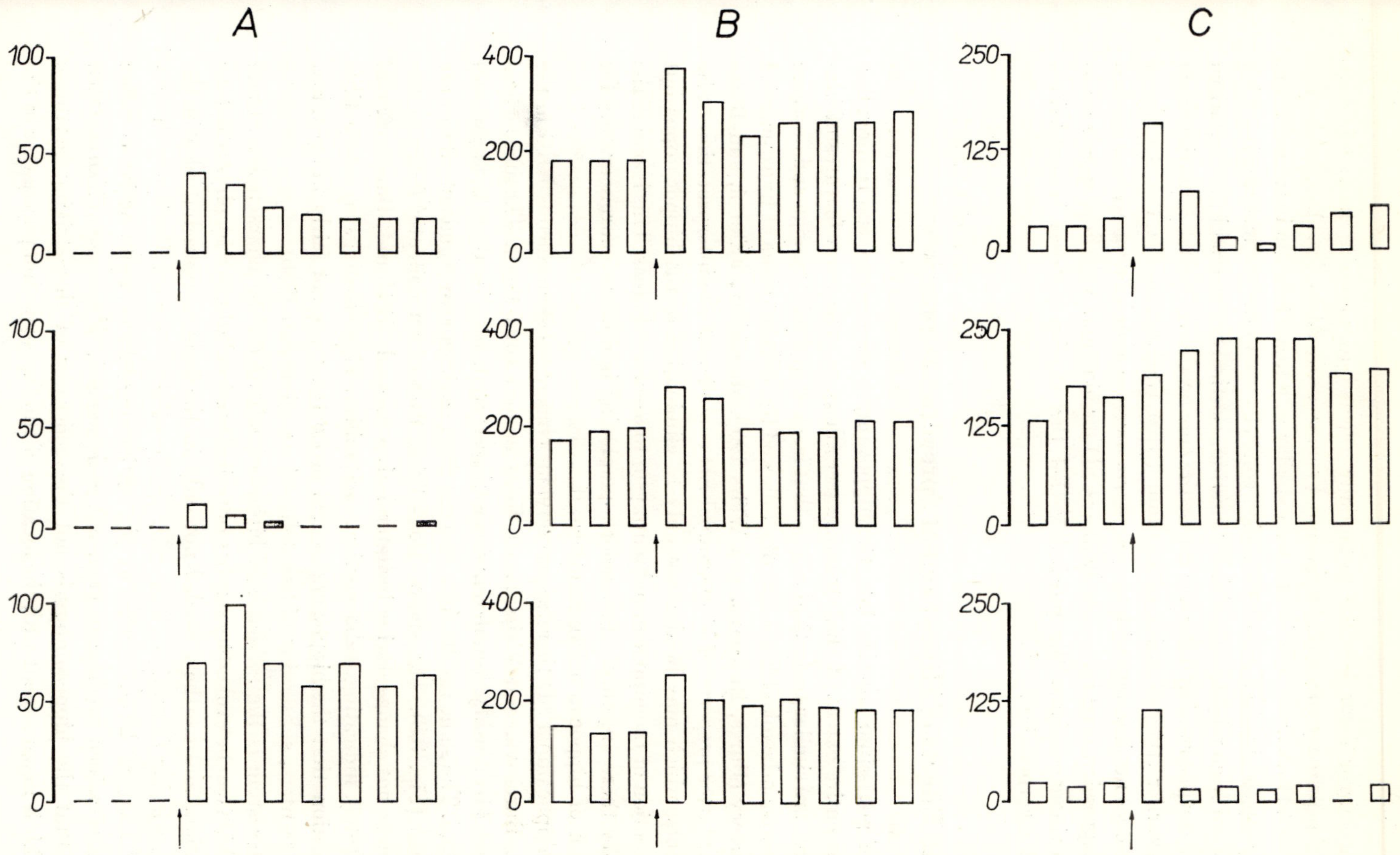

Fig. 8. 7. Changes of evoked activity of reticular neurons induced by CSD. Poststimulus histogram (*PSH*) due to sciatic nerve stimulation. Columns correspond to activity integrated at 10 consecutive 0.5-sec intervals. Ten responses were summated to construct one histogram. Above, middle, and below are before, during, and after CSD, respectively. *(A)* Reticular reaction decreased while spontaneous activity was absent. *(B)* Reaction decreased while spontaneous activity remained unchanged. *(C)* Reaction decreased while spontaneous activity increased (Bureš and Burešová 1964).

independent mirror focus is not substantially affected by CSD in the hemisphere containing the primary focus (Holubář and Fischer 1967, Atsev 1966).

Gartside (1971) used unilateral CSD in a similar way to analyse the increase of unit firing slowly developing in the cortical region contralateral to the cortical area in which the activity had been raised by anodal polarisation. Cortical SD evoked in the polarized cortex 1 hr after polarization did not decrease the enhanced activity on the unstimulated side. In an earlier study Gartside (1968) found that CSD evoked in the stimulated hemisphere does not interfere with the long-term increase of unit firing, which returned to the predepression level immediately after CSD termination. This finding was interpreted as evidence against the possibility that the activity increase is maintained by impulse reverberation.

3. Remote Effects of Hippocampal Spreading Depression

Injection of potassium chloride into the hippocampus evokes SD waves spreading through the entire extent of this structure (see Chap. 6). The main features of hippocampal SD are similar to cortical SD — that is, slow potential change and decrease of spontaneous and evoked EEG activity followed by different signs of hyperactivity during recovery (Bureš, Burešová, and Weiss 1960, Monakhov, Fifková, and Bureš 1962b). The latter property of hippocampal SD complicates the interpretation of its remote effects, which may be due not only to elimination of the hippocampus but also to projection of the hippocampal paroxysm to associated areas. This is one of the reasons, why there are only a few reports employing inhibitory neuronography for investigation of hippocampal connections.

During hippocampal SD there are no obvious changes of spontaneous EEG in the rat (Bureš, Burešová, and Weiss 1960, Weiss and Fifková 1960). The neocortical arousal evoked by sensory stimuli remains well preserved, and visual evoked responses are unaffected. The same results were also obtained during paroxysmal activity in the hippocampus (Fig. 8.8). The spontaneous firing rate of an epileptic focus in the neocortex does not change during ipsilateral hippocampal SD (Bureš, Burešová, and Janebová 1968), indicating stable cortical excitability. These findings are compatible with the notion that the hippocampus and neocortex represent fairly independent integration centers, subserving different functions (MacLean 1958).

More interesting is the influence of hippocampal SD on the characteristic theta activity, which can be evoked by sensory or reticular stimulation, or by physostigmine administration, and can be recorded not only in the hippocampus but also in the tegmental reticular formation, thalamus, and medial neocortex. During both unilateral and bilateral hippocampal SD physostigmine-induced theta activity in the tegmentum remained unchanged (Fig. 8.9, Bohdanecký, Weiss, and Fifková 1963) indicating that the hippocampus is not the generator of this striking rhythmic activity. This is in agreement with the location of the theta-rhythm pacemaker in the

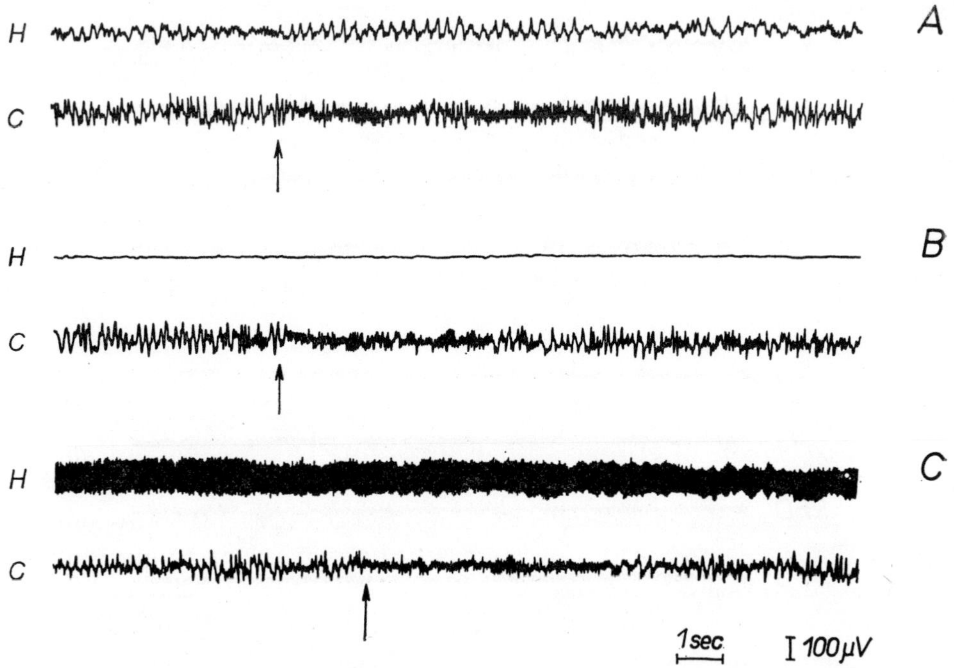

Fig. 8. 8. Cortical and hippocampal EEG activity during SD or seizure discharge in the hippocampus. Unanesthetized curarized rat. *H* is the bipolar recording from hippocampus; *C* is the bipolar recording from cortical surface. *(A)* Before hippocampal SD. External stimulus (arrow) elicits desynchronization in the cortex and theta rhythm in the hippocampus. *(B)* A marked decrease in activity occurred in the hippocampus during hippocampal SD, but the cortical arousal reaction remained unchanged. *(C)* Cortical arousal reaction was maintained even in the presence of a violent paroxysmal discharge in the hippocampus (Bureš, Burešová, and Weiss 1960).

septum (Petsche, Stumpf, and Gogolak 1962, Stumpf, Petsche, and Gogolak 1962). In contrast to the above findings, the amplitude of the slow irregular activity induced in the reticular formation by atropine is decreased to 40% of predepression level by bilateral hippocampal SD and to 15 % by bilateral cortical SD (Bohdanecký, Weiss, and Fifková 1964). Since the cortical slow wave activity evoked by atropine was not changed under the same conditions, the conclusion seems to be justified that the hippocampus is more closely related to the reticular formation than to the diencephalic synchronizing centers forming the main generator of the slow synchronous waves in the brain. Investigation of spontaneous activity of reticular units in unanesthetized curarized rats failed to reveal, however, any significant changes during unilateral hippocampal SD in more than 75 % of neurons (Bureš, Burešová, and Fifková 1961). Remote effects of hippocampal SD on unit activity in other brain regions have not yet been systematically studied.

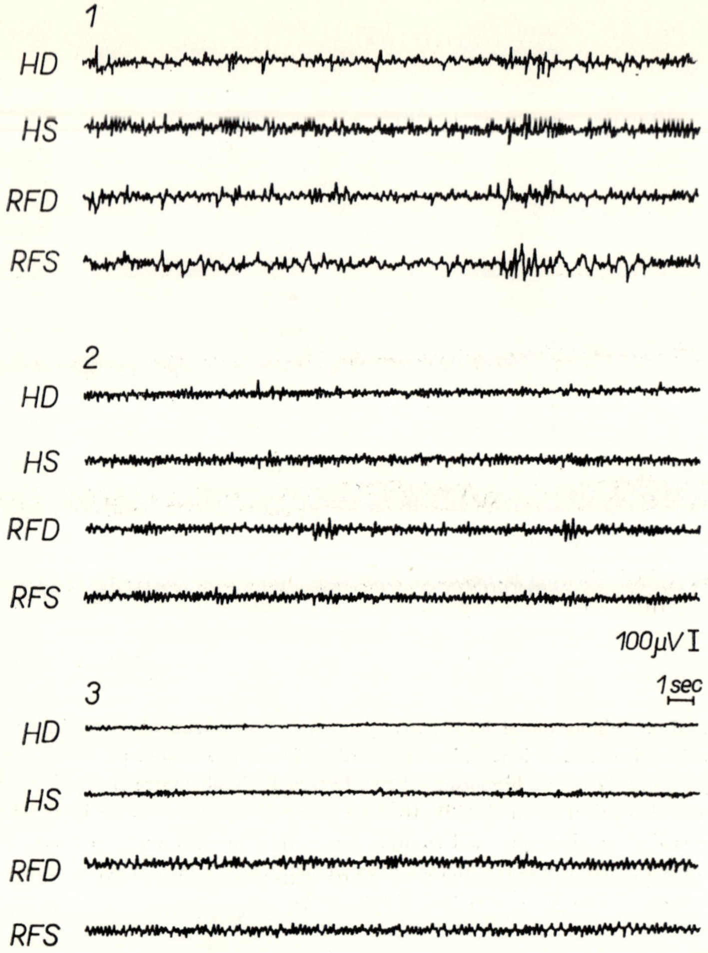

Fig. 8. 9. The influence of bilateral hippocampal SD in rat on the tegmental theta activity induced by physostigmine administration. Chronic experiment: (1) before physostigmine administration; (2) after physostigmine administration; (3) during bilateral hippocampal SD; EEG activity was recorded from both hippocampi *(HS* and *HD)* and right and left *(RFD* and *RFS)* tegmental reticular formation (Bohdanecký, Weiss, and Fifková 1963).

4. Remote Effects of Thalamic Spreading Depression

The discovery of SD in the thalamus of rats (Fifková 1964b, 1966a, see Chap. 6) made it possible to apply the principles of inhibitory neuronography in the study of the functional connections of this structure.

The SPC accompanying thalamic SD and the limits of spreading were described in Chap. 6. Since on the side of KCl application SD sometimes appears in nearby structures (mainly hippocampus) most observations on the remote effects of thalamic SD were made in the contralateral hemisphere, the thalamus of which was affected by the SD process alone (Bureš, Burešová, Fifková, and Rabending 1965, 1966).

Spontaneous and Evoked EEG Activity

After KCl injection into the right anterior thalamus (about 1.5 to 2.0 mm from the midline) no change in the EEG could be detected in the left hemisphere until the slow potential wave entered the left thalamus (usually after a delay of about 40 sec). The EEG was abruptly depressed, became irregular, and showed periods of complete silence alternating with isolated spikes or bursts of slow waves. The maximum effect lasted for 20 to 30 sec and full recovery was reached after 90 sec. With a row of electrodes applied in a rostrocaudal direction onto the cortical surface the EEG changes developed slightly earlier in the frontal than in the occipital leads (Fig. 8.10).

The rostrocaudal propagation of the cortical changes accompanying thalamic SD is still better expressed when recording evoked responses to different sensory modalities. Cortical evoked potentials to stimulation of the contralateral sciatic nerve were unaffected by SD in the contralateral thalamus, but as soon as the ipsilateral thalamus was invaded by the SPC they disappeared completely for approximately 30 sec and gradually recovered over the following 60 sec. Depression of sciatic evoked potentials coincided rather well with the decrease in spontaneous EEG activity. Auditory evoked potentials disappeared slightly later (10 to 20-sec delay) but were otherwise affected in the same way as the somatosensory ones. The visual evoked potentials were influenced in two distinct phases. During the decrease in spontaneous EEG activity, the amplitude of visual evoked potentials decreased over 20 to 30 sec to about two thirds of the predepression amplitude. After a shortlasting recovery (30 sec) the visual evoked potentials were decreased again and completely abolished for about 30 sec, even though the EEG in the rostral part of the hemisphere was already more or less normal (Fig. 8.10). The depression of visual evoked responses changed rapidly (over approximately 15 sec) into a phase of potentiation when both the positive and negative components of the cortical evoked potentials increased for approximately 30 sec to 170% of the predepression amplitude. In the interval following full depression, latent periods of both auditory and visual evoked responses were prolonged by 2.5 and 4.5 msec respectively, indicating increased synaptic delays and/or slower conduction through the radiation fibers (Fifková and Bureš 1966).

Contrasting with the effect on sensory evoked potentials, thalamic SD does not significantly influence responses in the motor cortex of rats (Bureš and Fifková 1968), evoked by antidromic stimulation of the pyramidal tract at the pontine level.

Results of over 100 experiments are summarized in Fig. 8.11. The recordings from different cortical areas were synchronized by the time the SPC in the rostral thalamus

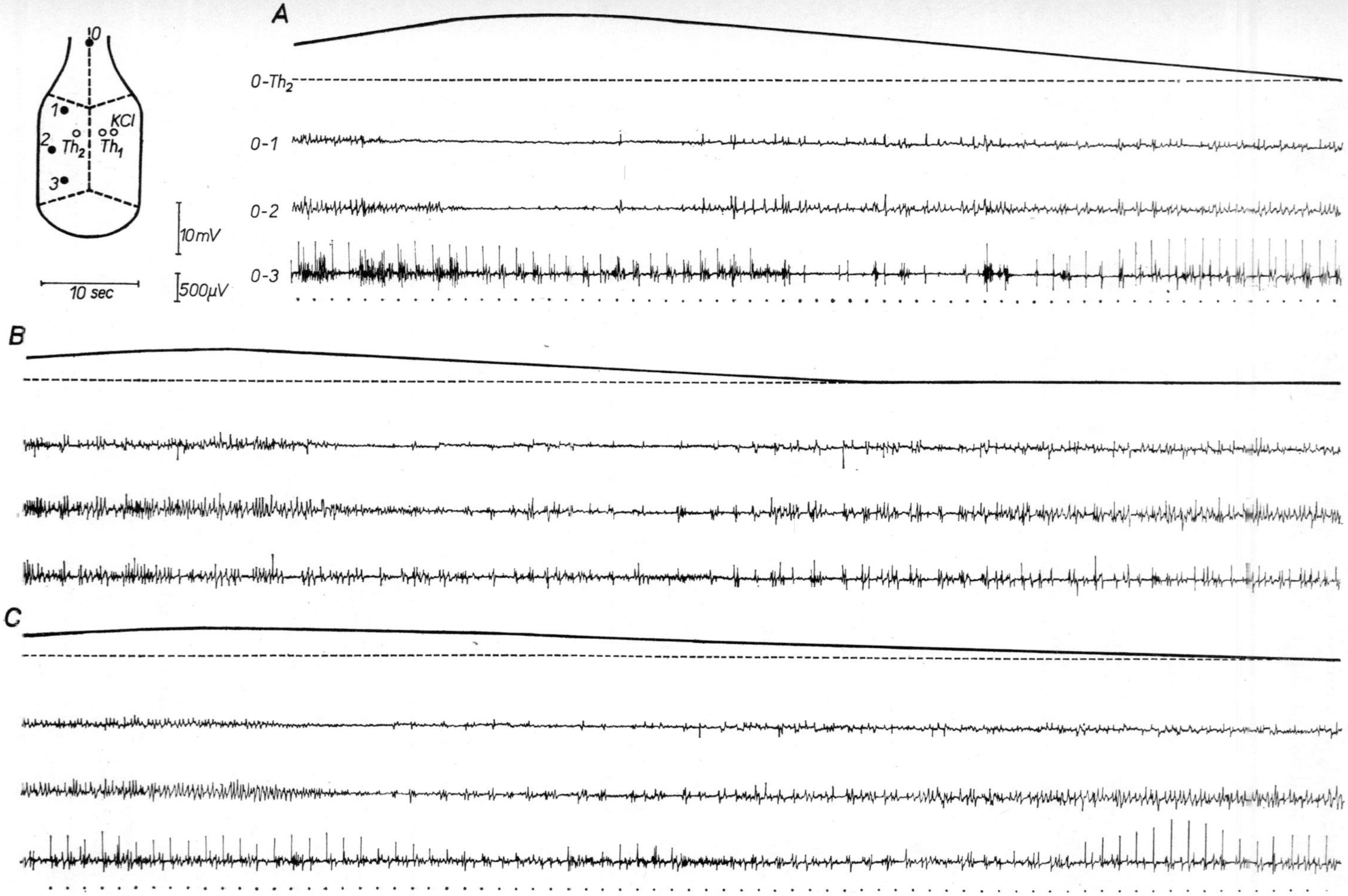

Fig. 8. 10. Changes of spontaneous EEG activity and of visual evoked responses during ipsilateral thalamic SD. *(A, C)* Recordings from two different rats during visual stimulation at 0.6/sec. *(B)* Same rat as in *(C)* without visual stimulation. Electrode position indicated in the inset diagram. Symbols: 0, reference electrode; 1, 2, 3, cortical electrodes for EEG recording; Th_1, Th_2, capillary electrodes for recording the thalamic slow potential; *KCl*, cannula for KCl application. Calibration: 500 μV for EEG; 10 mV for SPC. Upward deflection is positive in the EEG and negative in the SPC recordings. Stimulus application indicated by dots below the recordings. Note rostrocaudal propagation of EEG depression. The second phase of depression

underlying the cortical electrodes attained 50%. The surface positive components of the evoked responses were averaged in 10-sec intervals and expressed as percentages of the predepression amplitudes. The time course of the changes of evoked

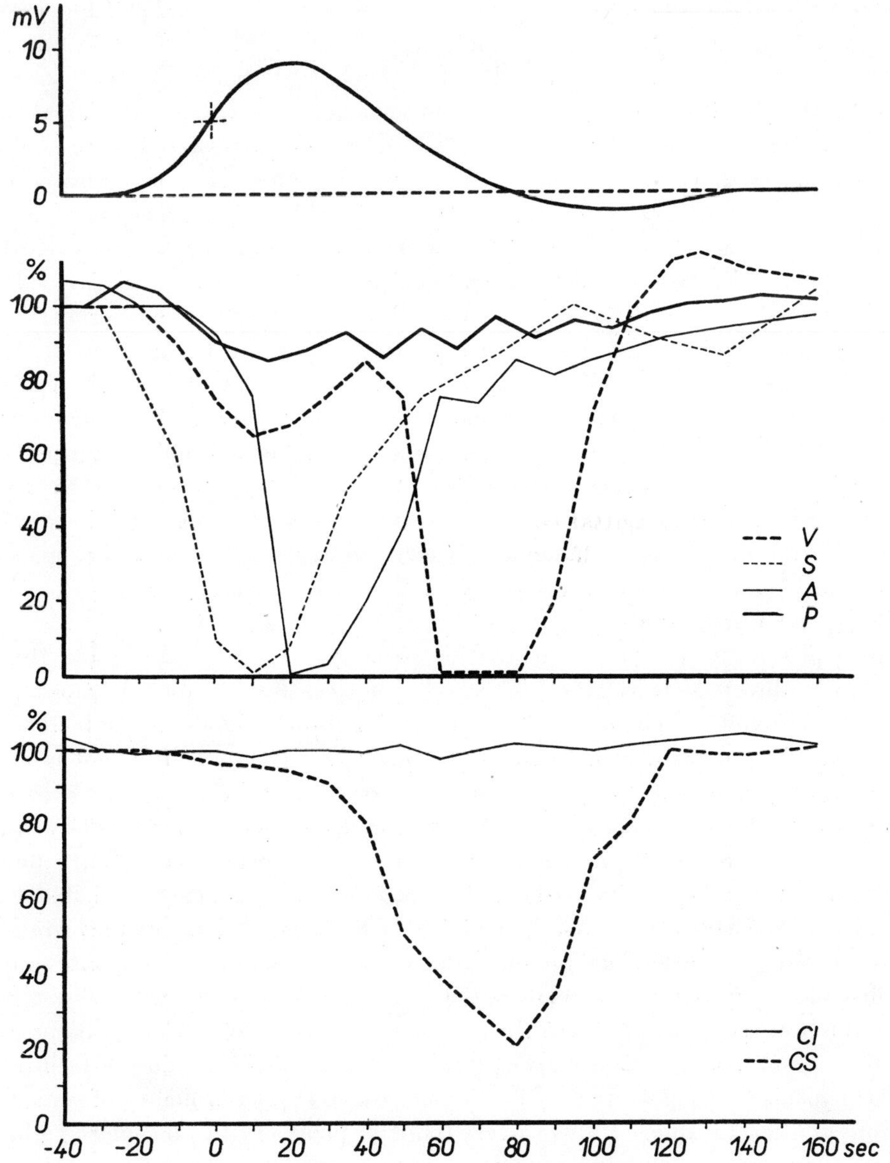

Fig. 8. 11. Average amplitude of auditory cortical *(A)* and collicular *(CI)*, visual cortical *(V)* and collicular *(CS)*, somatosensory cortical *(S)*, and antidromic pyramidal *(P)* evoked responses during thalamic SD (above). Curves represent mean amplitudes of the response in percentage of predepression values, averaged at 10-sec intervals. All changes were synchronized to the time when SPC in the ipsilateral thalamus attained 50 % of maximum negativity (zero of the time axis).

potentials is in agreement with the anatomical data. The dorso-latero-ventral aspect of the ventral nucleus relaying the sciatic volleys is approximately 1 mm nearer to the point of injection than the medial geniculate body and this distance accounts for the 10 to 15-sec delay between the depression of somatosensory and auditory-evoked responses. The long delay of the second phase of suppression of visual evoked responses is not due to distance, since the lateral geniculate body is actually closer to the point of KCl injection than the medial geniculate body, and SD should reach it sooner than the latter structure. Whereas the medial geniculate body is a direct continuation of the ventral complex, the lateral geniculate body is separated from the rest of thalamus by the lamina medullaris externa. This compact layer of myelinated fibers prevents direct spreading of SD into the lateral geniculate body, which can be entered by SD only when diffusion across the white-matter barrier raises the K^+ concentration to the threshold level. In about 50% of the experiments the threshold was never reached and the second phase was absent. In other rats thalamic SD invaded the lateral geniculate body directly, the first and second phase coinciding in the same time interval. This was usually the case in the injected thalamus (Burešová, Fifková, and Bureš 1966) where increased level of K^+ and a changed configuration of the SD wavefront facilitated penetration of SD across the white-matter barrier. A parasagittal cut along the medial surface of the lateral geniculate separated it from the rest of thalamus so effectively that the first partial suppression of visual evoked responses was almost never followed by the second complete blockade (Fifková and Bureš 1966).

The biphasic effect of thalamic SD on visual evoked responses shows that in addition to direct depolarization of the relay nucleus (second phase) transmission of the afferent volley is also affected by other mechanisms. Elimination of facilitatory influences of the depressed thalamus on the lateral geniculate body is not probable since the first depression wave was well preserved even when most connections between the lateral geniculate and the rest of thalamus were severed (Fifková and Bureš 1966). More important can be the decrease of cortical excitability due to elimination of the nonspecific thalamic influence on the visual cortex. Thalamic SD can also block conduction through the optic radiation fibers, where they are close to the posterior thalamus. The prolonged latencies of visual evoked responses during the first phase support such an explanation.

An interesting feature of SD in the lateral geniculate body is the postdepression potentiation of visual evoked responses in the cortex, obviously due to facilitation of the geniculate response. It may be an expression of supernormality of geniculate neurons at a certain stage of SD recovery (positive phase of SPC) but more probably is a mechanism analogous to post-tetanic potentiation. Depolarization of the presynaptic terminals of the optic tract fibers by the increased K^+ level may increase the rate of transmitter output and higher efficiency of the presynaptic volley becomes apparent as soon as postsynaptic elements are responsive again. Postdepression potentiation was not observed in somatosensory and acoustic pathways probably because post-tetanic potentiation is less pronounced in these structures and may be counteracted at the cortical level by the nonspecific effect of thalamic SD.

Collicular evoked responses to acoustic and visual stimuli are influenced by the thalamic SD in a different manner (Fig. 8.11). Whereas auditory evoked potentials in the inferior colliculus remained unchanged throughout the maximum depression of cortical evoked responses, visual evoked potentials in the superior colliculus were completely blocked when SD invaded the lateral geniculate body (Fig. 8.12), and their latency was slightly prolonged before and after disappearance of the response. Since thalamic SD does not reach the superior colliculus and since the retinotectal projection is not synaptically interpolated at the thalamic level, the suppression of collicular responses can only be due to a conduction block caused by a K^+ excess in the thin layer of optic tract fibers surrounding the lateral and dorsal surfaces of the lateral geniculate body (Fig. 8.27). The anatomical situation is quite different in the inferior colliculus, the acoustic afferents of which pass upwards and at no point come close to the thalamus.

Thalamic SD also interferes with transmission of nonspecific influences. Thus cortical arousal, elicited in unanesthetized curarized rats by electrical stimulation of the mesencephalic reticular formation (Fig. 8.13) was blocked at the height of thalamic SD (Bureš, Burešová, Fifková, and Rabending 1966). Instead of evoking cortical desynchronization, reticular stimulation sometimes accentuated the irregular slow wave pattern typical for the functionally deafferented cortex. These results confirm the assumption that reticular arousing influences reach the cortex through nonspecific thalamic nuclei.

The reduction of spontaneous cortical activity and blockade of cortical arousal are accompanied by a striking decrease of cortical excitability. This was shown by Bureš, Burešová, and Janebová (1968) in a series of experiments demonstrating the effect of thalamic SD on the activity of a cortical epileptic focus induced by topical application of metrazol or G-penicillin. Elimination of the thalamus caused complete cessation of spike generation for 20 sec on the average and evident slowing of the discharge rate for 40 to 60 sec (Fig. 8.14). Thalamic SD did not interfere, however, with the propagation of spikes to the contralateral hemisphere or to ipsilateral cortical areas. The results are summarized in Fig. 8.15, comparing the relative changes of the epileptic spike discharge rate with the duration of the arousal reaction. As follows from the comparison of the effects of thalamic and caudate SD (see p. 203) cortical excitability is mainly affected by nonspecific thalamocortical influences.

Thalamic synchronizing mechanisms are also affected. Since it is obvious that the recruiting response cannot be elicited by stimulation of the depressed thalamus, the SD effect can be demonstrated in a more clear way for the so-called caudate spindle (Laursen 1963) elicited by single electric shocks applied to the head of the caudate nucleus of unanesthetized, curarized rats. When thalamic SD remained limited to the thalamus contralateral to the stimulated caudate, the frequency of the waves constituting the spindle was considerably decreased in the deafferented cortex but

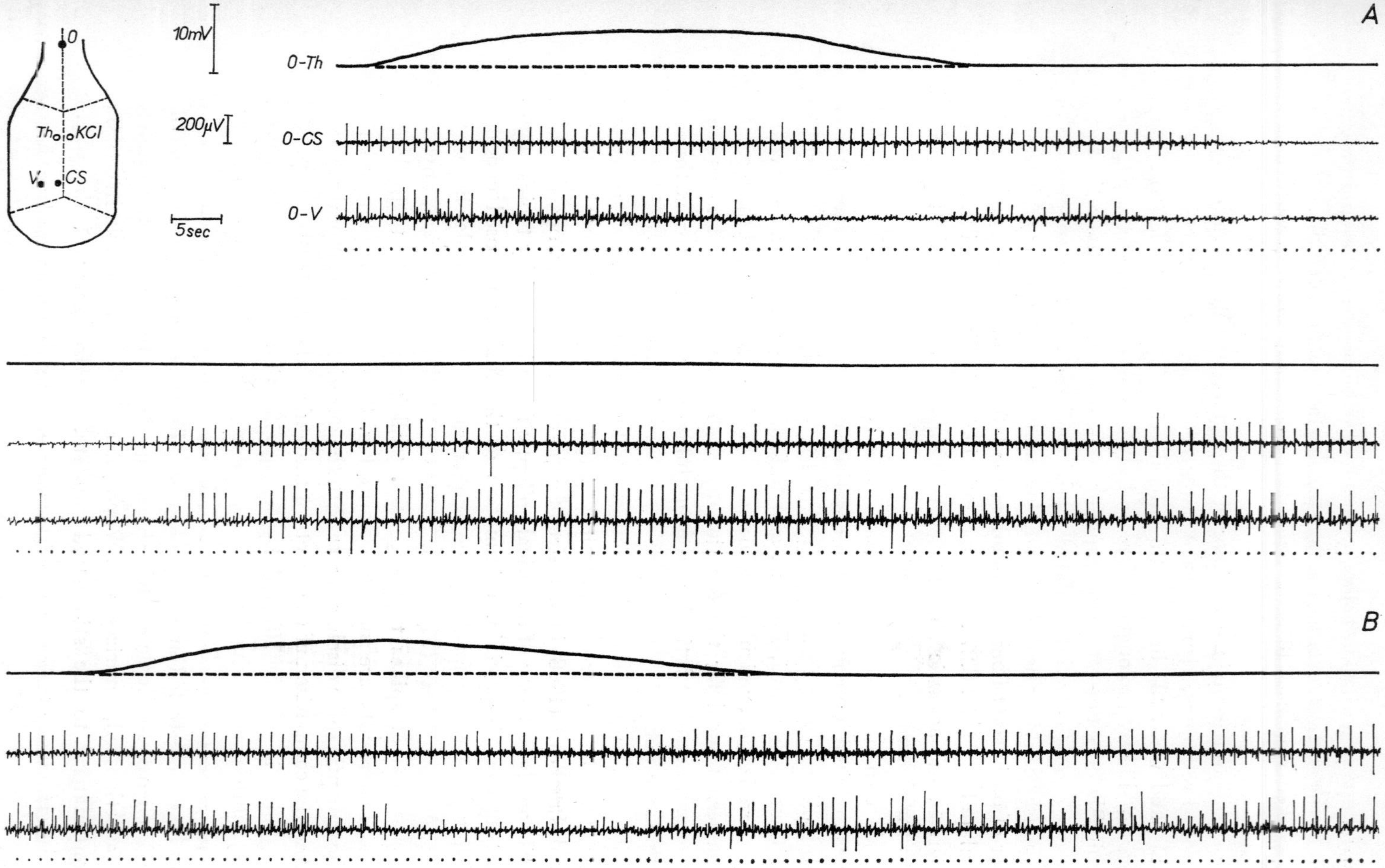

Fig. 8. 12. Biphasic *(A)* or monophasic *(B)* changes of visual evoked responses in the rat cortex during thalamic SD. Electrode location is indicated in the inset diagram. Symbols: *0*, reference electrode; *Th*, capillary electrode for recording the thalamic SPC; *KCl*, cannula for KCl application in the thalamus. *CS, V*, electrodes in the superior colliculus and visual cortex. Note that the collicular response disappeared during the second phase of the biphasic cortical reaction but that it was quite unaffected when there was no second phase of cortical suppression (Fifková and Bureš 1966).

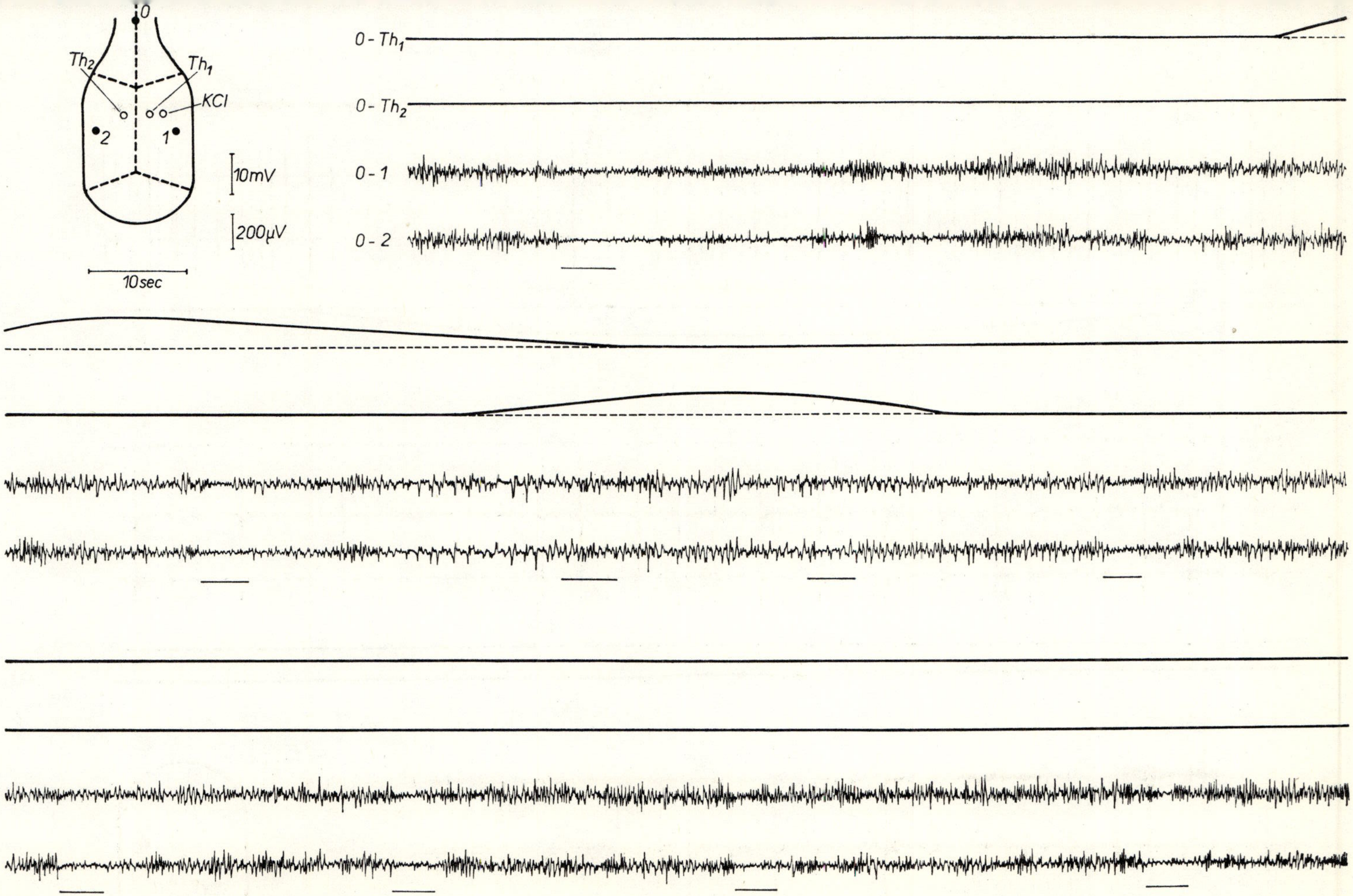

Fig. 8. 13. The effect of thalamic SD on the cortical arousal reaction evoked in unanesthetized curarized rats by 300/sec stimulation of the mesencephalic reticular formation. Position of electrodes is shown in the inset diagram. For symbols see Fig. 8. 10. Reticular stimulation is indicated by horizontal bars below the EEG recordings. Note decrease of EEG frequency and disappearance of the desynchronizing reaction during thalamic SD (Bureš, Burešová, Fifková, and Rabending 1966).

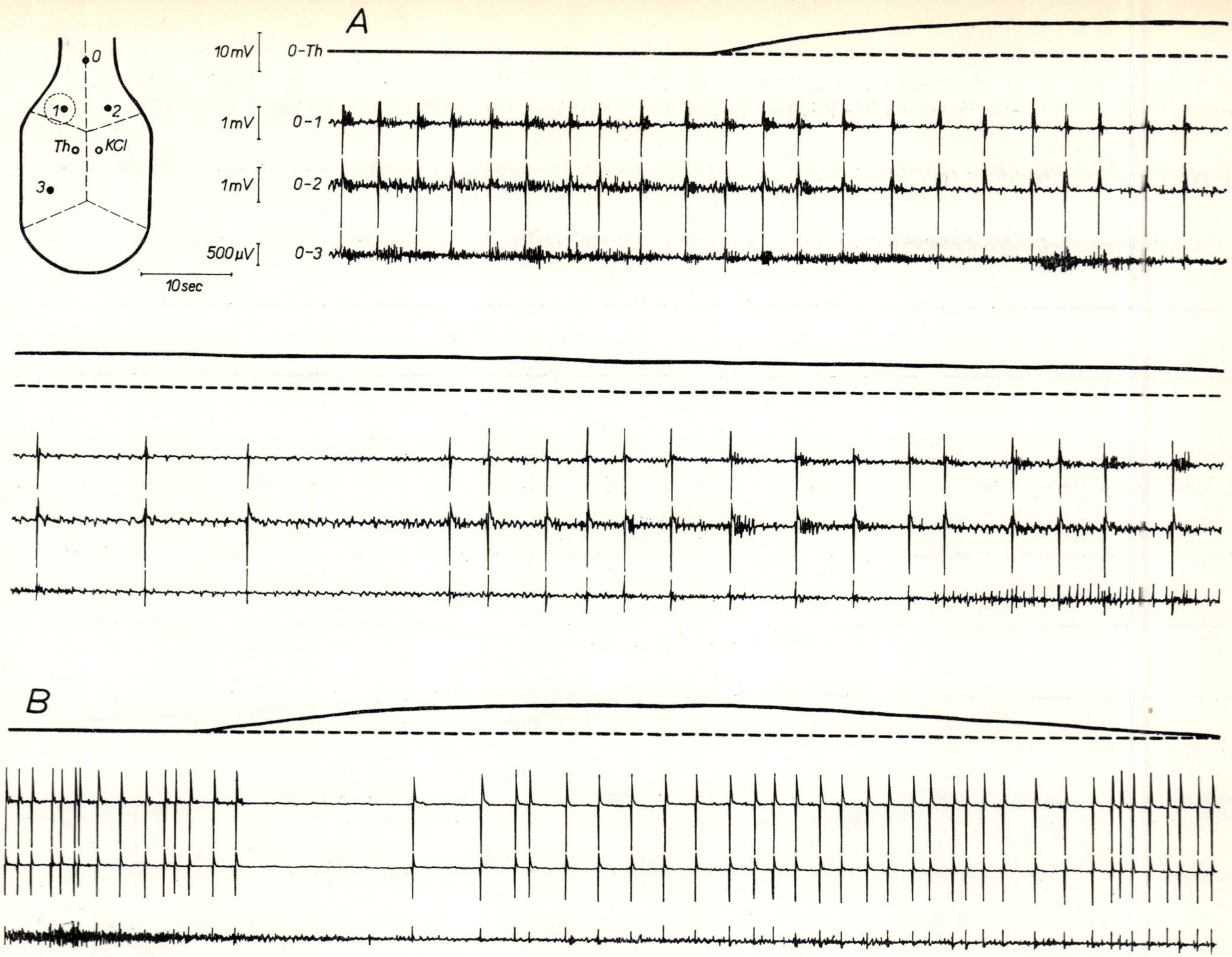

Fig. 8. 14. Effect of thalamic SD on the activity of a metrazol focus in the sensorimotor cortex. *(A)* Spikes followed by a spindle discharge. *(B)* Simple spikes. Electrode location shown in the inset diagram. For symbols see Fig. 8. 10. The region of metrazol application is circumscribed by

was unchanged in the normal hemisphere. As soon as the thalamic SD crossed the midline, caudate spindles disappeared in both hemispheres for approximately 1 min. This result is in good agreement with the assumption that caudate spindles are mediated by feedback circuits between cortex and nonspecific thalamic nuclei, which are activated by caudate stimulation. Essentially similar results were recently obtained in cats (Buchwald and Hull 1967, Trachtenberg, Hull, and Buchwald 1970); caudate spindles were blocked by SD evoked in the ventral lateral thalamic nucleus.

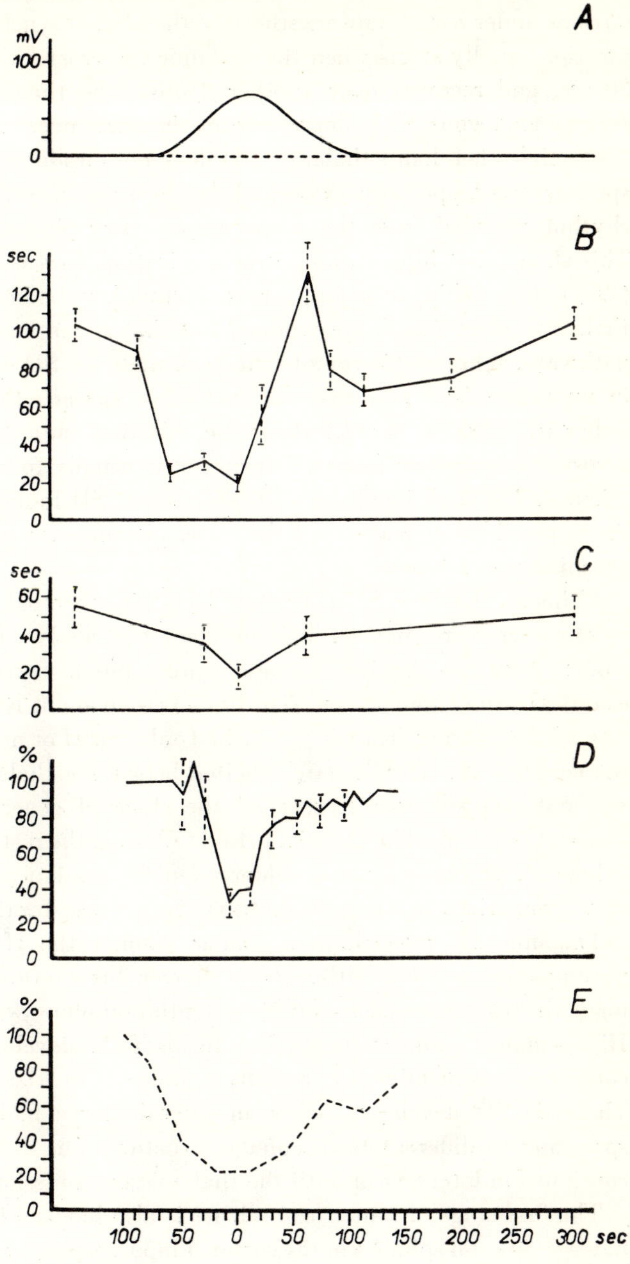

Fig. 8. 15. Effect of thalamic SD on the average duration of cortical *(B)* or hippocampal *(C)* afterdischarge, on the average discharge rate of a cortical epileptic focus *(D)* and on the relative duration of the cortical arousal reaction *(E)*. All recordings are synchronized with the maximum negativity of the thalamic SPC *(A)* (Aquino-Cias and Bureš 1966).

Much less is known about the effects of thalamic SD on the spontaneous EEG activity of subcortical centers. The caudate EEG is slowed and decreased in amplitude during thalamic SD in a similar manner to the cortical EEG (Aquino-Cias, Bureš, Fifková, and Popova 1966). The change can be detected in curarized rats but is more obvious under barbiturate anesthesia at the level of synchronized EEG activity. The depression usually starts when the thalamic SD crosses the midline, culminates within 30 sec, and recovers over another 2 min. The time course of the change closely follows analogous EEG depression in the thalamus.

On the other hand thalamic SD does not produce any clear-cut changes of the spontaneous hippocampogram and does not significantly influence the regular theta rhythm recorded from the hippocampus after physostigmine injection (1 mg/kg). This shows that hippocampal synchronization does not depend on an intact Papez (1937) circuit (hippocampus, fornix, mammilary bodies, anterior ventral nucleus of thalamus, cingulum, hippocampus) but that it can be maintained by extrathalamic pathways. Whereas the remote effects of thalamic SD on hippocampus are negligible, in unanesthetized rats thalamic SD often spreads to the overlying hippocampus either by diffusion of KCl along the injection cannula or by contiguity spreading across the brainstem fissure. Depression is usually followed by typical hippocampal seizures. The high incidence of hippocampal SD induced by thalamic SD seriously limits possible applications of the latter phenomenon in research into the functional organization of brain.

Although thalamic SD may start local hippocampal seizures, at the same time it blocks seizure irradiation. This problem was analyzed in detail in unanesthetized curarized rats by Aquino-Cias and Bureš (1967). Cortical afterdischarge evoked by electrical stimulation (20/sec, 5 to 10 sec) lasted about 100 sec on the average. Stimulation applied during thalamic SD elicited only a brief or no afterdischarge (Fig. 8.16). On the contrary an afterdischarge elicited before the thalamic SD had fully developed, was not stopped once it reached the stage of generalization. Effects of cortical stimulation, applied in the brief period following the restitution of thalamic SPC, were enhanced, probably by a postdepression facilitation at the thalamic level. Results are summarized in Fig. 8.15 showing the average duration of cortical afterdischarge.

Thalamic SD affected in a similar manner the afterdischarge evoked by hippocampal stimulation, although its shorter duration (55 sec) and greater variability made the results less clear-cut. No potentiation phase was seen in this case (Fig. 8.15). Hippocampal stimulation applied during fully developed thalamic SD was either completely ineffective or remained limited to the contralateral hippocampus. Thalamic SD developing after an afterdischarge had been initiated, modified its spreading to different telencephalic structures but did not stop the seizure, which continued in latent form until the thalamic transmission was restored.

The first stage of a metrazol seizure is also blocked by thalamic SD, which eliminates spikes and spindles in the cortex, hippocampus, caudate, and reticular formation for 100 to 120 sec. On the other hand fully developed grand mal seizures continue in spite of the thalamic blockade.

Thalamic SD interferes with the development of an epileptic seizure in several ways. In afterdischarge experiments it may reduce the excitability of the stimulated area. According to the unit activity findings, such an explanation applies to cortical

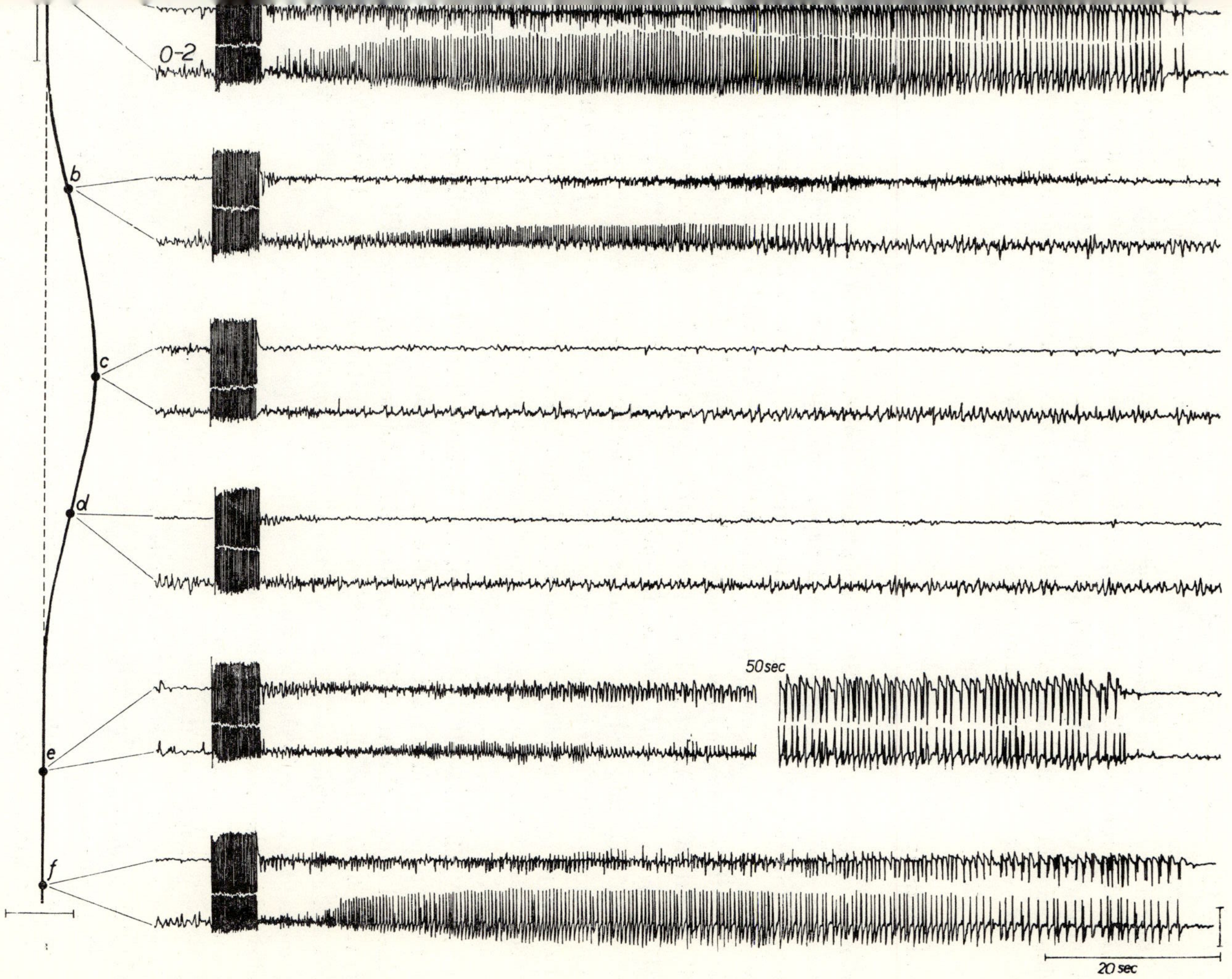

Fig. 8. 16. The effect of thalamic SD on cortical afterdischarge. Onset of cortical stimulation (frontal cortex, 20/sec, 1 msec, 5 sec) with respect to the development of thalamic SD is indicated by dots on the thalamic SPC recording (left margin). (0—1, 0—2) EEG recording from the occipital cortex contralateral or ipsilateral to the cortical stimulation. The afterdischarge is asymmetric in *(b)*, absent in *(c)* and *(d)*, and prolonged in *(e)*. Calibration ot the SPC recording: 10 mV, 20 sec (Aquino-Cias and Bureš 1967).

but not to hippocampal afterdischarge. Thalamic SD may also interfere with the propagation of the seizure, which finds most channels available for generalization blocked either by the primary depression in the thalamus or by its secondary remote effects. The feedback recruiting systems that seem to be essential for the process of seizure generalization are affected in the same manner. Since thalamic lesions prevent neither metrazol seizures (Machek, Saier, Desplan, and Naquet 1963, Starzl, Niemer, Dell, and Forgrave 1953) nor the propagation of afterdischarge to the contralateral hemisphere (Walker and Udvarhelyi 1965a, b, Udvarhelyi and Walker 1965), the elimination of the thalamus alone evidently plays a less important role in the overall blocking effect than the accompanying secondary changes.

Unit Activity

Remote effects of thalamic SD on spontaneous unit activity in functionally related structures were examined in several papers. Sokolov, Bureš, and Fifková (1966) recorded the activity of thalamic units during SD and found in 80 % of them a deep reduction of spontaneous activity (complete silence lasting 1.5 min), preceded in 55 % of the cases by a brief discharge. Units that remained unaffected by thalamic SD (less than 20 %) were probably located in thalamic nuclei not fully invaded by the SD process. A clear-cut decrease in spontaneous activity was found also in 80 % of the subthalamic and hypothalamic units. The increase-decrease type of reaction was less frequent than in thalamic neurons, however, and the onset of the activity decrease preceded full invasion of the thalamus. Most cortical neurons (62 %) were affected in a similar way (Fig. 8.17) but the average activity decreased to 25 % of the predepression activity only, and the duration of the change did not usually exceed 3 min (Aquino-Cias, Belcheva, Bureš, and Fifková 1966). The same distribution of different types of unit reactions and the same duration of the activity decrease were observed during thalamic SD in caudate units (Aquino-Cias, Bureš, Fifková, and Popova 1966). On the other hand 50 % of the reticular units were unaffected by thalamic SD and a moderate activity increase (to 154 % of predepression rate) was the most prominent reaction in the remaining ones. Hippocampal neurons were also not much affected by thalamic SD, the increase and decrease reactions being brief and equally frequent. The results are summarized in Fig. 8.5.

When interpreting the above results, the relationships between all interacting structures must be taken into account. As can be assumed from anatomical and physiological data, elimination of the thalamus should affect cortical, caudate, and hypothalamic activity much more than the activity of reticular and hippocampal neurons. Since reduction of spontaneous activity of cortical neurons results in decreased firing in the caudate and hypothalamus, the changes observed in these structures may be not only a direct consequence of thalamic depression but also a secondary effect of the changes observed at the cortical level. The same is true for reticular changes, which were similar in the relative incidence of increase and decrease reactions to the reticular effects of cortical SD and to changes in hippocampal activity.

The cortical consequences of functional ablation of the thalamus provide important information on the nature of thalamocortical interactions. The striking reduction of EEG activity observed after cortical deafferentation has been explained by elimination of facilitatory thalamocortical tone (Bremer 1958), by interruption of corticothalamic reverberation (Chang 1950), or by suppression of thalamic synchroniz-

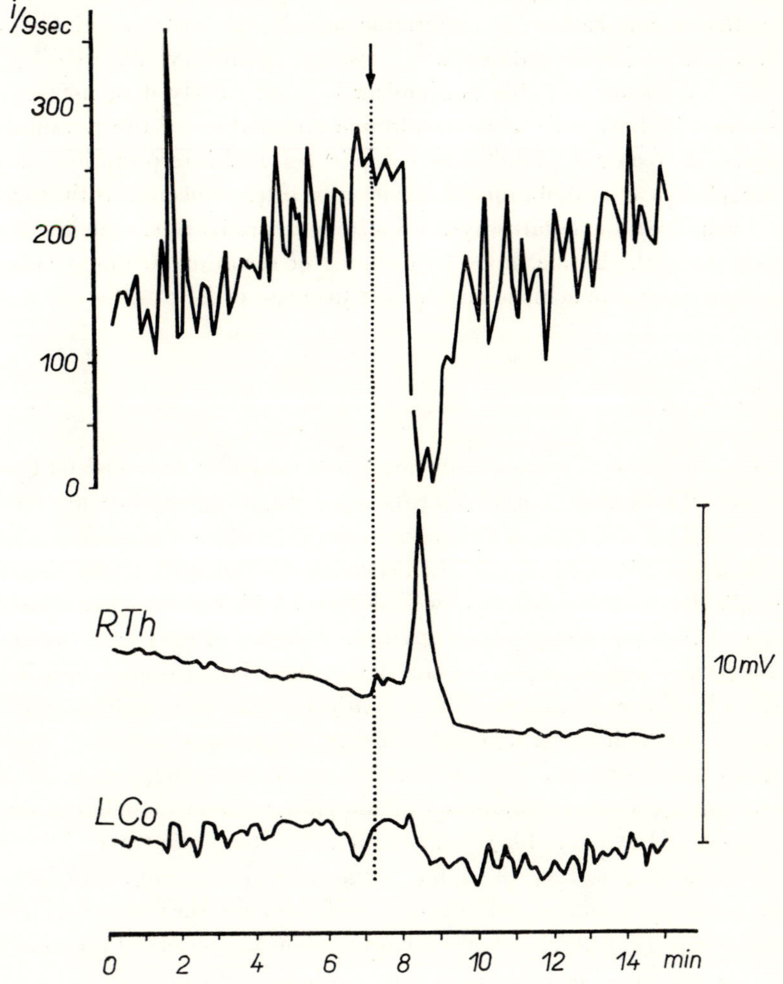

Fig. 8. 17. A typical example of the decrease of cortical unit activity during thalamic SD. (Above) Unit firing rate automatically integrated at 9-sec intervals; *RTh* and *LCo* are SPC recordings in the right thalamus and left cortex. The arrow indicates KCl injection into the left ventral thalamus. Calibration: 10 mV for SPC recordings (Aquino-Cias, Belcheva, Bureš, and Fifková 1966).

ing centers (Morrison and Dempsey 1942). Although the above mechanisms are not mutually exclusive, they all assume a predominantly excitatory thalamocortical influence. Further support for this view was obtained by intracellular recording from cortical neurons (Jasper and Stefanis 1965, Watanabe and Creutzfeldt 1966, Creutzfeldt, Watanabe, and Lux 1966a, b) showing a clear-cut preponderance of spontaneous and evoked excitatory postsynaptic potentials (EPSPs) over inhibitory postsynaptic potentials (IPSPs). It seems that cortical IPSPs induced by electrical stimulation of the central medial nucleus, ventrobasal thalamus, and caudate nucleus (Klee and Lux 1962, Lux and Klee 1962) are not due to activation of a thalamocortical inhibitory pathway but rather to antidromic activity in corticofugal fibers, which induces through recurrent collaterals a powerful inhibitory influence on cortical neurons. The significance of this mechanism is most clearly demonstrated by the IPSPs recorded in Betz cells after antidromic stimulation of the pyramidal tract. The presence of recurrent inhibition complicates the interpretation of changes induced by electrical stimulation of structures interconnected with the area of recording by bidirectional pathways. Inhibitory neuronography makes it possible to eliminate the orthodromic input to the area of recording without causing antidromic activation, and to achieve an absolute decrease of EPSPs.

Pupillary Paralysis

Cortical and subcortical SDs are usually not accompanied by any consistent peripheral manifestations. Thalamic SD in albino rats is an exception, since its presence can be reliably detected by a striking mydriasis starting immediately after KCl application, culminating about 90 sec later, and then slowly subsiding with a half time of about 5 min (Fig. 8.18). As the mydriasis is well developed in *encephale isolé* rats it cannot be due to activation of the sympathetic system but only to a dramatic decrement of the parasympathetic pupilloconstrictor tone. The mydriasis developed synchronously in both eyes even when KCl was injected 2.5 mm lateral from the midline and SD invaded the ipsilateral lateral geniculate body approximately 1 min earlier than the contralateral one. Such synchrony contradicts the possibility that the pupillary dilation is due to elimination of the photic reflex; the afferent link of this reflex is constituted by nerve fibers that branch from the optic tract to form a sheet around the caudal aspect of the lateral geniculate body and enter the superior colliculus. Although thalamic SD blocks conduction in these fibers (Fifková and Bureš 1966, see p. 191), the blockade cannot explain the observed pupillary dilation since the maximal effect is attained at a time when conduction on the contralateral side is still well preserved and the unilateral photic reflex maintains a nearly normal pupilloconstrictor tone. Remote influencing of the Edinger-Westphal nucleus by elimination of some tonic inflow is indicated by the early onset of mydriasis, which is detectable in some experiments within 10 sec after thalamic injection, that is at

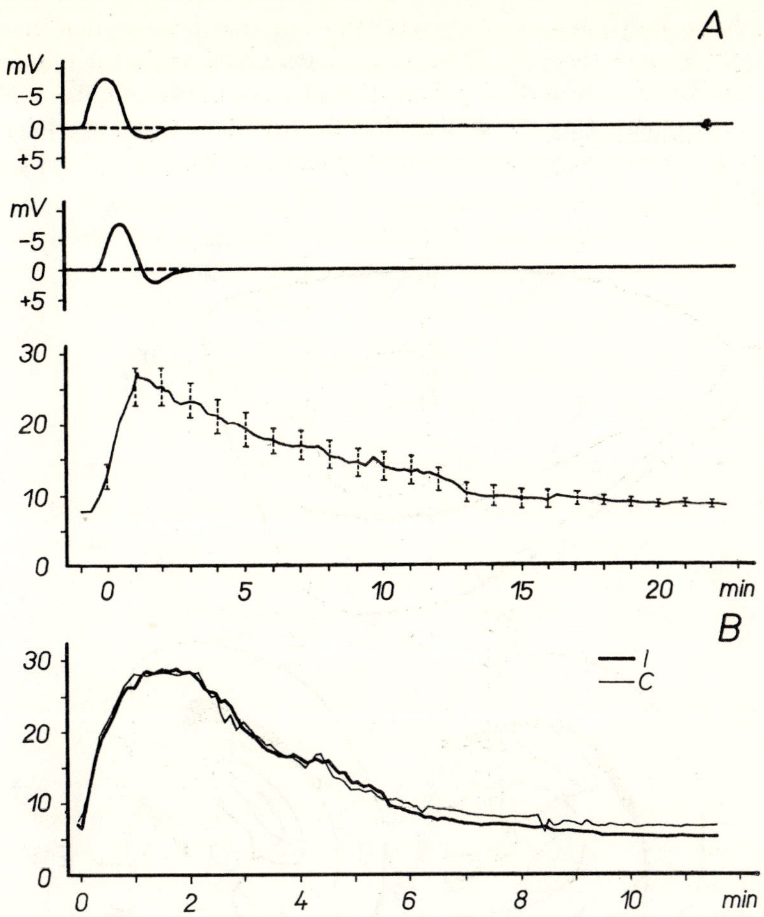

Fig. 8. 18. Mydriatic response to thalamic SD. *(A)* Thalamic SPC ipsilateral (upper curve) and contralateral (middle curve) to KCl injection; pupillary diameter (lower curve) in ocular micrometer units (six divisions equal 1 mm). Zero of the time axis corresponds to the time when SPC attains 50 % of maximum negativity in the contralateral thalamus. Vertical bars denote standard errors of the mean values. *(B)* Pupillary diameter of the right (ipsilateral, *I*) and left (contralateral, *C*) eye. Zero of the time axis corresponds to KCl application. Note the synchrony of the pupillary changes in both eyes (Burešová, Fifková, and Bureš 1966).

a time when thalamic SD is more or less limited to the nonspecific and somatosensory nuclei on one side. Cortical SD also has a slight initial mydriatic effect, which rapidly subsides, however, in spite of continuing EEG depression. But the remote changes cannot account for the complete pupillary paralysis developing at a time when the thalamic SD reaches the region of the isthmus and directly influences the Edinger-Westphal nucleus (Fig. 8.19). The maximum mydriasis due to thalamic SD resembles the pupillary dilation observed after aspiration of the Edinger-Westphal nucleus by King, Marchiava, and Moruzzi (1963). It seems therefore that thalamic SD either directly invades this part of the oculomotor nuclei or that it interferes with its efferent activity by causing a depolarization block of the output fibers. The latter explanation is supported by the finding that the mydriasis is not preceded by any miotic reaction corresponding to the excitatory phase of SD.

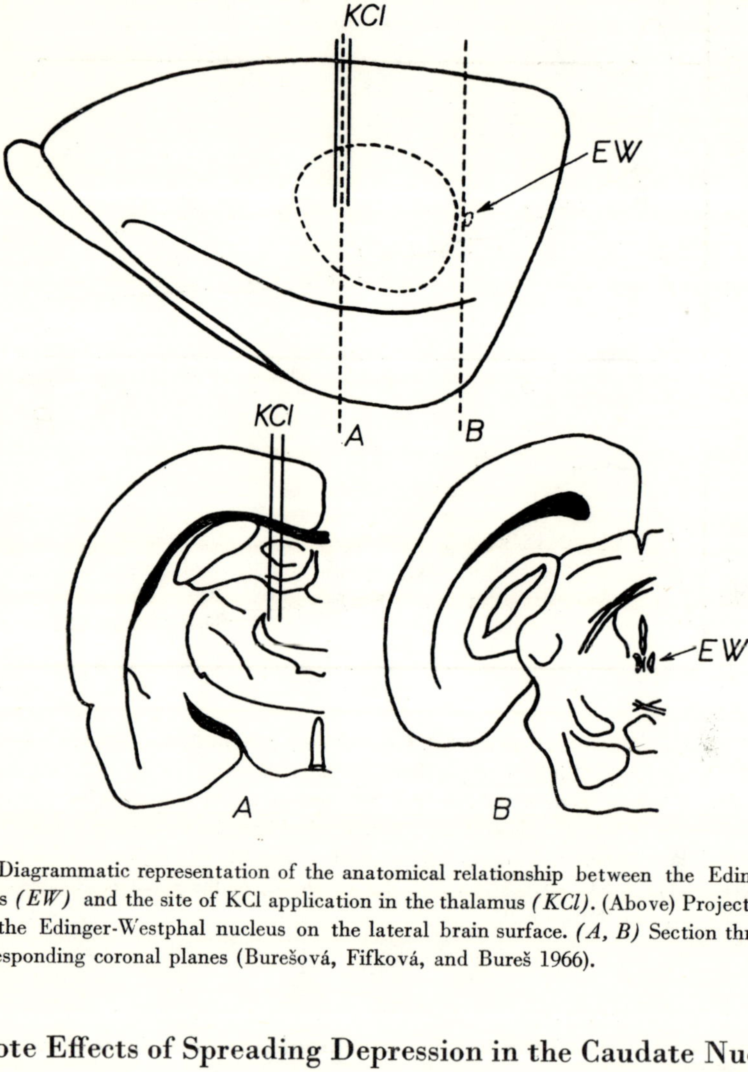

Fig. 8. 19. Diagrammatic representation of the anatomical relationship between the Edinger - Westphal nucleus *(EW)* and the site of KCl application in the thalamus *(KCl)*. (Above) Projection of thalamus and the Edinger-Westphal nucleus on the lateral brain surface. *(A, B)* Section through brain in the corresponding coronal planes (Burešová, Fifková, and Bureš 1966).

5. Remote Effects of Spreading Depression in the Caudate Nucleus

The possibility of eliciting SD in the caudate nucleus was first reported by Leão and Martins-Ferreira (1958) and the anatomical boundaries of the reaction in rats were studied in more detail by Fifková and Bureš (1964) and by Fifková and Syka (1964) (see Chap. 6). For purposes of inhibitory neuronography it is essential that the SD wave initiated in the head of the caudate nucleus enters all parts of the caudate-putamen complex, but does not reach the septum and globus pallidus. Approximately 40 % of SD waves enter the amygdala and spread from there to the neocortex, the parietal regions of which are invaded on the average after a 5-min delay. It is important therefore that possible spread to the ipsilateral cortex is monitored in all experiments and that the remote effects are evaluated only during the initial interval free of extrastriatal depression.

Spontaneous and Evoked EEG Activity

Unilateral SD in the caudate nucleus of rats causes no apparent changes of the spontaneous EEG activity in the overlying cortex (Bureš, Kozlovskaya, and Fifková 1964). Similarly it does not affect the spontaneous discharge of epileptic foci in the ipsilateral and contralateral sensorimotor cortex or in the ipsilateral visual cortex (Bureš, Burešová, and Janebová 1968). This failure to influence overall electrical activity does not indicate, however, that the basal ganglia do not influence the thalamocortical synchronizing mechanisms. Cortical recruiting responses evoked by unilateral stimulation of the nonspecific thalamus were clearly reduced as soon as SD invaded most of the caudate, and the change lasted for 3 to 4 min (Fig. 8.20).

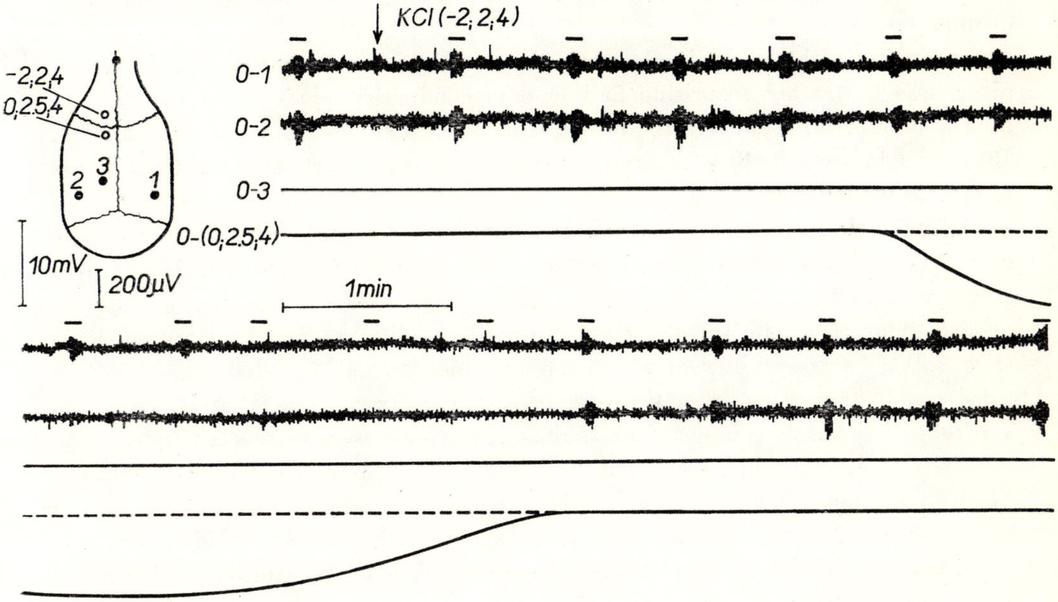

Fig. 8. 20. The effect of caudate SD on recruiting responses evoked by ipsilateral stimulation of the nonspecific thalamus. Symbols: (1, 2) Cortical electrodes for EEG recording; (3) cortical electrode for SPC; (0; 2.5; 4), capillary electrode for striatal SPC; 0, reference electrode; (—2; 2; 4), cannula for KCl microinjection. Horizontal bars above the EEG recording denote trains of thalamic stimuli. Calibration: 200 μV for EEG; 10 mV for the SPC (Bureš, Kozlovskaya, and Fifková 1964).

Synchronized spindles evoked by single thalamic shocks were affected in the same way. In this respect, remote effects of caudate SD resemble those of cortical SD (see p. 179) but are somewhat less marked in both intensity and duration (2.9 and 5.0 min, respectively).

The finding that caudate SD does not affect evoked responses in the specific thalamic relay nuclei but does cause a severe depression of the long-latency evoked responses in the nonspecific thalamic centers (Bureš, Hartman, and Lukyanova 1967) resembles the effects of CSD on these two types of thalamic responses (see p. 174). Caudate SD does not interfere with the projection of the recruiting responses toward the cortex, however, since with more intense stimuli, or with stimuli applied to the contralateral thalamus, recruiting responses can be obtained in the cortex overlying the depressed caudate nucleus even at the height of caudate depolarization.

Caudate SD can also be used to analyse the corticocaudate projection. Tolkunov (1970) recorded changes of gross responses evoked in caudate by cortical stimulation during caudate SD in rats. Careful analysis of results made it possible to demonstrate in this way the spread of the responses within the nucleus. With KCl microinjection into the caudal part of the caudate nucleus, responses evoked by stimulation of frontal cortex remained unaffected in the head of the nucleus while they were suppressed in the tail. On the contrary responses to stimulation of occipital cortex were abolished simultaneously in the head and tail, indicating intracaudate conduction of impulses.

Contrasting with the weak effect of caudate SD on the nonspecific EEG mechanisms was the rather surprising finding of a conduction blockade in the capsula interna fibers (Bureš and Hartmann 1967, Bureš, Hartmann, and Lukyanova 1967, Bureš and Fifková 1968) with resulting disappearance of cortical evoked potentials of certain modalities.

The most clear-cut depression was obtained with somatosensory responses. The cortical evoked potential started to decrease abruptly when the negative SPC culminated in the middle and caudal parts of the caudate nucleus, was nearly abolished for 30 to 40 sec and then returned rapidly to the predepression level (Fig. 8.21). The possibility of a transmission blockade at the thalamic level was ruled out by recording from the somatosensory relay nucleus, that is, from the ventrobasal thalamic complex. The thalamic responses were unaffected by caudate SD even at a time when the cortical evoked potentials were completely blocked. Thus the disappearance of cortical somatosensory responses must be due to a failure of thalamocortical transmission caused by a conduction block in radiation fibers forming a part of the internal capsule. A conduction block in capsula interna fibers was demonstrated still more convincingly by blockade of the pyramidal pathway that passes through the entire brain without synaptic interruption. Both the motor cortex responses to antidromic stimulation of the pyramids at the pontine level and the orthodromic responses to stimulation of the motor cortex recorded at the level of the pons were nearly completely blocked during caudate SD. Suppression of pyrami-

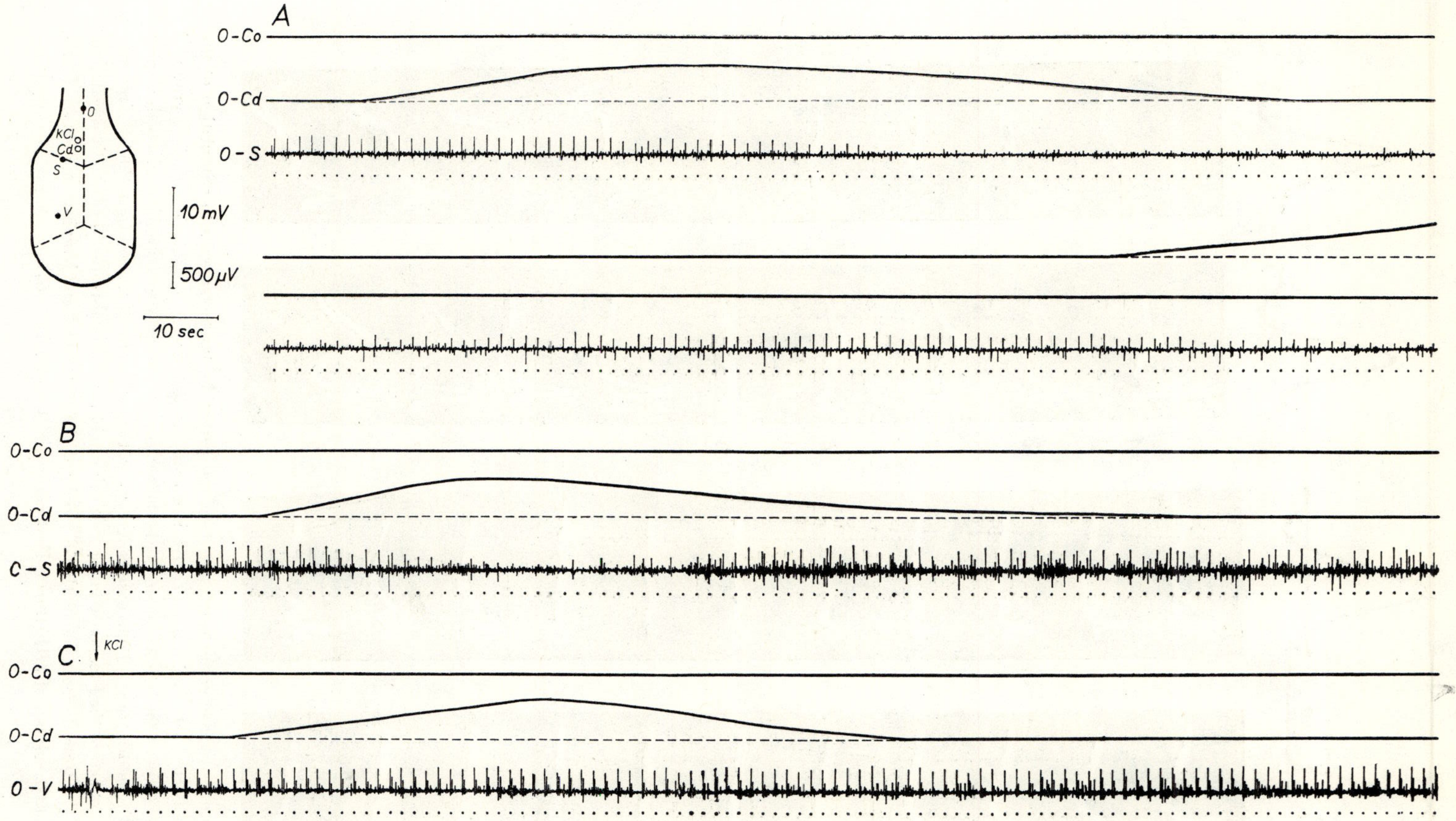

Fig. 8. 21. The effect of caudate SD on somatosensory *(A, B)* and visual *(C)* evoked responses in the cerebral cortex in rats. Electrode position shown in inset brain diagram. Symbols: (0), reference electrode; *(S,V)* electrodes in the somatosensory and visual areas; *(KCl)*, injection cannula; *(Cd)*, capillary electrode in caudate nucleus; (0—*Co*, 0—*Cd*), slow potential recording from the cortex or caudate, respectively; (0—*S*, 0—*V*), EEG activity in the somatosensory or visual cortical areas. Dots indicate application of stimuli. Calibration: 10 mV for SPC; 500 μV for EEG (Bureš and Hartmann 1967).

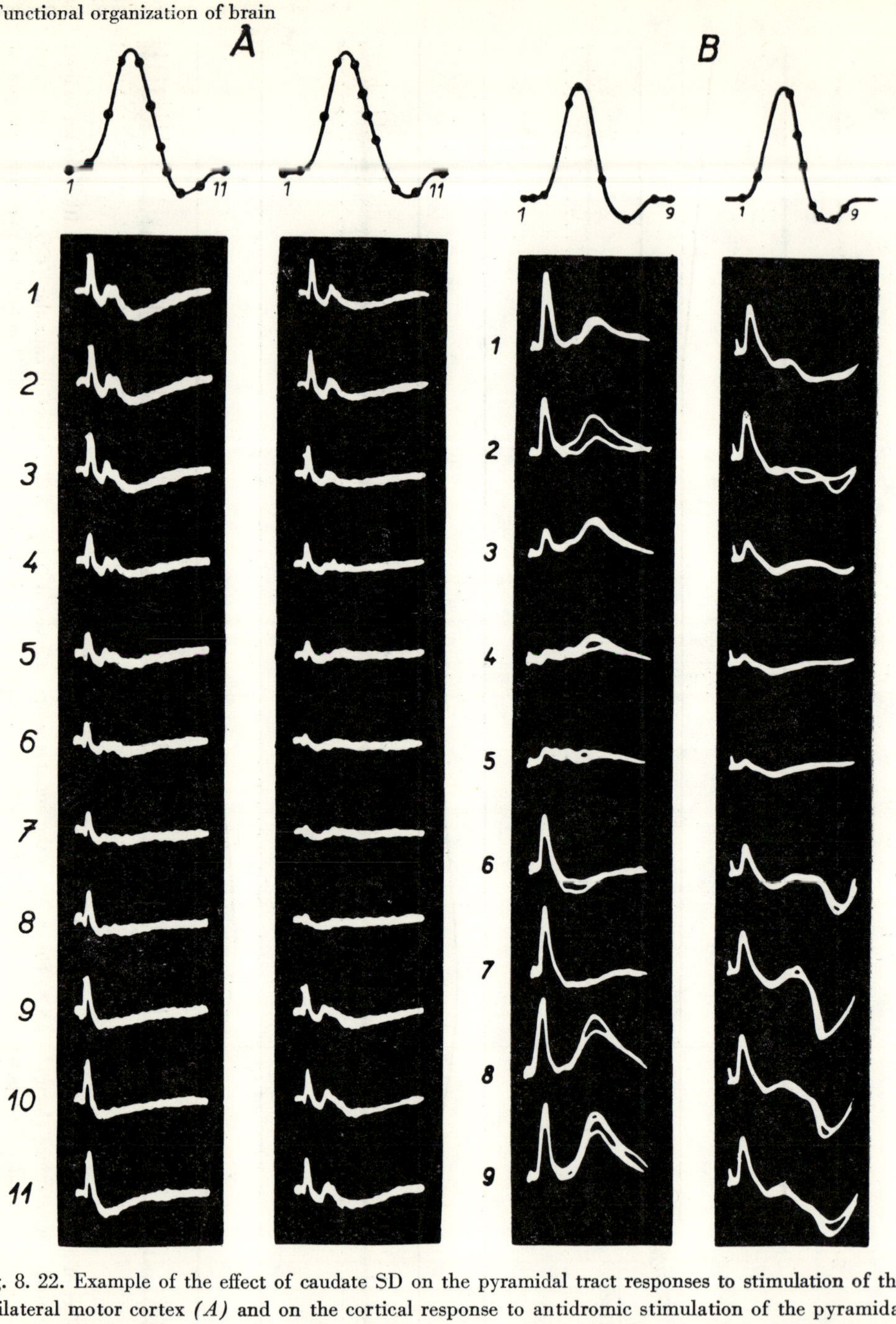

Fig. 8. 22. Example of the effect of caudate SD on the pyramidal tract responses to stimulation of the ipsilateral motor cortex *(A)* and on the cortical response to antidromic stimulation of the pyramidal pathways *(B)*. Figures at the left margin indicate the position of the individual oscillograms with respect to the caudate SPC shown above. Time base is 20 msec in the oscillograms and 2 min in the SPC records. Note the slow recovery of the I response in the first column of *(A)*, probably due to gradually developing CSD. Also note the time dissociation of the blockade of the pyramidal and lemniscal responses clearly expressed in the first column of *(B)* (Bureš, Hartmann, and Lukyanova 1967).

dal responses usually preceded blockade of somatosensory evoked potentials by 20 to 30 sec. This could be clearly seen in experiments in which pontine stimulation activated not only the pyramidal pathway but also the lemniscal fibers. The pyramidal antidromic responses (latent period of 2 to 3 msec) could be easily distinguished from the orthodromic lemniscal responses (latent period of 6 to 8 msec) recorded from the same cortical point. As shown in Fig. 8.22 disappearance and recovery of pyramidal responses preceded similar changes of the lemniscal responses by 20 to 30 sec.

In contrast to the above results, caudate SD did not affect the visual evoked responses and caused only a short lasting (30 sec) and incomplete decrease of auditory evoked responses in the cerebral cortex. Average changes of different evoked potentials caused by caudate SD are summarized in Fig. 8.23. In all experiments SD was evoked by KCl microinjection into the head of the caudate nucleus and the recordings were synchronized by the maximum negative SPC in the caudate at the level of the bregma. The latent periods of the blockade indicate that the SD wave moving in a rostrocaudal direction first blocks the pyramidal pathway, then the somatosensory

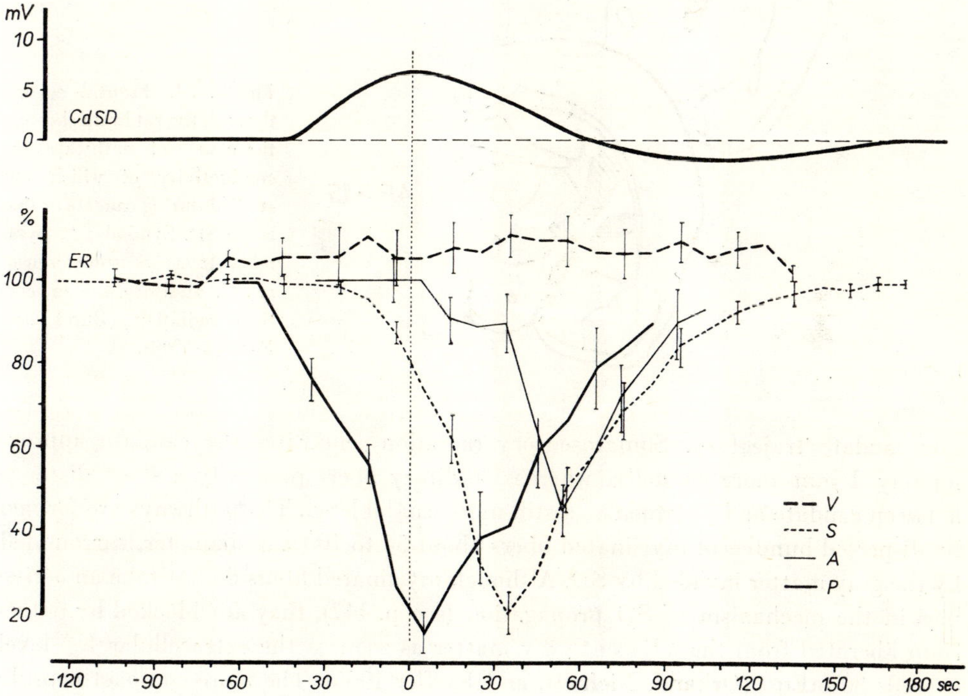

Fig. 8. 23. Mean amplitude (percentage of the predepression value) of evoked cortical responses *(ER)* in rats to antidromic stimulation of bulbar pyramids *(P)* and to somatosensory *(S)*, acoustic *(A)*, and visual *(V)* stimuli during caudate SD *(CdSD)*. Average curves were obtained by synchronizing individual recordings with respect to the maximum negativity of the SPC in the caudate nucleus. Vertical bars denote standard errors of the mean values (Bureš and Fifková 1968).

radiation, and finally slightly alters the auditory radiation, while leaving the visual projection unimpaired (Bureš and Fifková 1968). These results are in agreement with the anatomical course of the individual pathways as revealed by degeneration studies. As shown in Fig. 8.24 the pyramidal pathway is most rostral and has the longest

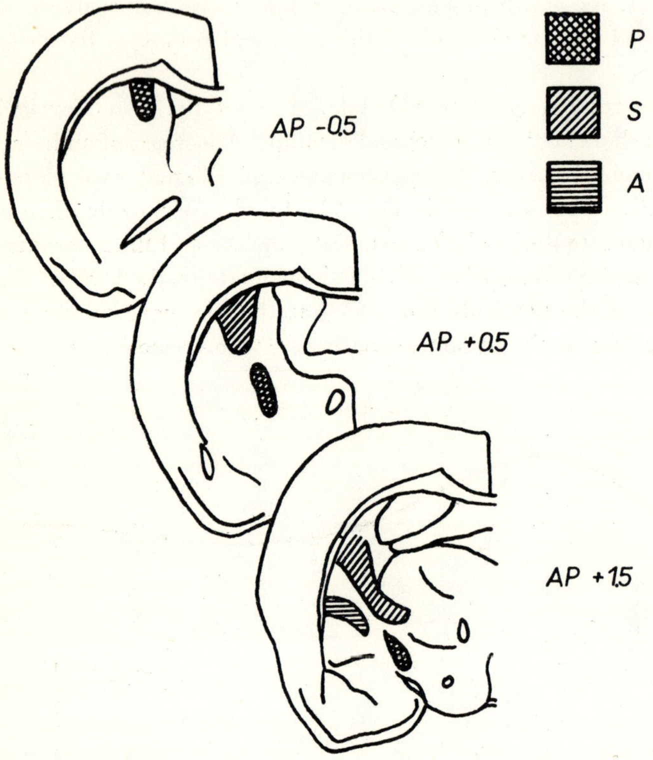

Fig. 8. 24. Frontal section through the rat brain showing the course of pathways the conductivity of which was studied during caudate or thalamic SD. Symbols: *P*, pyramidal tract; *S*, somatosensory; *A*, auditory thalamocortical radiation (Bureš and Fifková 1968).

intracaudate trajectory. Somatosensory radiation penetrates the caudate approximately 1 mm more caudally, whereas auditory fibers pass only a short distance between caudate and putamen at a still more caudal level. The pathways are formed by dispersed bundles of myelinated fibers about 50 to 100 μ in diameter, surrounded by the gray matter invaded by SD. Although myelinated fibers do not take an active part in the mechanism of SD propagation (see p. 147), they are blocked by potassium liberated from the adjacent gray matter as soon as the extracellular K^+ level exceeds 30 mEq/l (Orkand, Nicholls, and Kuffler 1966). The more compact capsula interna cannot be blocked in the same manner in cats. The otherwise puzzling finding by Trachtenberg, Hull, and Buchwald (1970) that unit activity remained preserved or was even enhanced in cat caudate nucleus invaded by SD can perhaps be explained as due to recording activity of bundles of myelinated fibers unaffected by depolarization.

Unit Activity

Remote effects of caudate SD were most marked in the spontaneous activity of thalamic neurons (Bureš, Kozlovskaya, and Fifková 1964). About 80 % of thalamic units decreased their activity to 10 to 20 % of the predepression firing rate. The activity decrease developed simultaneously with the caudate SPC and lasted for 4 min on the average. When caudate SD reached the cortex with the usual 4 to 5-min delay, thalamic neurons often displayed two distinct phases of inhibition, corresponding to the subsequent functional elimination of the two structures.

Less clear effects of caudate SD were found in the cortex and in the reticular formation (Tolkunov, Burešová, Bureš, Kutnetsova, and Fifková 1965). Cortical units reacted to caudate SD similarly as to thalamic SD (Fig. 8.5), but the inhibitory reactions occurred less frequently, were short lasting (1 to 2 min), and were less intense. The reactions observed in about 50 % of reticular units were also short lasting (1 min) and not very pronounced. Whereas the relative incidence of excitatory and inhibitory reticular reactions is three to one during cortical SD, it was one to two during caudate SD ($p < 0.01$) indicating different mechanisms of the two effects. Similar results were recently reported by Tolkunov (1969) who found during caudate SD inhibition in 50 % and excitation in 23 % of cortical neurons and in 45 % and 17 % of reticular neurons, respectively. Tolkunov (1969) analyzed not only spontaneous activity; he also established changes of single neuron responses to electrical stimulation of the sciatic nerve (Fig. 8.25) using computer processing of unit activity. According to the poststimulation histograms, changes of unit responses closely parallel the modification of spontaneous activity. The reactions were found to be abolished or decreased in 53 % of cortical and 40 % of reticular units, whereas they were increased in 25 % of cortical and 26 % of reticular neurons. Sometimes the effect of caudate SD could only be revealed by using more sophisticated analytic procedures, for example, autocorrelation function and expected densities (Poggio and Vierenstein 1964). In most neurons in which sciatic stimulation induced reproducible modifications of the discharge, caudate SD tended to restore the unstimulated activity pattern.

The picture of the intercentral relationships of the caudate nucleus based on the inhibitory neuronography is considerably different from the conventional one, according to which the caudate is an important part of the prosencephalic inhibitory system. This claim was supported mainly by results of caudate stimulation, which causes suppression of conditioned reactions (Buchwald, Wyers, Lamprecht, and Heuser 1961, Kurayev 1967), inhibition of cortical evoked potentials (Demetrescu and Demetrescu 1962, Krauthammer and Albe-Fessard 1965), and appearance of inhibitory postsynaptic potentials in cortical neurons (Spehlmann, Creutzfeldt, and Jung 1960, Hull, Buchwald, and Vieth 1967). The caudate spindles were also interpreted as a manifestation of an inhibitory influence (Heuser, Buchwald, and Wyers 1961). In a critical discussion of the experimental evidence Buchwald and Hull

(1967) point out that all these findings do not convincingly prove the inhibitory role of the caudate output, passing mainly via the globus pallidus and substantia nigra, since stimulation of the former structure fails to elicit spindles. Intracellular recordings from the putamen, globus pallidus, and nucleus entopeduncularis revealed early excitatory events during low-frequency caudate stimulation but predominantly

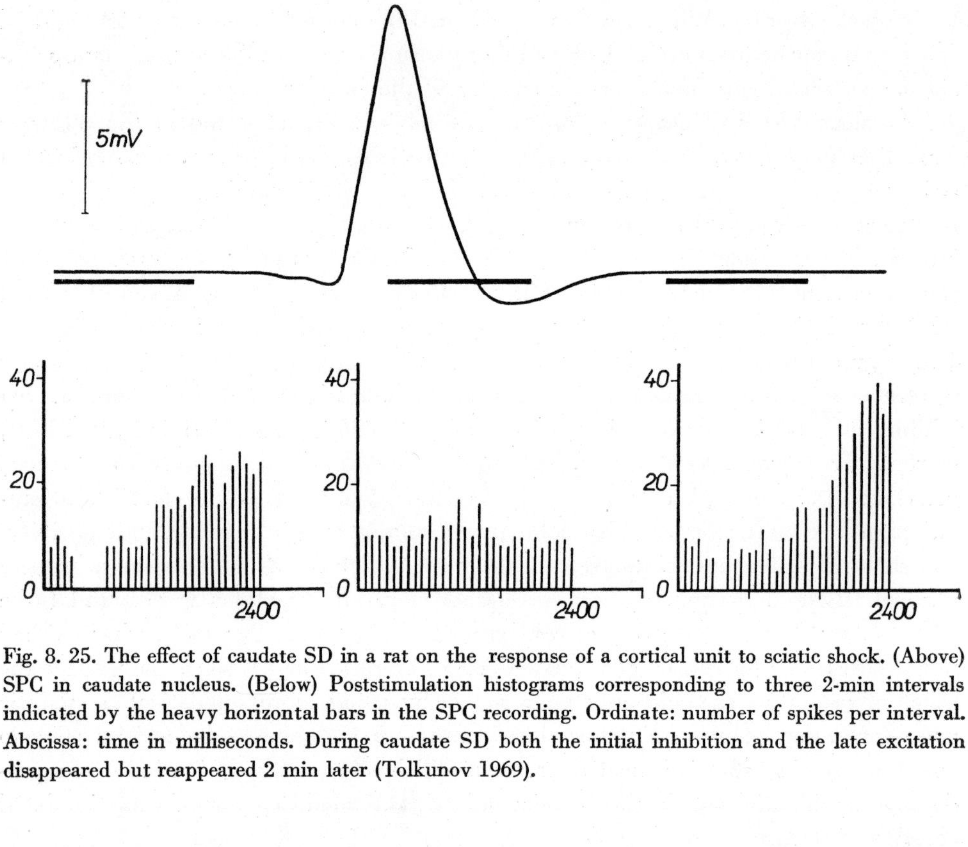

Fig. 8. 25. The effect of caudate SD in a rat on the response of a cortical unit to sciatic shock. (Above) SPC in caudate nucleus. (Below) Poststimulation histograms corresponding to three 2-min intervals indicated by the heavy horizontal bars in the SPC recording. Ordinate: number of spikes per interval. Abscissa: time in milliseconds. During caudate SD both the initial inhibition and the late excitation disappeared but reappeared 2 min later (Tolkunov 1969).

inhibitory effects during high-frequency stimulation (Malliani and Purpura 1967). It is quite probable therefore that the cortical inhibition and spindling are due to stimulation of nerve fibers passing through the caudate or to antidromic stimulation of corticocaudate fibers terminating in the caudate nucleus, and that the different phenomena do not necessarily share the same pathways. This conclusion was supported by experiments in which injection of KCl into the ventral lateral nucleus of the cat thalamus abolished the spindling but not the inhibition of cortical unit activity evoked by stimulation of the subcortical white matter. On the contrary caudate SD abolished cortical unit inhibition evoked by stimulation of the ventral lateral thalamus but did not affect spindling elicited by the same stimulus (Buchwald and Hull 1967).

The remote effects of caudate SD are devoid of any clear-cut signs of excitation and are more compatible with the assumption of a facilitatory rather than an inhibitory caudate output. Such a conclusion must be accepted with caution, however, since some of the remote effects might be due not only to elimination of caudate but also to blockade of the penetrating pathways. Thus thalamic consequences of caudate SD could be due to interruption of corticothalamic connections coursing through the capsula interna. Elimination of caudatothalamic and corticothalamic influences may both contribute to the overall effect of caudate SD on thalamus. A conduction block in corticopetal fibers may also explain the disappearance of unit reactions to sciatic nerve stimulation in the temporoparietal cortex of rats during caudate SD (Tolkunov 1969). The decrement of unit reactions in the reticular formation observed by Tolkunov (1969) can also be due to interruption of corticoreticular feedback, the importance of which was demonstrated in similar experiments by Bureš and Burešová (1964). On the other hand blockade of the capsula interna does not much affect the nonspecific thalamocortical influences, since the EEG activity and excitability remain unimpaired in cortical regions in which evoked responses to peripheral nerve stimulation were completely abolished by caudate SD.

Blockade of the pyramidal pathway during caudate SD may clarify the nature of the short-lasting excitatory reactions evoked in 60 % of reticular neurons during cortical SD. This conspicuous reaction was interpreted either as disinhibition due to elimination of some inhibitory corticoreticular influence or as excitation caused by the brief discharge of cortical neurons preceding the actual depression and transmitted through excitatory corticoreticular connections. Most corticoreticular fibers pass through the capsula interna and are blocked during caudate SD. The absence of clear-cut excitatory reactions in the reticular formation during caudate SD speaks against the inhibitory nature of the corticoreticular influence. Since blockade of fibers is not preceded by the brief excitation typical for SD passage through gray matter, the elimination of the excitatory corticoreticular influence is smooth. The weak effect of caudate SD on reticular neurons indicates that the tonic influence exerted by the cerebral cortex on the reticular formation is not very strong under resting conditions. It seems that the corticoreticular connections respond more to an increase than to a decrease of cortical activity.

6. Remote Effects of Striatal Spreading Depression in Birds

Detailed study (see Chap. 6) of the anatomical limits of SD evoked in the hyperstriatum and neostriatum of pigeons (Bureš, Fifková, and Maršala 1960, Shima, Fifková, and Bureš 1963) and chickens (Ookawa and Bureš 1969) made it possible to apply the technique of inhibitory neuronography to the analysis of the functional organization of avian brain.

The changes that take place in the directly depressed striatum of unanesthetized curarized pigeons were shown to be identical with those described in the mammalian neocortex (Burešová, Shima, Bureš, and Fifková 1963). Spontaneous unit activity of all examined neurons was abruptly depressed to zero and then recovered gradually to the predepression frequency, which was attained after approximately 6 min. Initial bursts of spikes preceding the actual depression were only rarely seen. It may be concluded, therefore, that striatal SD eliminates nearly 80 % of the volume of the hemispheres, corresponding to the highest level of the pigeon brain, by invading hyperstriatum and neostriatum.

Remote effects of the functional ablation of the striatum were described by Shima and Fifková (1963) and by Burešová, Shima, Bureš, and Fifková (1963). The results are summarized in Fig. 8.26. The most marked changes were recorded in the ipsila-

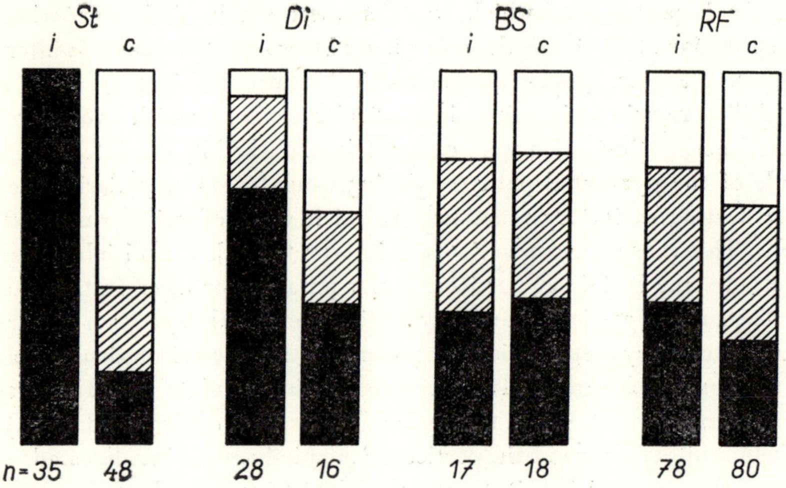

Fig. 8. 26. Survey of changes of spontaneous activity of striatal *(St)* and diencephalic *(Di)* units and of neurons in the bulbar sensory nuclei *(BS)* and in bulbar reticular formation *(RF)* evoked by striatal SD in the pigeon. Recording side with respect to the depressed striatum is ipsilateral *(i)* or contralateral *(c)*. Inhibitory reactions are black; excitatory reactions are shaded; no reactions are white. Sample size indicated by the *n* values below the columns (Shima and Fifková 1963).

teral diencephalon (nucleus ovoidalis, nucleus rotundus, nucleus dorsolateralis, nucleus posteroventralis). Ipsilateral SD decreased activity in nearly 70 % of the examined neurons to 50 % of the predepression rate, and the decrease lasted for 3 min on the average. Functional elimination of contralateral striatum was less effective; nearly 40 % of the neurons remained unaffected and the incidence of the decrease reactions was lower. A relatively high percentage of increase reactions (40 %) was obtained in a group of identified units in the brain stem reticular formation. The decrease reactions were equally frequent and there was no difference between the effect of ipsilateral and contralateral SD. Less complete data were obtained for units in the bulbar sensory nuclei, cerebellar cortex and nucleus dentatus, but the results were essentially similar to those in reticular neurons. In the combined brain stem data, contralateral SD seemed to be slightly less effective than the ipsilateral one, but the difference was small. Least affected by unilateral striatal SD was the contralateral striatum, where the activity of nearly 60 % of neurons remained unchanged.

In spite of the anatomical differences between mammalian and avian brains, the functions of bird hyperstriatum are roughly analogous to those of the mammalian neocortex. This view is supported by the finding that a decrease of unit activity is the most common diencephalic reaction both to ipsilateral cortical and striatal SD. The less marked effect of SD in contralateral diencephalon, indicating pronounced lateralization of nerve connections at this level, were also found in both cases. It seems therefore that the striatum resembles the neocortex in exerting similar excitatory influences on the activity of ipsilateral diencephalic neurons. On the other hand the prevalence of increase over decrease reactions, so typical for corticoreticular relationships, is substituted by rather equilibrated excitatory and inhibitory striatoreticular influences in the pigeon. Lack of direct connections between striatum and reticular formation in birds, which would be comparable to the pyramidal pathway in mammals, may account for the poor transmission of the excitatory component of SD to the lower brain stem. Striatoreticular interaction seems nevertheless to be quite important, since only 20 to 25 % of reticular neurons are unaffected by striatal SD. Nearly equal ipsilateral and contralateral effects at this level are probably due to the fact that the reticular formation reacts as a whole. The sagittal separation is much more marked at the diencephalic and particularly at the telencephalic level, where most of the changes induced by contralateral striatal SD seem to be an indirect consequence of the secondary effects at lower levels.

7. General Comments on the Principles of Inhibitory Neuronography

The above review of the applications of SD in research into the functional organization of the brain shows both the advantages and drawbacks of the method. Although essentially confirming the predominantly inhibitory nature of the primary process, it warns against oversimplifying conclusions. The following paragraphs summarize some of the prerequisites for a meaningful application of inhibitory neuronography and for correct interpretation of results.

(a) Single SD waves monitored by slow potential recording must be carefully compared with the time course of the remote change. The volume of the depressed tissue can be estimated from the SPC only when SD is always triggered from the same focus. Since the excitatory effects accompany the initial phase of SD the primary suppression culminates in the 1 to 2 min following the maximum depolarization. If the eliminated structure is not too large (less than 10 mm across) and if KCl injection is made close to its center, it is usually possible to get an interval of pure depression, the duration of which satisfies the purpose of the method. In some cases SD evokes abnormal activity (paroxysmal discharges) instead of functional ablation (Trachtenberg, Hull, and Buchwald 1970). Remote effects of the resulting disorganization of neural function must be interpreted with caution.

(b) The results of inhibitory neuronography are decisively influenced by the character of the connections between the depressed region and the investigated remote structure. In addition to the excitatory or inhibitory nature of the projection, other factors must be taken into account. First it must be pointed out that we can only see the average reaction of the elements in the investigated area. Remote inhibition can be due not only to elimination of an excitatory influence, affecting more or less uniformly the entire population, but also to increased excitation addressed to inhibitory interneurons in the target structure, the activation of which accounts for the overall effect. Similar considerations apply to the assumption of an inhibitory influence exerted by the depressed region on the remote center. Any statements on the excitatory or inhibitory influence of one structure on another based on inhibitory neuronography are purely operational and cannot be immediately identified with the underlying synaptic mechanisms. An important factor is the damping of the remote network. Structures like the reticular formation often respond to a single sensory stimulus by activation lasting for many seconds. It is conceivable that the brief initial excitation, accompanying the onset of functional ablation triggers an afterdischarge in the target structure that may prolong the secondary change considerably beyond the duration of the primary excitation. This would be particularly true in the case of structures with autochtonous activity (for example reticular formation) that are relatively insensitive to elimination but intensively responsive to activation of any excitatory input. On the contrary in highly damped networks (for example, the thalamus) the brief excitation fails to elicit any appreciable effect and the overall change mainly reflects the suppression phase of the primary process. Damping is often mediated not only by circuits contained in the target structure but also by intercentral feedback circuits that might be disrupted by the primary process.

(c) The primary process seems to exert no antidromic effects on the remote areas, but a conduction block in fibers coursing through the depressed region or close to it must always be considered (Fig. 8.27). Pure elimination uncomplicated by any signs of excitation characterizes this influence. The possibility of comparing the effects of functional ablation of the origin of a given pathway with the effects of the conduction block in the same pathway provides important information on the significance of the excitatory component of the primary process in the generation of the secondary effect (c. f. the effects of cortical and caudate SD on the activity of reticular units).

(d) In a system of tightly interlaced connections, it is often impossible to separate the secondary effect from the tertiary or higher-order effects, especially when the structures concerned cross-influence each other. It can only be surmised that the intensity of the remote change corresponds to the directness and importance of the connections. In principle, tertiary effects disappear when the critical secondary change is eliminated or when pathways mediating the tertiary change are blocked.

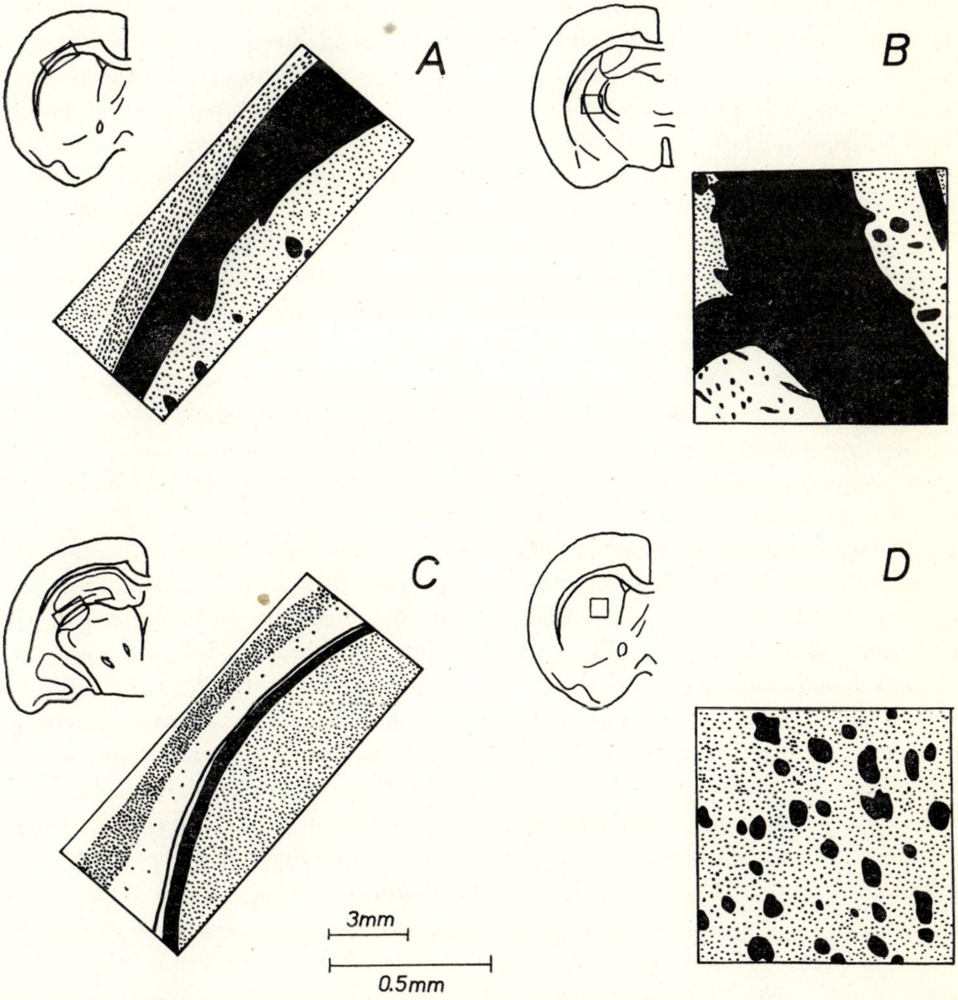

Fig. 8. 27. Diagrammatic representation of the relationship between gray and white matter in cases when SD induces (bottom) or does not induce (top) blockade of conduction in the adjacent white matter. *(A)* Callosal fibers in tangential contact with the dorsolateral surface of the caudate nucleus. *(B)* Capsula interna fibers in tangential contact with the thalamic reticular formation. *(C)* Retinotectal fibers in tangential contact with the dorsolateral surface of the lateral geniculate body. *(D)* Bundles of capsula interna fibers passing through the gray matter of corpus striatum. Location of the magnified section indicated in the frontal sections. Scale: 3 mm and 0.5 mm for the low and high magnifications (Bureš and Fifková 1968).

Unfortunately there are only few instances when it is feasible to perform such analysis using stereotaxic lesions or sections at different vertical levels (c. f. effect of cortical SD in cerveau isolé preparation).

(e) In unit activity experiments the relative incidence of increase or decrease reactions in the target area does not correspond to the relative number of excitatory or inhibitory fibers connecting the depressed region with the investigated remote structure, but rather to the internal organization of the latter. Even when the influence reaching the target structure is uniform, it is immediately transformed into a pattern of excitation and inhibition depending only on the functional relationships among the individual elements of the remote center. Thus stimulation of the reticular formation by various stimuli always results into an excitation-inhibition ratio of three to one. The inhibitory reactions are probably due to recurrent inhibition, activation of inhibitory interneurons, presynaptic inhibition, and similar factors.

It is obvious that inhibitory neuronography alone cannot provide sufficient information on the functional relationship of any two structures and that it only can be used in connection with other physiological and morphological methods. Being complementary to all techniques using stimulation for mapping neural connections, it may serve as an independent source of data, which should agree with the general framework described by a working hypothesis. Activation and elimination of the same input does not necessarily evoke symmetrically reciprocal effects in the target structure, which may be influenced more and longer by excitation than by inhibition. Since inhibitory neuronography eliminates tonic influences, it can only be directly compared with stimulation techniques revealing tonic interactions.

In spite of all the above reservations the results of inhibitory neuronography are sometimes so striking that they can be interpreted without difficulty (for example the effect of cortical SD on thalamus and caudate). Taken together the results of inhibitory neuronography support the assumption that brain centers are mainly connected by excitatory pathways, whereas the inhibitory neurons do not usually extend beyond the limits of the region in which they originate. Such a principle of functional organization assumes predominance of facilitatory interaction between distant structures whereas overexcitation by positive feedback is prevented by local braking mechanisms, mainly of the recurrent-inhibition type.

Chapter 9

The Application of Spreading Depression in Behavioral Research

1. Introduction

Understanding the intimate nature of processes underlying the highest functions of the human brain is the ultimate goal of any neurophysiological research. Formulations of new concepts of brain functions as well as modest improvements in experimental techniques eventually contribute to this aim. Spreading depression may serve as an interesting illustration of this assertion.

Before Leão's (1944a) discovery similar phenomena were observed by Dusser de Barenne and McCulloch (1938a, b, 1941), Hines (1936), Gedevani (1943), and others and considered as manifestations of neural inhibition which plays an important integrative role in normal brain function. Attempts to identify SD with Pavlov's irradiation of inhibition remained spurious, but the initially purely descriptive terms "suppression" and "suppression strips" assumed through inadequately substantiated concepts an erroneous meaning, which considerably influenced neurological thinking in the late forties and survived in leading textbooks of neurophysiology for nearly 20 years. After the identity of "suppression" and "spreading depression" was convincingly demonstrated by Sloan and Jasper (1950) and by Druckman (1952) SD was recognized as an artificial or even pathological phenomenon that cannot conceivably participate in neural coordination under normal circumstances. The only example of plausible hypothesis ascribing to SD a limited biological purpose is the suggestion by Van Harreveld and Stamm (1954b) that the electrical silence terminating an electrographic epileptic paroxysm is a manifestation of a diffusely initiated SD that protects cortical neurons from exhaustion by excessive activity.

A few years later SD entered behavioral research from a different direction — not as a brain mechanism but as a physiological method. Its application in animal experiments was prepared by two approaches.

Classical research into the physiology of the central nervous system, based on behavioral manifestations of morphologically controlled ablation and stimulation experiments, was more recently supplemented by electrophysiology. Electrophysiological techniques are used either to detect electrical signs of a given behavioral act or to deliminate the behavioral repertoire compatible with a well-defined electrophysiological state. The first approach, taking behavior as the independent variable and brain potentials as the dependent variable, is more typical for psychology, whereas the second more physiological approach attempts to establish how behavior depends on well-defined physiological processes (independent variable). Epileptic foci and epileptic afterdischarges, or changes of electrical activity induced by drugs, were used in this way. As SD seemed to be superior to most of these interventions, its application in this context was quite obvious.

The other line of research leading to application of SD in behavioral research consisted of attempts to develop a reversible functional ablation technique devoid of the disadvantages of a surgical lesion. Local cooling and local application of anesthetics were used from the end of the nineteenth century with variable success in suppressing the activity of circumscribed brain regions. The cooling technique in particular was considerably improved by modern technology (cryogenic probes using expansion of liquid gases or the Peltier effect, planar cooling with arrays of probes) and was successfully used by several investigators in acute animal experiments. Problems of spatial temperature gradients, together with the difficulties encountered adapting the cooling devices for application in freely moving animals, prevent at the present stage a wider use of this method. After the basic properties of SD were established, the possibility of using it as functional ablation procedure was obvious. In particular the prolonged impairment of cortical function evoked by application of suprathreshold chemical stimuli onto the exposed brain surface put into the hands of investigators a simple, reproducible, and fully reversible functional ablation technique that rapidly came into wide use.

The increasing application of SD in behavioral research is illustrated in Fig. 9.1. The first papers describing the behavioral effect of SD appeared in 1956 (Burešová 1956, Bureš and Burešová 1956c). Since 1960 the method has been used in other

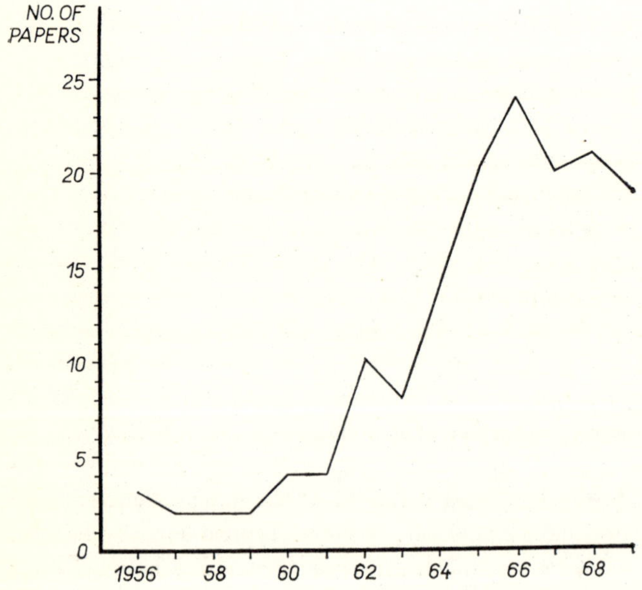

Fig. 9. 1. An increasing number of papers concerned with behavioral applications of spreading depression in the period 1956—1969.

laboratories. By 1965 the number of papers on behavioral SD applications reached 20 and remained at this level in the following years. The main attraction of SD was simplicity of application, which made it possible to approach many problems without using difficult and traumatic surgical techniques. Although the functional ablation technique could be used in the same way as surgical decortication in many experiments, the most important results in its applications came from taking full advantage of the reversibility of this ablation procedure, that is, the ablated region is eliminated during a particular stage of the experimental procedure but is normally used later.

Wide use of the SD technique in behavioral research occasionally lead to applications that did not fully respect the necessary conditions for reliably eliciting SD. As such omissions may cause controversial results, special attention is paid in the next section to the technical aspects of the use of SD in behavioral research.

2. Spreading Depression in Unanesthetized, Freely Moving Animals

The first prerequisite for application of SD in behavioral research was the knowledge that this phenomenon exists in freely moving animals. The early experiments by Leão (1944a, b) were concerned with the mechanism of SD and were performed therefore in anesthetized animals, mainly rabbits. Marshall (1952), working with anesthetized cats and monkeys, found it difficult to obtain SD reliably and suggested that exposure, dehydration, and cooling of the cortical surface are necessary factors in eliciting SD. This conclusion was criticized by Van Harreveld and Stamm (1951) who reported for the first time that SD evoked from a small trephine opening may pass through the enclosed rabbit cortex to a remote cortical region exposed by another burr hole. Although the facilitatory role of brain pathology for eliciting SD is beyond any doubt (see Van Harreveld and Bogen 1956), it is equally true that at least in some species SD can be evoked by appropriate stimuli in the intact normal brain. Similar results were reported later in anesthetized rats (Bureš 1954a) and in unanesthetized rats (Bureš 1954b) and rabbits (Magun and Ross 1954). Chronically implanted electrodes were successfully used for eliciting and recording SD in curarized rabbits, cats, and monkeys (Van Harreveld, Stamm, and Christensen 1956) and in freely moving rats (Bureš and Burešová 1960b, Huston and Bureš 1970, Carew, Crow, and Petrinovich 1970) or rabbits (Ochs, Hunt and Booker 1961, Suzuki and Uneoka 1966, Megirian and Bureš 1970). Steady potential and EEG changes indicated that the spreading rate and other features of the SD process are not different from those established in acute experiments.

Attempts to use SD in behavioral research can be divided into two groups, that is, experiments (a) with or (b) without direct electrophysiological checking of the development of the SD process. Technical difficulties made the first group very small in comparison with the second one. As reduction of EEG amplitude cannot be easily detected in aroused animals, the most reliable indicator of SD is the steady potential change. Implanted silver-silver chloride electrodes were used to record changes of cortical steady potentials accompanying chemically and electrically evoked SD and to correlate them with bar pressing in rats (Bureš and Burešová 1960b) and rabbits (Suzuki and Uneoka 1966, Megirian and Bureš 1970). These experiments demonstrated convincingly that the behavioral effect of SD is due to invasion of definite cortical regions by SD (see p. 238) but they did not satisfactorily resolve the problems of repetitive stimulus application and reliable SD initiation.

A recent improvement of the chronic technique is due to Janebová (1971) who elicited SD by intracortical (1 mm deep) electrophoretic injection of K^+ from glass capillaries filled with potassium-saturated ionex gel (Fig. 9.2). Anodic currents (0.5 to 1.0 mA for 5 to 20 sec) reliably elicited SD. The threshold amount of injected K^+ was 0.6 μg, that is, 25 to 50 times less than the threshold amount required with surface application of KCl (4 mm trephine opening, 5 to 10 μl of 0.6 % KCl). Freedman and Bureš (1972) and Huston and Bureš (1970) modified the technique by filling the cannulae (Fig. 9.2) with 3 M KCl and by using an adjustable mandrel

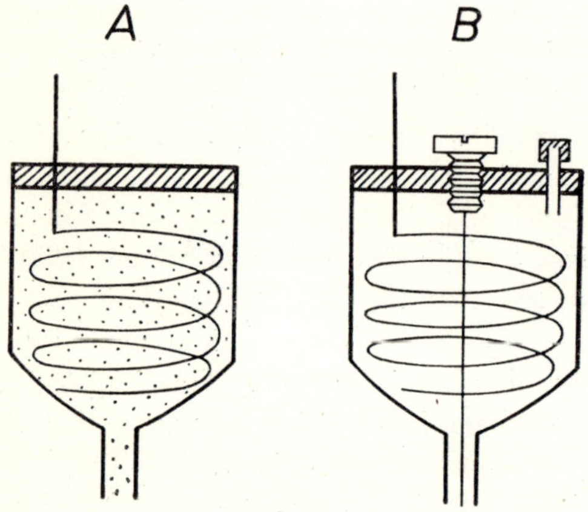

Fig. 9. 2. Examples of chronically implanted cannulae used for electrophoretic injection of K^+ into the cerebral cortex. *(A)* Cannula filled with KCl-agar gel. *(B)* Cannula filled with KCl solution, which can be changed after removing the screw and opening the air outlet. The screw-mounted mandrel can be used to remove clogs in the tip of the cannula.

to prevent obliteration of the cannula orifice. Silver-silver chloride electrodes coiled inside the cannula were used to supply current. The tip was inserted 1 mm below the cortical surface and the system was fixed to the skull bone with anchoring screws and acrylic resin. The SD wave could be elicited at predetermined intervals (starting from 4 min), if necessary, simultaneously in both hemispheres. With occasional refilling of the KCl solution 10 to 20 SD per day could be evoked for 2 weeks without excessive increase of the threshold.

The second approach takes advantage of the small variability of SD parameters (constant spreading rate and duration, constant stimulus threshold). This made it possible to use two groups of rats of the same strain and age in which SD was evoked by stimuli of the same intensity and applied in the same way. Average times of onset and duration of the behavioral changes in the freely moving group were compared with the averaged electrophysiological data obtained in the restrained group. Since its first application in 1956 (Burešová 1956) this technique has been used in the overwhelming majority of SD experiments and has brought important results. Unfortunately in some laboratories the correlation of electrophysiological and behavioral data was never retested for the particular conditions of stimulus application used, which might lead to serious errors. We shall therefore discuss these problems in more detail.

The most convenient stimulus for evoking SD in behavioral experiments is local application of drugs onto the exposed cortical surface. An SD focus established by a single application of a suprathreshold chemical stimulus generates a train of SD waves, the frequency and overall number of which depend on the concentration and volume of the applied drug, on the area of contact between the applied solution and the underlying cortex, on the permeability of dura, and on the physiological conditions of the exposed cortical tissue (see also p. 31). The original procedure (Burešová 1956) adopted later in other laboratories, consists of preliminary surgery followed after an appropriate recovery period by the actual drug application. The surgery is performed in rats anesthetized with ether. The frontoparietal bones are exposed by 3 cm long midline incision of the scalp. The incised skin is reflected from the area of trepanation and an opening 4 to 5 mm in diameter is made into the skull bones using a circular hand trephine with a central point. Great care is taken to avoid cutting the dura, damage of which may cause brain edema. This is best achieved by holding the trephine at a slightly oblique angle toward the skull surface. When the bone is completely cut through at two thirds of the trephine hole circumference and considerably thinned in the remaining segment, the bone can be easily broken out by sharp strong forceps. It is essential that there are no signs of subdural bleeding or brain edema and that the exposed cortical surface has a normal, clean appearance. In all dubious cases it is preferable to discard the animal at this stage before too much work is spent in further experimentation which may give unreliable results under such conditions. After the trephine openings are revised, the skin is replaced on the skull and fastened by one to two loose sutures, placed in such a way that they can be easily cut. The animal is allowed 4 to 24 hours for recovery from the surgery before the trephine openings are exposed again. This is usually made without anesthesia, restraining the rat by hand, cutting the sutures, and opening the skin flaps. The skull bones and the exposed brain surface are rinsed with Ringer's solution and carefully cleaned of coagulated blood and tissue debris. After the excess fluid has been taken up by dry cotton, a filter paper 3 by 3 mm soaked with about 5 µl of an appropriate solution is applied onto the exposed cortex. The skin around the exposed area is kept open in order to prevent displacement of the filter paper by movement of the scalp against the skull and dilution of the drug by the serous exudate accumulating in the slitlike space between skin and skull.

The above procedure can be modified in different ways. A simple improvement was introduced by Schneider and Behar (1964) and later modified by Burešová, Lukaszewska, and Bureš (1966). The retracted skin flaps are sutured to the rim of a plastic ring (12 mm internal diameter, 10 mm high) completely covering the skull surface with the trephine openings (Fig. 9.3). After completion of the surgery, a cotton pledget soaked with saline is placed into the plastic well which is then closed by a screw-shaped lid fitting into the threaded upper part of the ring. Before drug application, the lid is unscrewed, the cotton is removed and the trephine opening is revised. After removing any excess fluid, the filter paper with the drug is applied onto the exposed brain surface and the lid is replaced. The closed chamber formed in this way not only prevents mechanical displacement of the filter papers, it also protects the brain from desiccation and excessive cooling.

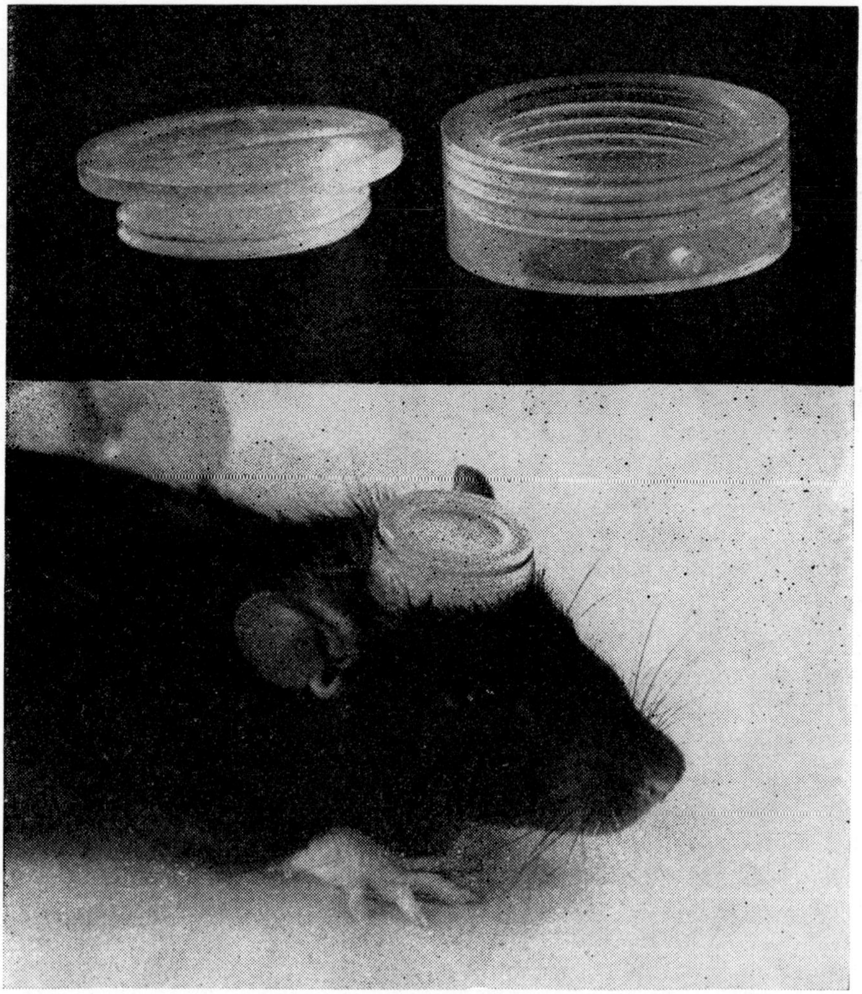

Fig. 9. 3. Plastic ring with a screw cap. The holes in the base serve for suturing the ring to the scalp.

Other modifications of the SD technique use application of drugs through implanted cannulae. Mogenson's method (Mogenson and Peterson 1966) represents an intermediate link between the open surface and intracannular application of drugs. A 4 to 5 mm high layer of methacrylate anchored to bone by screws is placed over the occipital cortex around a short piece of polyethylene tubing, so that a skull area 4 mm in diameter is left exposed. A few days later an opening is drilled through the bone at the bottom of the methacrylate well, which is then packed with cotton moistened in physiological saline. The plug is removed and the well is cleaned before the filter paper soaked in the drug solution is applied to the dura.

Cannulae fitting into prepared trephine holes were used for the first time by Russell and Ochs (1961). Cylindrical plastic cups 11 mm high and 5 mm wide with a 2-mm hole at the base were placed into a trephine opening 2.5 mm in diameter (Fig. 9.4). They were cemented into place with acrylic resin which bound them to jeweler's screws inserted in the skull around the trephine hole. A close-fitting plunger was inserted in the cups to minimize dehydration of dura. The plug was replaced during the actual experiment by a cotton pledget soaked in the drug solution. Tapp (1962) used polyethylene cannulae 11 mm long with an internal diameter of 2 mm. One end was slightly flared by heating and slipped gently between skull and dura into holes 3 mm in diameter. Self-tapping eyeglass screws and dental cement were used to fix the cups to the bone. Cotton soaked in Ringer's solution was inserted into the tubes as protection against foreign matter and changed daily. Before the actual experiment, the cotton was removed, the remaining fluid was extracted with a hypodermic needle cut to a length of 10 mm and replaced by 30 μl of the drug solution. After the experiment the tubes were flushed with Ringer and the cotton was reinserted.

A similar principle was used by Paolino and Levy (1970), whose cannula assembly consists of two parts: a nylon nut permanently mounted on the skull above the 3-mm trephine opening, and a reusable cannula which screws into the nut. A stainless steel inlet tubing in the cannula is

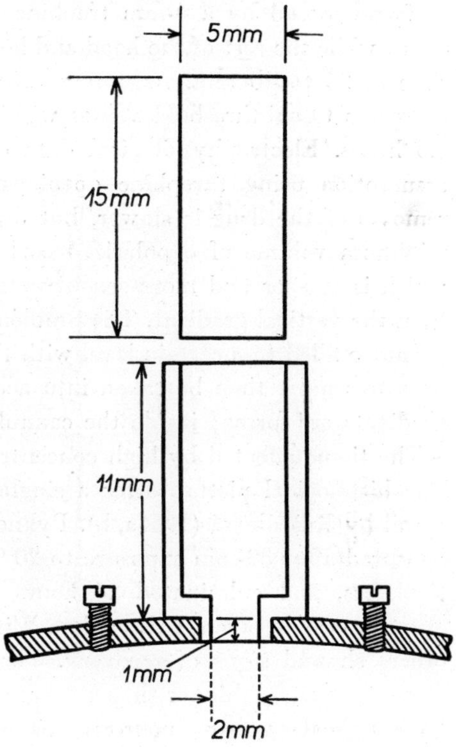

Fig. 9. 4. Diagram of the cannula and plunger, giving details of the dimensions and method of attachment to the skull (Russell and Ochs 1963).

connected by means of a sufficient length of flexible polyethylene tubing with a remote injection syringe. A short outlet tubing provides for the overflow. The system minimizes handling of the animals and improves timing of the KCl treatment.

With the above techniques, the contact area ranges from more than 15 to 3 mm² and the volume of the applied solution from 5 to 30 μl. Because the threshold of a chemical stimulus is within certain limits indirectly proportional to the area of stimulus application (see p. 31) the same stimulus applied onto a small area of cortical surface induces a shorter-lasting impairment of behavior than when using a large trephine opening. Thus 25 % KCl caused an impairment of comparable avoidance tasks lasting for 5 hours when applied into 4-mm trephine holes (Bureš, Burešová and Záhorová 1958) and only 1.5 hours with 2-mm cannulae (Tapp 1962), although a larger volume was applied in the latter case. Bondarenko (1964) used still smaller trephine openings (0.8 mm in diameter) and with applications of 1.3, 2.6, and 5.2 μl of 25 % KCl obtained EEG depression lasting for 6, 11, and 20 min, respectively.

The relationship between contact area, threshold concentration, concentration and volume of the applied solution, and duration of behavioral impairment is not simple, however. Large contact area facilitates removal of the applied drug by circulation. Burešová (1956) used ^{42}K to estimate the rate of K^+ removal from a cortical focus established by application of 5 μl of 25 % KCl onto the cortical surface exposed by a 4-mm trephine opening. Radioactivity measured above the focus, while the rest of the head and body was heavily screened, decayed with a half time of 25 to 40 min. Assuming exponential decay, the 25 % KCl concentration decreases to subthreshold values within five to six half-times, that is, over 2.5 to 4.0 hours. Electrophysiological data on SD duration are in agreement with this assumption using threphine openings of comparable size. With small openings removal of the drug is slower, but duration of impairment is shorter because the minimum volume of depolarized cortex is then attained by tangential diffussion, which is steeper and more sensitive to concentration changes in the area of focus than the vertical gradient. The problem becomes still more complicated when using cannulae filled to a certain level with the applied solution. Hydrostatic and osmotic pressures must then be taken into account. If no stirring is provided, important gradients are formed inside the cannula.

The tissue affected by high concentration of the drug may be seriously changed. The histological picture after a single application of 25 % KCl was described in detail by Ruščáková (1964a, b). Pyknosis of nuclei and vacuolization of cytoplasm appeared after 30-min exposure to 20 % KCl in nerve cells throughout the cortical thickness, and culminated 24 hours later by complete karyolosis and cytolysis of many cells in layers 1 through 4. Within a week most of these elements died while others showed signs of recovery. Three weeks after KCl application the treated cortex was 10 % thinner than the control one. All these results indicate that during KCl application many neurons in the treated area are permanently or reversibly injured. When with the decay of the focus (see also p. 32, Fig. 2.3) the threshold concentration shifts closer to the center of the area of drug application, the tissue in this region may already be nonresponsive. While diffusing across the inactive tissue, the drug is absorbed into the circulation at such a rate that it does not reach beyond the limits of the damaged cortex a concentration that would initiate SD. This factor becomes especially important when the drug is repeatedly applied onto the same cortical area. Damage amounting to 10 % of the cortical surface and affecting the whole thickness of the cerebral cortex was reported by Tapp (1962). Similar results were described in more detail by Hamburg, Best, and Cholewiak (1968). Hull, Buchwald, and Ling (1967) found 1 hour after 4-μl injection of 25 % KCl into the caudate nucleus of cats an unstained area 1 to 2 mm in diameter surrounding the point of injection. With the development of the cortical or subcortical lesion, the applied solution becomes separated from the intact cortex by an ever thicker barrier of tissue without neurones but with proliferating glia. The thickening of dura also slows down the penetration of the topically applied drugs into the brain. It is easily understandable therefore that the same chemical stimulus applied at daily intervals evokes behavioral impairment of decreasing intensity. Not only is the overall duration of depression reduced but also the intervals between the individual slow potential waves are prolonged. Unpredictable periods of partial recovery make the depression of cortical function incomplete and unreliable. The development of the lesion is often associated with appearance of paroxysmal activity in the EEG which might eventually lead to seizures or to lethargy (Russell and Ochs 1963). For all these reasons SD evoked by 25 % KCl is not suitable for chronic experimentation. Results must be carefully checked for duration and depth of depression if this solution is applied more than twice to the same area during a period of several days.

Attempts to improve the reversibility of the changes in the focal area and to develop a reliable chronic technique are few. The most obvious approach is to use isotonic KCl solutions in order to prevent lesions caused by hypertonicity. Because isotonic KCl is approximately double the threshold concentration, the concentration gradient must be maintained by a continuous supply of the drug by some kind of perfusion, which is rather impractical in freely moving animals. It is more desirable to use a drug that is more efficient in evoking SD than KCl, so that even its highly suprathreshold concentration does not exceed isotonicity. Ouabain was used for this purpose either in substance (100 μg) or in solution (Janebová, unpublished data). No osmotic damage was found in the area of drug application but higher dosages caused both local and general toxic effects.

Decreasing reliability of SD increases the significance of techniques designed for directly checking the presence or absence of depression. Whereas electrophysiological methods cannot be easily used in freely moving animals, cortical SD can be recognised by simple neurological tests, based on examination of cortical postural reactions. Cortical integration of the so-called placing and hopping reactions was described in rats by Brooks and Peck (1940). Most suitable for routine testing are the following reactions:

(a) The chin of the animal touches the edge of the table — both forelimbs are placed on the table beside the chin.

(b) The back side of the forelimb touches the edge of the table — the forelimb is placed on the table.

(c) The hindlimb or the forelimb hangs over the edge of the table — the limb is immediately lifted back onto the table.

These reactions are lost on the side contralateral to cortical SD evoked by 25 % KCl for 4 to 5 hours, that is, for the time corresponding to the impairment of conditioned reflexes (Burešová 1956). Some authors recommend modifications of the above tests. Best and Hamburg (1969) test placing responses by lightly rubbing a pencil over the back of the limb. According to Albert (1966a) a particularly useful indication of SD is failure to bring the forepaw on the insensitive side back to its normal position when it is moved under the chest. He also observed a tendency to allow the forepaw, and occasionally the hind leg to hang through the grid floor of the testing box. A similar observation was made by Mogenson (1965), Carlson (1967) and Carew, Crow, and Petrinovich (1970). Carlson (1967) also reported that rats under bilateral CSD would often walk off the edge of a table and when turned over on their backs would seldom struggle to right themselves. This finding is in good agreement with the potentiating effect of CSD on animal hypnosis (Bureš and Burešová 1956d) and on the duration of anesthesia (Bureš 1955, Bureš and Burešová 1956a) — both measured by suppression of righting reflexes.

The prerequisites for successful application of CSD in behavioral experiments can be summarized in the following two points:

(a) Cortical SD must be evoked in such a way that the rate of slow potential waves maintains cortical functions impaired for the required time.

(b) Impairment of cortical functions must be checked by appropriate electrophysiological or behavioral tests.

As none of the available techniques is quite satifactory for evoking CSD in chronic experiments from the same area repeatedly and reliably, the semichronic experiments are preferable for most applications. A search for efficient chronic techniques of reversible ablation remains an important task for all investigators in this field.

3. Mechanisms of the Behavioral Effects of Cortical Spreading Depression

Onset of Impairment

In early experiments (Burešová 1956, Bureš, Burešová, and Záhorová 1958) CSD was used in order to establish the exact localisation of presumed cortical links of different conditioned reactions. It was expected that invasion of the projection area of the conditioned stimulus (CS) or unconditioned stimulus (UCS) would suppress the respective conditioned behavior. The results obtained did not confirm the above assumption when using general motor behavior. In the first study (Bureš, Burešová, and Záhorová 1958) a 5-sec CS (buzzer) was followed by 15-sec CS-UCS (buzzer + foot-shock). The animal could avoid or escape the shocks by jumping on the wire mesh that formed one of the four vertical walls of the apparatus. The avoidance behavior was preserved during the first minute after application of 2 or 25 % KCl onto the parieto-occipital cortex and disappeared only during the second minute. The impairment occurred approximately at the time when motor and auditory cortices were invaded by CSD started from the parietooccipital cortex, but was directly related to neither of these events, since CSD elicited from temporal or frontal loci suppressed the avoidance reaction with the same latency. Because an area of 6 to 7 mm in diameter, invaded within 1 minute, covers the whole visual, acoustic or sensorimotor cortex, none of these projections is indispensable for the performance of the above avoidance reaction. More important than the stimulation locus is the total area of cortex depressed. Cortical SD elicited in one of the above regions will reach the other two within 2 minutes, but avoidance reactions disappear a little earlier, when the depression attains in each hemisphere an area of more than 10 mm in diameter.

The results are in agreement with Lashley's (1929) principles of equipotentiality and mass action; no particular part of the cortex in rats seems to be specific for the performance of the avoidance reaction, which disappears abruptly after the depression has involved over 60 to 70 % of cortical surface. Exact estimation of the minimum depressed area leading to avoidance impairment is difficult because the depressed surface grows at an accelerating rate, which reaches an increment of approximately 20% per 20 sec after invasion of 50 % of cortex.

In contrast to the above results there are other conditioned reactions with more discrete cortical representation that are blocked by invasion of a definite cortical area. Suzuki and Uneoka (1966) examined the effect of CSD on operant behavior in the rabbit. An animal was trained to press a bar with its nose or mouth to obtain food on a fixed reinforcement (FR) schedule. Bilateral CSD induced by electrical stimulation of the occipital areas impaired bar pressing with a latency of 5 min, whereas CSD elicited in the frontal regions did so within 2 min. The authors point out that this finding is incompatible with the mass-action principle, according to which the latency for bar-pressing suppression should be virtually constant irrespective of the position of the CSD focus. From the position of the recording and stimulating electrodes the motor and probably also the somatosensory areas seem to be essential in mediating bar pressing. Exact localization is complicated by the bilateral representation of bar pressing, which stops completely only when active regions are depressed on both sides. An asymmetry of CSD march through both hemispheres may thus lead to localization errors. Short-lasting reduction of bar-pressing rate caused by unilateral CSD is less expressed but more suitable for determining the relevant cortical regions.

Similar results were reported earlier by Bureš and Burešová (1960b). Rats stopped bar pressing when the slow potential elicited by KCl application onto the occipital cortex reached the frontoparietal regions. Since the sites of KCl application and slow potential recording were not varied, these experiments did not convincingly rule out the mass-action mechanism of the CSD effect.

Principles of CSD use in localization studies were recently discussed by Megirian and Bureš (1970) who examined the effect of CSD on the classically conditioned eye-blink reaction in the rabbit. In the hemisphere contralateral to the blinking eye, CSD evoked from either frontal or occipital cortex caused a complete suppression of the conditioned reaction when the negative SPC invaded a cortical region at the level of the bregma (Fig. 9.5).

The onset of impairment, coinciding with the penetration of SPC into a given area, for example, corresponding to the placement of the recording electrode, indicates that the focus lies on the perimeter of a circle with the center in the point of injection and a radius corresponding to the injection-recording distance. When the behavioral blockade coincides with SPC developing in the same cortical area even for CSD waves evoked from opposite directions, for example, from frontal and occipital cortex, this area corresponds to the point of contact between the two hypothetical circles and necessarily lies on the connecting line of their centers. Foci situated more laterally can be located by finding the intersection of the two circles circumscribed around the two injection points with radii corresponding to the respective injection-impairment latencies (Fig. 9.6). Assuming that performance is proportional to the intact surface of the critical region, its extent in the direction perpendicular to the CSD wavefront can be estimated from the time between the onset and culmination of impairment.

The latency separating KCl application from the onset of behavioral impairment in rats answers another important question. Application of a highly hypertonic KCl solution onto the dura often elicits a short-lasting painful reaction of the animal (attempts to remove the filter paper, squealing, and struggling) which might be suspected to interfere with performance of the conditioned behavior by external inhibition or distraction. This is evidently not the case since the animal readily reacts to CS applied within 20 to 30 sec after KCl application when the pain is maximal. Controls for the effects of pain caused by application of 25 % KCl to exposed muscle (Kupferman 1966) as well as elimination of pain by anesthesia of dural receptors, by employment of isotonic drug solutions, or by anoxic activation of subthreshold foci (Bureš and Burešová 1960a) did not reveal any significant role of pain in the behavioral effect of CSD.

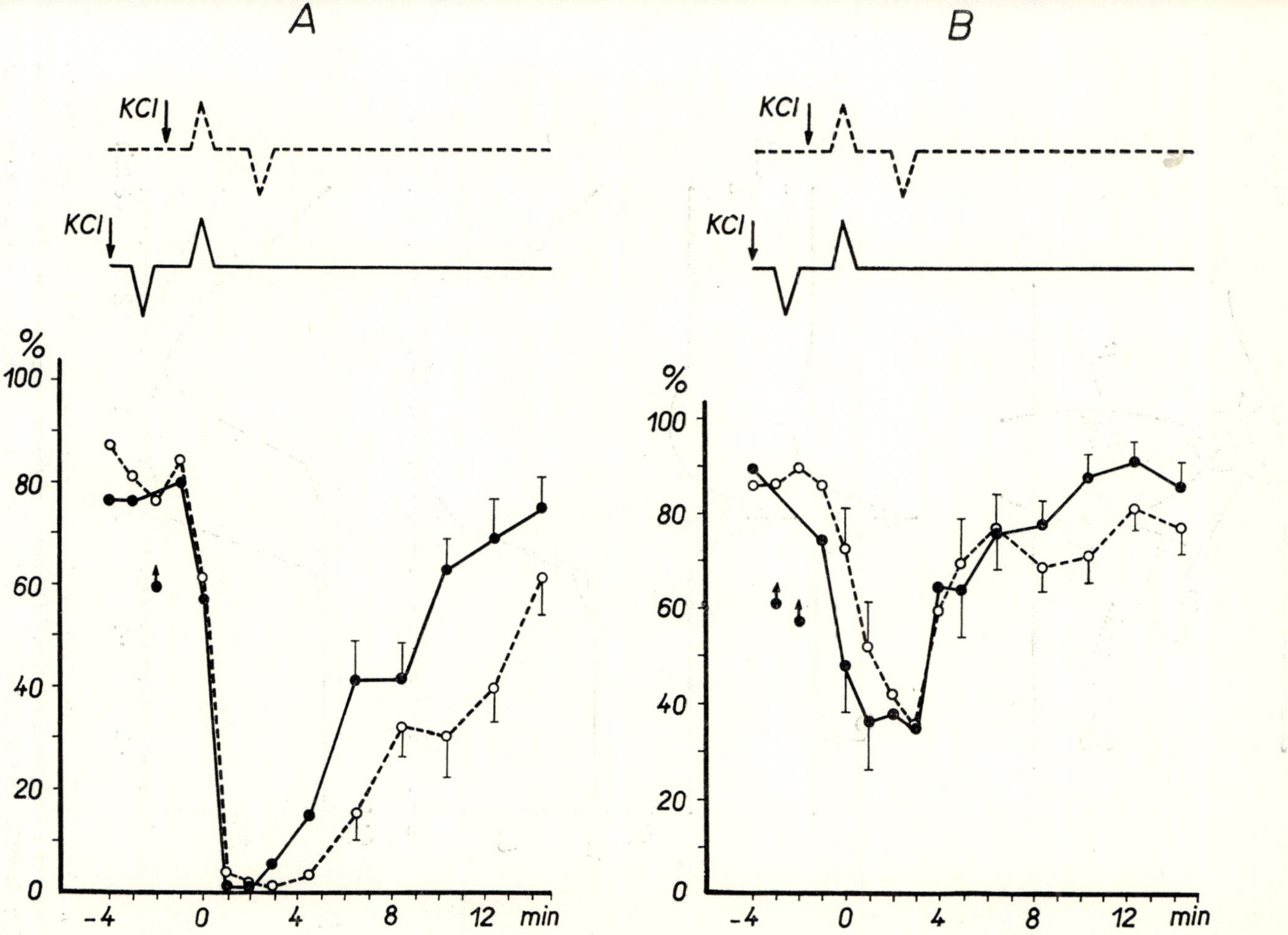

Fig. 9. 5. The effect of CSD evoked from the frontal (dashed line) or occipital (full line) cannulae in the left *(A)* or right *(B)* hemisphere on the average performance of the conditioned eye blink in the right eye of a rabbit. The upper curves show schematically the time of KCl application and the time course of SPC in bipolar recording (frontal negativity upward). Zero of the time axis corresponds to the negative maximum of SPC at the level of bregma. Dots with upward pointing arrows correspond to the performance impairment, probably caused by distraction of the animal (Megirian and Bureš 1970).

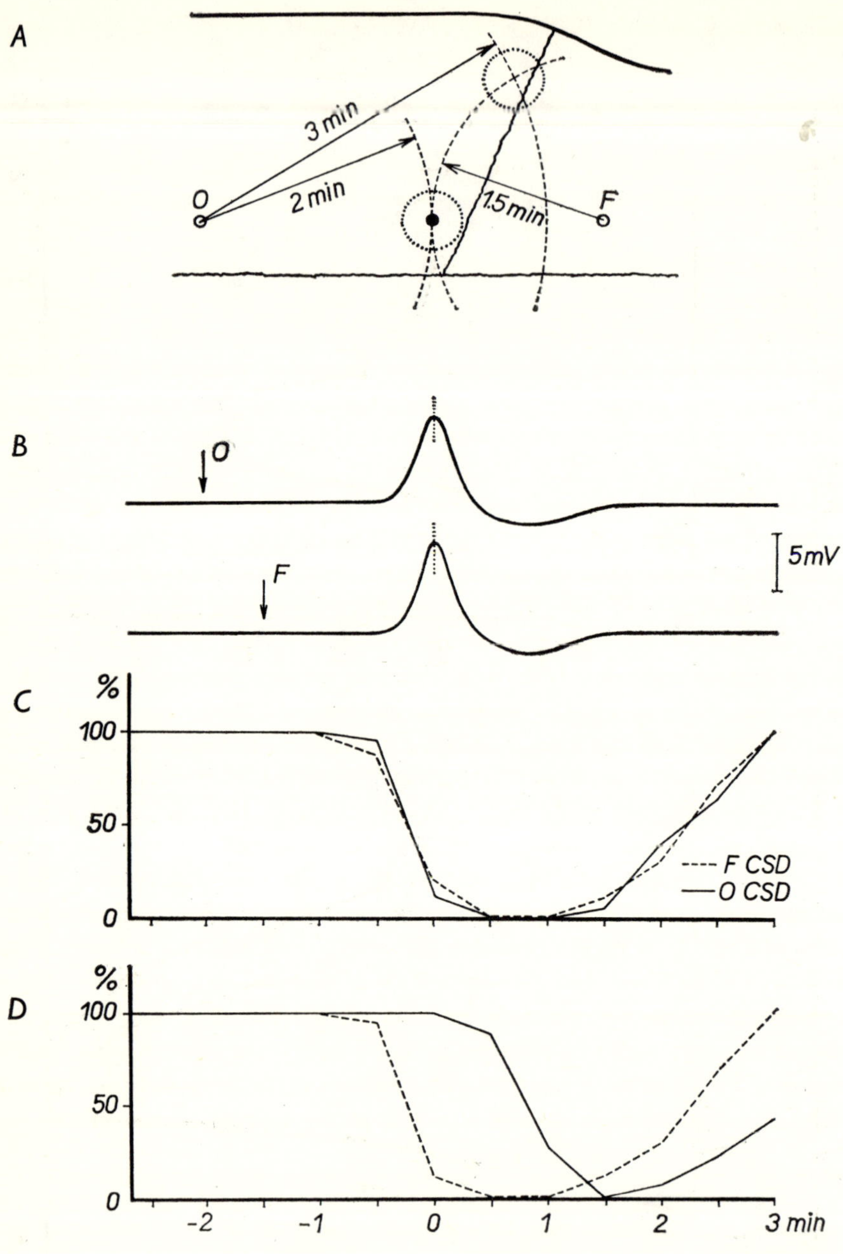

Fig. 9. 6. Schematic illustration of the use of CSD for location of cortical areas indispensable for performance of a conditioned reaction. *(A)* Position of the injection cannulae *(O* and *F)* and of the recording electrode (dot). Arrows indicate radii of the area depressed 1.5 min or 2 min and 3 min after CSD has been triggered from points *F* or *O*. Dotted circles correspond to the cortical regions that are suspected of playing a role in the examined reaction. *(B)* SPC from the recording electrode with CSD evoked from cannula *O* (arrow) or *F* (arrow). Both recordings are synchronized by the maximum

Duration of Impairment

Whereas the blockade of conditioned reactions begins abruptly and the dispersion of latencies is small, the overall duration of the impairment is much more variable. The recovery is a gradual slow process, depending in addition to other factors, on the depth and duration of the preceding impairment and on the conditioning and testing procedures. It is preferable therefore to discuss the effects of a single CSD wave and of a train of CSD waves separately.

Most relevant for assessing the effect of a single CSD wave are the experiments of Suzuki and Uneoka (1966) who recorded SPC in the cortex of freely moving rabbits. A single wave of CSD, elicited by electrical stimulation simultaneously in both hemispheres, impairs bar pressing for a food reward over 5 to 12 min. Recovery is rapid, the transition from complete absence of bar pressing to the predepression rate being attained in less than 1 min. Similar results were obtained by Megirian and Bureš (1970) for the conditioned eye-blink in the rabbit. When using electrical stimulation of the skin as the CS, a single CSD wave in the hemisphere contralateral to the blinking eye abolished the conditioned reaction for 4 to 5 min and full recovery was attained after 10 to 15 min. The recovery rate was slower when the critical motor area was affected not only by SD but also directly by the injected KCl solution in the case of frontal injections (Fig. 9.5). Different results were obtained in the same behavioral task with visual CS (Gutmann, Brožek, and Bureš 1971). After a single CSD wave elicited from the frontal cortex, full recovery of the conditioned eye blink took 30 min on the average, evidently because the detection of the weak visual signal required a more complete recovery of the cortical projection area than was needed for adequately processing somatosensory or auditory signals.

Until recently similar data were not available for rats, since most behavioral experiments were performed without simultaneous recording of the electrical concomitants of CSD. It is highly probable, however, that asphyxia activation of subthreshold KCl foci (Bureš and Burešová 1960a) produces only a single CSD wave. Under these conditions an avoidance reaction was abolished for 6 to 8 min in most animals but recovery could be retarded in this case by the aftereffects of asphyxia. Application of 2 % KCl to the cortical surface elicits up to three slow potential waves following each other with an interval of 5 min on the average (Bureš, Burešová, and

---

of SPC negativity. *(C, D)* Changes of the CR performance (percentage of correct reactions on the ordinate) due to CSD evoked from frontal *(FCSD)* or occipital *(OCSD)* cannulae. Records of behavioral changes are synchronized with the respective SPC recordings *(B)*. In *(C)* the conditioned reactions disappear as soon as the electrode is reached by the CSD wave from either direction. In *(D)* disappearance of the conditioned reaction coincides with the slow potential of the frontal CSD but with occipital CSD behavioral depression is delayed 1 min with respect to the SPC. The critical region must be located therefore at the intersection of the 1.5-min circle circumscribed from *F* and of the 3-min circle circumscribed from *O*.

Záhorová 1958). Avoidance reactions disappear in the second minute after KCl application and reappear in the eighth to twelfth minute. In some experiments this reappearance of response is followed by complete recovery, the rat never failing to avoid the electric shock over the next 20 min. In other experiments the recovery was only transient and was followed by another wave of extinction. Sometimes several waves could be detected with a recurrence period (time elapsed from the first recovered avoidance reaction through the following suppression period to the next recovered one) of 7.0 min. These periodic disappearance and reappearance of conditioned reactions evidently correspond to repeated waves of CSD. The average interval between periods of suppression of conditioned reactions is longer than the average interval between the slow potential waves. This is evidently due to an absence of behavioral recovery between slow potential waves separated by short intervals. With periodic suppression of avoidance reactions longer intervals occur with a higher probability than the short ones.

Behavior during periods of partial EEG recovery between consecutive CSD waves was studied by Freedman, Pote, Butcher, and Suboski (1968). The average inter-wave intervals after application of 10 % or 25 % KCl into Tapp's (1962) cannulae were rather long: 9.5, 8.4, and 7.6 min for different groups. Spontaneous activity of the animals was higher during high-amplitude phases of EEG activity than during marked EEG depression. Acquisition of a conditioned emotional reaction was impossible during the latter phase but proceeded more or less normally in the intervals of temporary EEG restitution. In another paper Freedman (1969) examined licking of sucrose solution and spontaneous activity or shock-motivated running in a wheel and found all these activities under similar conditions not totally depressed but displaying bursts of recovery alternating with periods of depression. The burst-to-burst intervals were 6.0 min for licking, 8.9 min for spontaneous and 6.9 min for shock-motivated wheel running after application of 10 or 25 % KCl to both cannulae. With 0.9 % NaCl the activity cycle ranged from 12 to 14.5 min probably corresponding to the physiological sleep-wakefulness cycle in rats (Roldán, Weiss, and Fifková 1963). Although interpretation of the above results is somewhat complicated by the unverified assumption of symmetrical development of CSD in both hemispheres, the data indicate that small trephine openings used by some authors (for example, Tapp 1962) and long interval between surgery and KCl application (48 hours) may not ensure a smooth EEG depression even when applying concentrated KCl solutions, and that the resulting incompleteness of functional decortication may considerably distort the results.

This problem was analyzed by Freedman and Bureš (1972) who generated the CSD waves synchronously in both hemispheres using iontophoretic injections of K^+ through implanted cannulae. With a 10-min interdepression interval, an overtrained one-way avoidance was partly blocked during the passage of the SPC across the cortex but fully recovered before the next CSD was triggered. With a 4-min interdepression interval, the blockade of avoidance behavior was almost complete and the impairment outlasted a train of 10 CSD waves for 20 to 40 min, probably because of cumulative effect due to metabolic exhaustion. Intermediate results were obtained with 6- and 8-min interdepression intervals (Fig. 9.7). Smooth behavioral impairment can be obtained with acute application of 25 % KCl into large trephine openings (4 to 5 mm diameter) because of a high CSD rate (initial interdepression interval less than 3 to 4 min). With repeated application of concentrated KCl solution to the same cortical region the damaged tissue interferes with K^+ diffusion to the intact cortex and prolongs the interdepression interval even when using the large-size trephine openings.

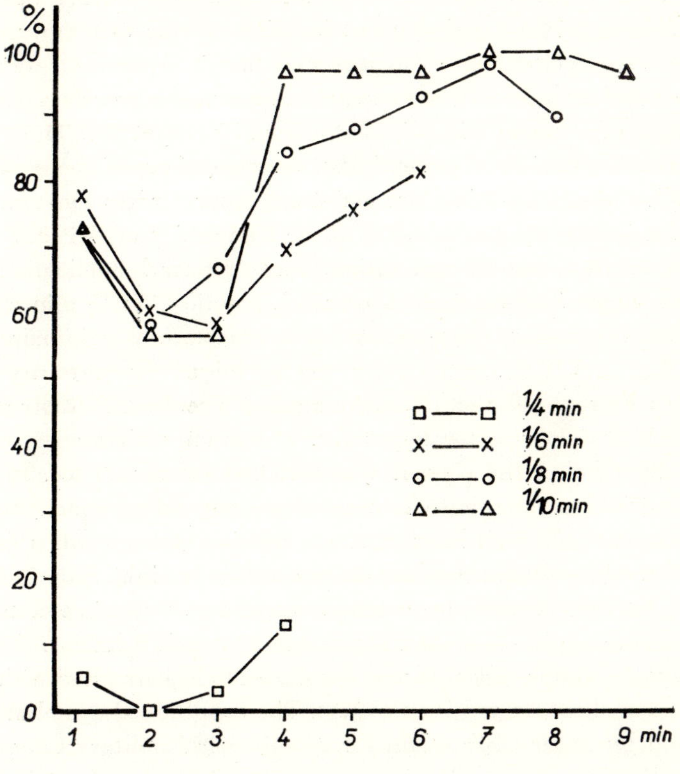

Fig. 9. 7. Percentage of the avoidance responses (ordinate) as a function of rate of electrophoretic generation of bilateral CSD waves and time following injection (abscissa) (Freedman and Bureš 1971).

Frequency of the slow potential waves gradually decreases to 50 % of the initial rate, but the conditioned reactions remain continuously suppressed evidently because repeated CSD waves exhaust the metabolic resources of the cerebral cortex (see Chap. 5). Complex habits reappear therefore only with a considerable delay after the last slow potential wave or after EEG recovery (Burešová 1956, Bureš 1959, Burešová and Bureš 1960) at a time when metabolic recovery is completed (Křivánek 1958). Removal of KCl by washing the cerebral surface with saline does not lead to immediate restitution of normal activity — the metabolic resources have to be restored first. This is a rather slow process, the duration of which is proportional to duration of the preceding depression. Supporting evidence for this statement was obtained in a recent study showing that the suppression of the cortical placing reactions outlasts the last of a series of slow potential waves by 30 to 60 min (Carew, Crow, and Petrinovich 1970). It is hardly possible to claim, however, that such results demonstrate a lack of correlation between CSD and behavior. They indicate rather that repeated waves of CSD affect conditioned reactions by two different mechanisms, the relative importance of which changes during the course of the experiment. The initial wave-dependent impairment due to temporary blockade of a large mass of neural elements changes smoothly into the late, wave-independent depression caused by a deep disorganization of metabolic processes (Chap. 5).

The duration of behavioral impairment caused by repeated CSD waves in different studies cannot be directly compared because conditions of focus may differ considerably. When these conditions are maintained more or less constant, the duration of impairment is directly proportional to the complexity of the task and indirectly proportional to the level of motivation. Thus bilateral application of 2 % KCl suppressed a simple food-motivated approach reaction for 45 min on the average, whereas a more complex approach-avoidance reaction was impaired for 72 min (Bureš and Burešová 1959). In the latter case the animal was prevented from drinking by the electric current (50 c/sec, 0.2mA) applied between the water in the drinking tube and the metal floor of the apparatus. It was only when an acoustic or visual signal was applied that the current was switched off for 20 sec. In the course of training, the drinking tube first changed from a natural approach stimulus into an avoidance stimulus and only later regained positive meaning when associated with sound or light. The complex mechanism of conditioned inhibition indispensable for correct performance of the above reaction evidently requires a more complete restitution of cortical function than the simple approach behavior. Differential CSD susceptibility of a simple task was recently shown to be correlated with the modality of CS (Gutmann, Brožek, and Bureš 1971). The conditioned eye-blink in the rabbit was depressed by single CSD waves for 20 min with auditory CS but for 30 min with visual CS.

Impairment of approach behavior can be estimated either by the absence of spontaneous reactions (for example drinking, feeding, bar pressing, and so on) or by unresponsiveness to conditioned stimuli, announcing the availability of reinforcement. In both cases no UCS is applied during the behavioral depression. On the other hand aversive behavior offers much more difficult problems. Escape response is not suppressed by CSD but deprived of its goal-directed, skilled components. In simple tasks the functionally decorticated animals usually succeed in reaching the goal after many random attempts to escape continuing electric stimulation. Escape latency gradually decreases with further testing (Bureš, Burešová, and Záhorová

1958) which might be due not only to subsiding depression but also to subcortical learning (see p. 238). In avoidance tasks absence of the conditioned response also leads to application of UCS and thus to some sort of learning. The UCS cannot be omitted during testing as this will especially in the phase of partial recovery of cortical functions, favor extinction of previously elaborated reactions. As the arousing effects of painful stimuli may significantly influence the overall duration of impairment, it is obvious that the frequency of testing becomes an important factor under these conditions. Nevertheless for long intertrial intervals (10 min) and tasks of comparable complexity, avoidance and approach are inhibited for approximately equal periods.

Since the cerebral cortex in the area of focus is more or less damaged by the highly hypertonic KCl solution, the question arises as to how significant is the localization of the focus with respect to the cortical representation of the CS or UCS. The experiments confirmed Lashley's mass-action hypothesis for simple approach or aversive reactions. The duration of impairment was independent of the location of the focus (Bureš and Burešová 1959, Tapp 1962). Anesthesia by novocaine of a cortical sensory area of the size of the focus did not influence reactions to the CS of the respective modality and deep thermocoagulation was only slightly more effective (Bureš and Burešová 1959). Sunenshine and Schwartz (1969) examined effects of bilateral lesions caused by repeated application of solid KCl to dura (on three consecutive days) on retention of the classically conditioned eyeblink in the rabbit. Although the cup-shaped lesions centered 1 mm anterior and 6 mm lateral to bregma ranged from 2.4 to 6.8 mm in diameter and from 0.9 to 4.8 mm in depth the performance of the animal remained close to 90 %. When CSD was evoked by KCl application onto the damaged region 1 hour prior to testing, the performance dropped to 55 %.

Similarly Freedman and Pote (1969) found no reduction of wheel running after ablation of the frontal cortex; the treatment of the frontal cortex with 25 % KCl usually caused a serious performance deficiency in rats. Focus position may be important, however, when using conditioned reactions with a well-defined cortical representation.

Spatially Limited Spreading Depression

The problems of cortical localization have also been approached in the SD studies from a different direction. The intactness of a certain cortical region can be considered a necessary and sufficient prerequisite of a definite behavior pattern only when two conditions are satisfied: (a) The reaction is eliminated by local destruction of the particular area, but (b) it survives total decortication sparing the same region (Sperry 1959).

Cortical SD can be confined to islands of cortical tissue prepared by subpial cuts penetrating through all cortical layers (Ochs 1962). Using this technique Ochs (1958) and Ochs and Hunt (1960) showed in acute experiments that CSD generated outside the island spreads all around it but does not enter it, and that CSD evoked within the island does not invade the surrounding cortex. The authors employed this technique to analyze the mechanism of the direct cortical response to electrical stimuli, but the same method can be also applied in behavioral experiments. The only attempt in this direction (Freedman and Pote 1969) probably failed because the cuts were too shallow (1 mm) and because with KCl application over the whole surface of the island, the diffusing potassium ions also elicited CSD in the outside cortex. No electrophysiological evidence was present that CSD remained limited to the island.

Islands of cortical tissue can also be protected against CSD by local treatment with divalent cations, which leave the spontaneous and evoked electrical activity in the treated areas more or less intact. Attempts to use this technique to achieve protection of the cortical links of different conditioned reactions were made by Burešová and Bureš (1960). Best results were obtained with a local reaching-for-food reaction used in experiments with "handedness". Rats trained to take small food pellets from a glass tube 14 mm in diameter prefer to perform this reaction persistently with the left or right forepaw. The movement is controlled from a circumscribed area of the contralateral sensorimotor cortex several cubic millimeters in volume (Peterson and Devine 1963). Cortical SD elicited by application of 2 % KCl onto the occipital cortex of the hemisphere contralateral to the preferred forelimb suppressed this reaction for about 40 min. Application of a filter paper soaked with 1.7 % $MgCl_2$ or 2.5 % $CaCl_2$ onto the motor cortex did not affect the reaching ability of the rat. Cortical SD elicited by 2 % KCl 20 to 30 min later caused none or only a short-lasting inhibition (less than 5 min on the average, Table 9.1). After a single application of 1.7 % $MgCl_2$, full protection could be observed for 5 hours and the protective effect disappeared only after 10 hours (Fig. 9.8).

Table 9. 1.

Duration of Impairment of a Discrete Operant Habit (Reaching for Food with One Forepaw) Due to CSD Evoked 30 min after Application of NaCl, $MgCl_2$, or $CaCl_2$ Solutions to Circumscribed Cortical Areas. (Unilateral CSD Elicited by 2% KCl Applied onto the Untreated Cortex)

Protective Solution (Percent)	Protective Solution Applied on: Frontoparietal Cortex (n)	Frontoparietal Cortex (min)	Occipital Cortex (n)	Occipital Cortex (min)
NaCl 0.9	17	40.5±7.1		
$MgCl_2$ 1.7	11	4.7±1.7	9	22.4±3.0
$CaCl_2$ 2.5	12	0.9±0.6		

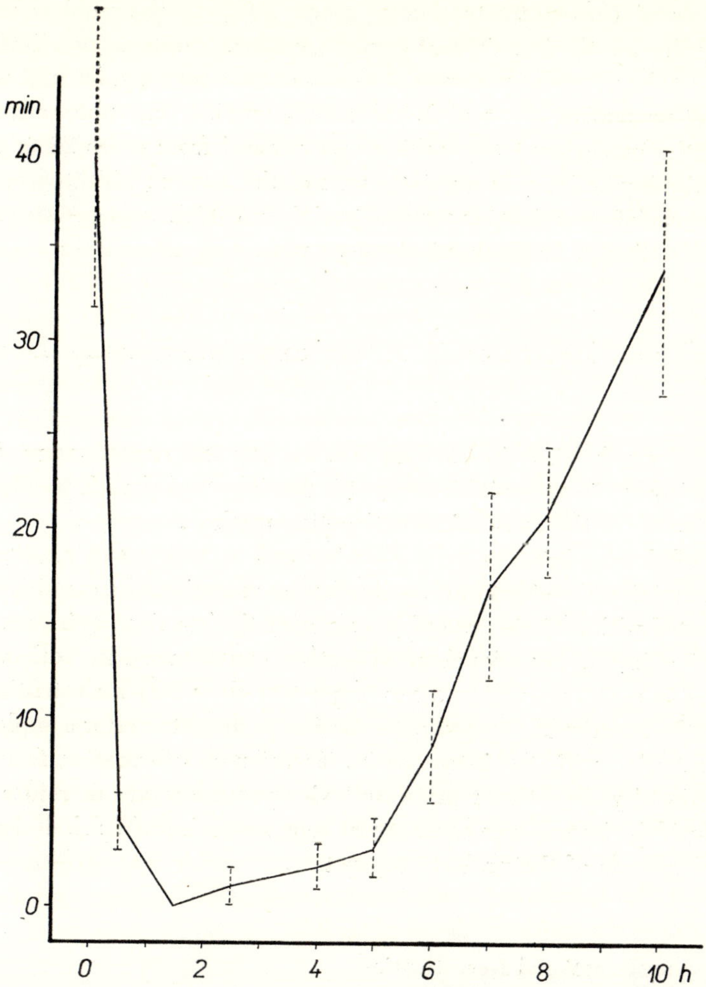

Fig. 9. 8. Protection of a local reaching-for-food reaction against the effects of CSD by a single application of a filter paper soaked with 1.7 % $MgCl_2$ on the contralateral sensorimotor cortex. Abscissa: time (in hours) from application of $MgCl_2$ to CSD initiation. Ordinate: duration of inhibition caused by 2 % KCl (in min). The dotted vertical lines give the standard errors of the means (Burešová and Bureš 1960).

The same treatment of the motor areas of both hemispheres by 1.7 % $MgCl_2$ only partly protected a runway avoidance reaction against the effects of bilaterally applied 2 % KCl, the duration of impairment being reduced from 37 to 21 min on the average (Burešová and Bureš 1960). This result is in good agreement with the earlier conclusion that the motor cortex is not indispensable for performance of general motor reactions, the impairment of which is more or less proportional to the area of depressed cortex. Protection of about 20 % of the cortical surface may considerably shorten the impairment caused by CSD. A diffuse contribution of wide cortical areas to local conditioned reactions was demonstrated in the case of "handedness" by the protective effect of 1.7 % $MgCl_2$ applied onto the occipital cortex. Duration of the impairment of reaching was reduced from 40 to 22 min, probably because continuing activity in a remote part of the cortex facilitated recovery processes in the crucial sensorimotor cortex. Possible role of the subcortical motivational centers in mediation of diffuse cortical effects will be discussed later.

4. Learning and Retention in Intact and Functionally Decorticated Animals

Although CSD can be used in the same way as surgical decortication, in a special class of experiments its reversibility makes it possible to deal with problems that are beyond the scope of the anatomical extirpation method.

The role of the cerebral cortex in learning and retention was classically studied either by examining the effect of decortication on retention of a conditioned reaction (CR) elaborated with brain intact or by comparing the learning abilities of normal and decorticated animals. Functional decortication can be used in both ways but in addition it can serve to explore a new aspect of the problem; retention of habits acquired by the functionally decorticated brain can be tested after complete recovery of cortical function with the intact brain. Transfer of information from the intact to the functionally decorticate brain and vice versa became therefore one of the areas in which the importance of CSD was soon recognized. We shall deal now with the different aspects of the problem separately.

Learning During Functional Decortication

As pointed out in the preceding section, retention testing under CSD may be confused with decorticate learning. It is essential therefore to characterize the learning ability of the functionally decorticated rats first. The possibility of elaborating a simple avoidance reaction under bilateral CSD was reported in one of the early CSD studies (Bureš 1959). In order to avoid electric shocks the rat was required to cross from one half of a rectangular apparatus into the other within 5 sec. When no partition separated the two halves, typical learning curves were obtained under CSD, although acquistion was slower than in normal rats. When the task was made more difficult by separating the start and goal by a partition with a 6 by 6-cm door, no signs of learning could be seen over a 30 min training period (Fig. 9.9). The notion that the difference in the efficiency of normal and decorticate learning increases with task difficulty was confirmed by other authors. Winokur (1965) gave functionally de-

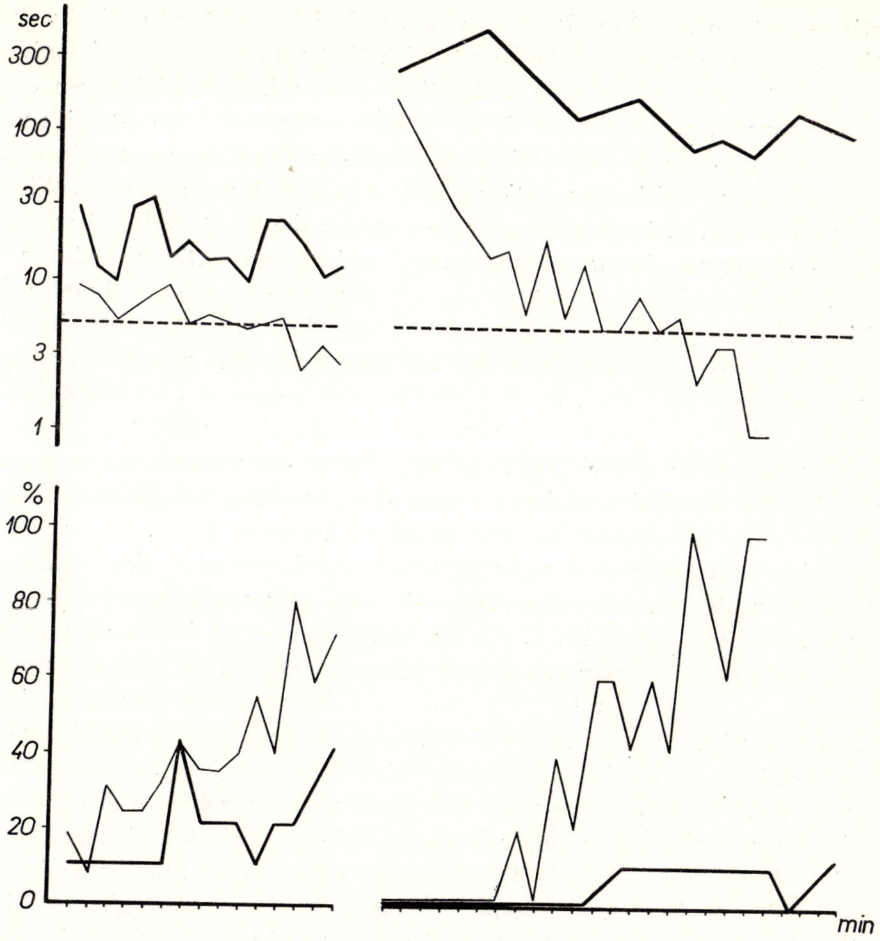

Fig. 9. 9. Elaboration of two types of avoidance reactions in control rats (thin line, $n = 12$) and in rats under bilateral CSD evoked by 25 % KCl (heavy line, $n = 8$). (Left) The rat is required to pass within 5 sec from the electrifiable floor in one half of the box to the other half. (Right) The two parts of the box are separated by a partition with a 6 × 6 cm door. (Above) Mean latencies of the avoidance or escape response. (Below) Percentage of avoidance responses. Abscissa: time in min (Bureš 1959).

corticate animals 30 trials in a one-way avoidance task. When the goal compartment was separated from the rest of the apparatus by two open doorways (each 15 cm wide) the rats achieved 40 % avoidances. Not a single avoidance was observed, however, when the safe compartment was only accessible through a small central opening (6 by 7 cm) situated 6 cm above the floor. In normal rats both tasks were equal in the acquisition rate measured by the number of to-criterion trials. Thompson and Hjelle (1965) studied one-way, two-way, and shuttle avoidance learning in a narrow runway and found the ratios of to-criterion trials in control and functionally decorticated rats to be 3.0 to 27.5, 9.1 to 31.2, and 22.5 to 60.0, respectively. In the shuttle avoidance task none of the 10 rats with bilateral CSD reached the criterion of nine correct responses out of 10 consecutive trials within 60 trials given during 2 hours of depression. Travis and Sparks (1963) were not able to establish under bilateral CSD one-way avoidance through the 10-by 10-cm door centrally located in the 40-cm long partition separating the start and goal compartments. Whereas normal rats took 7.7 trials on the average to reach the 9 out of 10 criterion, not a single avoidance reaction was found in the functionally decorticated animals over 40 trials. Significant improvement of escape performance was observed under these conditions, however, the mean escape latency dropping from 125 sec in the initial 10 trials to 16 sec in the last 10 trials. Similar results were reported by Russel, Plotkin, and Kleinman (1968). On the other hand Freedman and Lash (1966) found an increase instead of a decrease of average escape latencies (from 10 to 15 sec) over 40 trials performed by decorticate rats in a smaller one-way shuttle box (see p. 243).

Conditions for acquisition of the simple one-way avoidance habit described above (Thompson and Hjelle 1965) were analyzed by Thompson (1965). Under bilateral CSD 34 trials on the average were required to attain the criterion when using 30-sec intertrial intervals, whereas with 120-sec intertrial intervals the number of to-criterion trials dropped to 13. A similar relationship was found for intact brain learning, the respective to-criterion trials being 18 and 5. Plotkin (1967) reported that bilaterally depressed rats scored no successful responses over 20 avoidance training trials with intertrial intervals of 15, 30, 60 and 240 sec, but the average escape latencies were significantly shorter with the 15-sec interval than with the longer ones. This is opposite to what was found with controls in which the 15-sec intertrial interval resulted in longer latencies and less efficient avoidance learning. Decorticate learning also depends (Thompson and Hjelle 1965) on the discriminability of the conditioned stimulus. When only opening of the door served as the conditioned signal, over 50 % animals failed to attain the criterion within 60 trials applied during a single 2-hour session. Addition of a buzzer to the door opening decreased the number of to-criterion trials to 17 on the average.

Better results may be achieved with more prolonged training. Swenson and Goldowitz (1972) evoked bilateral CSD on 4 consecutive days and trained the depressed rats in a discriminated avoidance. With 40 trials per session, performance improved from 32 % avoidances on Day 1 to 84 % avoidances on Day 4. Significant discrimination started to appear on Day 2 and all animals reached criterion on Day 3. The results may be due to adaptation of the animal to the functional decortication or to the decreasing effect of the repeated CSDs (see p. 225).

An obvious conclusion from the above experiments is that functionally decorticate animals can learn simple avoidance reactions. The learning is much slower than in normal animals, however, the difference increasing with the difficulty of the task. No signs of approach learning were reported under bilateral CSD, evidently because of a deep inhibition of the hypothalamic drive centers (see p. 336).

Although the evidence for some kind of decorticate learning is convincing, it is less clear how long the acquired experience is retained and under what conditions it can be retrieved. In the experiments (p. 240) by Travis and Sparks (1963) an escape reaction was trained under bilateral CSD on two consecutive days without significant improvement of performance. On the other hand Thompson (1964) retrained a simple avoidance reaction 4.5 hours after the conclusion of the training session and found that the number of to-criterion trials decreased from 19 during original learning to 8 during retraining. The improvement cannot be considered as a conclusive proof of retention however since better performance during the second KCl application could also be due to decreased efficiency of the chemical stimulus. No adequate control experiments were made to rule out this possibility. In a later replication of the same experiments (Hjelle and Thompson, 1965) 26 trials were required during training and 16 trials during retraining but the difference was not statistically significant. When SD was maintained by repeated KCl application during the whole retention interval, retraining required 43 trials and did not significantly differ from the control group, which received first training after 5 hours of depression and required 50 median trials to criterion.

In other studies (Bureš 1964, Bureš and Burešová 1965, 1968a) preference of rats for the grid floor or wooden floor compartments of the training box was examined first. Then the animals were trained to avoid the grid floor and to stay on the wooden floor. On the next day, the preference was tested again. No change against the first preference testing was observed when all stages of the experiment were performed under bilateral CSD. It can be conceived therefore that the experience acquired during functional decortication decays so rapidly that it cannot be retrieved after longer intervals. This is in agreement with the data on learning in decerebrate animals in which short-lived conditioned reactions (Bard and Macht 1958) of the sensitization type are common.

There is some evidence, however, that classical conditioning of vegetative phenomena is not affected by CSD in the same way. Burgoyne, Pote, and Freedman (1967) elaborated cardiac acceleration to an acoustic CS followed by an electric shock in normal or in functionally decorticated animals on two consecutive days. Learning curves were similar for both groups, with a comparable improvement on the second day as compared with the first day. The authors conclude that cardiac conditioning does not depend on the availability of a functional cortex. A pseudoconditioning control in normal animals ruled out a sensitization interpretation of the above results.

Experiments of this kind indicate that the negative findings cannot be overestimated and that the absence of retention under bilateral CSD does not preclude any utilization of information acquired during functional decortication by the intact brain and vice versa. The following pages summarize the experimental evidence concerning this kind of transfer.

Transfer from Normal to Decorticate Brain

As already shown (Chap. 9, Sec. 3) conditioned reactions acquired with a normal brain cannot be retrieved during bilateral CSD. This statement requires some qualification, however. It is obviously true when the testing procedure cannot lead to relearning the task under CSD, that is, when we use conditioned reactions the elaboration of which in functionally decorticated animals is impossible, or when the number of testing trials is well below the decorticate learning threshold. The question remains, however, whether the experience acquired by the intact brain can influence the decorticate behavior at all. Thompson (1964) attempted to answer this problem by comparing elaboration of simple one-way avoidance under bilateral CSD in untrained animals and in animals that were trained in the same task 5 hours earlier with an intact brain. On the average, decorticate learning required 19 to-criterion trials in the untrained animals, but only 10 trials in the pretrained group, the difference being statistically significant ($p<0.01$). Similar results were obtained earlier by Bureš (1959,c. f. Fig. 9.9 and 11.1) who trained intact rats with a simple avoidance and immediately after reaching the criterion retrained them under bilateral CSD. Relearning in this group proceeded much faster than learning in untrained animals under CSD. Winokur (1965) also found in a similar one-way avoidance that pretraining intact rats increases from 12 to 17.5 the median number of avoidances made in 30 testing trials under functional decortication.

More complex tasks were examined by Kukleta (1966). In one of his experiments normal rats were trained in a maze to avoid electric shocks by entering the goal compartment within 10 sec. After six to-criterion training sessions over 3 days, retention was tested under bilateral CSD. Fifteen trials were given at 2-min intervals. If the animal did not escape the shocks within 1 min, it was removed from the apparatus and returned to the start only after another minute had elapsed. Although practically no avoidance reactions were seen under CSD, the depressed animals succeeded in 35% of the trials in reaching the goal or its close vicinity within 1 min. In a control group of unpretrained rats only 6% of the trials were successful. In the second experiment by the same investigator a maze with two goal compartments was used, the second of which was more easily accessible than the first one. Intact rats were trained in six sessions to make the more difficult avoidance to the first goal, the more accessible second goal being closed. During testing under bilateral CSD (15 trials) both goals were open. The pretrained animals escaped to the first and second goals in 33.3 and 8.2% trials, respectively, whereas in untrained animals the corresponding numbers were 4.6 and 14.4%, respectively. These results indicate that at least some of the functionally decorticated animals retain information on the spatial location of the goal previously acquired with the brain intact. The same conclusion was also supported by later findings (Kukleta 1968) demonstrating that the start-goal topography of a complex avoidance habit learned with a normal brain is partly remembered under bilateral CSD. Whereas untrained functionally decorticated rats failed in 62% of the cases to reach the goal of a U-shaped runway with the central partition removed, animals, that received 60 intact brain pretraining trials showed successful escape under bilateral CSD in 82% of the cases, with the form of the run resembling the original U-shape in nearly 70 % of the cases. Pretraining an active discriminated avoidance task for two days (Swenson and Goldowitz 1972) improves subsequent relearning of the same habit under bilateral CSD to 71 % avoidances and 75 % correct choices as compared with 32 % avoidances and 55 % correct choices in the naive depressed animals.

The most clear-cut transfer of information from normal to decorticate brain was demonstrated by Russell, Kleinman, Plotkin, and Ross (1969) for the passive avoidance response. In an apparatus consisting of a large, brightly illuminated compartment connected with a small dark enclosure, rats spent most of the 5-min exploration time (over 90%) in the small chamber (Fig. 9.10, group B). This preference, which is equally well expressed in normal and functionally decorticated rats, was reversed after intact animals had received several minutes of electric shocks in the small compartment. In retention tests performed 24 hours after learning, bilaterally decorticated rats (B) avoided the small compartment as efficiently as undepressed controls (A). The authors suggest that during classical conditioning the cortex acts as a passive mediating link transmitting information to subcortical storage sites (see p. 250). Retrieval of the stored information is possible without cortical participation if retention is expressed by modification of some continuing behavior in the presence of CS.

Contrasting with the above results are experiments by Freedman and Lash (1966) who found no significant positive transfer of simple one-way avoidance from normal brain to bilateral CSD. It must be pointed out, however, that these experiments are unusual because the mean escape latency was 10 sec at the onset of training and increased over the 40 trials performed under functional decortication to 25 sec. This might be related to the gradual development of CSD with the small trephine openings used for KCl application in this study, whereas 4 to 5-mm trephine holes were employed in the papers mentioned above.

Classical conditioning of the heart rate forms a separate subgroup of these studies. Mogenson and Peterson (1966) used a 3-sec buzzer as the CS, followed in 50% of the trials by a 2-sec grid shock. With 10 daily training trials, conditioned heart rate changes appeared consistently after 3 to 4 days. The heart rate increased from the prebuzzer frequency of 388/min to 421/min during the signal and to 452/min during the 5 sec after buzzer termination. Bilateral CSD evoked by 10% KCl reduced the background heart rate (369/min) but left the buzzer-dependent conditioned acceleration unaffected (402/min). The postbuzzer acceleration component was absent (396/min), however. In five rats a shuttle-box avoidance was established simultaneously with the conditioned cardiac reaction. Under bilateral CSD the rats continued to display the conditioned heart-rate acceleration (without the secondary acceleration component) but were seriously impaired in performing the avoidance reaction (only 1 avoidance in 50 trials).

Rather different results were reported by Hendrickson and Pinto-Hamuy (1967). A 5-sec increase of illumination served as the CS immediately followed by a 0.5 sec foot shock. With 10 to 20 trials per day a total of 90 to 120 pairings of CS and UCS were administered prior to testing under CSD. Although both accelerative and decelerative conditioned reactions appeared in the early stages of learning, the latter gradually became more prominent and the final conditioned response was a marked slowing of the heart observed in more than 70% of the trials. During bilateral CSD

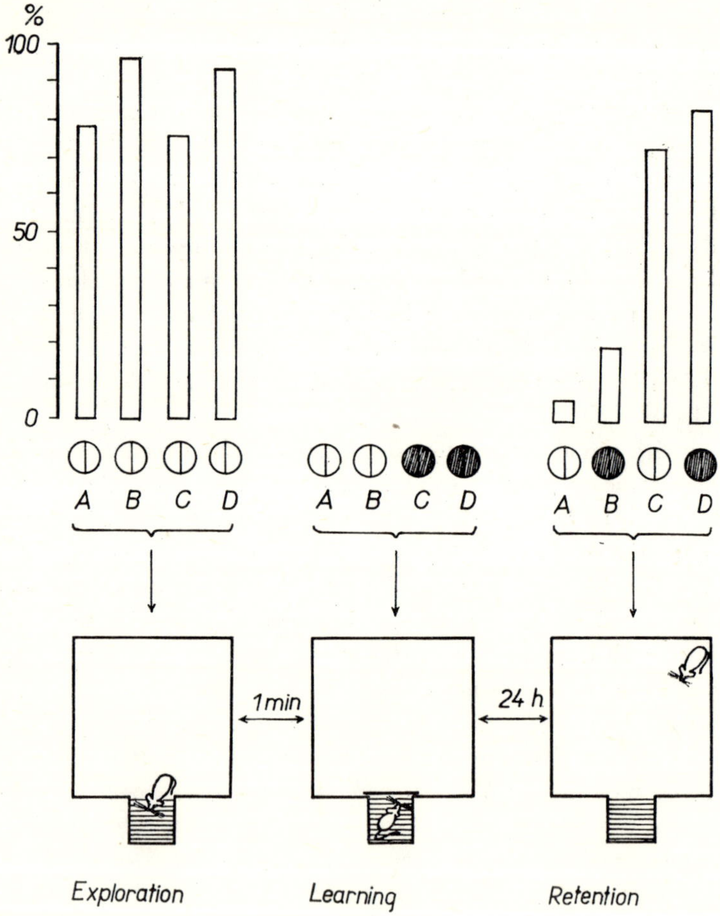

Fig. 9. 10. The effect of functional decortication on the acquisition and/or retention of a passive avoidance reaction in rats. The experimental paradigm is schematically shown below the respective columns. Ordinate: percentage of the total exploration time spent in the small compartment. Groups *A* and *C* from Bureš and Burešová (1963), groups *B* and *D* from Russell, Kleinman, Plotkin, and Ross (1969). For details see text.

the incidence of the conditioned reactions dropped to 6% and was thus even lower than in the first training session with an intact brain (20%). The authors suggest that the discrepancy between their results and the findings by Mogenson and Peterson (1966) is due to the sensitization nature of the accelerative heart reaction occurring during CSD in the latter study. As shown by Holdstock and Schwartzbaum (1965) pseudoconditioning causes accelerative heart rate responses that appear by the end of the first session and do not improve with further training whereas classical conditioning leads to a decelerative response that improves over sessions. As heart rate changes can be easily conditioned in surgically decorticate rats (Bloch-Rojas, Toro, and Pinto-Hamuy 1964) the blockade of the conditioned decelerative cardiac reaction in functionally decorticated animals is either due to some subcortical effects of CSD or it indicates that under normal conditions even the classical conditioning of vegetative functions is mediated by the cerebral cortex. Only when the cortex is eliminated, can memory traces be formed in the subcortical centers.

The classically conditioned eye-blink reaction in the rabbit is completely blocked during CSD in the hemisphere contralateral to the blinking eye (Megirian and Bureš 1970). Bilateral CSD also impairs the conditioned head shaking reaction, elaborated in young rabbits (aged one month) by pairing an acoustic CS with electrical stimulation of the neck skin (Malakhovskaya 1972). It seems that the degree of corticalization depends more on the character of the unconditioned reaction than on the conditioning paradigm.

The transfer from normal to functionally decorticate brain can be facilitated by a procedure essentially similar to a technique proposed by Meyer, Isaac, and Maher (1958), who found a complete loss of a brightness discrimination after bilateral removal of the visual cortex in rats. When the cortical ablations were performed in two stages separated by a 10-day interval and when the animals were trained during this period, the discrimination was not much impaired by the second operation, probably because the engram descended to and/or became retrievable from subcortical visual centers. Kukleta (1965a,b) first applied this principle in CSD studies. He used three one-way avoidance reactions differing in the accessibility of the goal, which was connected with the runway either through a small window located in the lateral wall well above the floor (apparatus No. 1), through a larger window forming the upper half of the front wall (apparatus No. 2), or finally through a large door occupying most of the front wall (apparatus No. 3). Rats learned the particular avoidance reaction first with right and 5 hours later with the left hemisphere. Immediately after the criterion was reached under right CSD, KCl was applied onto the left hemisphere and after 5 min, 10 to 15 retention trials were tested. Approximately 90 % of the rats were able to reach the 9/10 criterion on all three tasks, whereas only 1 of 10 rats with intact brain pretraining reached the criterion in the simplest task No. 3. Intermediate results were obtained when CSD was applied during pretraining to one hemisphere only.

Nearly identical results were reported by Schneider (1966) who trained rats with a simple one-way avoidance on 3 consecutive days. Animals learning the task on the first and second day with brain intact did not perform under bilateral CSD on the third day significantly better than untrained animals (more than 30 to-criterion trials). On the contrary, rats trained on the first and second day under unilateral CSD either in the same or alternate hemispheres required significantly less trials to relearn under bilateral CSD (14 and 11 to-criterion trials, respectively).

Also Best and Hamburg (1969) reported that unilaterally trained and contralaterally retrained brightness discrimination task transferred to the bilaterally decorticate state. The transfer was complete under escape and partial under avoidance conditions. The facilitatory effect of unilateral learning on formation of memory traces retrievable under bilateral CSD was confirmed by Carlson (1967) using a preference paradigm. On the first day this author allowed rats under bilateral CSD to explore an apparatus consisting of two compartments of equal size for 3 min; one compartment was painted black with a grid floor, the other was painted white with a wooden floor. The time spent in either compartment was recorded. On the second day rats were trained to actively avoid the black compartment to a 9/10 criterion and on the third day the preference under bilateral CSD was tested again. Whereas the original 70 to 90 % preference of the black compartment (first day) was also found on the third day in the group that was trained on the second day with brain intact, animals learning under unilateral CSD on the second day, displayed a marked preference for the white compartment (over 80 %) on the third day. The transfer from hemidecortication to decortication was better expressed in animals that showed signs of fright (urination, defecation, "freezing") while learning the task on the second day.

In another experiment by the same author rats were put on a 23-hour water deprivation schedule and after the initial preference testing, they were given on two consecutive days appetitive training (a 15 min confinement in the black compartment followed by 15 min confinement in the white compartment with a full water pot). Even when this confinement training was performed under unilateral CSD, testing under bilateral CSD did not reveal any change of the original black-side preference. The author concludes that "there is no appreciable subcortical storage of the emotional and cue components of an appetitive task".

Transfer from Decorticate to Normal Brain

Although transfer of experience from normal to decorticate brain and learning in decorticated animals are not specific to the functional ablation technique, transfer from decortication to the normal state can only be studied by using a reversible functional decortication procedure. As artificial and abstract as the problem appears, it might serve as an experimental model of certain real situations, for example, transfer of experience acquired during the early periods of postnatal development with an immature cortex, to the fully developed brain of adult animals (Campbell and Campbell 1962). Even without these analogies the theoretical interest of the problem is obvious.

In the early CSD studies the problem was not specifically examined. An attempt to train a passive avoidance reaction under bilateral CSD was reported by Bureš and Burešová (1963). Normal rats exploring an apparatus consisting of a small (10 by 10 cm) and a large (40 by 40 cm) compartment spent over two thirds of the 3-min test in the small compartment. When they were confined in the small compartment for 1 min and subjected there to painful foot shocks, the preference in another exploratory test performed 24 hours later was changed and the small box was nearly completely avoided (Fig. 9.10, group A). When the aversive electrical stimulation was applied during bilateral CSD, however, the small compartment preference remained unchanged, indicating either that no learning occurred or that the subcortically formed and stored engrams are unretrievable with intact brain (Fig. 9.10, group C). This finding was recently confirmed by Russell, Kleinman, Plotkin, and Ross (1969) who also tested retention of the above passive avoidance response 15 min after decorticate learning. In this short term retention testing they found marked avoidance of the small compartment. The same behavior was also observed in the pseudoconditioning group, however, which received shocks outside the apparatus. Well expressed preference for the small compartment in untrained functionally decorticated animals made it possible to perform meaningful retention testing under bilateral CSD evoked 24 hours after decorticate conditioning. As no retention was found in this group (Fig. 9.10, group D) the conclusion seems to be justified that absence of passive avoidance in intact animals was not due to cortical interference with the retrieval of subcortical engrams, but rather to the fact that no such engrams had been formed under bilateral CSD.

The validity of the above conclusion was specified in the recent application of CSD technique (Burešová and Bureš 1973) to the analysis of the conditioned taste aversion (for review see Garcia and Ervin 1968 and Rozin and Kalat 1971). Water deprived rats were offered 0.1 % saccharin (CS) for 10 min and made sick 30 min later by intraperitoneal injection of lithium chloride (UCS, 0.14 M, 2 ml/100 g). The animals associated the nausea with the taste stimulus and on the next day reduced considerably the saccharin intake. Bilateral CSD elicited 15 min after saccharin ingestion and maintained during the rest of the CS-UCS interval and during the most severe phase of lithium intoxication did not diminish the aversion. On the other hand no aversion developed with the same CS-UCS delay when saccharin was administered to bilaterally depressed rats by forced feeding (to overcome the CSD-induced adipsia). This result contrasts with the claim by Best and Zuckerman (1971) that saccharin aversion elicited by apomorphine injection can be established during several training sessions under bilateral CSD. It appears, however, that functional decortication was highly incomplete in these experiments since there was no impairment of spontaneous drinking after KCl application. The conclusion seems to be justified, therefore, that normal cortical function is a necessary prerequisite for the formation of a temporary subcortical engram which can be changed by association with a gastrointestinal distress into a permanent trace even under bilateral CSD.

Significant transfer of information from decorticate to normal brain was described first by Travis and Sparks (1963), who trained bilaterally depressed rats in a rather difficult one-way avoidance task on 2 consecutive days and did not obtain any avoidance response in 40 trials (see p. 240). On the third day these animals were significantly worse than untrained controls in relearning the task with brain intact. Negative transfer between escape training received under bilateral CSD and subsequent avoidance learning without CSD indicates that the subcortically stored fear of unavoidable shocks interferes after cortical recovery with rapid recognition of the avoidance solution of the situation.

Korányi, Endröczi, and Lissák (1965) were also unable to train bilaterally depressed rats to avoid electric shocks by jumping on an insulated bench, when a buzzer was used as the warning CS. Unsuccessful learning under CSD did not facilitate later acquisition of the same avoidance reaction by the intact brain. Decorticate learning results, nevertheless, in formation of memory traces that could be revealed under certain conditions. The above avoidance reaction was firmly established and then extinguished with a normal brain. Ten reinforced trials given under bilateral CSD yielded no avoidance responding, but a new retention test performed on the next day in intact animals disclosed full restitution of the extinguished reaction. Again the number of nonreinforced trials required to achieve extinction was the same as the first time.

A sensitive method for testing the transfer from decorticate to intact brain is the preference method (Bureš 1964, Bureš and Burešová 1965, 1968a, see p. 241). Rats were trained under bilateral CSD to avoid the grid compartment of a shuttle box. When they were allowed 24 hours later to explore the apparatus for 5 min, they reduced their preference for the grid floor from the original 90 % to approximately 50 %. As rats trained with intact brain displayed a nearly complete preference for the wooden floor, it is obvious that the transfer from decorticate to intact brain is not perfect (Fig. 9.11).

Another preference method was successfully used by Kukleta (1968), who taught functionally decorticated rats to escape from the runway through a lateral door at the goal end. Later retesting with a normal brain and with both lateral doors open revealed a marked preference for the side reinforced under bilateral CSD.

Less clear results were obtained when using to-criterion trials as the measure of transfer. Kukleta (1968) failed in the above experiments to find any improvement of intact brain escape learning by decorticate pretraining. Thompson (1964) was also not able to demonstrate any acquisition of a simple one-way avoidance task in animals pretrained under bilateral CSD (2.5 and 2.6 to-criterion trials in the pretrained and untrained rats, respectively). On the other hand the incidence of stereotyped reactions (returning from the door to the back wall before passing into the goal compartment) was higher in pretrained animals than in untrained ones (16.0 and 3.2%, respectively).

Kukleta (1966) gave bilaterally depressed rats 15 escape or avoidance trials in a simple runway with an elevated goal area, and tested retention under unilateral CSD 5 hours later. A criterion of five consecutive avoidances was reached after 4.7 trials in this group as compared with 11.7 trials in rats that received bilateral CSD but no training. In a later study Kukleta (1967) pretrained bilaterally depressed rats in the same apparatus and after 5 to 7 hours continued to train them under unilateral CSD to avoid or escape through openings in the lateral walls at the far end of the runway. Pretrained rats were not better than untrained ones in the first unilateral CSD training session (17.2±2.0 and 15.7±2.1 to-criterion trials, respectively), but they displayed significant interhemispheric transfer when tested with the opposite hemisphere 5 to 7 hours later. In another series of experiments (Kukleta and Libouban 1967) escape training in functionally decorticate rats decreased escape latencies and improved

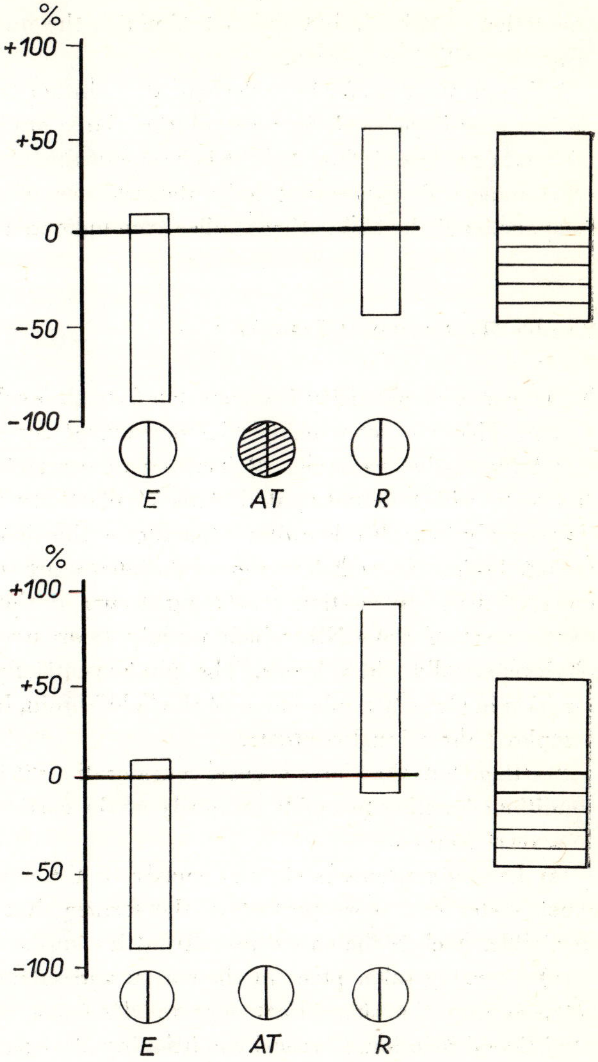

Fig. 9. 11. Intact brain retrieval of information acquired with a functionally decorticate brain. The columns denote the percentage of time spent by the rat in the grid floor or wooden floor compartments of the apparatus (diagram on the right), either during original exploration *(E)* or during the retention test *(R)*; *AT* is the period of avoidance training either under bilateral CSD (above) or with intact brain (below). Note that avoidance training under bilateral functional decortication reduced the preference for the grid floor significantly but less efficiently than intact brain training.

orientation of animals but did not diminish the number of to-criterion trials during relearning with intact brain.

Although the transfer from decorticate to intact brain depends considerably on the testing procedure used, in most of the above studies information acquired under bilateral CSD later influenced the behavior of the intact animal in some way. Whereas some papers demonstrated only the transfer of the emotional or motivational components of the task, other studies even indicated transfer of cue recognition.

Possible Mechanisms of Transfer

Some degree of plasticity is encountered at all levels of the nervous system organization. This was convincingly demonstrated by comparative physiology, which found impressive examples of learning in invertebrates, as well as by functional anatomy, which demonstrated signs of plasticity in the isolated spinal cord and increasingly complex learning capacity in the decerebrate and decorticate mammalian brain. Nevertheless the evolutionary arguments clearly indicate that the most efficient information processing occurs at the highest, phylogenetically most recent level of the CNS, which usually takes over most functions of the lower, phylogenetically older levels. The phylogenetically new superstructure can only function in close interrelation with the "old" brain, however, with which it maintains complex bidirectional contacts.

Starting from the above general considerations it is conceivable that under normal conditions learning proceeds primarily at the cortical level in rats. This may be due to several factors:

(a) Learning proceeds simultaneously in the cortex and subcortex, but it is so much faster and more perfect in the former that the subcortical contribution is negligible. Such is the case especially with complex learning tasks.

(b) Learning takes place in the cortex and subcortex at approximately the same rate, so that the subcortical engram alone can ensure good performance of the conditioned reaction. Classical conditioning of vegetative phenomena belongs to this category (Mogenson and Peterson 1966, Burgoyne, Pote, and Freedman 1967).

(c) Whereas in the previous cases cortical and subcortical learning is assumed to be mutually independent and subserved by parallel afferent and efferent pathways, in some instances formation of the subcortical engram may be facilitated by the availability of the cortex (Meyer, Isaac, and Maher 1958, Kukleta 1965, Schneider 1966, Carlson 1967, Russell, Kleinman, Plotkin, and Ross 1969).

(d) Finally, according to the classical view, availability of the cortex inhibits the subcortical storage mechanism, which is disinhibited or even activated by partial or complete decortication.

Since the above possibilities are not mutually exclusive, several of them may combine in each particular case. Experimental evidence indicates that the subcortical trace cannot be improved by extreme overtraining with an intact brain (Lashley 1929). This does not necessarily mean that subcortical learning is prevented by an active inhibitory process. The very fact that the task already has a successful solution at the cortical level decreases the probability that new engram will be formed during the overlearning trials. As will be shown later (see p. 263) pure performance does not induce formation of additional memory traces that would be unnecessary and superfluous when there already is an available engram. Evidently an important prerequisite for information storage is the active character of the learning process based on high motivation and arousal. After the cortical trace is established, the emotionality of the learning situation is considerably reduced and trial and error attempts to find other possible solutions are discontinued. They reappear, however, in decorticated animals, in which intense unconditioned stimuli maintaining the active search for an adequate solution of the task may result in subcortical storage of information that would not be subcortically stored otherwise (Carlson 1967).

The above point of view is somewhat at variance with data on enhanced formation of subcortical memory traces during unilateral CSD. More subcortical learning probably occurs because unilateral learning is significantly slower than the bilateral. Furthermore, during training the decorticated hemisphere may be guided by the intact one to find the correct solution more efficiently. Formation of the subcortical engram in the decorticated hemisphere while the same trace is available in the contralateral cortex is mainly due to the influence of the conditioned and unconditioned stimuli on subcortical centers deprived of the usual interaction with the cerebral cortex. According to Kukleta (1967) learning under unilateral CSD leads to bilateral information storage, which proceeds in the decorticated hemisphere more slowly than in the normal one. The subcortical part of the trace is again lateralized and independent of storage on the intact side.

In comparison with cortical engrams, the subcortical traces seem to be more short-lived or more susceptible to forgetting perhaps because of impaired consolidation in the decorticated brain. This is one of the reasons why the information stored under bilateral CSD is only partially retrieved both by functionally decorticated and intact brains. These results also indicate that training under bilateral CSD cannot be interpreted as a special case of state dependent learning (Overton 1964, Holmgren 1966) which would predict better retention under CSD than with brain intact.

The limitations of the subcorticocortical transfer of information are also due to the blurred, inexact character of the subcortical trace, which might represent a distorted reflection of reality. This is perhaps best illustrated by the experiments of Travis and Sparks (1963) in which unsuccessful avoidance pretraining under bilateral CSD caused slower avoidance learning with an intact brain, probably because the subcortical engram incorrectly interpreted the shocks as unavoidable. Sometimes the transfer of the emotional component alone may activate an extinguished preformed response (Korányi, Endröczi, and Lissák 1965) or accelerate acquisition of similar responses. It seems quite clear, however, that at least some recognition of simple cues, transferred from the decorticated to the intact brain (Carlson 1967, Bureš and Burešová 1968a, Kukleta 1967, 1968, Russell, Kleinman, Plotkin, and Ross 1969) can be demonstrated by adequate testing techniques.

The impaired performance of functionally decorticated rats has sometimes been attributed to a motor deficit (Tapp 1962, Mogenson 1965, Winokur 1965, Freedman and Lash 1966, Meyers and Stern 1966) rather than to impaired learning and/or retrieval. This problem was carefully analyzed by Russell, Plotkin, and Kleinman (1968), who separately measured the latency of exit from the start box and the actual running time across the 6-foot long runway during acquisition of an avoidance reaction. Bilateral CSD selectively prolonged start latencies but did not significantly affect running times, which were as short in depressed as in normal animals (about 2 sec). An occasional increase of running time in depressed animals was always due to presence of competing responses such as retracing and freezing. These results indicate that the motor requirements of most learning situations do not exceed the motor capacities of unilaterally or bilaterally depressed rats and that the deficits observed are due to poor acquisition or retrieval, weak motivation, low reactivity, sensory blockade, and so forth. Another factor that may obscure the existence of subcorticocortical transfer of information is the generalization decrement. Its importance was stressed by Schneider (1967) who perhaps overestimated the significance of this phenomenon for the interpretation of different transfer findings (see p. 279). It is obvious, however, that all cues acquired during decortication will appear as considerably changed to the intact brain and that further training is required to recognize them in a new context.

Chapter 10

Unilateral Cortical Spreading Depression in Behavioral Research

As pointed out in Chap. 2, CSD evoked by chemical stimuli in one hemisphere does not spread to the contralateral hemicortex if precautions are taken to prevent direct diffusion of the SD-evoking agent across the midline. This can be easily achieved by eliciting CSD from lateral trephine openings separated by a 3 to 4-mm wide strip of intact bone along the sagittal suture and by protecting the KCl-soaked filter papers from mechanical displacement. It is generally agreed that under such conditions even highly concentrated KCl solutions evoke only unilateral CSD. Reports to the contrary (Gollander and Ochs 1963, Cofoid 1965) are inadequately documented and cannot be regarded as sufficient proof of possible interhemispheric spread of CSD. Lateralization of CSD in rats was recently questioned by Crow, Petrinovich, and Carew (1973). Inspection of their recordings shows, however, that the abortive slow potential shifts (predominantly positive low amplitude waves) found in the hemisphere contralateral to KCl application are not due to interhemispheric propagation of CSD but rather to field potentials generated in the depressed cortex and picked up by the common reference electrode.

The lateralization does not mean, however, that the functions of the undepressed hemisphere remain unaffected. They are indirectly modified by the effect of unilateral CSD on the diencephalic and mesencephalic centers with bilateral cortical projections. Although the resulting changes of arousal, emotionality, and motivation may account for some peculiarities of behavior in functionally hemidecorticated rats, the basic ability of the undepressed hemisphere to acquire and retrieve information remains well preserved.

The behavioral applications of lateralized CSD are manifold. They will be systematically dealt with in this chapter, although some aspects of the problem are also discussed in other parts of the book.

1. Unconditioned Reactions in Unilaterally Depressed Rats

After an initial painful reaction due to stimulation of dural receptors, unilateral application of 25 % KCl evokes remarkably little behavioral manifestations. More careful examination reveals significant changes in motor and sensory functions and in the level of arousal and motivation, all of which are predictable consequences of the underlying neurophysiological mechanisms. It is obvious that in a nervous system with predominantly crossed projection of sensory pathways to the cerebral cortex, elimination of one hemisphere causes considerable neglect of the contralateral side of the body. The motor pathways controlling the cortically organized motor behavior are also crossed and their unilateral blockade results in disappearance of some specific localized reactions in the contralateral limbs. More general motor reactions (running, walking, eating, drinking, climbing, righting, bar pressing, and so on) are mainly integrated at the subcortical levels. Their overall character is therefore unaffected by unilateral CSD, although the threshold for eliciting such reactions may be changed. The intensity of the effect may range from zero to that due to bilateral CSD.

The disappearance of cortical postural reflexes on the side contralateral to CSD (Burešová 1956, Bureš and Burešová 1960 b — see p. 226) is a good example of the localized motor effects. A similar consequence of unilateral CSD is inability of the animal to use the contralateral forelimb for reaching or grasping (Burešová, Bureš, and Beran 1958 — see p. 236). General motor activity is changed less consistently. Nadel (1966) reported that unilaterally depressed animals displayed a decrease of exploratory activity approximately half way between undepressed controls and bilateral depression. On the other hand latencies of step down in the one-trial learning tests did not differ in unilaterally depressed and untreated rats (Schneider 1967). Bureš, Burešová, and Fifková (1964) found that rats under unilateral CSD displayed during a 3-min exploration of a two-compartment apparatus as much preference for the small dark compartment as control rats (see Fig. 9.10). Carlson's (1967) data also indicate that unilateral CSD does not decrease the preference of the animals for the black compartment.

Consummatory behavior is also affected to varied degrees. Burešová, Rüdiger, Bureš, and Fifková (1962) reported that unilateral CSD decreases the water intake during the first 8 min following 24 hours of water deprivation to 75 % of control values (Fig. 10.1). This finding was confirmed by Schneider (1965) who found that the impairment of water consumption

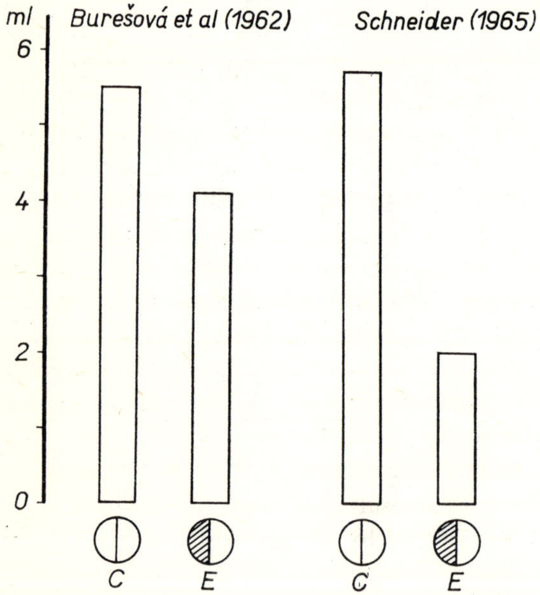

Fig. 10. 1. Unconditioned water consumption (in milliliters) during 8 min (Burešová, Rüdiger, Bureš, and Fifková 1962) or 3 min (Schneider 1965) of drinking under control conditions *(C)* and under unilateral CSD *(E)*.

was most marked in the first 3 minutes of the period of water access but diminished later. The total water intake under unilateral CSD approached the control level after 15 min. Similar initial impairment was also described for food intake (Burešová 1956)). Whereas normal rats, maintained on a 24-hour deprivation schedule consumed about 90 % of their daily ration during the first 30 min of the 1 hour food access time, unilaterally depressed animals ate only 30 % of their food during the same time (Fig. 10.2). This 60 % difference between normal and functionally hemidecorticate animals decreased towards the end of the 1 hour feeding period to 30 %.

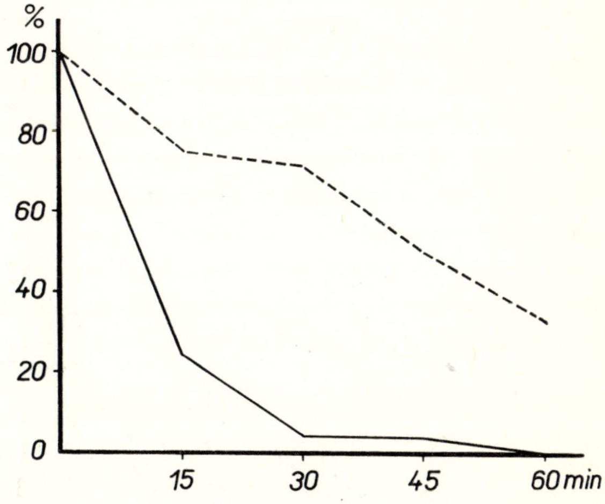

Fig. 10. 2. Consumption of the daily feeding ration (100 %) in normal (full line) and unilaterally depressed rats (dashed line). Ordinate: percentage of the daily feeding ration left. Abscissa: time in min (Burešová 1956).

Because the delayed improvement of consummatory behavior observed in the above experiments occurs at a time when cortical functions are still deeply impaired, its explanation must be sought in the gradual adaptation of the animal to the novel conditions caused by unilateral CSD. It is easily understandable that the rapid elimination of one hemisphere creates a most disturbing situation when many well known stimuli appear in an unusual context and some links of complex chain reactions are missing. This may cause distraction comparable to Pavlovian external inhibition, which subsides when the animal becomes habituated to the continuing hemidecortication. At the same time parallel neural circuits are activated to compensate for the eliminated ones.

The degree of disorientation caused by unilateral CSD is well illustrated in the experiments of Koppmann and O'Kelly (1966) who found that unilaterally depressed rats under free-choice conditions in a T maze prefer to turn to the side ipsilateral to the functionally decorticated hemisphere. This result, essentially similar to that reported earlier by Ellen (1963), cannot be explained by the contralateral muscular weakness but is evidently due to the inadequate perception of the visual and somesthetic stimuli received by the contralateral side of the body. Such explanation does not apply, however, to the other observation from the same investigators that functionally hemidecorticate rats facing a circular food container approached it from the side corresponding to the depressed hemisphere and ate with the side of the mouth contralateral to the unilateral CSD.

The physiological mechanisms of the perceptual asymmetry caused by unilateral CSD were analysed by Weiss and Bureš (1959) who demonstrated that lateralized somesthetic stimuli (puff of air directed to the pinna, sciatic nerve stimulation) applied to the side ipsilateral to CSD evoked a more prolonged arousal than contralateral stimuli of the same intensity (Fig. 10.3, see also p. 181). Electric shocks

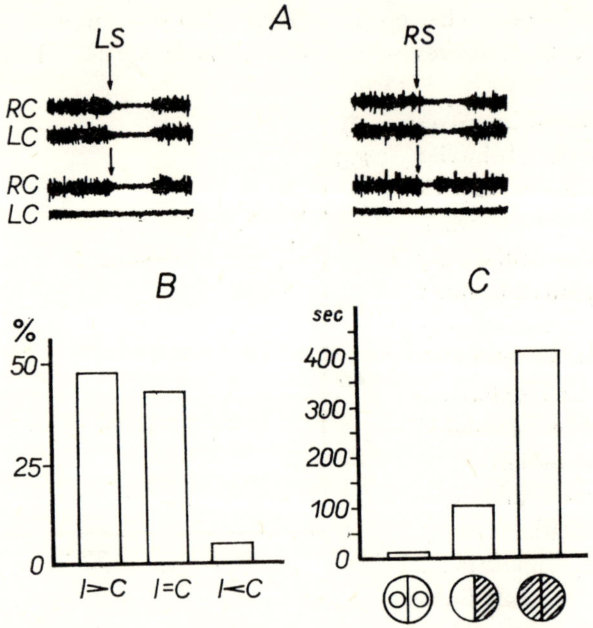

Fig. 10. 3. Effect of unilateral CSD on arousal in unanesthetized unrestrained rats. *(A)* EEG arousal reaction elicited by lateralized cutaneous stimuli. The upper recording was before CSD initiation; stimulation of the right and left side produced EEG desynchronization of the same duration. The lower recording was during CSD in the left hemisphere; the arousing effect of the stimuli applied to the right side of the body was decreased. *(B)* Percentage of experiments in which the stimulus contralateral to the depressed hemisphere was less *(I > C)* or more *(I < C)* effective than the ipsilateral one or when both were equally effective *(I = C)* (Weiss and Bureš 1959). *(C)* Average duration of animal hypnosis in control rats (trephine openings only) and in rats under unilateral or bilateral CSD (Bureš and Burešová 1956d).

administered to both feet through the conventional electrifiable grid floor elicit the threshold flinch response or the more general locomotor reaction in the unilaterally depressed rats at current intensities higher than in controls but lower than with bilateral CSD (Thompson and Enter 1967). This finding may reflect the fact that under conditions of random distribution of current to all four feet the stimulus often predominantly affects the hypesthetic side or that in case of a symmetric current flow the summation of the stimuli applied to the normesthetic and hypesthetic skin areas does not attain the effect found in normal rats. It may also be explained as a manifestation of a general decrease in reticular excitability, which can be demonstrated during unilateral CSD by other methods. Thus duration of the so-called animal "hypnosis" elicited in rats by abrupt rotation around the longitudinal axis of the body by 180 degrees, is prolonged from 10 sec in normal rats to over 100 sec after unilateral and to 420 sec after bilateral application of 25 % KCl (Bureš and Burešová 1956d; Fig. 10.3C).

Whereas most of the above effects are inhibitory in nature, Huston and Bureš (1970) demonstrated facilitation of drinking and eating in satiated animals during a brief period following the passage of a single CSD wave across one hemisphere. The mechanism of this effect is discussed elsewhere (see p. 340).

The above review of changes of spontaneous, unlearned reactions induced by unilateral CSD is by far not exhaustive. It should, however, draw attention of investigators to the necessity of taking such changes into account when planning, performing, and interpreting experiments with lateralized CSD.

2. Unilateral Retrieval of Bilaterally Learned Reactions

Many of the spontaneous reactions mentioned in the preceding section include learned components and natural conditioned reactions acquired during postnatal life which are affected by unilateral CSD in the same way as reactions deliberately established by specific training.

Thus, highly lateralized conditioned reactions acquired with intact brain in so-called handedness experiments (reaching for food pellets into a narrow tube, preferentially with one forelimb, Tsai and Maurer 1930) are blocked by CSD elicited by 2 % KCl in the hemisphere contralateral to the preferred forelimb for approximately the same time as by bilateral CSD, whereas elimination of the ipsilateral cortex does not impair the food seeking behavior in most cases (Burešová, Bureš, and Beran 1958) (Table 10.1). The striking difference in the duration of impairment

Table 10.1.

Suppression of the Lateralized Reaching-for-Food Reaction ("Handedness") by Unilateral CSD

		Duration of impairment	
		Right CSD	Left CSD
"Left-handed" rats	n	8	8
	Min	33.7±6.8	1.2±0.8
		$p < 0.01$	
"Right-handed" rats	n	9	9
	Min	5.0±4.3	46.5±12.2
		$p < 0.01$	

caused by contralateral and ipsilateral CSD is obviously due to the relation of the respective hemisphere to the efferent link of the conditioned reflex: about half the rats with contralateral CSD displayed clear-cut alimentary reactions in spite of the loss of coordinated movements in the preferred forelimb and attempted to get the food with jaws, muzzle or tongue. Some of these animals eventually succeeded in grasping food with the nonpreferred forelimb but returned to the original preference as soon as the brain was normal again (Fig. 10.4). In other rats, contralateral CSD elicited deep inhibition of alimentary behavior: the animals did not react to visual and auditory stimuli associated with placing food into the tube. In this case lateralization of the efferent link probably induced unilateral organization of other components of the conditioned reaction.

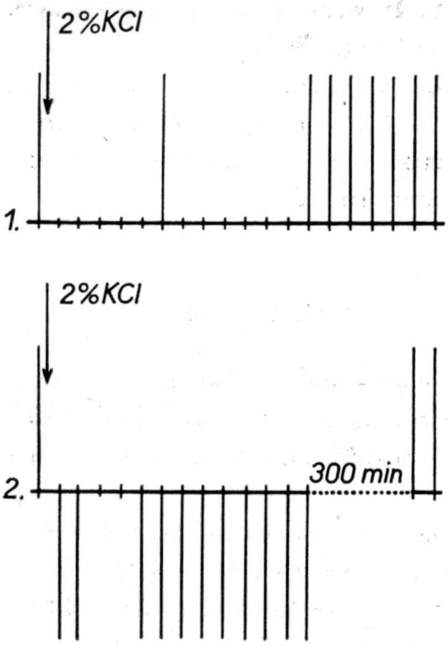

Fig. 10. 4. Change in "handedness" in the course of CSD evoked in the right hemisphere of a "left-handed" rat. Long vertical lines indicate reaching for food with the left (upward) or right (downward) forelimb. Short vertical lines indicate food left untouched. Time interval between stimuli was 3 min. On day 1 reaching for food was completely suppressed. On day 2 during depression the animal got food with the nonpreferred extremity but the original left handedness recovered 5 hours later (Burešová, Bureš, and Beran 1958).

Nonlateralized operant reactions are affected by unilateral CSD proportionally to their complexity (other factors, for example, the degree of overtraining, are probably also important but have not yet been adequately examined). Bar pressing — which is usually not a discrete response made with one paw but a complex reaction performed with the head, flank or both forelimbs — has bilateral cortical representation. After intact brain acquisition of bar pressing for food reward, rats were given extinction sessions either with brain intact or with unilateral CSD elicited by 25 % KCl (Russell and Ochs 1963). The habit was well retained with one hemisphere although the bar pressing rate was about 30 to 40 % lower than in intact animals. The same 35 % decrement was obtained during unilateral CSD in rats previously trained to bar-press for electrical stimulation of the brain (Rüdiger and Fifková 1963) (see p. 304). Suzuki und Uneoka (1966) also found only a slight reduction of food-rewarded bar-pressing during unilateral CSD elicited in rabbits after 20 to 30 sessions of intact brain pretraining.

Similar data were obtained for bilaterally acquired runway behavior. Rüdiger

(1962) and Burešová, Rüdiger, Bureš, and Fifková (1962) found after unilateral CSD only a brief inhibiton (15 min) of water-rewarded runway running, which would be suppressed by bilateral CSD for several hours.

Since the testing procedure may induce some relearning of the task with the intact hemisphere, it is often more correct to express unilateral retention of the bilaterally learned habits in savings scores. Kukleta (1965) found that unilateral relearning of a bilaterally acquired runway avoidance requires approximately the same number of to-criterion trials as the original learning (4 to 5 trials). The absence of savings is only an apparent one, however, since the relearning scores must be compared with learning in unilaterally depressed untrained rats which require three times as many trials (16 to 18) to reach criterion. A more difficult avoidance reaction (shuttle between two elevated retractable platforms) learned to a 9/10 criterion with an intact brain was not transferred to the functionally hemidecorticate brain at all (Burešová, Bureš, and Lukaszewska 1966), the performance during the retention test not being significantly different from that of untrained animals under unilateral CSD. The failure of transfer is probably due to the important role played in this particular reaction by spatial orientation according to visual cues. Elimination of one hemisphere results in a nearly complete blindness of the contralateral eye, so that the animal has to learn first how to use the lateralized visual input for solving the problem. It is understandable that this requires a fundamental reorganization of the memory trace. Some improvement of unilateral retrieval is achieved when testing starts only 1 hour after unilateral KCl application. In rats trained to differentiate moving targets from stationary visual stimuli (Bianki 1967) performance dropped to 35 % within 10 min after unilateral application of 2 % KCl onto the parietal cortex. Full recovery was attained after 90 min.

Conditioned reactions to time (food accessible for 10-sec periods separated by regular 62-sec intervals; the same visual CS rewarded or nonrewarded when following a 62- or a 20-sec interval, respectively) were impaired for 3 hours by unilateral CSD evoked by 25 % KCl in normal rats (Bianki 1967). Elaboration of such conditioned reactions to tone is considerably slower in callosotomized rats in which unilateral application of 2 % KCl causes a more prolonged impairment of performance than unilateral application of 25 % KCl to intact animals.

Bilaterally acquired passive avoidance reactions are retrieved under unilateral CSD nearly as efficiently as with the brain intact. This is especially true for the avoidance of the small shock compartment (Bureš and Burešová 1966a, see Fig. 9.10) whereas for the step-down avoidance (Schneider 1967) retention test latencies are approximately midway between those of untrained rats and intact trained animals.

The effects of unilateral CSD on bilaterally acquired multiple T-maze behavior were described by Burešová, Bureš, and Beran (1958). Under unilateral CSD evoked by 2 % or 25 % KCl, most rats were capable of correct orientation although the running time and number of errors were increased. Spies (1967) has shown that the number of to-criterion trials during relearning of a bilaterally acquired sixfold T maze is the same under unilateral CSD as with brain intact.

Limited transfer of experience from normal to unilaterally decorticated brain was also shown in reversal experiments. Bureš and Burešová (1960c) taught intact rats to go left in a spatial discrimination box and one hour later reversed this habit during CSD in the left hemisphere. Whereas intact animals took 36.5 trials to reach the reversal criterion, the functionally hemidecorticated rats required only 22.9 trials as compared with the 17.9 trials required by untrained hemidecorticated rats.

Several reports are concerned with the problem of whether the experience acquired by the intact brain is symmetrically represented in both brain halves. Burešová, Bureš, and Beran (1958) established at first a forelimb preference in rats, which were then taught a multiple T maze. Retention of the maze habit tested during unilateral CSD was the same irrespective of whether hemidecortication eliminated the hemisphere controlling the preferred forelimb or the other hemicortex (Fig. 10.5). This indicates that hemisphere "dominance" in rats is limited to motor control of the forelimb, whereas general motor reactions and complex habits are formed with symmetrical participation of both hemispheres. Burešová, Kozlovskaya, Fifková,

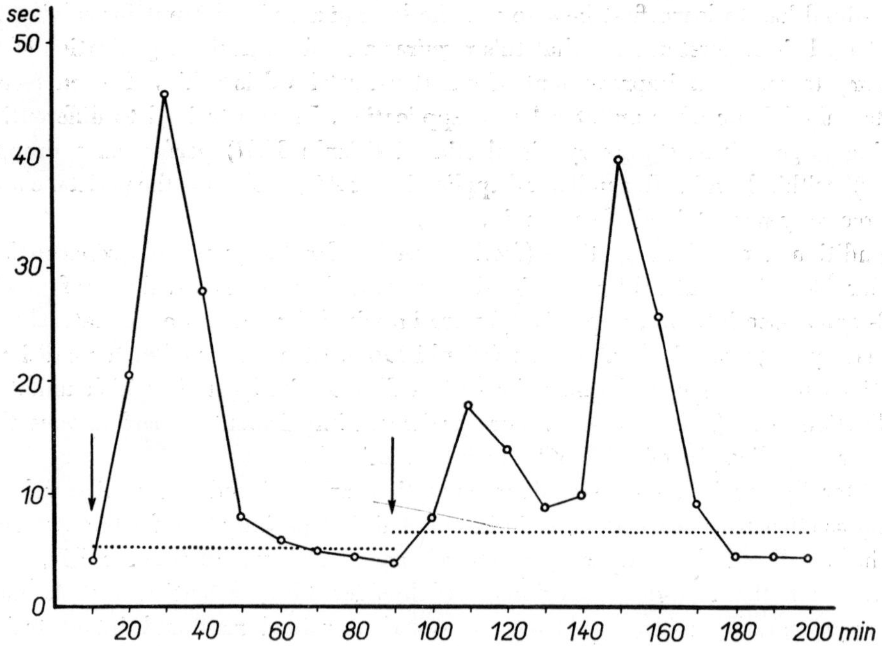

Fig. 10. 5. Influence of unilateral CSD on an overlearned maze habit. Application of 2 % KCl on the "dominant" or "nondominant" hemisphere indicated by arrows. Ordinate: time needed for the passage through the maze in seconds. Abscissa: time from the beginning of experiment in minutes. Dotted line shows a 50 % prolongation of passage as compared with the predepression level (Burešová, Bureš, and Beran 1958).

and Weiss (1961), Russel and Ochs (1963), Suzuki and Uneoka (1966), Lishman and Eayrs (1966) also found equal retention of bilateral engrams with CSD evoked in either hemisphere. Such findings are in agreement with Sperry's (1967) conclusion derived from split brain studies that engrams are typically formed in duplicate form in cats. Whereas brains of lower mammals are remarkably symmetrical in their learning capacities, monkeys show a certain concentration of learning in one hemisphere (Gazzaniga 1963). This trend ends in extreme asymmetry of language representation in humans, which is probably caused by the incapability of the callosal commissure to handle the information flow associated with the highest brain functions (Bogen and Bogen 1969).

Kunc (1964) is the only investigator who found with the CSD technique a significant left-right asymmetry of rat brain. According to this report CSD in the right hemisphere causes a more pronounced depression of feeding and drinking (20 % glucose) than left CSD. Functional decortication of the right hemisphere is also more efficient in prolonging the latencies of a runway esape induced by foot shocks (Kunc and Kukleta 1965) or by a heated floor (Kunc 1971) In all these experiments the asymmetry was rather marginal, however, and limited to some parameters only. It is quite possible that it was not due to an organic asymmetry of brain but rather to some unrecognized asymmetry of the experimental situation. In an attempt to verify Kunc's suggestion, Plotkin and Russell (1969c) failed to find evidence indicating a dominant hemisphere in rats.

Certain lateralization of engrams in intact brain can be achieved by limiting the sensory input to one hemisphere during learning. This technique, well known from the surgical split brain studies (Myers and Sperry 1958) was used in CSD experiments by Lishman and Eayrs (1966). Intact rats were trained a simple avoidance reaction using illumination of the start box as the CS and foot shock as UCS. Opaque contact eye-occluders and rubber membrane "boots" were used to limit the CS, UCS, or both to one side of the body during acquisition training. After the habit was well mastered, retention was tested under unilateral CSD but without sensory restriction. In the hemisphere contralateral to the trained side CSD elicited a more severe impairment than ipsilateral CSD only when both CS and UCS were lateralized to the same side during learning. The performance was 95 % with intact brain, 46 % with the untrained, and 25 % with the trained hemispheres depressed.

Whereas lateralization of CS or UCS alone did not result in significant engram lateralization in the above experiments, Nadel and Burešová (1968, 1969) and Burešová, Bureš, and Rustová (1971) succeeded in forming lateralized visual engrams by monocular training of brightness (black-white) or pattern (horizontal-vertical stripes) discrimination in hooded rats. During unilateral CSD in the hemisphere contralateral to the trained eye, retraining with the untrained eye required 30 to 40 % less trials than training of the unilaterally depressed untrained animals. Retention testing during CSD in the ipsilateral hemisphere revealed more significant savings (70 %). Intact brain overlearning of monocular discrimination improved the primary but not the secondary trace, the quality of which is probably limited by the capacity of the transcallosal information flow and of the ipsilateral visual projection in rats. Monocular training of the pattern discrimination task did not result in formation of a secondary trace in albino rats (Fig. 10.6). On the contrary callosotomy did not prevent formation of the secondary trace in monocularly trained hooded rats, probably because the uncrossed visual projection in the latter strain provided sufficient access to the ipsilateral hemisphere (Burešová and Bureš 1970b, 1971b).

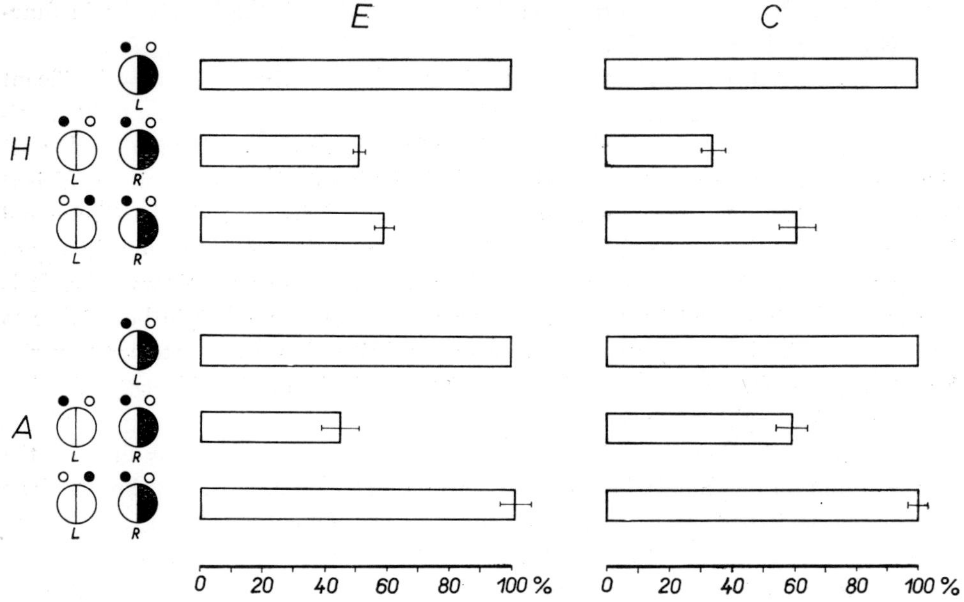

Fig. 10. 6. Primary and secondary engrams formed in the hooded *(H)* or albino *(A)* rats during monocular acquisiton of the horizontal-vertical discrimination task. *(E)*, callosotomized animals, *(C)*, control animals. The columns indicate the average number of to-criterion trials expressed in percentage of the learning scores in untrained hemidecorticate rats. Ten animals per group, SEMs indicated by horizontal bars. Conditions of the experiment are schematically shown in the brain diagrams. Spreading depression and eye occlusion indicated by black color. *(L)*, learning; *(R)*, relearning (Burešová and Bureš 1971b).

Formation of the secondary trace is markedly enhanced by the drug UCB 6215 (Piracetam), a compound selectively increasing the amplitude of callosal evoked responses (Giurgea 1970). Monocular learning of the pattern discrimination was faster under Piracetam than in control animals and generated a much stronger secondary trace. The savings found during unilateral CSD in the hemisphere contralateral or ipsilateral to the trained eye were both 70 %, that is, the secondary trace was improved to the level of the primary one. Since Piracetam did not facilitate learning with the uncrossed visual fibers, its effect is probably due to improvement of the transcommissural write-in mechanism (Burešová and Bureš 1971d).

Once the lateralized trace had been formed by monocular training, binocular to-criterion relearning of the discrimination did not equalize the primary and secondary traces (Burešová, Bureš, and Rustová 1971). It seems that binocular "readout" under these conditions does not initiate improvement of the engram in the initially untrained hemisphere (see p. 283). This may explain why a functional symmetry of the hemispheres valid for groups of rats does not imply exact symmetry of individual brains. In fact Russell, Plotkin, and Kleinman (1970) showed a surprisingly small correlation between learning performance of the left and right hemispheres both in to-criterion trials and running times. The range of the intraindividual and interindividual differences being approximately the same, the distribution corresponded to a random combination of two independent variables. Since untrained acquisition rates are influenced by the unknown previous experience of the animal, better performance of one hemisphere may be caused by a slowly developing disuse of the other hemisphere due to asymmetric sensory influx (unilateral otitis, peripheral injury, vision deficit, and so on).

3. Unilateral Learning and Retrieval of the Corresponding Engram with the Same or with Both Hemispheres

Learning under unilateral CSD usually proceeds two to four times more slowly than bilateral acquisition of the same task. This is illustrated for different kinds of escape or avoidance learning in Fig. 10.7 which reviews the results of six reports. Kukleta (1968b) found that unilateral CSD increased the number of to-criterion trials required for acquisition of an avoidance reaction from 4 to 13, but did not interfere with the elaboration of an anologous escape reaction. This finding was attributed to the differential effect of CSD on the integrative mechanisms of escape and avoidance learning. The general validity of such a conclusion was questioned by Plotkin and Russell (1969c) who found a marked hemidecorticate learning deficit on a simple escape task.

The learning deficit is evidently due to the reduced volume of cerebral cortex participating in the elaboration of the reaction. As pointed out by Russell (1969) such a result can be predicted from Lashley's concept of mass action (Lashley 1929), according to which efficiency of learning is related to the mass of participating cortex. The learning ability of hemidecorticated animals can be improved by increasing the CS duration and permitting the brain more time for processing the incoming information (Russell 1969, Plotkin and Russell 1969b). In a runway avoidance task, raising of the start door was accompanied by a buzzer, at the end of which a shock was delivered to the grid floor. With a 5-sec CS, hemidecorticate rats scored 6 to 7 avoidances in 20 acquisition trials, as compared with 14 to 15 in normal animals. With a longer CS, the performance of the unilaterally depressed animals gradually

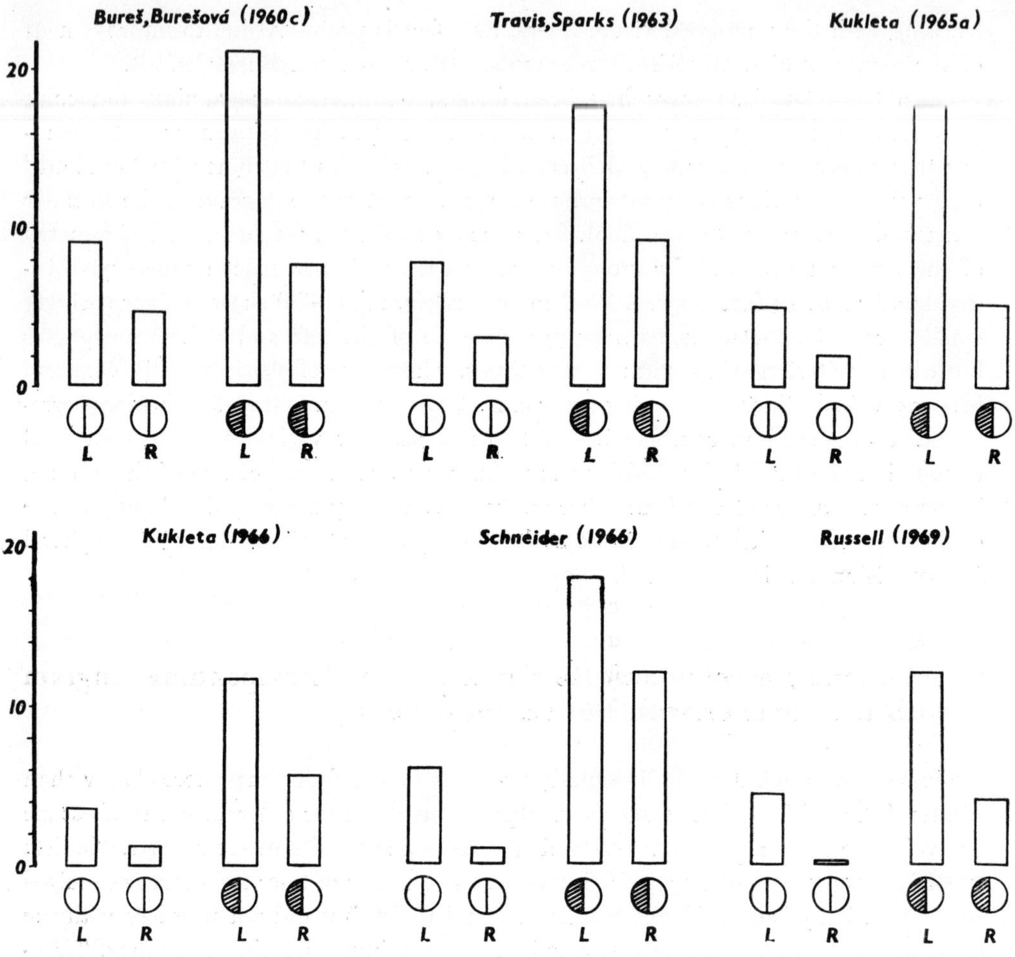

Fig. 10. 7. Comparison of learning and relearning rates of various escape or avoidance reactions in intact or functionally hemidecorticate rats. Columns denote the number of to-criterion trials during learning *(L)* or relearning *(R)*. The CSD is indicated by shading. The learning-relearning interval was 24 hours.

improved until it reached for a 30-sec CS 14 to 15 avoidances out of 20 trials. In intact animals a similar prolongation of CS resulted in deteriorated performance, evidently because the warning characteristics of the sound became more and more remote from the onset of the shock. These results indicate that hemidecorticate rats can handle the same information as normal animals, but require more time to get the correct result. On the other hand the unilateral learning deficit was independent of the intertrial interval in the range of 15 to 240 sec (Plotkin 1967, Plotkin and Russell 1969a) indicating that the hemidecorticate impairment is not due to slower information equilibration outside the learning situation (Estes 1955a, b). The above difference in learning rates in intact and hemidocorticate rats applies also for retrieval tested under the same conditions. As follows from data illustrated by Fig. 10.7, to-criterion relearning is again two to four times faster with an intact brain than under unilateral CSD. Relative savings expressed as percentages of the to-criterion trials during initial learning were similar for both groups. Plotkin and Russell (1969c) found the ratio of the mean to-criterion trials for normals to mean to-criterion trials for hemidecorticate rats to be 0.48 during acquisition and 0.52 during retention testing (criterion of nine successive escapes with a latency below 3 sec).

An adequate transfer of experience can be expected from the hemidecorticated into the normal state, since the lateralized memory trace can be used by the intact brain without much additional information. Travis and Sparks (1963) demonstrated, however, that bilateral relearning of an active avoidance acquired under unilateral CSD is only slightly better than learning of the same task in untrained animals with brain intact but worse than relearning in animals who received the first training with an intact brain. Similar data were obtained by Burešová, Bureš, and Lukaszewska (1966).

Evidently some generalization decrement explanation (Schneider 1967, see p. 279) applies to these findings. The information acquired during unilateral decortication cannot be immediately recognized and employed by the intact brain, which uses additional channels for perception and new ways of motor adjustment. As the unilaterally learned habit might be awkward and even maladaptative under conditions of intact brain activity, it has to be reorganized, the extent of the change being proportional to the complexity of the habit. From the neurophysiological point of view the reorganization corresponds to formation of a duplicate engram in the contralateral hemisphere and to development of a bilateral rather than a unilateral control of behavior. The unilateral behavioral pattern remains preserved, however, and can be used without further changes later. Some of these points are discussed in greater detail in connection with interhemispheric transfer (p. 273).

4. Lateralization of Engrams Acquired under Unilateral Cortical Spreading Depression

The most important aspect of learning under unilateral CSD is localization of the corresponding engrams. Such experiments may contribute to resolving the general problem of temporal and spatial organization of memories. Surgical techniques have yielded useful results, indicating which parts of the brain are necessary and sufficient for the storage and retrieval of a particular type of information (Lashley 1950, Sperry 1959) but the permanent mutilation of the nervous system caused by the surgical intervention prevents the engrams from forming or maintaining normal connections with other brain areas.

Is the information stored in the form of single or multiple traces? Is the engram formed during the actual learning stationary or does it grow or shrink after termination of training (for example, during consolidation or during forgetting)? Can the initially localized engram spread to other brain structures?

These questions, essential for an understanding of the intimate mechanisms of memory, cannot be fully answered by classical ablation methods. Their solution is only possible when the experimental procedure, employed for localizing the engram formation during learning, does not interfere with later growth or multiplication of the memory trace. The functional ablation technique is a powerful experimental tool well suited for analyzing some of the above problems.

Convincing evidence for duplicate storage of information was obtained in split brain experiments brought to perfection by Sperry (1961, 1964) and by other investigators. Their main results can be summarized in the following points.

(a) During learning, when relevant information is channeled through lateralized inputs to one hemisphere, engrams are formed not only there but also in the contralateral hemisphere.

(b) Formation of the duplicate trace is prevented when the corpus callosum and other commissural pathways are interrupted prior to learning.

(c) In the split brain preparation, lateralized inputs generate lateralized independent engrams; the two hemispheres behave as two separate minds competing for the control over the undivided remainder of the brain.

It is obvious that the problem of engram growth could be easily studied in a preparation in which the lateralized memory trace can interact with the other hemisphere through intact comissural pathways. This is possible with the functional ablation technique which achieves lateralization of memory traces by eliminating one hemicortex from learning but leaves the brain normal for later use. Whereas a lateralized input and section of commissures are necessary for producing lateralized engrams in the surgical split brain, in the so-called "reversible split brain" memory traces are only formed in the normally functioning hemisphere, the other hemicortex being impaired by CSD (Fig. 10.8). Thus although the two methods for trapping the engram and confining it to one hemisphere are different, they should give the same results within certain limit. However, since different species (predominantly cats or monkeys for the surgical split brain, almost exclusively rats for functional decortication) and different time scales (commissurotomy requires a long recovery, CSD acts immediately) are used,

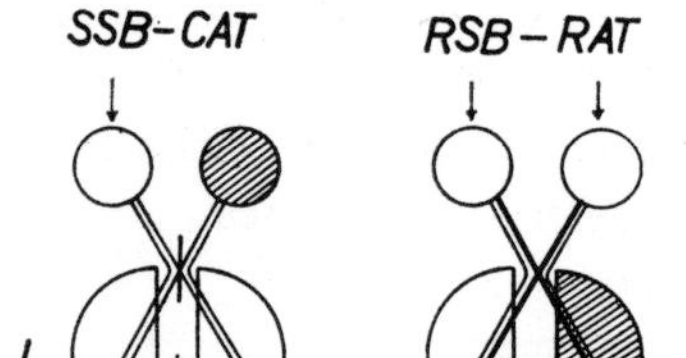

Fig. 10. 8. The surgical split brain (*SSB*) and reversible split brain (*RSB*). *L* indicates learning; *R* indicates retention testing.

the results obtained by the two techniques are not necessarily identical. Careful checking of the degree of engram lateralization is the necessary prerequisite for application of the functional ablation technique in the reunified split brain studies.

Engram lateralization in both surgical and reversible split brain animals is estimated by retention testing with that hemisphere which did not participate in the original learning. This is achieved by using the input connected to the untrained hemisphere in the first case or by eliciting CSD in the trained hemisphere in the second case (Fig. 10.8).

Some confusion in terminology is often due to the fact that both the reversible and surgical split brain experiments usually appear under the heading of "interhemispheric transfer studies". Although the term transfer is usually employed in a purely operational sense (transfer from learning to relearning, from one CS to another), in the above context it is sometimes given a more specific interpretation, implying that a memory trace initially formed in one hemisphere is transmitted or made available to the contralateral hemisphere by means of commissural systems. Such interhemispheric transmission can be demonstrated in the surgical split brain preparation when commissurotomy prevents formation of the secondary trace or indirect readout of the primary trace. All other cases when the secondary trace in the supposedly indirectly accessed hemisphere is formed in spite of commissurotomy through uncrossed sensory projection or by non-lateralized subcortical storage mechanisms, are better described as "incomplete lateralization" than as "partial transfer". This convention is adhered to throughout the present book.

There is another important difference in interhemispheric transfer as studied by the two methods. Commissurotomy performed after lateralized training reveals the degree of interhemispheric transfer that has taken place during intact brain acquisition, characterized by simultaneous formation of the primary and secondary traces. With the reversible split brain technique it is possible to form a strong lateralized memory trace in one hemisphere only and to examine its transfer to the other hemisphere in the intact brain later. The simultaneous and successive formation of the primary and secondary (or transmitted) traces must always be taken into account when interpreting results obtained with the two techniques.

Both methods here revealed complete lateralization of engrams, the acquisition of which required processing complex sensory information and mastering difficult motor reactions. Average learning and relearning curves for the two hemispheres were usually found to be strikingly similar, as was the number of to-criterion trials. Figure 10.9 summarizes data on comparable avoidance learning obtained in seven different laboratories using the functional decortication technique.

On the other hand memory storage of simple tasks cannot be completely lateralized by section of the neocortical commissures or by unilateral CSD. Thus obvious brightness discrimination can be interocularly transferred (Meikle and Sechzer 1960), whereas the more difficult threshold discrimination fails to transfer in chiasma and callosum sectioned cats.

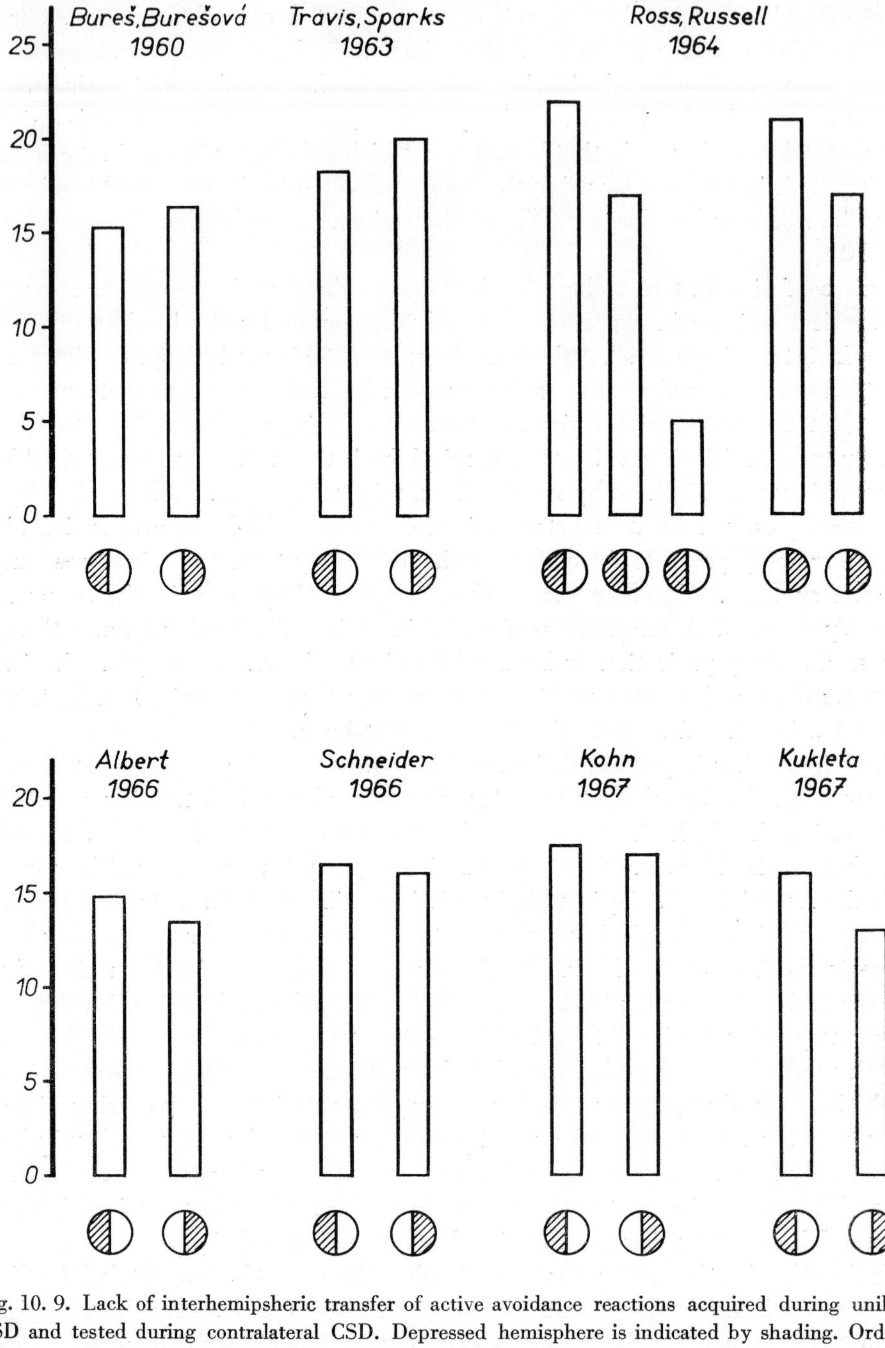

Fig. 10. 9. Lack of interhemipsheric transfer of active avoidance reactions acquired during unilateral CSD and tested during contralateral CSD. Depressed hemisphere is indicated by shading. Ordinate: number of to-criterion trials. Retention was tested after three acquisition sessions in the experiments by Ross and Russell (1964) and after a single learning session in the other studies.

Hall and Thompson (1971) trained unilaterally depressed rats in three brightness discrimition tasks of increasing difficulty: simple (0 vs. 8 ftc.); medium (1 vs. 8 ftc.); and difficult (2 vs. 8 ftc.). The mean trials to criterion for the three tasks were approximately 30, 60, and 90, respectively. Control animals tested with the same hemisphere showed an almost perfect retention for all three tasks. Retrieval with the contralateral hemisphere was indirectly proportional to the difficulty of the task, the savings being 90 %, 50 %, and 10 % for the simple, medium and difficult discrimination, respectively. Similarly relearning of the emotional and vegetative components of a conditioned reaction proceeds in the untrained hemisphere faster than the original unilateral acquisition (Meikle, Sechzer, and Stellar 1962). Learning under unilateral CSD does not result in complete lateralization of passive avoidance (Bureš, Burešová, and Fifková 1964, Carlson 1967, Schneider 1967, Russell, Kleinman, Plotkin, and Ross 1969) or its extinction (Bureš and Burešová 1966a). Retention tests performed after unilateral training with the contralateral untrained hemisphere reveal retention of the classically conditioned vegetative reactions (Ross and Russell 1967) and of habituation to a new environment (Squire 1966) (Fig. 10.10). Also the conditioned taste aversion acquired under unilateral CSD is perfectly retrieved with the contralateral hemisphere (Best and Zuckerman 1971, Burešová and Bureš 1973).

The degree of lateralization may also vary according to the testing procedure used. With the to-criterion relearning technique Albert (1966a), Carlson (1966) and Kohn (1967) demonstrated full lateralization of visual discrimination of two compartments, whereas Carlson (1966, 1967) found with preference testing under similar conditions partial retention in the untrained hemisphere.

Bianki (1968a) found in a group of 62 mice facilitation of contralateral relearning of the unilaterally acquired avoidance reaction (15 versus 10 to-criterion trials), but in another series of experiments failed to establish any correlation between the number of trials given to one hemisphere (0 to 100) and to-criterion learning of the same task in the other hemicortex.

Kukleta (1967) showed that contralateral retention of unilaterally acquired runway avoidance improved with overtraining of the original habit. Only insignificant improvement was found with to-criterion relearning, whereas marked savings were observed in escape latencies and in the preference for one of two available escape pathways. These findings indicate that tasks may differ according to the relative strength of the lateralized and nonlateralized engrams formed during acquisition and recovered during retrieval.

This assertion was borne out by Best and Hamburg (1969) who trained unilaterally depressed rats in a brightness discrimination in a T maze (illuminated alley positive) under escape or avoidance conditions. When the task was well mastered (after four to five daily sessions), retention was tested during CSD in the trained hemisphere. Both groups showed perfect retrieval of the brightness discrimination under escape conditions, but the animals trained to avoid had to relearn the avoidance reaction nearly completely. After the hemispheres were switched, the rats typically

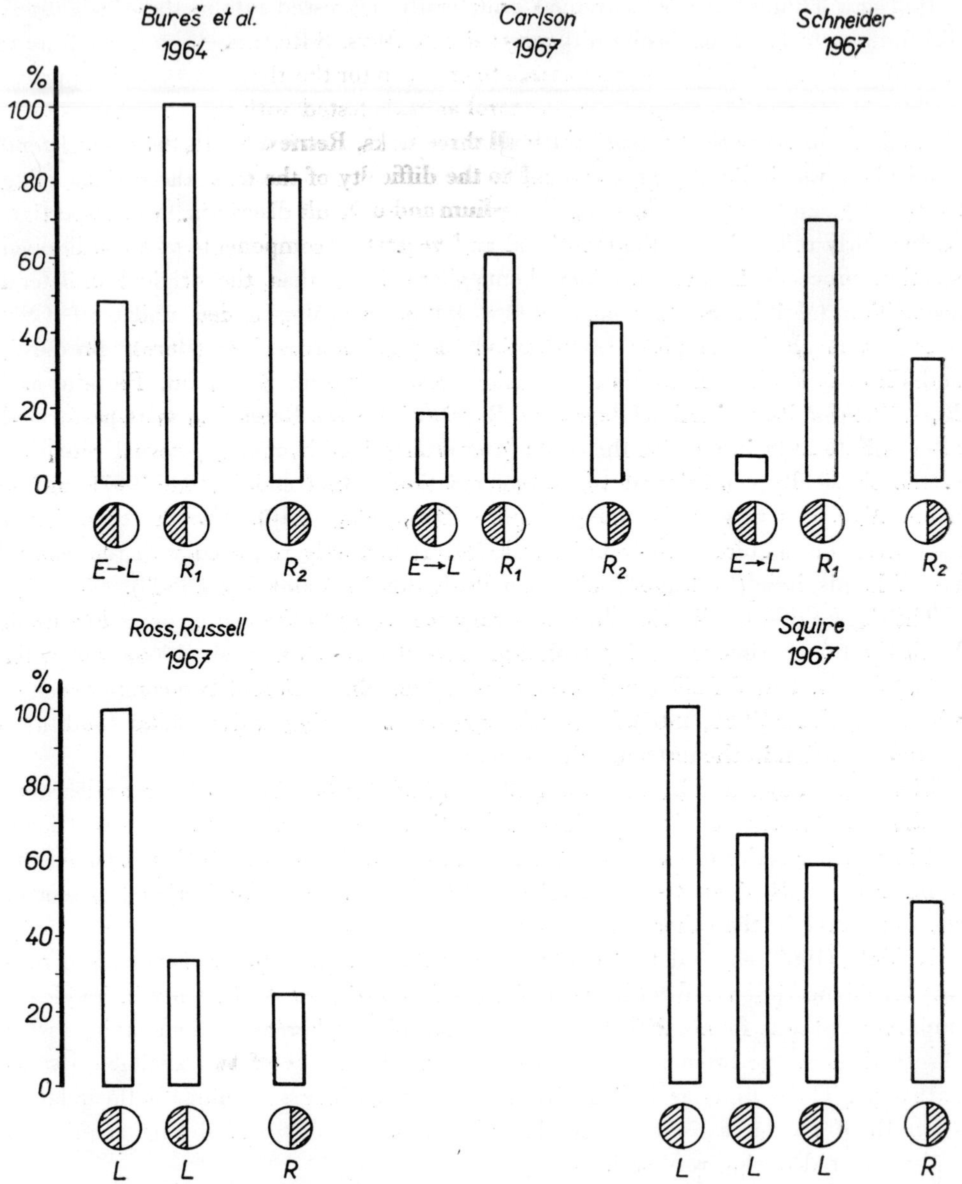

Fig. 10. 10. Examples of conditioned reactions that cannot be lateralized by using the split brain technique. (Above) Passive avoidance tasks. Spontaneous preference for one part of the apparatus, expressed as percentage of the total exploration time *(E)*, is changed by learning *(L)*. Retrieval of the new preference is better with the same (R_1) than with the opposite hemisphere (R_2). Different two-compartment tests were used by Bureš, Burešová, and Fifková (1964) and Carlson (1967) and a step-down test was used by Schneider (1967). (Below) To-criterion learning *(L)* and relearning *(R)* of a conditioned respiratory response (Ross and Russell 1967). Habituation of the orienting response in a maze expressed by the number of entered alleys (Squire 1966). First day performance was 100 %.

waited in the start area until the shock onset and then ran directly to the correct arm.

Intensity of the aversive stimulus may be another important variable. According to Best (1972) an active avoidance task acquired under unilateral CSD was fully lateralized when a 0.6 mA foot shock was used during both acquisition and retention training. Significant savings were found with a higher shock level (1.3 mA).

Russell, Plotkin, and Kleinman (1970) performed a careful analysis of one-way escape during original hemidecorticate training and following retraining with the contralateral hemisphere. Whereas frequency distribution of response times indicated complete lateralization of all instrumental components of the task, emotional responses during the retention test (lack of exploration, crouching, defecation) suggested non-lateralization of the classically conditioned fear component. Although the animal appeared to recognize some aspects of the situation with the new hemisphere, anticipation of the electric shock did not facilitate the acquisition of the escape reaction. Comparison of escape training and retraining with alternate hemispheres showed lack of correlation between the number of to-criterion trials for individual animals. The authors conclude that learning in each hemicortex is mediated by an independent stochastic stimulus sampling process.

The impossibility of lateralizing some types of conditioning in the anatomically split brain is evidently due to the fact that the unilateral input induces formation of bilateral engrams (probably at subcortical levels) or of unilateral engrams available for contralateral readout.

In CSD experiments an alternative possibility must be taken into account: the unilateral engram may spread to the contralateral hemisphere after the latter has recovered from the CSD impairment. This mechanism was ruled out in experiments in which the two hemispheres were never functioning simultaneously during the learning-retrieval interval (Bureš, Burešová, and Fifková 1964). Since contralateral retention of a unilaterally acquired passive avoidance reaction was the same irrespective of whether during the learning-retention interval both hemispheres were normal (allowing for transfer at the cortical level) or depressed (excluding such transfer), a bilateral engram was obviously formed during acquisition (Fig 10.11). Lateralization of the passive avoidance reaction acquired under unilateral CSD was not better in callosotomized than in normal rats (Bureš, Burešová, and Fifková 1964). The statement that engrams formed during learning do not spontaneously grow afterwards is still more clearly supported by experiments with fully lateralized memory traces. Although up to 2 weeks of intact brain function were available for transfer of the lateralized engram to the untrained hemisphere, the latter consistently displayed no retention (Russell and Ochs 1963).

Thus the first conclusion derived from the reversible split brain studies is that unilateral engrams formed during learning with one hemisphere do not spontaneously spread during the learning-retrieval interval to the untrained hemisphere. This is intuitively unexpected since we might predict that highly emotional experiences are repeatedly subjected to "internal rehearsal". The lack of spontaneous interhemispheric transfer of lateralized engrams in rats may, therefore, indicate either that such internal recall mechanisms are poorly developed in this species or that such internal rehearsal alone is inadequate for multiplying and expanding the original memory trace. This distinction becomes important in the light of further experiments in which the conditions of interhemispheric transfer have been specified.

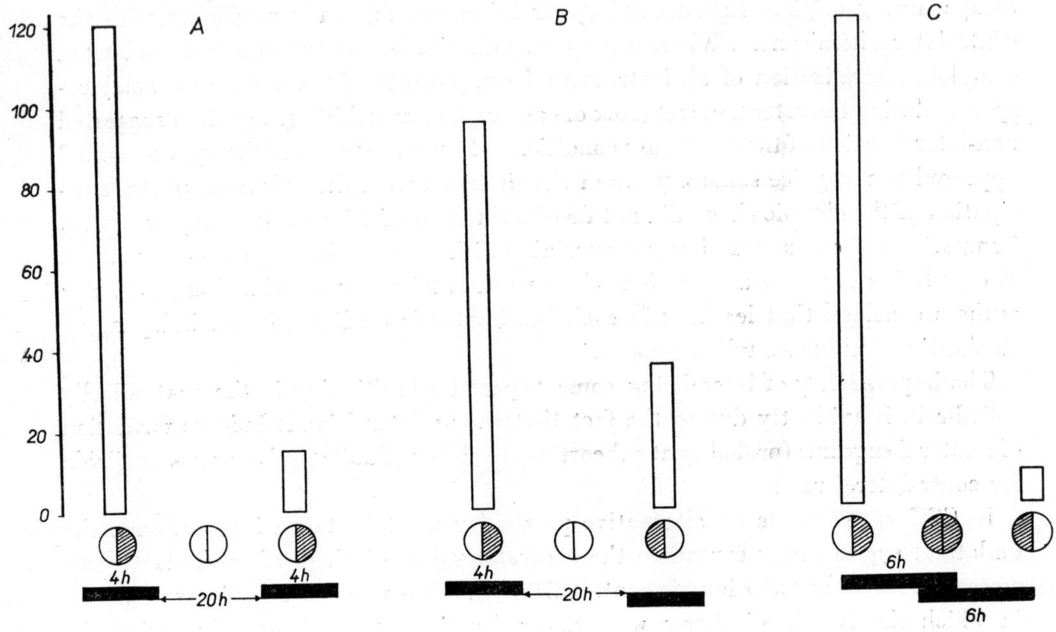

Fig. 10. 11. Nonlateralization of a passive avoidance habit acquired during unilateral CSD. Ordinate: time (in seconds) spent in the small compartment of a two-compartment apparatus during the original 3-min exploration test and during the 3-min retention test. The rat received a 1-min foot shock immediately after the original exploration. Functional elimination of one hemisphere is indicated by shading; duration of CSD in the respective hemisphere is indicated by the horizontal black bar. Note that the degree of retention was similar when identical *(A)* or alternate *(B)* hemispheres were used during learning and retrieval. The same results were obtained even when there was no interdepression interval of intact brain activity between learning and retention (C) (Bureš, Burešová, and Fifková 1964).

Lateralization of engrams also has important implications for the hypothesis about the chemical transfer of engrams (Quarton 1967). It seems that such transfer should be better expressed between two hemispheres sharing the same genetic background and chemical environment than between individuals of the same or even of different species. The absence of spontaneous interhemispheric transfer of lateralized engrams indicates that the hypothetical macromolecules which have encoded the information, are not free to migrate in the brain and to reach the untrained hemisphere. To induce chemical transfer Albert (1966c) removed a part of the trained hemisphere (he claims that the avoidance response is chemically stored in the medial cortex of rats) and injected it intraperitoneally to the same animal. Retention test performed on the next day with the trained hemisphere depressed revealed marked savings (5.0 to-criterion trials as compared with 18.4 to-criterion trials). In an attempt to repeat this surprising result Burešová (1966) left the destroyed cortical tissue in situ, assuming that this may facilitate the access of the untrained hemisphere to the information macromolecules. Relearning with the untrained hemisphere was faster, but similar facilitation was observed when the lesion was made in the untrained hemisphere. It seems that the nonspecific factors associated with brain damage (changes of circulation, temperature, stress) can improve the performance of the untrained hemisphere. Evidence for a specific chemical transfer between the hemispheres remains as inconclusive as it is for the chemical transfer of engrams between different brains.

5. Interhemisperic Transfer of Lateralized Engrams

Lateralized memory traces may facilitate formation of the same engram in the opposite hemisphere when several transfer trials are performed with an intact brain in the period between unilateral acquisition and contralateral retrieval. Since its first demonstration (Bureš and Burešová 1960b, c, Bureš 1959), this phenomenon has been repeatedly confirmed using both appetitive and aversive tasks and different testing methods (Russell and Ochs 1961, 1963, Dorfman 1963, Travis 1964a, Ross and Russell 1964, Ray and Emley 1964, 1965, Bivens and Ray 1965, Albert 1966a, Beach 1966, Schneider 1966, Kohn 1967, Burešová and Bureš 1968). These studies made it possible to examine some factors involved in interhemispheric transfer more systematically and to contribute to a better understanding of the underlying physiological mechanisms.

A typical interhemispheric transfer experiment consists of three phases—unilateral learning, intact brain transfer trials, and contralateral relearning — which are separated by intervals of various length. According to the assumption that during the transfer (interdepression) trials information is passed from the originally trained hemicortex to the untrained one, the two hemispheres are termed "transmitting" and "receiving", respectively.

Strength of the Transmitted Engram

It is obvious that with increasing amounts of interdepression training the result of the retention test becomes independent of the original learning and asymptotically approaches the bilateral acquisition — unilateral retrieval situation. On the other hand transfer is best expressed when elicited by a single transfer trial (Russell and Ochs 1961, 1963, Albert 1966a, Ray and Emley 1965, Bivens and Ray 1965, Kohn 1967) which alone does not significantly facilitate the subsequent unilateral learning. Under these conditions the strength of the unilateral engram in the transmitting hemisphere is the most important variable. Both factors were systematically examined by Travis (1964a) who used three levels of original learning (accumulation of 0, 3, or 15 avoidances) and four levels of interdepression learning (accumulation of 0, 1, 5, or 10 avoidances). Relearning with the recipient hemisphere 30 min after the interdepression training indicated that with one or five trials transfer is best expressed in rats that achieved 15 avoidances in the original learning. With ten interdepression trials performance of the recipient hemisphere was no longer significantly influenced by the original learning. Data from other sources (Bureš and Burešová 1960b, Schneider and Hamburg 1966) fit well into the same picture (Fig. 10.12). Interdepression trials can also influence relearning in the recipient hemisphere in an adverse way. Travis (1964a) obtained such negative transfer with weak original learning (three avoidances) followed by one or five interdepression trials. This finding was confirmed by Bianki (1968a) in mice in which five or ten interdepression trials facilitated contralateral relearning of an avoidance reaction trained with the first hemisphere to a criterion of nine correct out of ten consecutive trials, but impaired it if the criterion of two consecutive avoidances was used in the original learning.

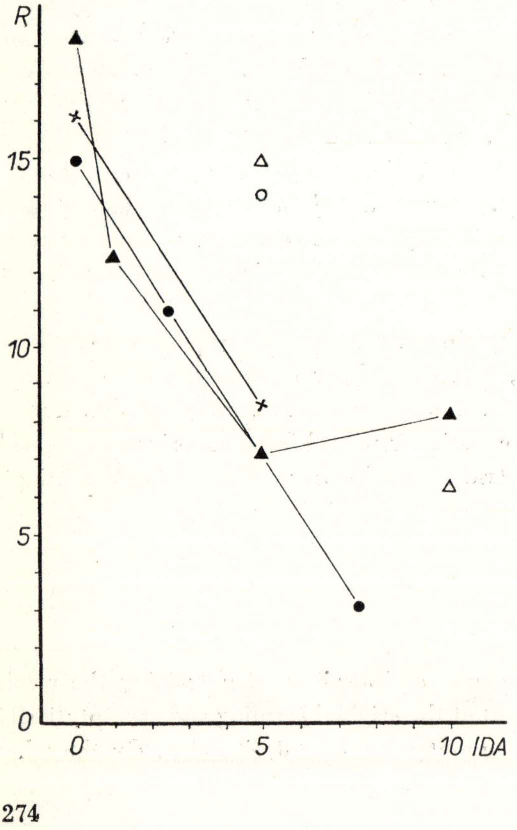

Fig. 10. 12. Interhemispheric transfer of active avoidance induced by interdepression training. Ordinate: number of to-criterion trials during relearning with the recipient hemisphere *(R)*. Abscissa: number of interdepression avoidances *(IDA)*. Approximately equal to-criterion training of the transemitting hemisphere preceded the interdepression trials in the groups represented by full triangles and circles or by crosses, whereas no such training was applied in the control groups (empty triangles and circles) (Bureš and Burešová 1960b-circles; Travis 1964-triangles; Schneider and Hamburg 1966-crosses).

Time Factors

Another important variable is the time required for the completion of transfer. It may be that formation of the transferred trace involves influences originating in the trained hemisphere and outlasting the actual performance of the interdepression trials. Elimination of the transmitting hemisphere by CSD before the transmission of information to the untrained hemisphere is completed may thus interfere with information transfer. In most transfer experiments, however, thirty or more min elapsed between the interdepression trials and relearning under CSD in the trained hemisphere. This seems to exceed considerably the minimum transmitting time (Fig. 10.13). In experiments with successive brightness discrimination

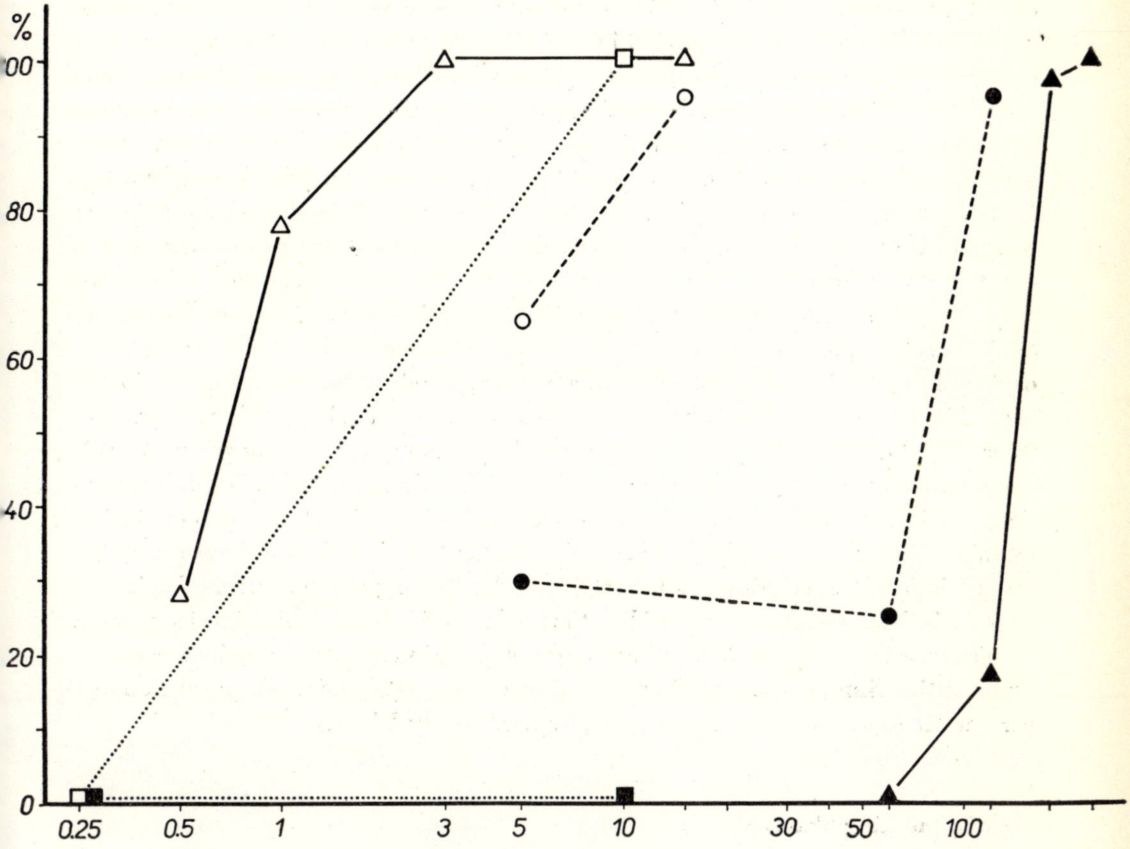

Fig. 10. 13. Transmitting time (empty symbols) and consolidation time (full symbols) in interhemispheric transfer experiments. Ordinate: performance during retention test. Performance of animals not subjected to CSD within 24 hours after transfer trials corresponds to 100 %. Abscissa: time (in minutes) from the last transfer trial to KCl application onto the transmitting (empty symbols) or recipient (full symbols) hemisphere (Burešová and Bureš 1968-circles; Albert 1966a-triangles; Ray and Emley 1965-squares).

Ray and Emley (1965) evoked CSD in the transmitting hemisphere 15 sec or 10 min after a single transfer trial and tested retention with the recipient hemisphere 4 hours later. The transfer was absent in the 15-sec group and complete in the 10-min group. In simple runway avoidance experiments Albert (1966a) established complete transfer after 3 min but only minimal signs of transfer after 30 sec. Transmitting times shorter than 5 min were also reported for a delayed spatial alternation habit by Burešová and Bureš (1968).

Time plays a still more important role in the consolidation of the transferred trace. The memory-disturbing effects of bilateral CSD are described in Chap. 11. In the interhemispheric transfer experiments CSD can be applied to interfere more specifically with consolidation of memory traces in the recipient hemisphere alone. Using this approach Ray and Emley (1965) reported complete or partial disruption of the transferred trace when CSD in the untrained hemisphere was evoked 15 sec or 10 min after the transfer trial. Bivens and Ray (1965) found no transfer when CSD was elicited in the recipient hemisphere 1 hour after the interdepression trial and Albert (1966a) reported disruption of transfer when less than 2 hours were allowed for consolidation. This finding was confirmed by Mayes (1973) who made the additional observation that there is partial recovery of the transferred engram over 15 days which is proportional to the duration of the transfer trial-disruption treatment interval. Albert (1966b) also reported that the amnesic effect was proportional to the duration of depression, but his other findings (disruption by weak cathodal polarization of medial cortex, restitution of the consolidation process by anodal polarization) are rather puzzling and need independent confirmation. Interhemispheric transfer of delayed spatial alternation (Burešová and Bureš 1968) is suppressed when CSD is evoked in the recipient hemisphere 15 min or 1 hour, but not 2 hours after the transfer trials (Fig. 10.13). Under these conditions CSD seems to evoke prolonged retrograde amnesia similar to or even exceeding that described with bilateral functional decortication. Rapid formation of the transferred trace makes it possible to use this method to examine the early consolidation phase of complex tasks which cannot otherwise be trained in a few trials. More important for understanding the general mechanism of learning is the possibility of subdividing the total transfer time into the time component required for the recipient hemisphere to develop an independently maintained trace (transmitting time, about 1 min) and the time component required for formation of a permanent engram (consolidation time, approximately 1 hour).

Stimuli Inducing Transfer

Interhemispheric transfer induced by several interdepression trials can be interpreted in different ways. In addition to the straightforward transfer hypothesis, which assumes transcallosal facilitation of the formation of the duplicate trace in the symmetrical region of the contralateral hemisphere, other mechanisms must also be taken into account. The trained hemisphere may simply guide the animal to the correct solution of the task and thus considerably shorten the trial-and-error phase of learning in the untrained hemisphere. The transfer would not be mediated through commissural pathways in this case, but through an extracerebral event recorded by sensory channels of the recipient hemisphere. The existence of such extracerebral transfer was recently reported in the split brain monkeys by Johnson and Gazzaniga (1970). After a lateralized engram had been established by monocular overtraining, the untrained eye was allowed to observe 40 perfect trials performed by the trained eye and hemisphere. Subsequent testing with the untrained eye revealed complete transfer in spite of the absence of commissural pathways. Observation learning underlying such extracerebral transfer mechanisms seems to be less important in rats. A lateralized engram established by monocular overtraining was not transferred to the untrained side by binocular experience even in intact rats (Burešová, Bureš, and Rustová 1971). Section of corpus callosum prevented interhemispheric transfer of a simple active avoidance reaction (Mayes and Cowey 1973) and of pattern discrimination under indirect access conditions (p. 285). There are other arguments in favor of the commissural nature of the transfer process. The guidance or observation hypothesis implies that only correct responses can induce interhemispheric transfer. Although this was originally believed to be the case (Bureš and Burešová 1960b, Russell and Ochs 1963), later experiments, attempting to determine which components of the learning situation are relevant to the transfer, proved that correct performance is not an obligatory condition of transfer.

Russell and Ochs (1963) considered reinforcement crucial for transfer. In their experiments rats were trained to bar-press for food with one hemisphere and then tested under extinction conditions either with the trained or untrained hemisphere. A single reinforced trial performed with both hemispheres intact greatly increased the subsequent extinction score of the recipient hemisphere above the basal operant level. On the other hand 10 to 25 nonreinforced bar presses with brain intact did not induce any signs of transfer.

The interhemispheric transfer interpretation of these experiments was questioned by Schneider and Ebbesen (1967) and Schneider (1967) who found in a similar situation a considerable increase of bar pressing with the recipient hemisphere not only when the unilaterally trained rat was given a bilateral transfer trial, but also when it was allowed to perform a single reinforced bar press with the recipient hemisphere alone. The unilateral one-trial learning explanation does not apply, however, to experiments in which this possibility was checked by adequate controls, or in which transfer was induced by nonreinforced trials.

Ray and Emley (1964, 1965) failed to find a difference in transfer of a successive brightness discrimination for animals rewarded or not rewarded on the interdepression trial. Still more interesting is their observation that bilateral exposure to one of the two cues induces transfer of the total discrimination pair, although the recipient hemisphere never experienced the second cue. Also Kohn (1967) reported good transfer of appetitively motivated simultaneous brightness discrimination by a single nonreinforced trial.

The possibility of achieving transfer by application of the isolated unconditioned stimulus was investigated by Schneider and Hamburg (1966) (Fig. 10.14). After unilateral elaboration of a runway avoidance he applied either five avoidances or 3 min of unescapable shocks to the intact animal. Since tranfer was the same in

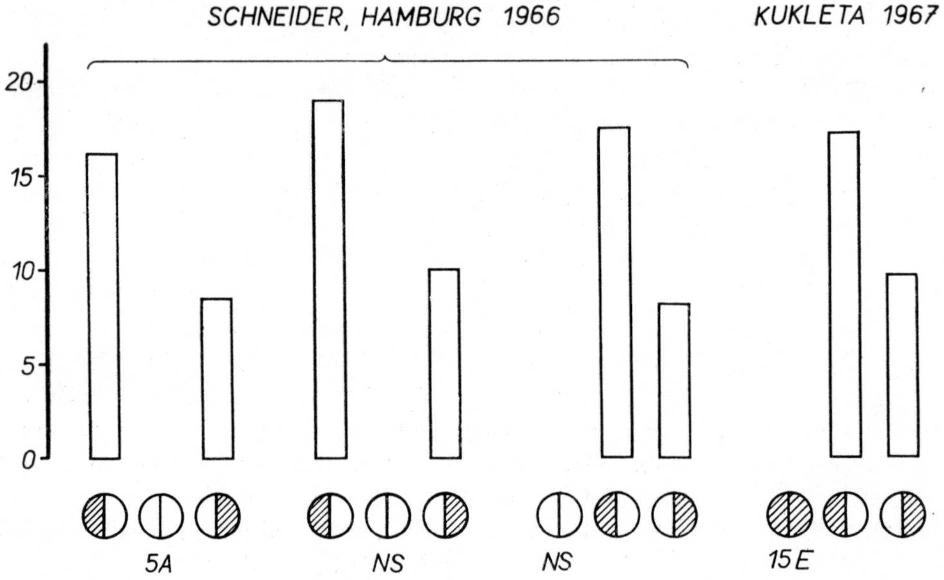

Fig. 10. 14. Interhemispheric transfer induced by nonspecific interdepression facilitation of the predepression experience. Ordinate: number of to-criterion trials during learning (first column) and reiearning (second column) of a simple runway avoidance. Conditions of transfer: *5A*, 5 avoidances; *NS*, unescapable electric shocks applied between or prior to the two CSDs; 15*E*, 15 escape trials applied under bilateral CSD prior to the first unilateral training.

both groups, it would seem that activation of the emotional component of the task may induce transmission of the engram. A similar result was also obtained, however, when the unescapable shocks had been applied prior to the first unilateral training. Although the latter finding is interpreted by Schneider as supporting his generalization decrement hypothesis, it may simply indicate that the nonlateralized subcortical component of the memory trace formed by unescapable shocks constitutes a bridge between the two hemispheres mediating later transmission of more specific unilaterally acquired engrams.

This conclusion is supported by Kukleta's (1967) finding that 15 escape trials given in a simple runway under bilateral CSD facilitated subsequent interhemispheric transfer of a more complex avoidance task (Fig. 10.14).

The most detailed analysis of the conditions required for successful transfer was performed by Kohn (1967). This author elaborated a simultaneous brightness discrimination with one hemisphere and then exposed the intact animal to a single transfer trial. Transfer occurred not only when the animal was allowed to make a correct reinforced response but also when it was exposed to locked positive, negative, or unpainted doors and even when the passage through the unlocked negative door was reinforced by food. Significant transfer was also observed when the animal found no goal box (and no reinforcement) after opening the correct panel. On the other hand transfer was not induced by an interdepression trial in which the stimulus panels were removed and the rat had free access to the reinforcement in the goal box or in which the stimulus panels as well as the goal boxes were removed. In another experiment Kohn (1967) trained unilaterally depressed rats to avoid a black compartment and go to a white compartment, or vice versa. Twenty four hours after to-criterion learning with one hemisphere, the intact rat was given a single transfer trial during which the escape or avoidance either corresponded to the original learning or to its reversal. In both cases retraining of the original task with the recipient hemisphere was facilitated. On the other hand reversal training with the recipient hemisphere was considerably impaired by a positive and unaffected by a reversed transfer trial.

The above experiments indicate that interhemispheric transfer occurs even when there is considerable difference between the conditions of the initial training and of the transfer trials. Some minimum resemblance to the original situation appears to be necessary, however, for activation of the experience stored in the transmitting hemisphere. Further study of the selectivity of this reminder effect, which is remotely analogous to the perceptual activation of human reminiscences, may shed light on the role played in the mechanism of recall by the stimulus generalization phenomenon, that is by the ability of the animal trained under a definite set of stimuli to respond with the same reaction to more or less different sets of stimuli.

Generalization Decrement Hypothesis

The stimulus generalization phenomenon was used in a different context by Schneider (1967) to interpret some of the reversible split brain results. In a series of papers (Schneider 1966, 1967, Schneider and Hamburg 1966, Schneider and Ebbesen 1967, Schneider and Kay 1968) this author advocated a view according to which learning under unilateral CSD leads to formation of bilateral subcortical engrams. The absence of savings in a retention test performed with the contralateral hemisphere is not due to the inavailability of the engram but to a generalization decrement, that is, to the inability of the brain to recognize the old cues in the new context. According to this interpretation, which resembles in many respects the hypothesis underlying so-called "state dependent learning" (Overton 1964) the transfer trials help to bridge the gap between the two unilateral CSD states by facilitating the transfer of the conditioned response from one set of stimuli to another via a stimulus generalization process. Although the generalization decrement may play a role in some CSD experiments (it may explain why after unilateral learning retrieval with the same hemisphere may be better than bilateral retrieval — Schneider 1967, Burešová, Bureš, and Lukaszewska 1966), it seems hardly possible that this phenomenon would account for complete absence of savings. On the contrary perfect interocular transfer (Sheridan 1965) in rats makes the generalization decrement hypothesis extremely improbable. It may even be guessed from the easy generalization and difficult differentiation between stimuli applied to symmetrical receptors (Bykov 1924) that unilateral CSD would resemble contralateral CSD more than bilateral decortication or an intact brain. Schneider and Kay (1968) came to a similar conclusion in experiments in which they reinforced bar pressing during unilateral CSD but not during bilateral CSD or with an intact brain.

Schneider's hypothesis does not satisfactorily explain why the same cues are correctly recognized by the untrained hemisphere when used as CS during unilateral training of a classically conditioned vegetative reaction (Ross and Russell 1967), of a passive avoidance task (Carlson 1966), of a conditioned taste aversion (Best and Zuckerman 1971, Burešová and Bureš 1973), or during habituation (Squire 1966), and why they remain lateralized when associated with active avoidance or approach conditioning. As pointed out by Hall and Thompson (1971) the stimulus generalization decrement hypothesis would have predicted an equal degree of lateralization or of interhemispheric transfer for easy as well as for difficult tasks, since the change of stimuli resulting from switching CSD between hemispheres would be always the same. Examples of transfer between intact and bilaterally decorticated brain and vice versa (Thompson 1964, Bureš and Burešová 1968, Russell, Kleinman, Plotkin, and Ross 1969) and between unilateral or bilateral decortication states (Carlson 1967) are also at variance with the generalization decrement hypothesis. The significance ascribed by Schneider (1968) to the kinesthetic stimuli generated by CSD contrasts with the relatively easy transfer of conditioned reactions between curarized and intact animals (Solomon and Turner 1962) or from bulbocapnine catalepsy to normal activity (Beck and Doty 1957).

While stressing the purely behavioral aspects of the problem, Schneider (1968) has proposed a very improbable explanation of its physiological mechanism. He assumes that during unilateral training, storage is displaced from the cortex to the subcortex of the depressed hemisphere and that this storage remains undetected when depression is shifted because of the stimulus change produced by the shift. Although some subcortical storage of information evidently takes place during lateralized learning (Thompson 1965) it must be stressed that subcortical learning is highly inferior to cortical and that the more complex tasks especially can only be mastered with cortical participation. Cortical storage of lateralized engrams was proved beyond any doubt in surgical split brain experiments (Sperry 1967) and also the manifestations of cerebral dominance in man are evidently due to lateralization of storage rather than to a generalization decrement. The generalization decrement hypothesis does not account for disruption of transfer by CSD evoked shortly after the transfer trials in the transmitting and particularly in the receiving hemisphere (see p. 276). Since the latter disruptive effect is evidently caused by CSD interference with engram consolidation in the recipient hemisphere, it is scarcely possible to maintain that the transfer is due to stimulus generalization at the subcortical level. Schneider (1968) attempts to explain this argument by suggesting that the greater disruption of transfer by CSD evoked in the receiving hemisphere is due to neural aftereffects of the initial CSD, which persist even after 24 hours, when the transfer trials are given, and potentiate the amnesic effect of CSD applied to the same hemisphere. Schneider's suggestion was experimentally tested by Mayes (1973), who applied the interdepression training three days after the initial hemidecorticate learning. Amnesia caused by unilateral CSD elicited in the recipient hemisphere 30 min after the transfer trial remained undiminished although any aftereffects of the original unilateral CSD were likely to dissipate during the long interval. Schneider (1972) used unilateral CSD to disrupt consolidation of a bilaterally acquired step-through task. He found partial amnesia with a 3-min but not with a 15-min acquisition-disruption interval. When retention in the 3-min group was tested under unilateral CSD on the next day, retrieval was better with functional hemidecortication ipsilateral rather then contralateral to the hemisphere depressed during consolidation. This is contrary to the prediction of the generalization decrement hypothesis since in animals trained with normal brain, unilateral CSD in either hemisphere should cause the same generalization decrement. In his last articles Schneider (1968, 1972) seems to accept that some lateralization of storage is involved in the interhemispheric transfer phenomena.

Schneider's generalization decrement hypothesis was critically disputed much along the lines adopted in this book by Squire and Liss (1968) and somewhat uncritically reviewed by Deutsch (1969) who is rather sceptical about the possible use of SD in memory studies: "Spreading depression has never been a tool of choice for studying such phenomena and one may confidently say it never will be". We feel that scientific problems are more efficiently settled by experiments than by precognition. The proposal to explain interhemispheric transfer by generalization decrement and the ensuing discussion with the proponents of the memory-confinement view may only be useful when it leads to more convincing evidence. It has already stimulated new experimental work attempting to test the stimulus generalization hypothesis by examining transfer between different KCl concentrations applied during learning and retention on one or both hemispheres. Reed and Trowill (1969) did not find any difference in to-criterion relearning of an avoidance task when the same hemisphere was treated with 15% KCl during training and with 10, 15, or 20 % KCl during retention, but the total duration of the shock received was decreased most in the 15 % - 15 % group. It seems questionable that the animal can distinguish between 10 and 20 % KCl which have similar initial effects when applied to large trephine openings (4 to 5 mm in diameter), however, with the 2 mm trephine holes used in this study the two solutions probably differed in the rate of SD waves generated. Langford, Freedman, and Whitman (1971) found in similar experiments that performance during retention correlates better with the absolute KCl concentration than with the similarity of KCl solutions employed during learning and relearning.

The crucial predictions of the stimulus control hypothesis were experimentally examined by Mayes and Cowey (1973). With a simple active avoidance task transfer from the normal brain to unilateral CSD was better than transfer between two identical hemidecorticate states. Also, contrary to the stimulus control hypothesis, rats trained under unilateral CSD relearned faster with normal brain than under CSD in the same hemicortex. In another experiment interdepression training failed to induce transfer of the above avoidance reaction from the trained to the untrained hemisphere in callosotomized rats. The memory confinement view is also supported by the evidence that interhemispheric transfer of pattern discrimination learning depends on the intactness of corpus callosum (Burešová and Bureš 1971b, see p. 285).

Imperative and Facultative Transfer

Another interesting approach to the problem of interhemispheric transfer is offered by a combination of unilateral CSD with a lateralized sensory input. Nadel and Burešová (1968, 1969), Burešová and Nadel (1970) trained hooded rats under unilateral CSD in a pattern discrimination task. On the next day 10 transfer trials were given with both hemispheres intact but with vision restricted to one eye. Since the optic nerves in rats are nearly completely crossed (Lund 1965), the eye contralateral to the trained hemisphere has a direct access to the original engram that is available to the ipsilateral eye either indirectly, through the visual cortex of the untrained hemisphere and through callosal fibers, or directly, through the few ipsilateral fibers. It is obvious that the transfer trials performed with the contralateral eye do not directly involve the recipient hemisphere which is not indispensable for correct performance. Participation of the recipient hemisphere in the transfer process is therefore a facultative one. On the other hand the use of the ipsilateral eye in the transfer training makes the participation of the recipient hemisphere an imperative condition. Retention testing with the untrained hemisphere on the third day revealed good transfer in the imperative (indirect-access) transfer group but practically no savings under facultative (direct-access) transfer conditions (Fig. 10.15). Neither group deviated significantly from randomness during the transfer trials but when no training was given during CSD on the first day, the interdepression trials alone did not significantly influence the relearning on the third day. Similar results were obtained with a black-white discrimination.

The mechanism underlying the above examples of transfer can employ various processes involving (a) transcommissural "write-in" activated from the trained hemisphere by sensory input directed to that hemisphere; (b) transcommissural "readout" of the trace in the trained hemisphere by the sensory input directed to the untrained hemisphere; (c) transcommissural "write-in" initiated by stage (b); (d) comparison of the transmitted traces formed during stages (b) and (c) with the direct sensory input.

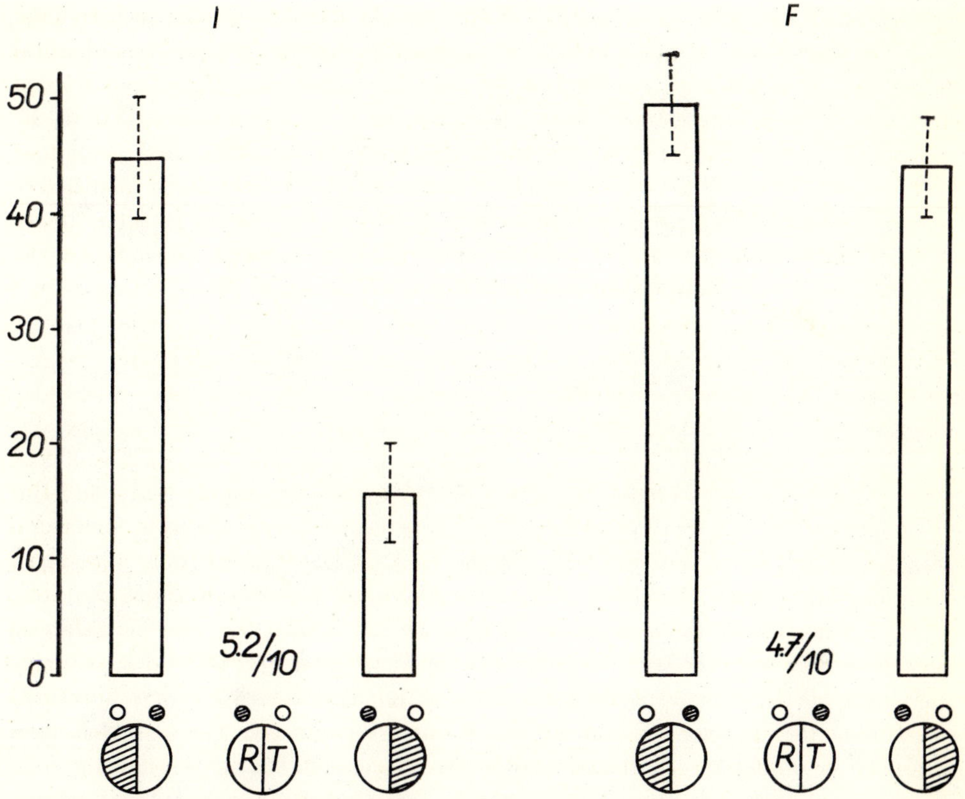

Fig. 10. 15. Imperative *(I)* or facultative *(F)* conditions of interhemispheric transfer. Ordinate: number of to-criterion trials. Shading indicates the covered eye and depressed hemisphere. *R* is the recipient hemisphere; *T* is the transmitting hemisphere. The numbers indicate the ratio of correct responses to all interdepression trials (Nadel and Burešová 1968).

Whereas only stage (a) participates in the facultative transfer, stages (b), (c), and (d) combine under imperative transfer conditions. Better transfer achieved by directing the monocular input to the untrained hemisphere may be due primarily to simultaneous matching of the transcallosally mediated image with the sensory input. Only when the two sets of information agree is a memory trace recorded in the recipient hemisphere. Such a mechanism may be of general biological importance, as it would enable the brain to ignore false information generated by spontaneous neural activity (for example, during dreaming). It is well known, however, that in animals with a completely lateralized visual input, transcallosal engrams are formed during monocular learning (Myers 1957, Myers and Sperry 1958). Thus the inferiority of transfer under facultative transfer conditions resembles the poor quality of the secondary trace formed during monocular learning. We can really consider the interdepression trials in a typical facultative transfer experiment as equivalent to the acquisition stage of an interocular transfer study (see p. 261). This assumption implies that the transferred trace formed under direct-access conditions cannot be better than the secondary trace formed in the hemisphere contralateral to the intact eye under interocular transfer conditions. On the contrary the retrieval stage of interocular transfer resembles indirect-access transfer. The lateralized primary trace is read indirectly through the ipsilateral eye while mechanisms (b), (c), and (d) are activated. Together with the already existing secondary trace, this results in an immediate high-level performance of the untrained eye and in rapid improvement of the secondary trace to the perfection of the primary one (Burešová, Bureš, and Rustová 1971). The latter process takes place because direct readout of the transferred engram is evidently more efficient than transcallosal communication, and the principle of parsimony requires the brain to employ the simplest solution available.

In further experiments (Nadel and Burešová 1970) direct- or indirect-access transfer was studied under reversal conditions. Under unilateral CSD rats were trained a visual descrimination task with the eye contralateral to the depressed hemisphere. On the second day, intact brain animals were given five to ten trials with the stimuli reversed, using either the trained or untrained eye. Relearning with the untrained hemisphere and eye was tested on the third day. In spite of the reversed transfer experience, the transferred trace facilitated contralateral relearning of the original task. Unlike the unreversed transfer trials, the reversed ones caused more significant transfer under direct- than under indirect-access conditions (Fig. 10.16). This rather unexpected finding may be due to disagreement between the direct sensory input and the stored engram, which under indirect-access conditions limits the transcallosal readout (process b) and prevents activation of the transcallosal write-in (process c). On the contrary direct-access transfer under reversal conditions is extremely arousing for the animal. This can account for a rapid formation of the transferred trace, the strength of which probably does not exceed the secondary trace limit postulated above. Support for the above explanation was obtained also in the reversal transfer studies by Nadel (1971) and Burešová and Bureš (1972). The effect of nonspecific interdepression training is less clear, however. According to Nadel (1971) a lateralized brightness discrimination can be transferred to the other hemisphere by brief interdepression training on a pattern discrimination only under direct-access conditions. On the other hand, interdepression training of a brightness discrimination failed to induce transfer of a lateralized pattern discrimination habit both under direct- and indirect-access conditions (Burešová and Bureš 1972).

The assumption that interhemispheric transfer of visual information is mediated through the corpus callosum was borne out by Burešová and Bureš (1970b, 1971b). The indirect-access transfer of a horizontal-vertical discrimination was completely

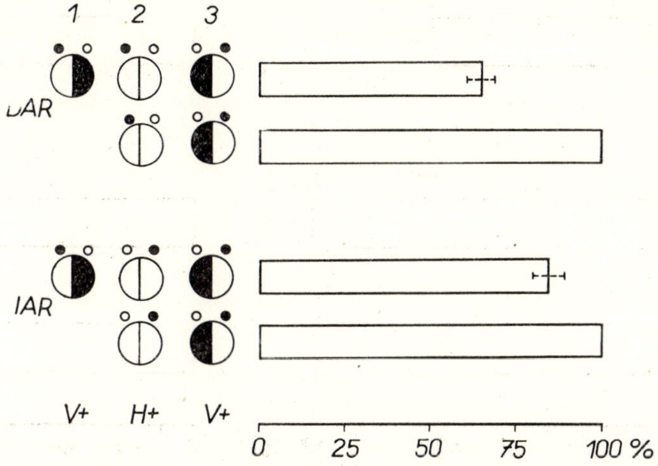

Fig. 10. 16. Interhemispheric transfer induced by reversed interdepression experience. The experimental paradigm is shown in the diagrams on the left margin. Symbols: *DAR*, direct access reversal; *IAR*, indirect access reversal; *H*+, horizontal positive; *V*+, vertical positive. Mean to-criterion trials during relearning of the original task expressed as a percentage comparison, using data for the control group as 100 %. Note that with reversed interdepression training facultative transfer results in more savings than imperative transfer (Burešová and Nadel 1970).

absent in callosotomized hooded rats trained with CSD in one hemisphere and retrained with CSD in the other hemicortex. Significant transfer of black-white discrimination was still observed under these conditions but it was considerably weaker than in unoperated animals (Fig. 10.17). These results prove that the role played by the corpus callosum in the transfer mechanism corresponds to the memory confinement view but can hardly be reconciled with Schneider's (1967, 1968) generalization decrement hypothesis (see p. 279). On the other hand callosotomy does not prevent interocular transfer of pattern discrimination. This is in agreement with similar findings by Sheridan (1965). It seems that callosotomy interferes less with the interhemispheric readout (stage b) than with the ensuing write-in (stage c).

Besides the callosal transfer interpretation, the role of the ipsilateral optic nerve fibers and of subcortical visual centers must also be considered. In the experiments by Nadel and Burešová (1969) no learning was found in rats given 25 black-white discrimination trials with one hemisphere depressed and with the ipsilateral eye occluded. Similarly, no improvement was seen in a retraining test given under the

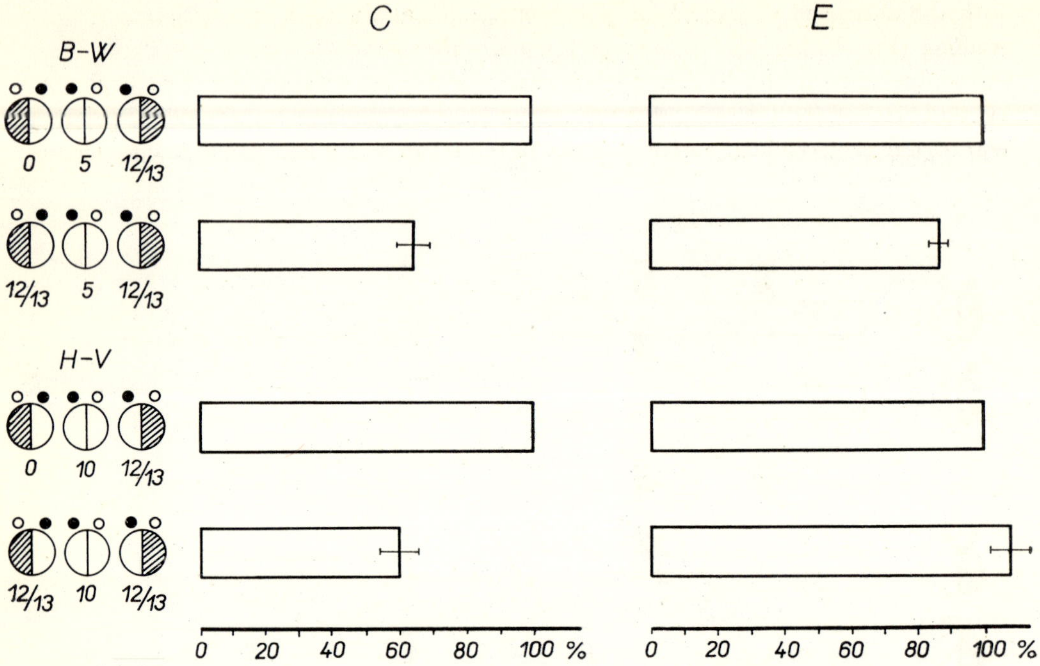

Fig. 10. 17. The effect of callosotomy on the interhemispheric transfer of black-white *(B—W)* and horizontal-vertical *(H—V)* discrimination learning in the hooded rat. The experimental paradigm is indicated at the left margin. Numbers denote the learning criteria used and the number of inter-depression trials. *C* indicates intact animals and *E* indicates animals with section of corpus callosum. Results are expressed in percentage of the control group receiving no training on the first day (Burešová and Bureš 1971b).

same conditions 24 hours later. A black-white discrimination learned during unilateral CSD with the eye contralateral to the intact hemisphere also could not be retrieved under the same CSD conditions with the ipsilateral eye. This indicated that neither subcortical storage nor ipsilateral visual projections are physiologically significant with the above experimental paradigm. Somewhat different results were obtained by Burešová and Bureš (1971b). Whereas functionally hemidecorticated albino rats were unable to learn within 200 trials a horizontal-vertical discrimination when using the eye contralateral to the depressed hemisphere, hooded rats under the same conditions mastered the task but needed considerably more to-criterion trials than when using opposite eye and hemisphere (Fig. 10.18). An engram established in an intact animal with both eyes could be retrieved in a functionally hemidecorticate rat even with the eye ipsilateral to the functional hemicortex, but retraining required about twice as many trials as when using the contralateral eye. Pattern discriminations formed through crossed or uncrossed visual projections during monocular occlusion and contralateral or ipsilateral CSD were completely lateralized, since relearning with the untrained eye and hemisphere proceeded at the same rate as the original training (Fig. 10.18). On the contrary black-white discrimination trained with the eye contralateral to the depressed hemisphere can be partly retrieved by the untrained eye and hemisphere. Comparison of albino and hooded rats indicates that the ipsilateral visual projection is more important in the latter strain and that it can be more

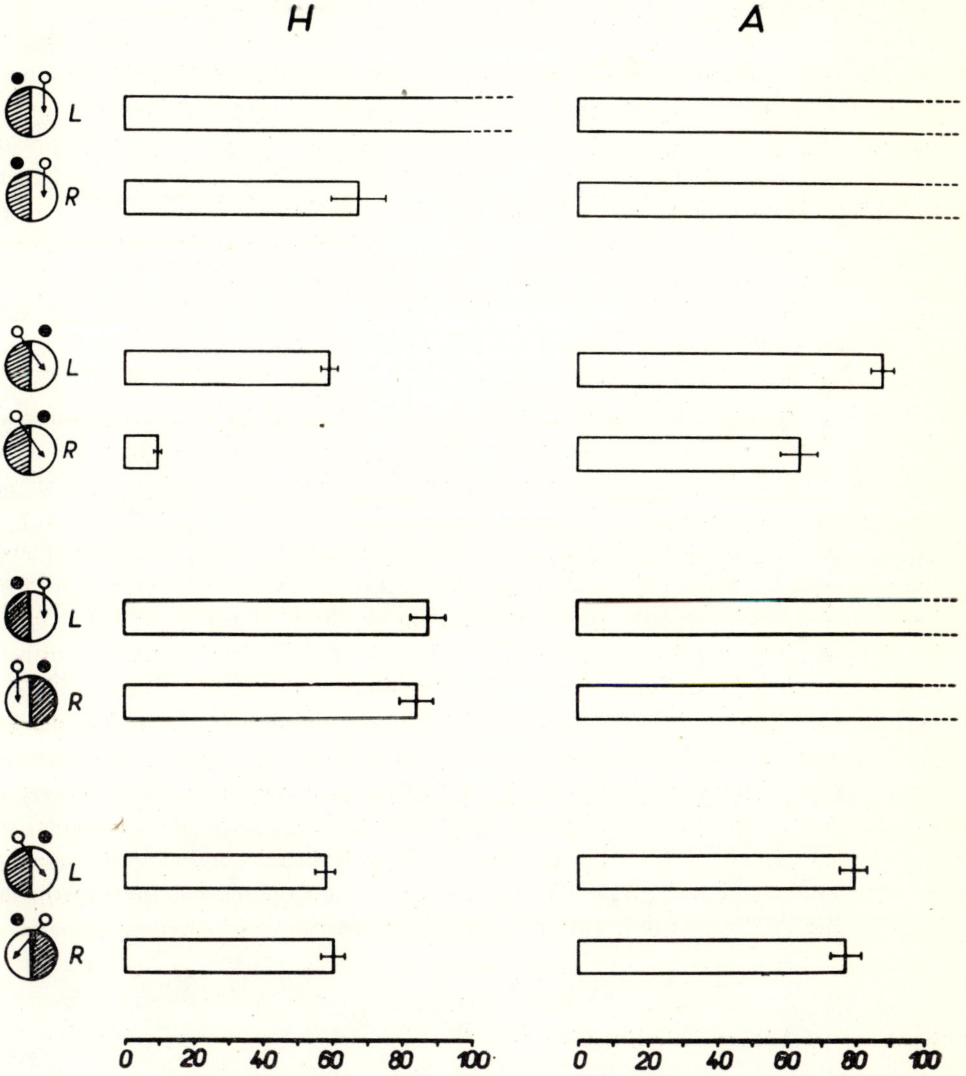

Fig. 10. 18. Significance of the ipsilateral visual pathways for learning and retrieval of pattern discrimination habits in hooded and albino rats. The experimental paradigm indicated by the brain schemes. *H* indicates hooded rats and *A* indicates albino rats. The columns indicate the number of trials to the 12/13 criterion. Other description as in Fig. 10. 17 (Burešová and Bureš 1971c).

efficiently used for retrieval than for acquisition. Whereas pattern discrimination learning is highly corticalized, brightness discrimination acquired with the ipsilateral eye and hemisphere is partly stored at subcortical levels.

6. Interhemispheric Synthesis of Lateralized Engrams

Analysis of lateralized engram formation under unilateral CSD, and of the conditions for interhemispheric transfer of such engrams, lead logically to the problem of interhemispheric synthesis. In preceding sections a single experience was examined; but the split brain technique makes it possible to store two independent memory traces, one in each hemisphere. Mutual interference of the separately stored experiences is prevented by the absence of commissures in the surgically split brain (Trevarthen 1962, Sperry 1964) and by the lack of spontaneous interhemispheric transfer in the reversibly split brain (Bureš and Burešová 1960c). Any of the two engrams can be separately used later when reading out through lateralized sensory inputs in the first case, or during unilateral CSD in the second case. A different situation arises, however, when the split brain animal with the two independent sets of information is exposed to stimuli simultaneously activating both engrams. As pointed out by Sperry (1967) the only means remaining in the bisected brain for interhemispheric communication "are indirect and not unlike those by which one person informs another of something that he has experienced". Beside this mechanism the reversible split brain also has all commissural pathways available for an internal interhemispheric information flow and internal synthesis of the separated engrams into a newly integrated entity. The main objective of the interhemispheric synthesis experiments is to contribute by studying the differences between intrahemispheric and interhemispheric integration to a better understanding of the architecture of the logically constructed engram assemblies.

The typical interhemispheric synthesis experiment proceeds in three stages; (a) acquisition of experience A with the first hemisphere, (b) acquisition of experience B with the second hemisphere, (c) synthesis of A and B with the brain intact. According to the character of tasks A and B and to the synthesis situation, the experiments may be classified as synthesis of antagonistic or synergistic experiences.

Synthesis of Antagonistic Experiences

Although the possibility of using CSD technique to store conflicting experiences in both hemispheres and to maintain their separate coexistence in the intact brain was described in the first interhemispheric transfer experiments (Bureš and Burešová 1960c, Bureš 1959), the results of the collision of two opposite tendencies were experimentally analyzed only much later (Burešová, Votava, and Bureš 1966, Gerbrandt, Burešová, and Bureš 1968, Burešová and Bureš 1969a).

In the simplest case (Burešová and Bureš 1969a) rats are taught with the left hemisphere to go left and 24 hours later with the right hemisphere to go right in a T maze. On the third day both arms of the T maze are open and the animals are allowed to choose between them freely. When the two engrams are well balanced in strength, the left and right choices occur at random as in an untrained animal. This randomness is not due, however, to mutual annihilation but rather to mutual equilibration of the two engrams. If on the third day retention is tested not by free choice but by relearning one of the tasks, considerable savings are found as compared with untrained animals.

The relearning experiments clearly demonstrate the essential difference between interhemispheric synthesis and normal learning. In intact brain, learning task B as directly opposed to previously acquired task A necessarily results in reversal, that is, the animal learns not only to go right on the second day but also to inhibit the tendency to go left. Relearning of task A on the third day is then a new reversal, which usually requires more to-criterion trials than the original learning (Fig. 10.19).

With lateralized learning, acquisition of task B does not imply inhibition of task A, both engrams remaining equally available for the synthesis experiment. The sequence of tasks A—B—A on the first three days does not lead, therefore, to reversal learning on the third day but to relearning of task A with considerable savings. Of the two engrams, that which corresponds better to the requirements of the synthesis test is used. However, the advantages of the separate memory storage are lost by completion of the synthesis. A new switching to task B requires more trials and does not differ from reversal of bilaterally learned task A (Fig.10.19). This is not the case in commissurotomized animals since the capability of split brain monkeys to facilitate reversal learning by selective use of the more appropriate of two conflicting responses, stored separately in the opposite hemispheres, is not deteriorated by simultaneous activation of both brain halves (Johnson and Gazzaniga 1971).

The absence of reversal learning in the reversibly split brain can be interpreted as due to substitution of common sequential or successive learning by parallel learning. Under normal conditions, each experience is given a definite time label. This is not only important for a chronological ordering of events, but also for evaluating their significance for decision making. When there are different possible solutions of the problem, the simple hypothesis is usually adopted that the response which was correct the last time, will also be correct the next time. Thus of two conflicting experiences the recent one will have a decisive influence on the behavior of the animal. This is not the case when learning is lateralized by CSD. It seems that time labeling of unilaterally acquired engrams is lost or at least so weakened that no one of them is the first or the second as far as the animal is concerned. The engrams are there, but the bonds connecting them with the whole system of memories are loose and waiting for a more definite integration.

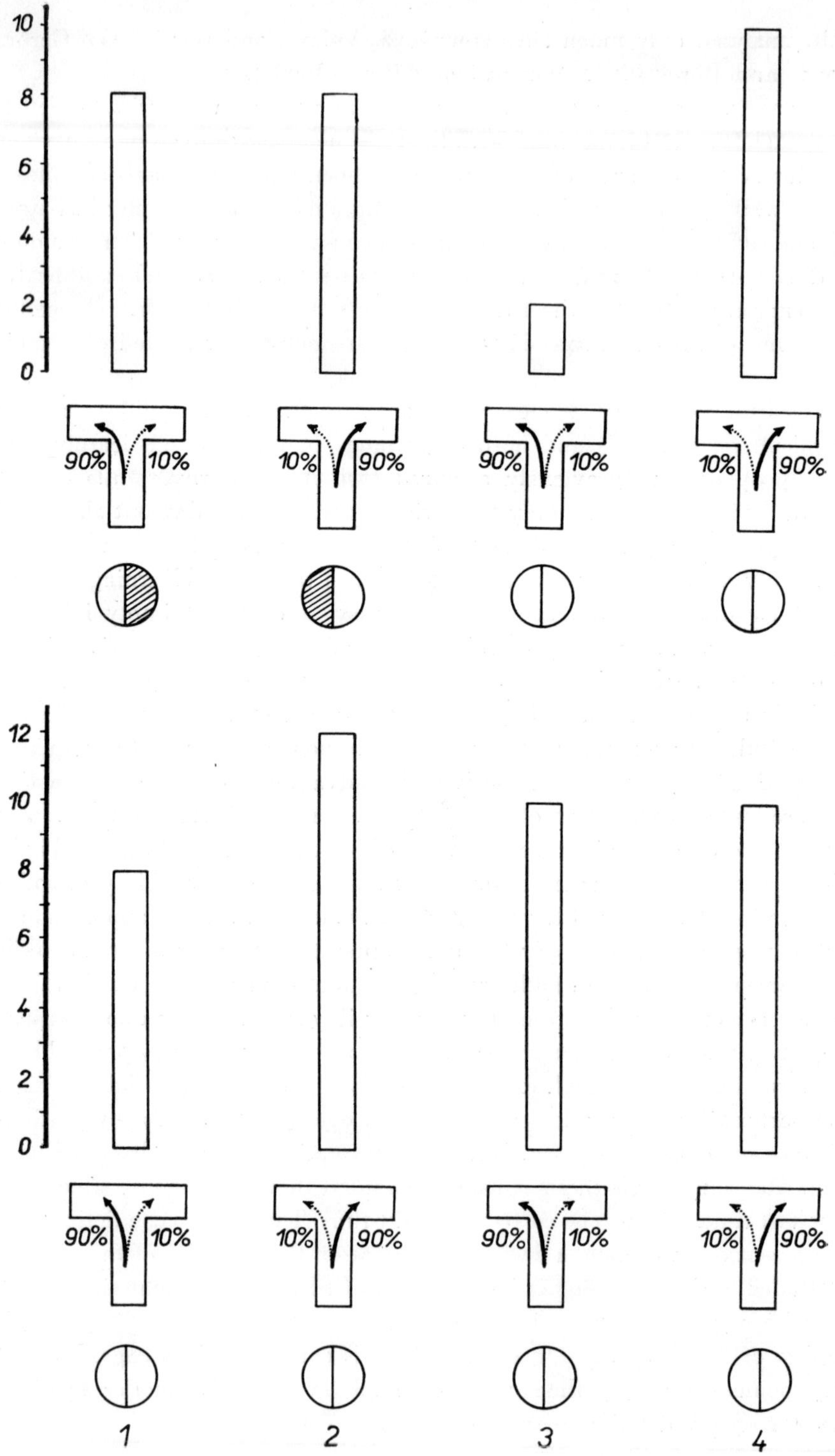
10
8
6
4
2
0
90%
10%
10%
90%
90%
10%
10%
90%
12
10
8
6
4
2
0
90%
10%
10%
90%
90%
10%
10%
90%
1
2
3
4

When conflicting tendencies are not well balanced, the behavior of the animal is determined by the more powerful experience. Interhemispheric synthesis can be used for testing the strength of memory traces acquired under different conditions of learning and with a different motivational background. Fig. 10.20 illustrates a

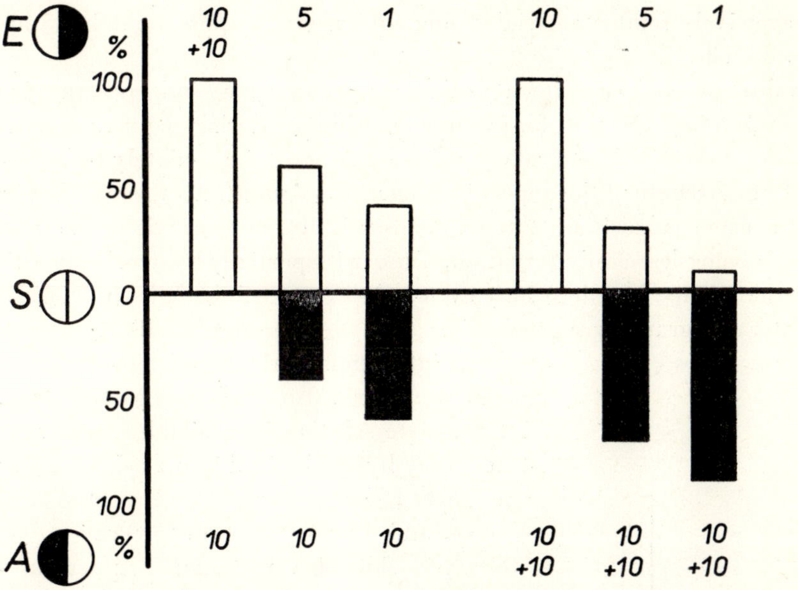

Fig. 10. 20. Competition between aversively and appetitively motivated conflicting experiences, stored separately in the left and right hemispheres. Columns indicate the percentage of left (white) or right (black) choices in the T maze during the synthesis stage of the experiments *(S)*. The numbers above and below the columns indicate the amount of escape or avoidance training to the left *(E)* and of the appetitive training to the right *(A)* previously given to the left and right hemispheres, respectively. For details see text (Bureš and Burešová 1970).

comparison of the strength of appetitive and aversive memory traces. Rats learned with the left hemisphere to escape electric shocks through the left arm of a T maze, and with the right hemisphere to get water in the right arm of the same maze. These habits were mastered to a different extent: criterion of nine correct choices

---

Fig. 10. 19. Comparison of parallel learning in the reversible split brain preparation (above) with the sequential learning in intact rats (below). Columns denote the number of to-criterion trials when the rat learns the left- or right-side orientation in the T maze (criterion level and direction indicated in the diagram below the columns). Note that sequential acquisition of the two conflicting experiences on first or second days leads to prevalence of the last experience on the third day indicated by the absence of savings on the new reversal. With parallel learning on the first and second day, relearning of the first task is facilitated on the third day. Learning of the opposite task on the fourth day already has the character of a normal reversal (Bureš and Burešová 1966b).

out of ten consecutive trials (10) in some groups followed by ten overlearning trials (10 + 10), criterion of four correct choices out of five consecutive trials (5) or one (1) reinforced trial. On the next day with both hemispheres intact the animal was placed at the start of the T maze and its behavior at the choice point was recorded. The results indicate that aversive learning is much more efficient than appetitive learning, 1 to 5 aversively reinforced trials being equivalent to approximately 15 appetively reinforced trials.

In evaluating such experiments other factors that may influence the final result must be taken into account, for example, motivation during acquisition and motivation during retention. If the rats are given 5 ml water immediately before the retention test, the strength of the appetitive engram is significantly decreased (Fig. 10.21). The sequence of acquisition of the two tasks is also not negligible, the more recent experience being less easily forgotten. Tasks with partially bilateral subcortical storage (simple escape learning) may even induce weakening of the previously formed contralateral engram by a mechanism akin to reversal (Fig. 10.21).

The interhemispheric conflict is not necessarily resolved by prevalence of one partial task. If an intermediate solution is available, the two memory traces may by synthetized into a behavioral act which was never before performed by the animal. Burešová, Votava, and Bureš (1966) taught rats to avoid the white left side of a rectangular apparatus with the left hemisphere, and to avoid the black right side

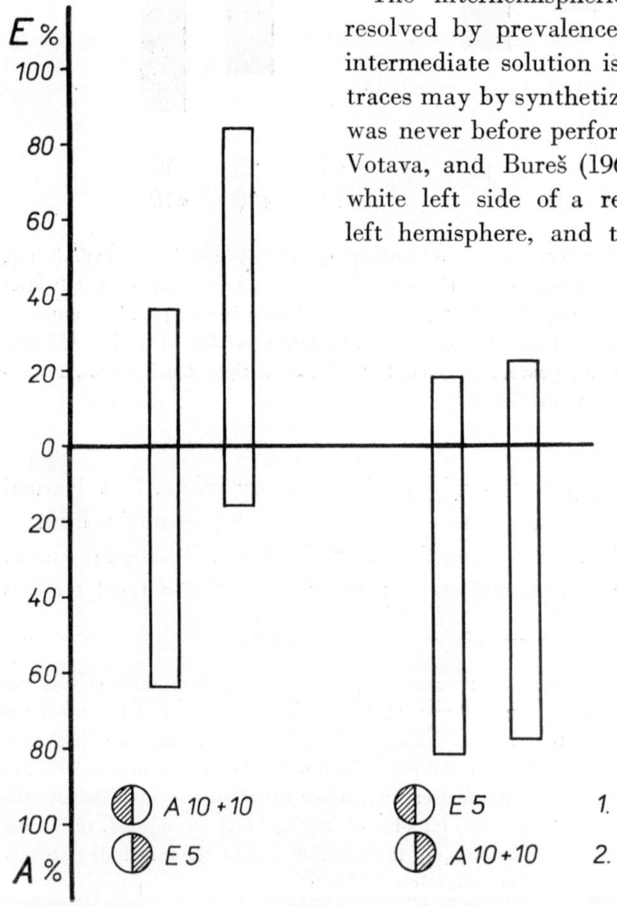

Fig. 10. 21. Competitive synthesis of lateralized engrams: the role of the sequence of the partial experiences and of motivation level during retrieval. Columns indicate the percentage of left (upwards) or right (downwards) choices during the synthesis stage of the experiment. The conditions of training on the first and second days are given at the bottom (*A*10 + 10, appetitive training to the right; *E*5, escape training to the left). The right columns of each pair represent groups that were allowed to drink 5 ml of water before the retention testing (Bureš and Burešová 1970).

with the right hemisphere (Fig. 10.22). When allowed to explore the apparatus with both hemispheres intact, about 40 % of the animals preferred to stay in the center. This behavior (distinctly different from that of untrained animals, which displayed a marked preference for corners) was evidently due to some kind of subtraction of the two opposing avoidance gradients. In the remaining animals one of the engrams was clearly prevalent with a significant bias for the black sidecfield 5).

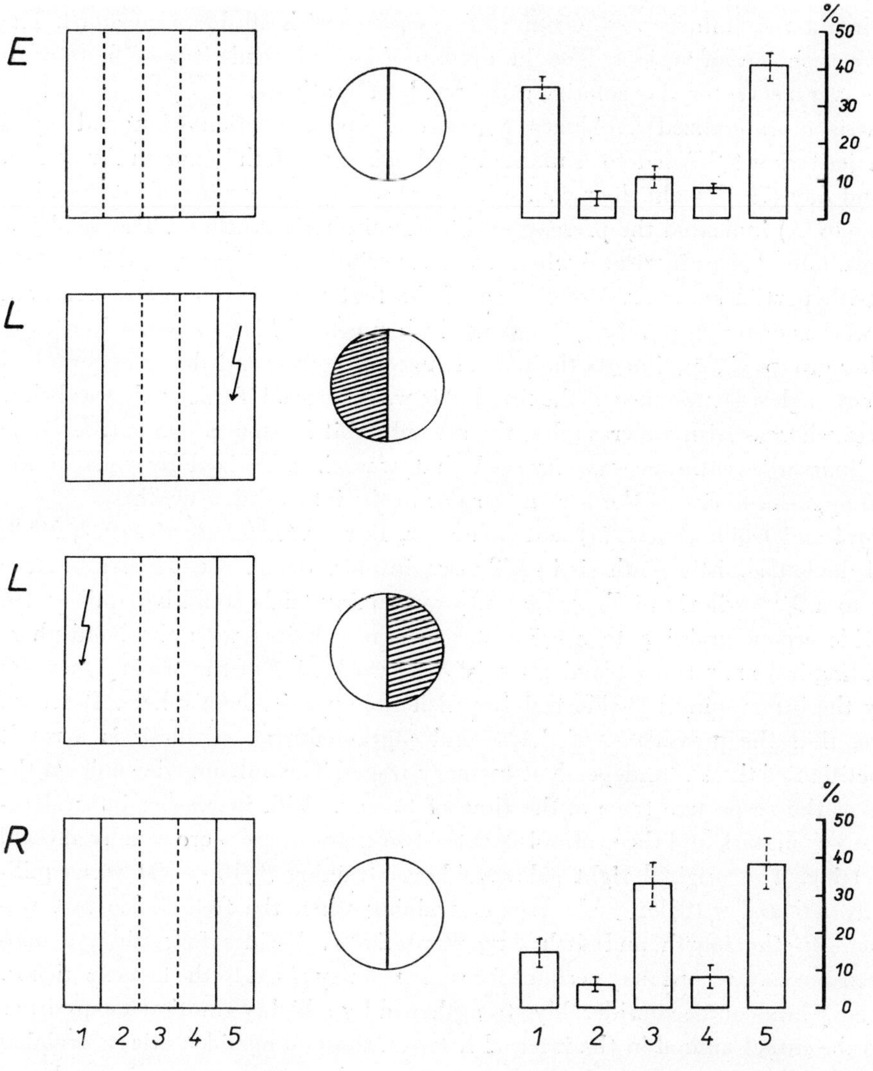

Fig. 10. 22. Exploratory behavior of rats before *(E)* and after *(R)* painful electric shocks were applied in fields 1 and 5 *(L, L)* during CSD evoked in the left and right hemispheres, respectively. The columns indicate the percentage of the 5-min exploratory period spent in each of fields 1 to 5. For details see text (Burešová, Votava, and Bureš 1966).

Some of these problems were analysed in detail by Bianki, Pokrovskaya, and Voyevodenkova (1969) and Bianki 1971). Experiments were performed in albino mice using a semicircular avoidance box with the start in the center and nine doors on the perimeter (spaced at intervals of 22.5 angular degrees). On the first day avoidance reaction was established to the extreme left door with CSD in the right hemisphere. On the second day CSD was evoked in the left hemisphere and the animals were trained to avoid through the extreme right door. On the third day with both hemispheres intact the animals were given 20 free choices with all doors unlocked. The frequency of choices of various doors in a group of animals made it possible to compute the average vector characterizing the result of synthesis.

Synthesis of lateralized avoidance reaction of opposite orientation and equal strength (criterion 9/10) led to a marked predominance of the engram formed on the second day (79 % right door choices), whereas only a few runs of intermediate direction (16 %) indicated the presence of interhemispheric synthesis. The incidence of intermediate choices increased when a weaker criterion (2/2) was used for establishing both partial engrams. Dominance of the first memory trace was observed when a weaker criterion (2/2 or 1/1) was used when establishing the second engram. In another group of experiments the partial engrams corresponded to runs oriented at different angles. Dominance of the first habit was observed if this angle was below 45 degrees whereas with wider angles, the second habit became prepotent. In some cases a "mirror" synthesis was observed that was characterized by runs in the direction opposite to one of the partial tasks or to the intermediate synthesis.

Burešová and Goldowitz (1971) and Goldowitz, Burešová, and Bureš (1972, 1973) analyzed the antagonistic synthesis in a T maze in more detail. Right-side avoidance training to a 9/10 criterion followed by 30 overtraining trials could be equilibrated by left-side escape training to a 3/3 criterion. Free choices with the hemisphere participating in the first-day training revealed no weakening of the original memory trace by the intervening left-side training with the opposite hemisphere. It seems, therefore, that the prevalence of the second engram during synthesis is a result of competition of the two independent memory traces. The outcome depends on the strength of the respective trace at the time of testing. With increasing interval between the second task and the synthesis test the two engrams are more equally affected by forgetting. The original right side avoidance training (9/10 + 30) was equilibrated by 5/6 and 9/10 left side escape training when the free choice test was performed on the fourth and fifth day, respectively. Besides forgetting, a nonlateralized recency record may account for some priority given to the last experience. This recency link can be considerably strengthened by a highly emotional experience given to the intact animal in the interval between the two hemidecorticate training sessions. Thus 30 min swimming preceding by 2 hours left side escape training almost completely restored the correct time relationships of the two lateralized engrams and increased the left side choices to 80 %, that is, to the level corresponding to reversal learning with intact brain. It appears that the emotional experience serves as an outstanding reference event in the bilateral time record which can re-establish the proper sequence of the lateralized engrams the formation of which preceded or followed the swimming.

Synthesis of Synergistic Experiences

Not only antagonistic, but also synergistic engrams can be used for interhemispheric synthesis (Burešová and Bureš 1965b, Burešová, Lukaszewska, and Bureš 1966, Burešová, Votava, and Bureš 1966). To answer the question whether new complex behavior can be directly synthetized from partial information independently stored in the left and right hemisphere, an escape reaction (jumping on an elevated platform) was elaborated with the left hemisphere (Burešová and Bureš 1965b). On the next day a conditioned emotional response was established in the right hemisphere (an acoustic signal of 10-sec duration coincided during the last 5 sec with unescapable electric shocks). On the third day these partial habits were used to synthetize an avoidance reaction (jumping on the elevated platform on the sound alone). Synthesis in control group A (Fig. 10.23), which learned both the escape and the conditioned emotional reaction with the intact brain, was slightly better expressed than in control group B, which learn-

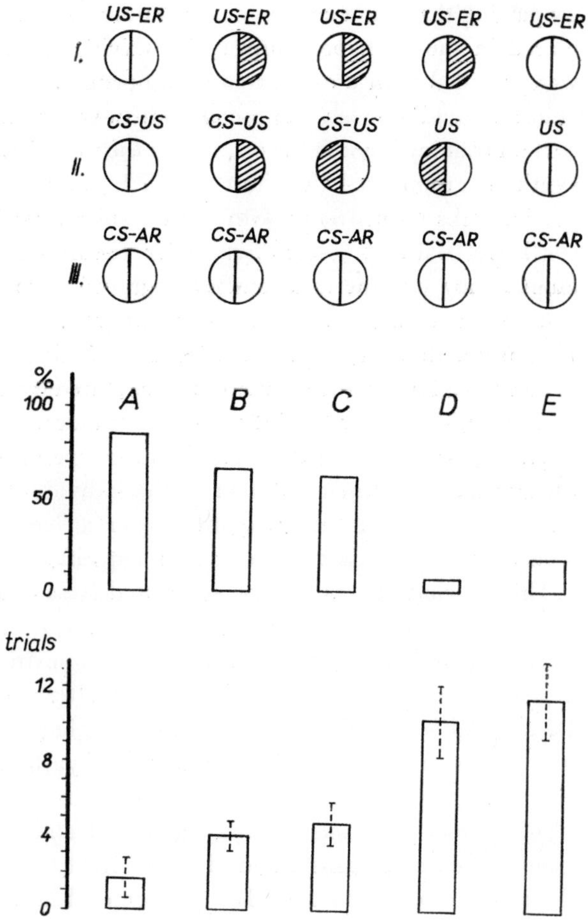

Fig. 10. 23. Interhemispheric synthesis of memory traces. (Top) Experimental arrangement in groups *A* to *E*. Symbols: *ER*, escape reaction; *AR*, avoidance reaction; *CS*, buzzer; *US*, shocks from the electrifiable grid floor; I, II, III, experimental days 1, 2, 3. (Middle) Incidence of the avoidance reactions in three nonreinforced synthesis trials. (Below) Number of to-criterion trials in avoidance learning (Burešová and Bureš, 1965a).

ed both partial tasks with the same hemisphere. Essentially similar results were obtained in the interhemispheric synthesis group C, which performed the avoidance task much better than animals in which no conditioned emotional reaction was elaborated (group D and E).

Unfortunately the above experiments cannot be regarded as conclusive proof of interhemispheric synthesis, the most important prerequisite of which is complete lateralization of the partial engrams. This condition is not satisfied in the case of the conditioned emotional reactions (see p. 269). Only strictly lateralized instrumental reactions were used therefore in further experiments, which lead to the rather unexpected conclusion that under certain conditions interhemispheric synthesis may be more efficient than the usual intrahemispheric synthesis. In one of these experiments (Burešová, Votava, and Bureš 1966) rats learned with one hemisphere to avoid or escape electric shocks in a U-shaped runway (Fig. 10.24). On the next day the animals were trained with the contralateral hemisphere in another apparatus to escape from the grid floor compartment into the safe compartment by passing through a curtain-covered door. On the third day the animals were again placed in the U-shaped runway in which the partition separating the two alleys was provided with a curtain-covered opening. By passing through this opening the animals could shorten the escape pathway by about 70 %. Animals that had no curtain training ignored the opening in the partition completely. The interhemispheric synthesis group used the short cut 17.1 times and the control group (learning the partial tasks sequentially with both hemispheres intact) only 11.2 times out of 30 synthesis trials. It seems that under conditions of interhemispheric transfer, the animal may use the independent engrams more efficiently than a normal animal can use the same, but sequentially acquired, experience.

The fact that the synthesis situation highly resembles task A probably induces in normal animals with sequentially structured memory some inhibition of B engrams and decreases the probability of their readout. Absence of such quasi-antagonistic relationships between the undated and independent partial engrams and their loose fitting into the memory system of the individual thus creates at least in some behavioral situations, better conditions for a "creative" unusual combination of previous experiences then the common sequential learning.

This conclusion was further supported by analogous results of another synthesis experiment (Burešová, Lukaszewska, and Bureš, 1966). The procedure consisted of two preliminary stages (Fig. 10.25): I, acquisition of a left-right alternation habit in a T maze to a criterion of 9 correct alternations out of 12 consecutive trials. II, acquisition of a simple platform jumping reaction to a criterion of 9 escape reactions with latencies below 5 sec. In the synthesis stage (III) the animal was given 100 trials in which it was required to alternate jumping escape reactions between two identical platforms located to the left and right of the starting place. Control group A, learning tasks I and II with intact brain, displayed a rapid acquisition of these conditioned reactions but performed below the chance level in the synthesis

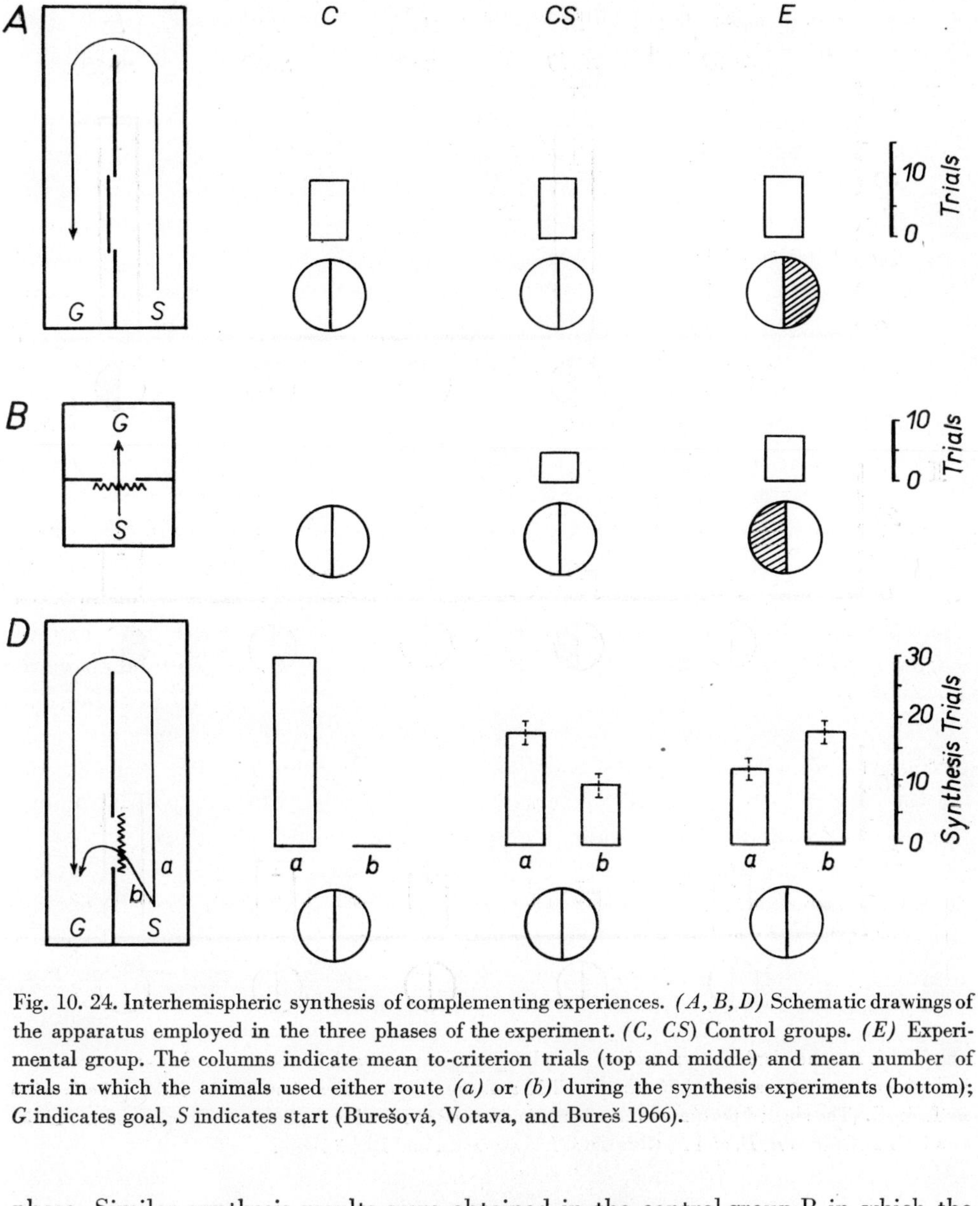

Fig. 10. 24. Interhemispheric synthesis of complementing experiences. *(A, B, D)* Schematic drawings of the apparatus employed in the three phases of the experiment. *(C, CS)* Control groups. *(E)* Experimental group. The columns indicate mean to-criterion trials (top and middle) and mean number of trials in which the animals used either route *(a)* or *(b)* during the synthesis experiments (bottom); *G* indicates goal, *S* indicates start (Burešová, Votava, and Bureš 1966).

phase. Similar synthesis results were obtained in the control group B in which the preparatory learning was restricted to the left hemisphere. Acquisition of tasks I and II was somewhat slower in this group probably because less brain tissue was available for learning. Also control groups C and D which received no preliminary training did not exceed the chance level performance over the 100 jumping alternation trials. Contrasting with all control experiments the interhemispheric synthesis group E performed well above the chance level in the jumping alternation, indicating

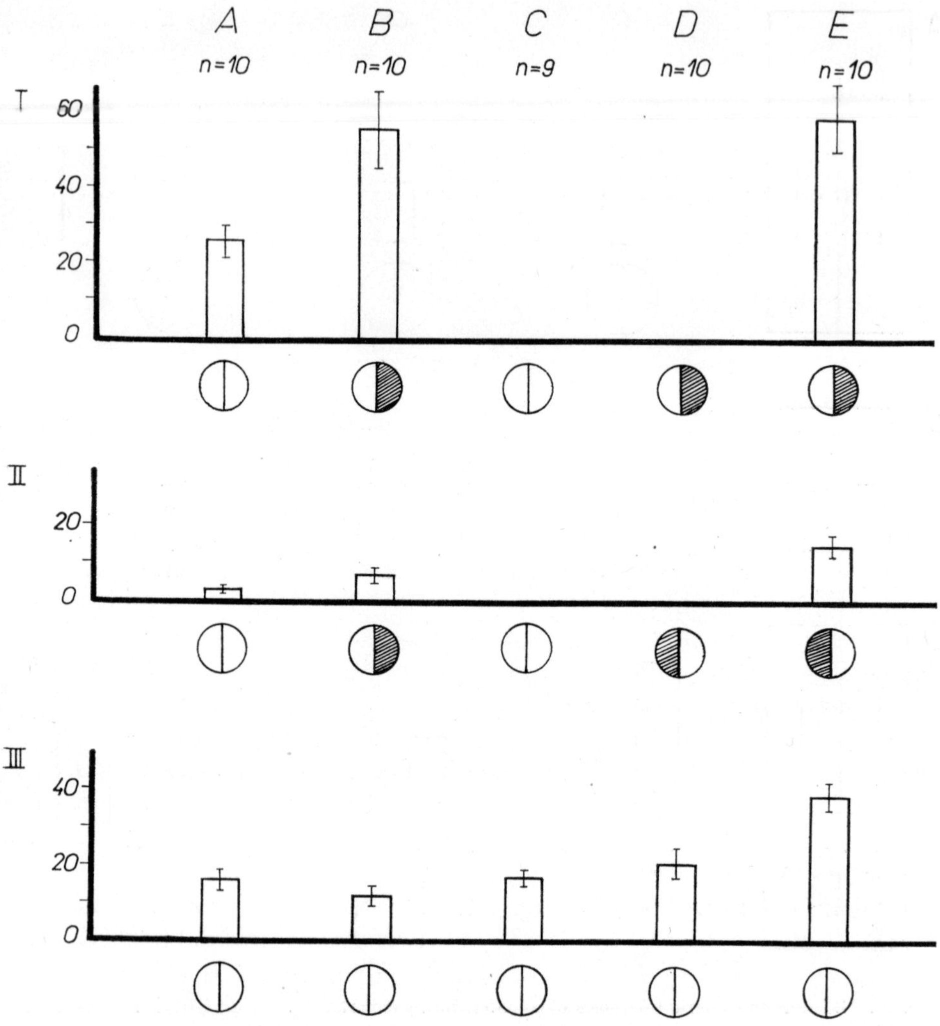

Fig. 10. 25. Interhemispheric synthesis of complementing experiences. Number of trials to reach criterion in both component reactions in Tasks I and II and number of alternations in the 100 synthesis trials in Task III. (The shaded portion of the schematic drawing of both hemispheres under each column indicates CSD in Groups *B, D,* and *E*) (Burešová, Lukaszewska, and Bureš 1966).

positive transfer of experience from stage I to stage III. The absence of such transfer in control groups A and B is probably due to mutual interference of the sequentially acquired tasks I and II.

True interhemispheric synthesis is always restricted to the first few trials performed with both hemispheres intact. After transferred secondary engrams are formed in the contralateral hemisphere, the synthesis may adopt an intrahemispheric rather than interhemispheric character. The first interhemispheric synthesis trials are therefore the most important ones, since their result may considerably influence the further course of the experiment.

7. Combined Use of Unilateral Lesion or Stimulation and of Unilateral Cortical Spreading Depression

The remarkable symmetry of brain functions in laboratory animals makes it necessary to use bilateral lesions in analyzing the role of subcortical centers in learning, motivation, emotionality, and so on. Unilateral lesions usually have no apparent effects, the lost functions being effectively compensated by the remaining paired centers. The split-brain technique makes it possible, however, to investigate the learning abilities of each brain half separately and to reveal any hidden asymmetry induced by the lateralized lesion. The surgical split brain was used in this way by Sperry (1964), who was able to demonstrate in monkeys that animals trained with an amygdalectomized hemisphere displayed emotional changes typical of bilateral lesions, but behaved quite normally when using the intact brain half. Section of the deeper commissural pathways in the surgical split brain may enhance the lateralization of the unilateral lesion effect by limiting the influence of the intact center to the normal hemisphere only. The functional split brain technique can be applied in the same way with some advantage since it leaves the communication between the two hemispheres at the subcortical levels well preserved. Because CSD eliminates primarily the cortical component of learning, its combination with a lateralized subcortical lesion can be used to reveal the degree of lateralization of the corresponding cortico-subcortico-cortical connections.

Using this technique Burešová, Kozlovskaya, Fifková, and Weiss (1961) and Bureš, Burešová, Weiss, Fifková, and Bohdanecký (1962) investigated the role of lateralized corticothalamic, corticohippocampal, and corticohypothalamic connections in elaboration of a simple runway avoidance. Unilateral electrolytic lesions, about 2 mm in diameter, were made in the anterior thalamus, dorsal hippocampus, and posterolateral hypothalamus approximately 8 to 12 days before the actual experiment. One experimental paradigm required the lesioned animals to learn the avoidance habit under CSD in one hemisphere on the first day and to relearn it under CSD in the other hemisphere on the second day. In another series of experiments lesioned animals acquired avoidance with both hemispheres on the first day whereas retention was tested under CSD in alternate hemispheres on the second and third days. Since the task could be completely lateralized, learning rates and savings in both hemispheres were identical under control conditions and any departure from symmetry was considered a consequence of the lateralized subcortical lesion. The results are summarized in Table 10.2 which shows the average number of to-criterion trials in various experimental groups.

Table 10.2.

Influence of Unilateral CSD on Elaboration of Avoidance Reaction in Rats with Unilateral Lesions In Different Brain Structures

Unilateral Lesion	n	Number of Trials To-Criterion		
		Ipsilateral CSD	Contralateral CSD	Difference
Cortex	12	16.1	17.1	1.0±2.3
Thalamus	10	14.8	27.0	12.2±2.1
Hypothalamus	7	20.3	20.5	0.2±2.7
Hippocampus	8	30.0	30.0	—
		Escape latencies (sec) in trials 21 to 30		
Hippocampus	6	9.0	40.0	31.0±15.3

Unilateral damage to the nonspecific thalamus did not significantly affect the learning rates of otherwise intact animals. The asymmetry of the brain functions could be revealed, however, when testing retention during unilateral CSD; the normal hemisphere displayed clear-cut savings, while no signs of relearning could be obtained with the lesioned hemisphere. Similarly, untrained rats learned with the normal hemisphere approximately as fast as normal animals, but were unable to reach the 9/10 criterion within 30 trials in most cases when working with the thalamectomized hemisphere.

Rats with a unilateral hippocampal lesion learned considerably more slowly than controls. Retention tests performed under unilateral CSD demonstrated that most of the learning took place in the intact hemisphere, which displayed marked savings, whereas the performance of the lesioned hemisphere did not differ from that of untrained rats. Untrained rats with a unilateral hippocampal lesion reached the 9/10 avoidance criterion during neither ipsilateral nor contralateral CSD, although the escape latencies over trials 21 to 30 were shorter with the intact hemisphere (9 sec) than with the lesioned one (40 sec, Table 10.2). Both results indicate that the hippocampal damage affects not only the lesioned hemisphere, but that it interferes with functions of the contralateral hemisphere, which is probably influenced by irritative manifestations of the hippocampal scar.

A unilateral hypothalamic lesion caused a slight prolongation of avoidance learning with either hemisphere, but did not elicit any clear-cut asymmetry, evidently because lateralized corticohypothalamic circuits are not essential for this particular conditioned reaction.

Control experiments finally indicated that the cortical damage caused by electrode tracks did not induce any appreciable asymmetry of cortical function.

The above results are in agreement with anatomical and electrophysiological data. Thalamic damage deprives the overlying hemisphere of many important connections and thus seriously limits its participation in conditioning. Although the hippocampocortical connections are more indirect, lateralization of the hippocampocortical effects remains preserved. Perhaps connections between neocortex and hippocampus originating in the cingular region or passing through the pyriform and entorhinal area may be important in this respect.

Whereas lateralized hypothalamic damage did not evoke any asymmetry of avoidance learning, the same type of lesion caused a marked lateralization of appetitive learning. Burešová, Rüdiger, Bureš, and Fifková (1962) trained rats with unilateral lesion of the hypothalamic drinking center (Montemurro and Stevenson 1957) to approach the drinking tube located at the end of a runway. After the habit had been firmly established, unilateral CSD was elicited by application of 25% KCl either onto the normal or onto the lesioned hemisphere. Elimination of the cortex overlying the normal hypothalamus impaired the conditioned approach reaction for a much longer time (105 min) than functional decortication of the lesioned hemisphere (45 min). In control animals with an intact hypothalamus CSD evoked in either hemisphere impaired the conditioned drinking reaction for only 15 min. Unconditioned water intake was affected in the same way (see p. 254).

Rats with unilateral hypothalamic damage are affected by unilateral functional decortication more than normal controls, evidently because the reduced drive mechanisms are less resistant to interference. The asymmetry of the effect can be due either to an asymmetric representation of the conditioned reaction at the cortical level or to an asymmetric influence of CSD on hypothalamic centers. Although the two explanations are not mutually exclusive, the second is in agreement with the results of electrophysiological experiments, which showed that during unilateral CSD spontaneous EEG activity is reduced (Weiss and Fifková 1961b) and unit activity decreased (Burešová, Bureš, Weiss, and Fifková 1961, Rüdiger, Burešová, and Fifková 1962, Bureš, Burešová, Fifková, Olds, Olds, and Travis 1961) in the ipsilateral hypothalamus more than in the contralateral one (Fig. 10.26).

Similar conclusions also apply to experiments with a unilateral lesion of the hypothalamic thermoregulatory center at the border of area hypothalamica lateralis and area hypothalamica anterior (Rüdiger and Seyer 1965). In a shuttle box consisting of a cold (2 °C) and a warm (30 °C) chamber interconnected by a short runway, the normal animals crossed from the cold to the warm side within 10 to 12 sec. When the temperature gradient between both chambers was gradually reversed, rats left the previously warm chamber when its temperature dropped to 12 to 14 °C (Fig. 10.27). Unilateral hypothalamic lesion did not significantly change this behavior even when combined with ipsilateral CSD. On the other hand functional decortication of the intact hemisphere resulted in a complete loss of thermotropic behavior, the animal remaining in the cold chamber for the entire 5-min observation period. The same impairment was also evoked by bilateral hypothalamic damage or by bilateral CSD.

The combination of lateralized hypothalamic and cortical ablations offers interesting possibilities for analyzing the role of these structures in motivational and associative components of behavior. According to the classical point of view, the first are mainly represented in hypothalamic centers whereas the second prevail at the cortical level.

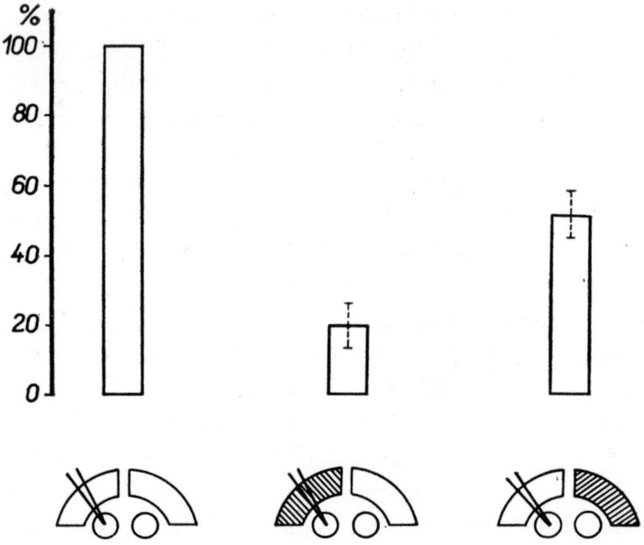

Fig. 10. 26. Lateralized corticohypothalamic influences revealed by the asymmetric effect of CSD on the spontaneous activity of hypothalamic neurons. Columns denote the change of firing rate with respect to the predepression level. The brain schemes show the experimental arrangement.

Isolated unilateral elimination of corresponding structures impairs either component only insignificantly. The striking effect obtained when hypothalamic lesions and CSD are located in opposite hemispheres but not when they are confined to the same side indicates that the associative and motivational aspects of learning are not independent. It is obvious that the hypothalamic drive centers are under permanent tonic influence from the cerebral cortex, which is indispensable for maintaining activity at the diencephalic level. Cortical interpretation of environmental stimuli generates influences increasing or decreasing the excitability of hypothalamic drive centers in a more specific way.

The cortical gustatory area can be an important part of the latter mechanism. Janebová (1967) has shown that unilateral ablation of the gustatory cortex in rats increases the quinine threshold in the two-bottle test ($20 \cdot 10^{-6}$ M Benjamin and Pfaffman 1955) only slightly, but that contralateral CSD decreases gustatory discrimination to the level found in bilaterally decorticate animals ($160 \cdot 10^{-6}$ M quinine

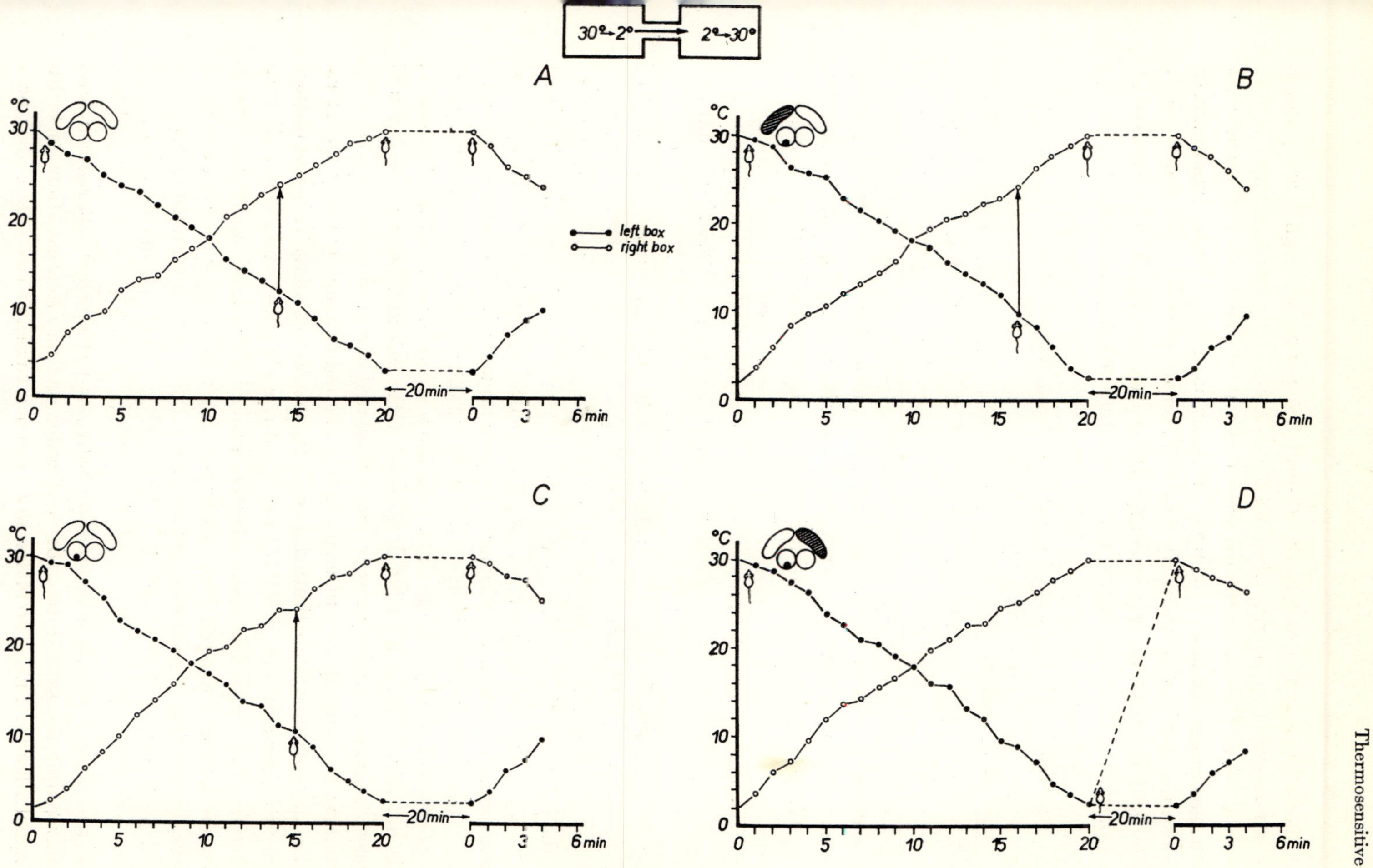

Fig. 10. 27. Typical experiment illustrating the effect of unilateral CSD in thermosensitive behavior. *(A)* Intact animal; *(C)* unilateral hypothalamic lesion; *(B)* ipsilateral lesion and reversible decortication; *(D)* contralateral lesion and reversible decortication. Only in the last case was the thermosensitive locomotion completely abolished. Arrows indicate moment of crossing from the now colder part into the warmer compartment. Broken line indicates that the rat was put by the experimenter from cold to warm compartment (Rüdiger and Seyer 1965).

solution). Total fluid intake during the 15-min test period was significantly lower during contralateral than during ipsilateral CSD, probably because the lesioned hemisphere could not maintain the drinking drive at the same level as the normal one. Both effects are mediated by predominantly uncrossed corticohypothalamic connections maintained under participation of other diencephalic and limbic structures. The significance of the neocortex for appetitive motivation is also borne out by the impairment of unconditioned intake reactions during bilateral CSD (see p. 336).

Although motivation is essential for learning, the influence exerted by the hypothalamus on the association-forming process in the neocortex is less clear. It is conceivable that a weaker memory trace is formed in the hemicortex deprived of the ipsilateral drive center than in the normal one. Unfortunately this is difficult to prove, since retention testing under unilateral CSD is affected by the persisting hypothalamic lesion in the same way as by the predicted asymmetry of the cortical engram. Functional elimination of one side of the hypothalamus during intact cortical learning and unilateral CSD with an intact hypothalamus during retention testing is a solution that will perhaps become feasible with further improvement of functional ablation techniques.

Asymmetry due to partial isolation of the neopallium of one hemisphere was demonstrated by Mysliveček, Hasmannová, and Springer (1962, 1964). These authors cut most connections between the cortical mantle and the brain stem on one side of the brain in 5-day old rats. Adult rats were trained in a maze and the effect of unilateral CSD on maze performance was established. Whereas functional elimination of the isolated cortex did not cause any substantial impairment of maze performance, CSD in the intact hemicortex had nearly the same effect as bilateral CSD in intact control rats. Although disruption of corticosubcortical connections on the operated side is not complete (peripheral stimuli can trigger evoked potentials in the deafferented cortex), the above results indicate that participation of the lesioned hemisphere in higher nervous functions is negligible. It is also possible, however, that the isolated cortex is not normally invaded by CSD, since Grafstein and Sastry (1957) found a decreased CSD susceptibility in chronically isolated cortex in cats.

Asymmetry of motivational mechanisms can be induced not only by unilateral lesions but also by unilateral stimulation of the respective centers. This was demonstrated by Rüdiger and Fifková (1963) for hypothalamic self-stimulation. Unilateral CSD elicited in the hemisphere contralateral or ipsilateral to the stimulating electrodes in the lateral hypothalamus reduced the bar pressing rate to 65 or 37 % of the intact brain level, respectively, probably because excitability of the stimulated region is decreased by ipsilateral CSD more than by contralateral. This conclusion was supported by results of another series of experiments in which electrical stimulation of the hypothalamus was used to interfere with bar pressing for water. Each lever press delivered at the same time a drop of water and an electrical stimulus to the lateral hypothalamus. The current intensity causing the same decrease of bar pressing rate (interference threshold) was increased to 157 % during ipsilateral but only to 105 % during contralateral CSD. In another paper (Rüdiger 1962) the hypothalamic interference threshold was established in a different way, that is, as the current intensity (0.5-sec trains of 50/sec shocks applied at 1.5-sec intervals) stopping the actual drinking reaction of the animal. During ipsilateral CSD the interference threshold increased to 189 % whereas contralateral CSD raised it only to 123 %. When the interfering stimulus was applied to the mesencephalic reticular formation, the interference threshold was increased by ipsilateral and contralateral CSD to approximately the same extent (183 and 161 %, respectively). The threshold of the escape reaction evoked from the same mesencephalic locus (Rüdiger and Bureš 1962) was increased by unilateral CSD in the same, nonlateralized manner (121 and 119 %).

These results are in agreement with electrophysiological findings indicating that both EEG activity and unit firing at the diencephalic level are more affected by ipsilateral than by contralateral CSD, whereas the mesencephalic activity is influenced by unilateral functional decortication in a more or less symmetrical manner.

The CSD effect on electrical activity of the limbic structures is also poorly lateralized (Burešová, Bureš, Fifková, Vinogradova, and Weiss 1962). This may account for the failure of Levitt and Krikstone (1968) to find an asymmetry in the modification of cholinergic thirst by unilateral CSD if drinking was elicited by implanting crystalline carbachol into the lateral septal nucleus. Although bilateral CSD abolished cholinergic drinking completely, ipsilateral and contralateral CSD blocked drinking in 24 and 38 % of cases, respectively. It is also possible that a chemical stimulus applied near to the midline (0.75 mm) can affect the symmetrical centers in the contralateral hemisphere, the physiological significance of which increases proportionally to the damage caused in the ipsilateral centers by the implant.

A combination of unilateral CSD with lateralized visual stimulation was used to produce hemispheric asymmetry by Bianki (1968b, 1970), Bianki and Makarova (1970), and Bianki and Trubacheva (1970). The visual stimuli were flashes of 36 or 12 joules applied from a 20 cm distance to one or both eyes of a restrained mouse at a frequency of 2/min. Unilateral CSD was evoked 10 min after the visual stimulation was completed, and a simple avoidance reaction was trained. The procedure was repeated on the next day with CSD in the other hemisphere. The number of to-criterion trials was decreased by preliminary exposure to bilateral flashes from 16 to 9.Monocular flashes decreased the number of to-criterion trials in the contralateral hemisphere to 12 and increased it to 21.5 in the ipsilateral hemisphere. This effect was the same on the first and second day of training with alternate hemispheres, but was significantly less marked in callosotomized rats. The asymmetry induced by visual stimulation was only seen when 30 or 35 flashes were applied but could not be demonstrated with less (2 to 30) or more (40 to 100) flashes. The effect outlasted the visual stimulation for about 3 hours.

Lateralized flash stimulation applied before the interdepression training (10 or

5 trials) facilitated transfer when the recipient hemisphere was contralateral, but blocked transfer when it was ipsilateral to the flashes. It was suggested that lateralized visual stimuli elicit a dominant focus (Rusinov 1965) in the contralateral hemisphere the presence of which may facilitate learning in this hemisphere and inhibit it in the other. Such an interpretation is partly supported by Robertson and Evans (1965) who found that an increase of unit activity in cortical neurons induced by a single high power flash may last for hours.

Chapter 11

Further Behavioral Consequences and Effects of Spreading Depression

1. Behavioral Consequences of Spreading Depression in Nonneocortical Structures

Although SD can be evoked in different nonneocortical structures, it has seldom been used to explore their role in the mechanism of learning. The main limiting factor is unreliability of the technique. With microinjection of threshold volumes of 25 % KCl (0.2 to 0.5 μl) initiation of SD must be ascertained by electrical recording, whereas with a larger volume the probability increases that the applied KCl solution will spread along the cannula to the overlying tissue (that is, to the neocortex in most cases). Since recording of the electrical SD manifestations is impractical, the simplest alternative is to use larger volumes of KCl in the deep structures and to evoke SD deliberately in the overlying cortex by additional KCl application. The effect of subcortical SD can then be obtained as the difference between the consequences of pure CSD and CSD combined with subcortical KCl administration.

The technique used for eliciting subcortical SD requires preliminary preparation of the animal. A piece of injection needle tubing about 10 mm long and tightly fitted into the small trephine opening is stereotaxically inserted into the brain to the region of the target structure. A shoulder limits insertion of the guiding needle so that the part protruding above the skull surface is always of the same length. The cannula is then cemented to the roughened bone, with anchoring eyeglass screws. Mandrels of appropriate size lubricated with liquid paraffin or silicone oil are used to prevent obstruction of the cannulae by blood and proliferating tissue. Only immediately before the actual injection are the mandrels removed and an adapted injection needle is inserted into the guide so that it slightly protrudes into the brain. The injection needle can either be connected with polyethylene tubing to a microinjection device or small quantities of solid KCl (or other drug) can be placed in the tip and allowed to diffuse out. Oblong KCl crystals can be pushed through the guiding needle into the target structures using the mandrel as a piston. The methodological problems of intracranial injection of chemicals were recently reviewed by Routtenberg (1972).

Caudate Nucleus

As shown by Fifková and Syka (1964) CSD may spread through the amygdalar region to the ipsilateral caudate nucleus (see p. 125). Penetration of CSD into the basal ganglia can be prevented by a shallow cut made in the temporal cortex 1 mm above and parallel to the rhinal fissure. Although CSD was unaccompanied by caudate SD in the operated animals, it impaired the previously acquired avoidance to the same extent as in normal rats (Bureš 1964). The memory disturbing effect of CSD is thus probably not due to invasion of caudate, since CSD applied immediately after passive avoidance training elicits a significant impairment of retention even in animals with temporal slits (Kupferman 1966). These results indicate that the short-lasting and infrequent SD waves in the caudate nucleus do not contribute particularly to the behavioral consequences of CSD. Little is known of the behavioral correlates of caudate SD. According to Weiss and Fifková (1963) and Stille and Sayers (1969) microinjections of 1.5 μl 25% KCl into one caudate nucleus elicited circling movements lasting for 10 to 20 sec and directed to the contralateral side of the body. Similar circling movements can be induced by lateralized electrical stimulation of the caudate (Forman and Ward 1957), whereas unilateral caudate lesions cause circling to the ipsilateral side (White and Himwich 1954). It seems therefore that circling is probably triggered by the brief wave of excitation preceding the actual depression of caudate function, which does not manifest itself as clearly. Hull and Buchwald (1968) injected 4 μl of KCl solution into the caudate nucleus or internal capsule of cats. In animals trained to bar press, injection into brain sites contralateral to the pressing paw stopped this behavior within 1 min. Ipsilateral injections were less effective. As the authors were unable to find a direct correlation between the electrophysiological signs of SD and the behavioral inhibition, the latter seems to be partly due to diffusion of the injected KCl.

A clear-cut effect of caudate SD was recently described by Stille and Sayers (1969). Catatonia induced in rats by intravenous injection of reserpine (2.5 mg/kg) or by intraperitoneal injection of SUM—3170 (4 mg/kg) was blocked by bilateral injection of 0.5 to 1.0 μl 25% KCl into the head of the caudate nucleus. Ten to 20 sec after injection the rats started to move and over 1 min developed considerable locomotor activity, including sniffing, searching and compulsive gnawing. Ptosis and rigor disappeared, skeletal muscles were limp and posture flat. After 4 to 6 min striatal SD terminated and catatonia suddenly reappeared. The disinhibitory effect coincided with suppression of caudate EEG activity. Cortical SD did not influence the catatonia until it entered the caudate nucleus, 4 to 5 min after KCl application on the occipital cortex. Abolition of the striatal activity led to motor excitation also in animals untreated with the neuroleptic drugs, but the effect was less pronounced. For pertinent discussion of the above results see Stille (1971a, b).

Hippocampus

More data are available for hippocampal SD evoked in rats or cats by implantation of a small KCl crystal into the dorsal hippocampus (Bureš 1959, Bureš, Burešová, and Weiss 1960, Bureš, Burešová, Weiss, Fifková, and Bohdanecký 1962). Several slow potential waves were induced, hippocampal activity being impaired for 1 hour on the average. The record of low voltage activity alternated with seizure discharges while cortical activity remained normal. Rats with bilateral hippocampal SD fell into a stuporous state, characterized by a marked reduction of reactivity to external stimuli. Postural and locomotor reactions remained intact, however, and undirected jumping or aggressive behavior was elicited by strong nociceptive stimuli. A simple avoidance reaction, elaborated immediately before application of KCl to the hippocampus, disappeared completely, and even the reaction to electric shocks was so decreased that it was sometimes difficult to force the animal to leave the electrified part of the floor. The avoidance could be relearned only several hours after KCl injection into the hippocampus. Although the possibility must be considered that in some cases KCl could spread to the overlying cortex and elicit CSD, occurrence of the latter reaction cannot account for the above behavioral effects, since bilateral CSD impairs the same avoidance to a much smaller degree (Fig. 11.1). It seems that hip-

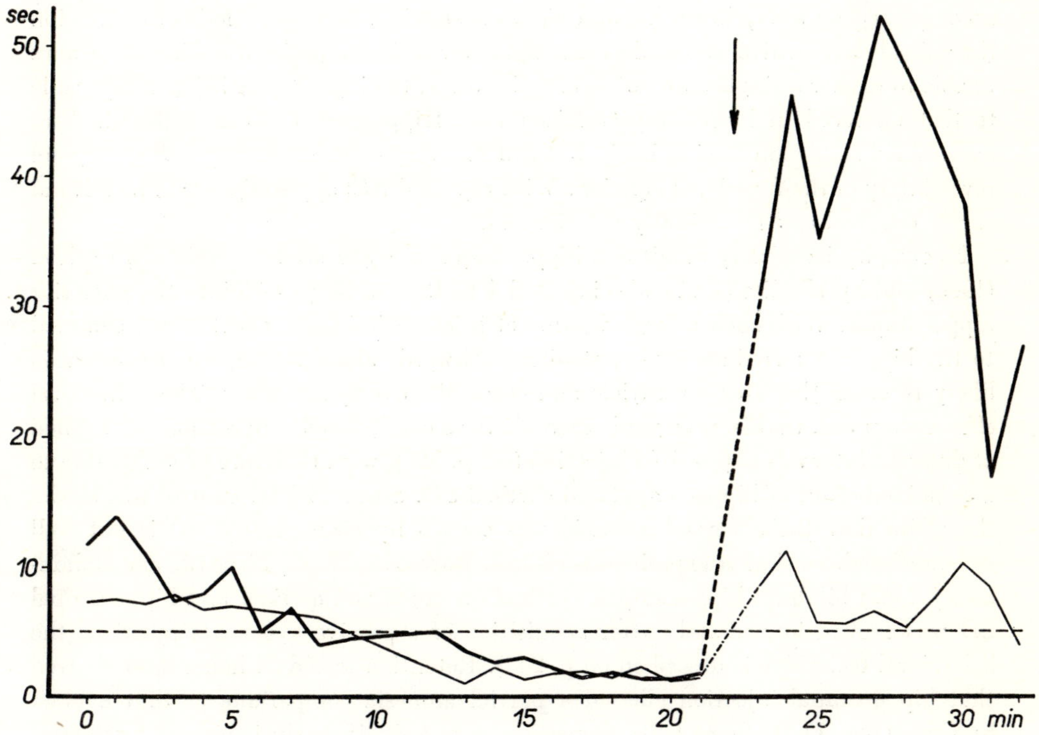

Fig. 11. 1. The average latencies of escape or avoidance reactions in the course of learning in intact rats and in rats under bilateral cortical (thin line, eight rats) or hippocampal SD (thick line, nine rats). Ordinate: latency in seconds. Abscissa: time in minutes. Arrow denotes the initiation of SD. Dashed line corresponding to the 5-sec warning interval separates the escape and avoidance reactions (Bureš 1959).

pocampal SD causes a more serious disturbance of behavior than functional decortication.

Similar results were obtained in cats, in which hippocampal SD can be evoked without the danger of concomitant CSD. An overlearned alimentary conditioned reaction disappeared for several hours after KCl application, which evoked a generalized motor inhibition.

Hippocampal injection of solid potassium chloride was reported by Grossman and Mountford (1964) to cause only a slight impairment of a black-white discrimination. These results cannot be directly compared with those of Bureš, Burešová, and Weiss (1960), mainly because the KCl quantities applied (1 to 6 μg) were insufficient to evoke SD, typical signs of which were lacking in the EEG records. Repeated application of KCl on 20 consecutive acqusition days favored the development of an irritation lesion, the presence of which may account for both the electrophysiological and behavioral findings. Greene (1971) elicited hippocampal depression by inserting through implanted cannulae probes packed with 10 μg of solid KCl. A stuporous condition was observed only during the hippocampal seizures, which were usually accompanied by heavy breathing and vigorous shaking. During periods of depression the animals were active and could learn and reverse simple position habits. They were unable to master a single alternation task, however, the impairment being comparable to that observed in hippocampectomized rats. Hippocampal SD also abolished an overtrained single alternation habit, but full recovery on the next day indicated good reversibility of the functional ablation. With repeated KCl applications, the behavioral effects declined and reversibility deteriorated.

Electrophysiologically monitored hippocampal SD was used by Avis and Carlton (1968) and by Hughes (1969) who injected 4 to 12 μl of 25 % KCl into the posterior hippocampus. With such a large volume of injected fluid, the effect is not confined to the hippocampus since KCl spreading backwards along the injection cannula is likely to enter the lateral ventricle and reach the overlying cortex. The behavioral effects observed, that is, retrograde amnesia for a conditioned suppression established at different intervals before KCl injection (see p. 327), were therefore probably due to a combined effect of hippocampal and cortical SD. Since no CSD control was made, the claim that the observed amnesia was caused by hippocampal SD is not well substantiated. In similar experiments (Bureš, Burešová, Weiss, Fifková, and Bohdanecký 1962) bilateral hippocampal, cortical, or combined cortical and hippocampal SD was evoked immediately after acquisition of a passive avoidance reaction (the behavioral technique is described on p. 244). Retention tested 24 hours later showed that hippocampal injection elicited a partial amnesia comparable to that evoked by CSD (Fig. 11.2). Since CSD amnesia was not significantly increased by hippocampal SD, it seems that participation of the neocortex and hippocampus in consolidation of memory traces is highly occlusive. The alternative explanation is that the amnesia caused by hippocampal injection of KCl was evoked not by hippocampal SD but by the concomitant CSD that probably developed in most cases.

The same reasoning applies to the observation that small acute brain puncture reaching the dorsal hippocampus of mice produced amnesia in a step-through task if applied up to 1 hour after or 1 hour before learning, but not if the treatment preceded or followed learning by more than 6 hours (Bohdanecká, Bohdanecký, and Jarvik, 1967). In a later study Dorfman, Bohdanecká, Bohdanecký, and Jarvik (1969) compared the amnesic effects of bilateral punctures limited to cerebral cortex or involving cortex and hippocampus in mice. Both treatments impaired retention of the step-through passive avoidance in a similar way when the punctures were made immediately after learning, but cortical injury was ineffective when inflicted 1 hour after acquisition.

Dissociation of the effects of cortical and hippocampal SD on memory consolidation was recently achieved by Kapp and Schneider (1971), who elicited SD by insertion of injection needle tubing packed with 14 μg of KCl crystals into the target structure through implanted cannulae. After 3 min the probe was removed and replaced with recording electrodes. When electrical activity was not disrupted for at least 30 min additional injections (usually 2 to 5) were given until this condition was met. Hippocampal SD elicited in the above way 10 sec or 24 hr after acquisition of a conditioned suppression similar to that used by Avis and Carlton (1968), caused a complete block of retrieval in a retention test perform-

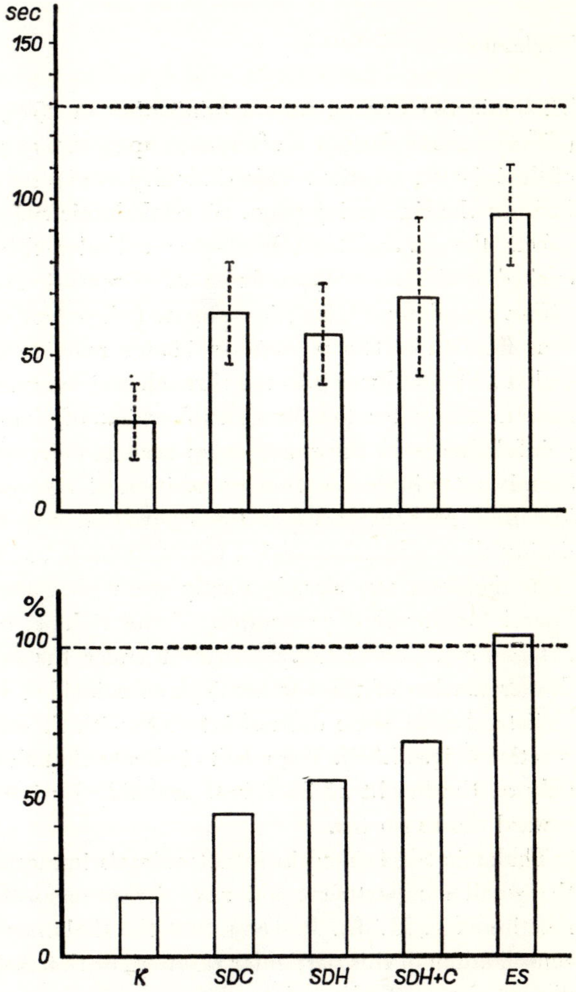

Fig. 11. 2. The influence of ECS *(ES)*, cortical *(SDC)*, hippocampal *(SDH)*, or combined cortical and hippocampal *(SDH + C)* SD evoked immediately after learning on retention of a passive avoidance reaction. *(K)* control group without amnesic treatment. (Above) Time spent in the small chamber. (Below) Percentage of animals spending more than 15 sec in the small chamber. The dotted line represents the average values of untrained animals (Bureš, Burešová, Weiss, Fifková, and Bohdanecký 1962).

ed 4 days later. Cortical SD evoked at the same intervals after training had no disruptive effects.

Functional ablation of hippocampus is not yet satisfactory. Improvement of technique is the crucial prerequisite of the efficient and reliable use of SD for this purpose.

Thalamus

Thalamic SD evoked by microinjection of 25 % KCl into the thalamic complex (Fifková 1964b, 1966a) is often accompanied by cortical SD due to backward spread of the injected solution. This difficulty can be circumvented by deliberately evoking CSD on the side of injection. Since thalamic SD spreads across the midline, it also affects the contralateral hemisphere. Under these conditions behavioral changes evoked by thalamic SD are due to deafferentation of the intact hemicortex. Burešová, Fifková, and Ross (1965) investigated the effect of thalamic SD on acquisition and consolidation of the passive avoidance reaction (Fig. 11.3). In one group of rats 1 μl of 25 % KCl was injected through an implanted cannula into the right thalamus immediately after the 3-min exploration of the apparatus and 90 sec before the painful shocks in the small compartment (Fig. 11.3C). A retention test performed 30 min later indicated that acquisition of the passive avoidance reaction was not impaired, probably because the whole thalamus was not simultaneously depressed during the stimulation period (SD culminated in left thalamus at a time when the right thalamus was already partly recovered). On the other hand in rats with unilateral functional decortication of the right hemisphere acquisition of the same reaction was considerably impaired under the same conditions, probably because deafferentation of the left hemisphere coincided well with the shocks (Fig. 11.3A). Unilateral CSD alone did not interfere with the acquisition of the passive avoidance reaction (Fig. 11.3B). The results indicate that thalamic SD interferes with learning only at the height of its effect, probably by interrupting the flow of information toward the neocortex.

Thalamic SD evoked in intact animals immediately after a 1-min stimulation in the small compartment did not disrupt consolidation of the passive avoidance reaction (Fig. 11.3E). It seems that the thalamus does not play an essential role in consolidation of this particular reaction, or that a single wave of thalamic SD cannot disrupt the newly formed engrams effectively.

Avian Striatum

Little information is available on the behavioral effects of SD in submammalian species, although the phenomenon was demonstrated in the brain of birds and reptiles (see p. 133). The highly developed avian striatum subserving highest level functions in birds seems to be especially suitable for this purpose. The electrophysiological

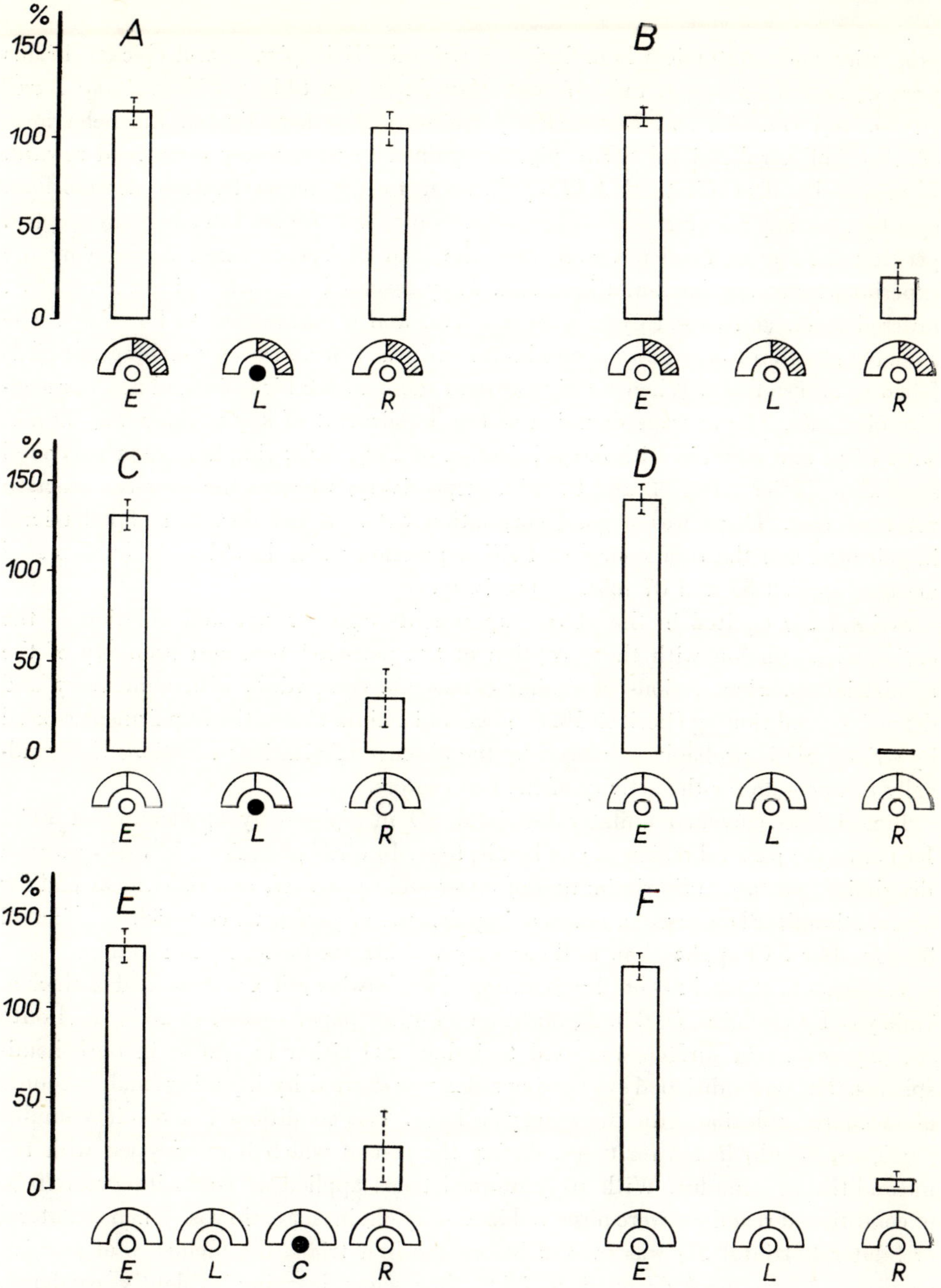

Fig. 11. 3. The influence of thalamic SD on learning and consolidation of the passive avoidance reaction. Columns indicate the time (in seconds) spent in the small chamber before *(E)* and after *(R)* the painful experience. Schemes in groups *(A)* to *(F)* illustrate the functional state of the cerebral hemispheres (CSD indicated by shading) and of thalamus (black circle denotes thalamic SD) in various phases of the experiment. For details see text. Symbols: *E* exploration; *L* learning; *C* consolidation; *R* retrieval (Burešová, Fifková, and Ross 1965).

properties and anatomical boundaries of striatal SD in pigeon and chicken brains were described by Bureš, Fifková, and Maršala (1960), Shima, Fifková, and Bureš (1963), and Ookawa and Bureš (1969). Shima (1964) investigated the behavioral effects of bilateral striatal SD in pigeons trained to peck a key for a food reward. Immediately after bilateral KCl application to the hyperstriatum accessorium, spontaneous key pecking was still present. Some 30 to 60 sec later pigeons stopped pecking the key and did not even take the food that was offered to them by the experimenter at regular 2-min intervals. They assumed a posture with a bent back, lowered head, and closed eyes, were inactive, and often seemed to be asleep. The aversive reaction toward an approaching hand was lost and even touching the birds failed to arouse them. When walking around the box, the birds seemed not to recognize obstacles. The average duration of the impairment of key pecking was 39 min with 1.5 μl and 100 min with 3.0 μl injection of 25 % KCl; simple feeding recovered somewhat earlier (after 32 and 87 min, respectively) whereas the aversive reaction returned first. There was a good correlation between the duration of behavioral impairment and the time course of EEG depression which lasted with the two KCl dosages applied 33 and 87 min, respectively.

Striatal SD elicited in the above experiments causes functional ablation of the entire telencephalon with the exception of the paleostriatum and probably of the archistriatum. Since lesions of similar extent are compatible with alimentary and defensive conditioning (Beritoff 1926, Tuge and Shima 1959), the impairment caused by striatal SD is probably enhanced by the absence of vicarious functions that gradually compensate for the activity of the lost centers.

Bianki (1967) evoked unilateral striatal SD in pigeons by application of 20 % KCl onto the parietal region of one hemisphere. In birds pretrained in various visual discrimination tasks (discrimination of lower and upper, left and right, near and far visual stimuli) SD caused a marked impairment of performance which culminated 30 min after KCl application. Full recovery was attained after 90 to 120 min.

The effect of striatal SD on the conditioned swallowing reflex was studied in chicken embryos by Sedláček (1964). Application of filter paper soaked in 25 % KCl onto the exposed brain surface was used to induce SD either in one or in both hemispheres. The unconditioned swallowing reflex was elicited by injecting small amounts of saccharin solution into the embryo's beak. The conditioned acoustic stimulus (3000/sec, 68 db) lasted for 6 sec, during the last of which it overlapped with the unconditioned stimulus. With 10 reinforced trials applied at 1-min intervals 70 % of conditioned reactions were observed in 21-day old intact embryos. When unilateral or bilateral striatal SD was evoked before the first trials, the incidence of positive conditioned responses dropped to 35 % but some learning evidently persisted. In 20-day old chicken embryos KCl application did not impair the acquisition of the conditioned swallowing reaction, perhaps because in the less mature brain the depression did not spread though the entire striatum or because the relationships between striatum and lower brainstem are different.

2. Effect of Cortical Spreading Depression on Consolidation

As shown in the preceding chapter the reversibility of CSD makes it possible to separate decorticate and intact states in time (decorticate learning - intact retention and vice versa) or in space (reversible split brain). An obvious alternative application is to insert CSD between intact brain learning and intact brain retention in order to test its effect on memory.

Before describing the actual experiments it is necessary to point out that in research of this kind several tightly interconnected processes are investigated — acquisition of experience, formation of the corresponding engrams, retention of the relevant information and its availability for retrieval. The existence of a particular engram can only be ascertained by successful retrieval, but failure to retrieve some supposedly acquired information may be due to inadequate acquisition, poor consolidation, decay of the trace in time, or inaccessibility of the trace. Cortical SD applied after acquisition but prior to retrieval may interfere not only with consolidation but also with the preservation of the consolidated engrams or even with the readout mechanism. Unfortunately many of the experiments on the amnesic effect of CSD were not planned in such a way as to make it possible to differentiate between the above alternatives.

In most studies CSD was used to disrupt the consolidation process by inducing functional decortication at different intervals after learning. The experimental paradigm was similar to that in analogous ECS studies. In complex tasks, the acquisition of which requires long training, the experience acquired during early trials may consolidate more than the experience immediately preceding criterion. The estimation of the consolidation time is then uncertain. This difficulty is avoided in one-trial learning procedures, in which the information is introduced into the brain within a brief and well-delimited interval. This evidence will be reviewed first.

One-Trial Learning

Pearlman and Jarvik (1961) reported a disrupting effect of CSD applied within 10 min after a single step-down avoidance trial. The experiments were described in greater detail in a later paper (Pearlman 1966). The rat was placed on a small platform, elevated 18 cm above the table. The platform was then lowered to the table and as the rat stepped off the platform, it completed a circuit and received a 1.5 mA shock. Bilateral CSD was evoked by applying 25 % KCl to both occipital cortices 1, 5, 10, and 15 min after the foot shock. As soon as CSD developed (as indicated by cessation of the cortical placing reaction), KCl was removed and the area of application was washed with saline. The author points out that only a single CSD wave was generated under these conditions since normal activity was restored about 10 min after KCl removal. Retention was tested 21 hours later by again placing the rat on the platform and recording the time before stepping off with all four paws. Untrained controls stepped down within 2 to 3 sec, shocked controls after 19 sec. Cortical SD elicited 1 and 5 min after foot shock caused complete amnesia, the average step-down latencies being 1 and 5 sec, respectively. Partial amnesia was seen with the 10-min acquisition-disruption interval (11-sec step-down latency), whereas after 15 min the memory trace was not affected by CSD (20-sec step-down latency). Administration of ether (saturated vapors for 1 min) at the same intervals after foot shock caused approximately the same degree of amnesia. No direct comparisons of the CSD and ECS effects were made, but other studies using similar one-trial passive avoidance techniques indicate that ECS has a more pronounced amnesic effect than ether (for example, Bureš and Burešová 1963). The assumption seems to be justified, therefore, that the CSD technique used by Pearlman (1966) is less disruptive than the standard ECS.

Kupferman (1966) confirmed the above findings using a slightly different step-down task; the rat was placed on the wooden platform and when it stepped on the grid floor, it was shocked until it stepped back on the platform and stayed there for 1 continuous min. Immediately after this criterion was reached (usually in less than 3 min), CSD was evoked by 25 % KCl. Retention was tested 24 hours later by measuring the total time spent on the platform during a 300-sec observation period. Untrained controls spent 36 sec there, shocked controls 159 sec. Bilateral CSD reduced the stay on the platform to 59 sec. A test for the amnesic effect of the pain associated with KCl administration (application of KCl onto exposed bone and muscle) failed to reveal any memory disturbance (140 sec on the platform). Kupferman (1966) also attempted to find out whether the amnesic effect of CSD is due to subcortical spread by repeating the above experiments in rats with transcortical incisions approximately 1 mm above the rhinal fissure, which prevent CSD from entering the amygdala, entorhinal cortex, and caudate nucleus (Fifková and Syka 1964). It seems that CSD induced less amnesia in the operated animals, but a large scatter in the data makes this evidence rather inconclusive.

Bureš and Burešová (1963) used bilateral CSD to disrupt consolidation of the one trial passive avoidance reaction described in Chap. 9 (p. 244). The rat was allowed to explore the two-compartment apparatus for 3 min and the time spent in the big and small chambers, respectively, was measured. Then the animal was confined in the small compartment and exposed there to intermittent electric shocks for 1 min. After the painful stimulation, CSD or ECS were administered at different intervals. Since filter papers soaked in 25 % KCl were left on the exposed cortical surface, functional decortication lasted for several hours. Retention was tested 24 hours later by a new 3-min exploration; whereas untrained rats preferred to spend about two thirds of the exploration period in the small compartment, the trained animals displayed a clear-cut avoidance of the small compartment, 82 % of them spending less than 15 sec there.

When applied immediately after learning ECS wiped out the memory trace almost completely. Cortical SD also impaired memory but the deficit was somewhat less expressed. Both procedures caused severe memory loss also when applied 2 hours after learning. With prolongation of the acquisition-disruption interval to 6 hours, the amnesic effect of CSD and ECS was reduced but still remained statistically significant. Ether anesthesia elicited immediately after learning and maintained for 5 min did not interfere with consolidation of this passive avoidance reaction (Table 11.1).

Table 11.1.

Retention Loss Caused by Different Memory Disturbing Procedures applied Immediately after Learning a Pasive Avoidance Response

Group	*n*	Time Spent in Small Compartment during 3-min Retention Test (sec)	Rats Spending 15 Sec or More in Small Compartment (Percent)
Controls	22	27 ± 13	18
Ether anesthesia	10	29 ± 20	20
CSD	18	$62 + 17$	61
Electroshock	10	94 ± 17	100
Untrained Rats	60	135 ± 4	97

Using a similar training procedure Rabedeau (1966) compared the amnesic effects of CSD applied 1,16, and 156 min after a foot shock (10 sec, 3 mA) in the small compartment. A retention test performed 48 hr later revealed amnesia only in the 16 min group, whereas no disruption was found with the 1 min shock-CSD delay. This unexpected result was confirmed by Paolino and Levy (1971) in a replication study, employing a slightly modified passive avoidance situation and an implanted cannula for KCl application to free-moving rats (Paolino and Levy 1970). It was suggested that CSD evoked immediately after learning facilitates a temporary storage of the memory trace at a subcortical level until recovery of normal cortical function makes permanent fixation possible. Onset of the cortical storage process rapidly eliminates the subcortical trace and consolidation becomes sensitive to CSD disruption. This interpretation was supported by the finding that a second KCl application, following 4 hr after the 1-min delay CSD treatment, produced a retention deficit not significantly different from that caused by a single KCl application with the 16-min shock-disruption interval (Paolino and Levy 1971).

The passive avoidance reaction is either due to a generalized conditioned emotional reaction (freezing, suppression of motor activity) or to a more specific avoidance of the punished response. To decide between these two possibilities Black, Suboski, and Freedman (1967) used a one-trial discriminated avoidance technique. An open field in the shape of a right triangle had two small chambers cutting off the acute angles, one painted white with a circular opening, the other painted black with a rectangular opening. The animal was placed in the open field and allowed to enter one of the small chambers. On the next day the chamber chosen on the previous occasion was closed so that the animal was forced to enter the other small compartment. A total of four alternated free and forced single daily trials were given in the pretraining phase. In the actual experiment the grid floors of both chambers were electrified and the rat received foot shocks until it left the chamber. After 5 min a 33% KCl solution was applied to both cortices and left there for 45 min. Retention was tested 24 hours later by giving the animal another free choice in the apparatus. The choice latency and the number of boli was recorded. During the retention test the no-shock saline controls entered the same compartment in 80% of the cases with an average latency of 5 sec. In 80% of the cases the shocked animals entered the compartment not associated with the painful experience, but the latency of the choice was increased over 600 sec. Shock followed by CSD was less well remembered; the latency of the first choice was 260 sec and only 53% animals reversed from the chamber in which they had been shocked. The results indicate that CSD impaired retention of the nonspecific fear component of the task, whereas disruption of the discriminative component was not statistically significant. Cortical SD probably also affected retention of conditioned suppression, disrupted according to Avis and Carlton (1968) by hippocampal SD (see p. 310).

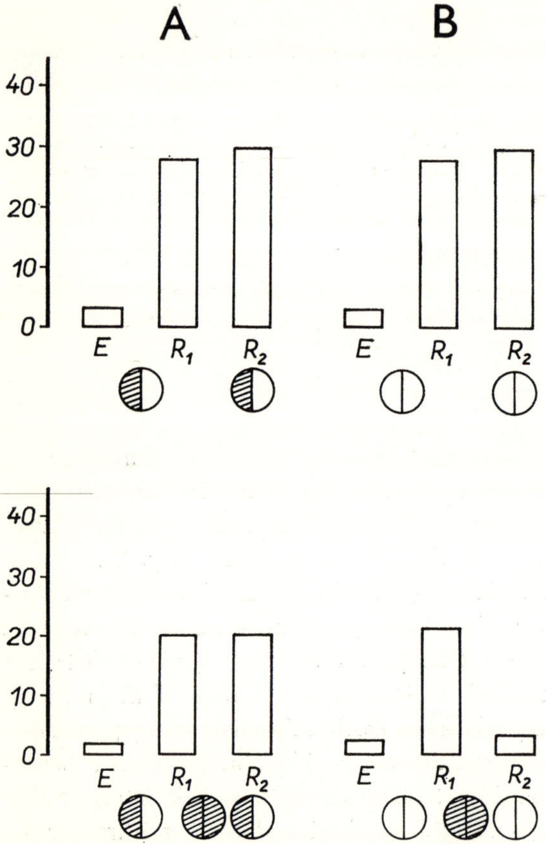

Fig. 11. 4. The effect of bilateral CSD on retention of a passive avoidance reaction acquired with intact brain *(B)* or under unilateral CSD *(A)*. Control groups above, experimental groups below. Ordinate: median step-down latencies (sec) during initial exploration *(E)* and during the first *(R_1)* and second *(R_2)* retention test performed 30 sec and 4 hr after the footshock, respectively. Brain schemes indicate conditions during learning and retention testing. Bilateral CSD was elicited immediately after the first retention test(Schneider 1967).

An interesting observation is that of Schneider (1967) who trained rats in a simple passive avoidance reaction (a step down situation) either with brain intact or with unilateral CSD and tested retention under the same brain conditions 4 hours later (Fig. 11.4). Bilateral CSD evoked immediately after training caused an almost complete amnesia in the group trained with brain intact, but only partial amnesia in rats trained under unilateral CSD. This may indicate that the subcortical memory trace formed during unilateral CSD training is more resistant to the amnesic effect of bilateral CSD than the information stored predominantly at the cortical level. Schneider (1967) also confirmed the weak amnesic effect of unilateral CSD following intact brain learning mentioned by other investigators.

The results of all the above experiments indicate that CSD disrupts consolidation of passive avoidance reactions. The amnesic effect depends on the intensity and duration of CSD, but it is usually less pronounced than that of ECS applied at comparable intervals after learning. The decrement of the amnesic effect with an increasing learning-disruption interval points to interference with consolidation rather than to impaired retrieval.

Giurgea (1972) demonstrated the significance of the cerebral cortex of rats for the plastic changes at the spinal cord level using the technique developed by Chamberlain, Halick, and Gerard (1963). Unilateral lesion of vermis elicits an asymmetry of tonus in the hindlimbs which persists after transection of spinal cord performed 45 min after lesion and recovery from anesthesia. The asymmetry is not preserved when the spinal cord is transected earlier (35 min after recovery from anesthesia). Cortical SD elicited by application of 2 % KCl onto the occipital region of the hemisphere ipsilateral to the lesion immediately after arousal from the anesthesia prolongs the "spinal fixation time" from the usual 45 min to 75 min. Contralateral CSD is without effect. Giurgea (1972) concluded that cerebral cortex facilitates the fixation of this particular experience in the spinal cord.

To-Criterion Learning

Complex information cannot be introduced into the brain by a single trial. If consolidation of each quantum of information is to be affected in the same way, the memory-disturbing procedure must follow each trial. Duncan (1949) used ECS in this way to disrupt maze learning. Although his classical experiments were later criticized because of the lack of adequate control for ECS aversiveness (Coons and Miller 1960, McGaugh and Madsen 1964) the approach remains a valid possibility. It was used by Doolittle and Thompson (1966) to test the effect of topical posttrial application of different drugs on maze learning. The animal received one daily trial in a 6-unit U maze. The rat was removed 30 sec after it entered the goal box and the epidural cannulae (according to Tapp 1962) were cleaned and filled with 25% KCl, 0.01% pentylenetetrazol, 0.01% strychnine sulphate or saline. The mean number of errors over the 10 days of training was 33.4 for saline, 32.8 for KCl, 32.4 for strychnine, and 22.8 for pentylenetetrazol. Although interpretation of these experiments is somewhat obscured by the decreasing efficiency of KCl over the ten daily applications, motor impairment and aphagia developing after each KCl administration indicated the presence of CSD which evidently failed to cause a significant disruption of the maze habit. The facilitatory effect of pentylenetetrazol application contrasted with the absence of KCl amnesia, but discussion of this finding is beyond the scope of this chapter.

Kupferman (1965) failed to disrupt a food-reinforced pattern discrimination by CSD. His rats learned in a single session to discriminate between horizontal and vertical stripes, until the criterion of six consecutive correct responses was reached. Cortical SD was evoked immediately afterwards. Retention was tested by retraining the animal to a criterion of 9 correct out of 10 consecutive responses 24 hours later. The number of errors to reach criterion in the control and CSD groups, respectively, was 16.2 and 15.5 on original learning and 1.8 and 2.2 on relearning. It was suggested that absence of CSD amnesia may be due to positive reinforcement used in these experiments, but this view is not supported by other evidence.

Table 11.2.

Effect of CSD and Electroshock on Retention of a Left-Right Discrimination

Group	n	First Day	Second Day	
		Trials to Reach Left-Side Criterion*)	Right Choices in Free Choice Situation (Percent)	Trials to Reach Right-Side Criterion*)
Control	10	4.4±1.5	0	65.8±7.4
Electroshock**)	10	4.4±1.0	10	11.2±1.7
Spreading Depression**)	10	3.1±0.5	10	43.3±5.3

*) The 10 trials in which the criterion was reached are not included.
**) Memory-disturbing procedure applied 1 min after learning.

Burešová and Bureš (1969a) found that bilateral application of 25% KCl immediately following to-criterion acquisition of an aversively reinforced left-right discrimination does not impair consolidation. Bureš and Burešová (1963; Table 11.2) compared the effects of ECS and CSD on consolidation of an overtrained left-right discrimination (to-criterion learning + 20 overlearning trials). Retention was tested 24 hours later by allowing the animal to perform three choices with both alleys of the discrimination box open. The control animals as well as the CSD and ECS rats clearly preferred the side reinforced during the original learning.

Some amnesic effects of CSD could be detected in these experiments when using a different retention test. After the free choice trials, the original spatial discrimination was reversed. The criterion of reversal was rapidly reached in the ECS group (11 trials) as compared with control animals (66 trials). Cortical SD had an intermediate effect (43 trials). Cortical SD and ECS did not eliminate the memory trace, the continuing existence of which accounted for savings during relearning and side preference in the free-choice test. The memory-disturbing procedures reduced the strength of the engram and rendered it less resistant to reversal.

The amnesic effects of CSD and ECS are more expressed when reversal is used during both learning and retention testing. Bureš and Burešová (1963) taught rats to escape electric shocks through the left alley of a left-right discrimination box. After the criterion of 9 correct out of 10 consecutive choices was reached, 20 overtraining trials were added. After an hour's interruption, the discrimination was reversed and training was continued until the animal made 9 correct right side choices in 10 consecutive trials. Bilateral CSD or ECS was applied 1 min or 2 hours later. Retention was tested after 24 hours by offering the animal 3 free choices (with both alleys open) and reversing the discrimination once more. Whereas the original learning took only four to-criterion trials on the average, the first reversal required from 23 to 41 trials in the different groups. In control animals the free-choice test revealed a complete retention of the reversed discrimination, 100% of choices being to the right side. The next reversal also proved to be difficult and required 42 to-criterion trials. Both ECS and bilateral CSD applied immediately after the first reversal caused pronounced memory impairment. The free-choice retention test (Table 11.3) revealed a preference for the originally reinforced side in the ECS group

Table 11.3.

The Effect of CSD and ECS on Retention of a Reversed Spatial Discrimination

Groups	n	1 day		2 day	
		Trials to Reach Left-Side Criterion	Trials to Reach Right-Side Criterion	Right Choices in Free-Choice Situation (%)	Trials to Reach Left-Side Criterion
Controls	10	4.1±1.0	36.5±4.6	100	42.1±2.7
ECS applied					
1 min	9	4.1±1.0	27.7±2.8	22	5.6±2.9
2 hours	10	4.6±1.3	40.9±4.9	47	16.9±3.0
after first reversal					
CSD applied					
1 min	9	3.5±0.8	23.2±4.3	44	13.6±4.3
2 hours	10	3.5±0.7	34.8±4.9	74	36.0±5.9
after first reversal					

(78% of left-side choices) and an equal probability of both choices in the CSD group (56% of left-side choices). The random choice was not due to elimination of both right-and left-side engrams but to a weakening of the left-side discrimination which now only balanced the original right-side tendency. This was demonstrated by the outcome of the second reversal, which required 13.6 to-criterion trials in the CSD group as compared with 5.6 to-criterion trials in the ECS group. Applied 2 hours after the first reversal, CSD did not significantly influence retention, and also the amnesic effect of ECS applied with this delay was considerably decreased (Table 11.3).

The amnesic effect of ECS in the above experiments resembles that described for a similar situation by Duncan (1948). In a later study Burešová, Bureš, and Gerbrandt (1968) analysed different situational and organismic factors influencing the ECS amnesia under reversal conditions. Although the absolute number of to-criterion trials required for reversal was considerably lower in the replication study than in the original paper, the main results of the latter were essentially confirmed; ECS affected a reversed spatial discrimination habit much more than a simple one. This may indicate that the ECS-sensitive link is the inhibitory component of reversal. The animal learns two different things during the reversal: the new spatial discrimination habit and at the same time suppression of the original one. If ECS (and CSD as well) mainly affects the differential suppression of the first habit, the two conflicting discriminations would be equilibrated and the equilibrium would be indicated by a random distribution of free choices.

Gerbrandt, Burešová, and Bureš (1968) and Burešová, Bureš, and Gerbrandt (1968) attempted to test this assumption by comparing the ECS effect on two conflicting memory traces acquired either under conditions of conventional reversal training or under conditions of interhemispheric conflict. In the latter case rats were trained under CSD in the left hemisphere to go to the right and 24 hours later under CSD in the right hemisphere to go to the left in a T maze. Such a procedure does not lead to reversal of the first habit but to a separate storage of the two tasks, the first in the right and the second in the left hemisphere (see Chap. 10). When applied immediately after attaining the criterion of the second discrimination, ECS did not weaken the corresponding experience. When tested with both hemispheres intact, equilibrium of the two conflicting tendencies was indicated by random distribution of left and right choices both in the control and in the ECS group. If all stages of the above experiment were performed with an intact brain, a typical reversal learning was obtained. On the testing day the last experience clearly prevailed, the most choices being to the left. When applied immediately after completion of left-side learning, ECS suppressed the reversal, and free-choice testing revealed randomness (Fig. 11.5). Whereas the two procedures are essentially identical as far as timing of learning and testing is concerned, the lateralized discrimination learning is not accompanied by inhibition of the first habit, the memory traces of which are suppressed by CSD. This may account for the different effect of ECS in both cases. Thus the results support the assumption of a greater susceptibility of inhibitory connections to memory-disturbing procedures. There is some evidence that reversal memory can be selectively affected not only during consolidation but also during retrieval. Hart and Geyer (1971) trained and immediately reversed a position habit in rats. On the next day, animals tested under bilateral hippocampal SD chose the initially trained side whereas the undepressed controls preferred the reversal side.

The failure to disrupt consolidation of operant tasks by ECS or CSD may have different reasons. It is possible that consolidation of these engrams is so rapid they attain a stage of considerable resistance during the to-criterion learning. Complex habits acquired in a single trial (or in a few trials) as in the interhemispheric transfer experiments are susceptible to the amnesic effect of CSD and their consolidation times are comparable to those established by other methods (see Chap. 10). An alternative possibility is that ECS or a single application of 25% KCl is not powerful enough to interfere with later phases of consolidation.

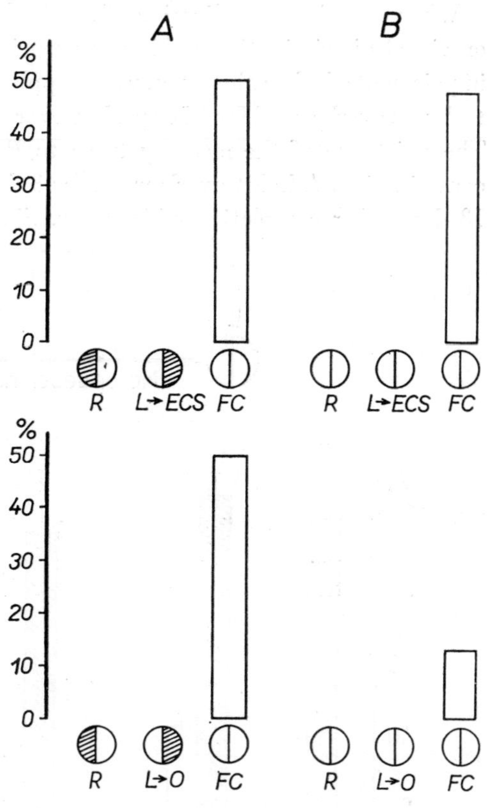

Fig. 11. 5. Effect of ECS on conflicting lateralized memory traces *(A)* and on sequentially acquired nonlateralized engrams *(B)*. Left—right discrimination in a T maze (ten animals per group). Symbols; *R*, to-criterion training to the right; *L*, to-criterion training to the left; *ECS*, electroconvulsive shock applied immediately after attaining the left-side criterion; *O*, no amnesic treatment; *FC*, retention expressed in percentage of right choices in the three free choices.

Graded Amnesic Effects of Cortical Spreading Depression

Whereas a maximal ECS seizure is an all or none phenomenon that cannot be easily graded, CSD has an amnesic effect depending on the duration and intensity of the treatment. One or two waves of CSD evoked by application of 2 % KCl cause a much weaker retrograde amnesia than a long-lasting train of CSD waves evoked by 25 % KCl (Bureš and Burešová 1963, Albert 1966a). Burešová and Bureš (1969b, 1971a) have recently shown that repeated application of 25 % KCl at five 1-hour intervals (so-called "prolonged" CSD, PCSD) may affect even those stages of consolidation, that are fully resistant to a single application of 25 % KCl.

Rats were taught a simple spatial discrimination in a T maze or a visual pattern discrimination. Different levels of overtraining were obtained either by giving additional trials after reaching the 9/10 criterion on the first day or by repeating the to-criterion learning on several consecutive days. In addition to the level of training the interval between learning and PCSD and the interval between PCSD and the retention test were varied. Single applications of 25 % KCl and of saline were used in the control experiments.

Whereas a single application of 25 % KCl did not decrease retrieval of the spatial or visual discrimination habit acquired in a single session, PCSD caused a severe impairment of relearning even when applied after 3 days of overtraining. When the task was overlearned for 14 days, however, retention remained unaffected (Fig. 11.6). The resistance of the memory trace to PCSD also increased with the duration of consolidation. A habit overlearned for 3 days remained unaffected by PCSD applied 13 days after completion of learning. Six days after the last training trial, PCSD

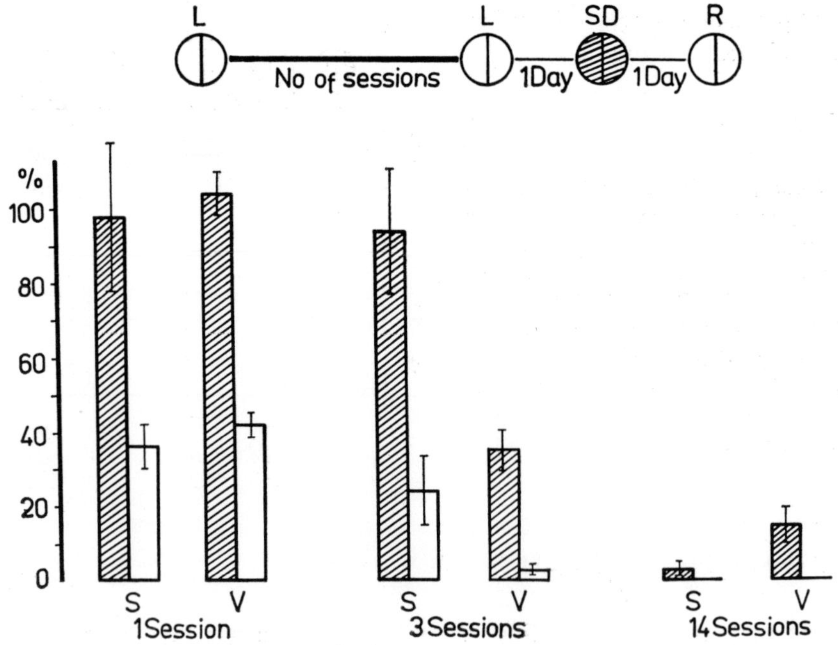

Fig. 11. 6. Effect of PCSD on retention of a spatial *(S)* or visual *(V)* discrimination habit overlearned to different extents. Shaded columns indicate PCSD experiments; white columns indicate single application of 25% KCl. Ordinate: number of to-criterion trials during the retention test expressed in percentage of the original to-criterion training. In the scheme of the experimental paradigm: *L*, learning; *SD*, SD or PCSD treatment; *R*, retention testing; SEM indicated by vertical bars.

evoked amnesia of intermediate intensity (Fig. 11.7). Although the time scale is much extended, these data resemble other consolidation studies. The consolidation was completed between 7 and 14 days and its duration seemed to be dependent on the intensity of the original training. After a certain level of learning was reached (three training sessions) consolidation improved the resistance of the engram with the same efficiency as continued overtraining.

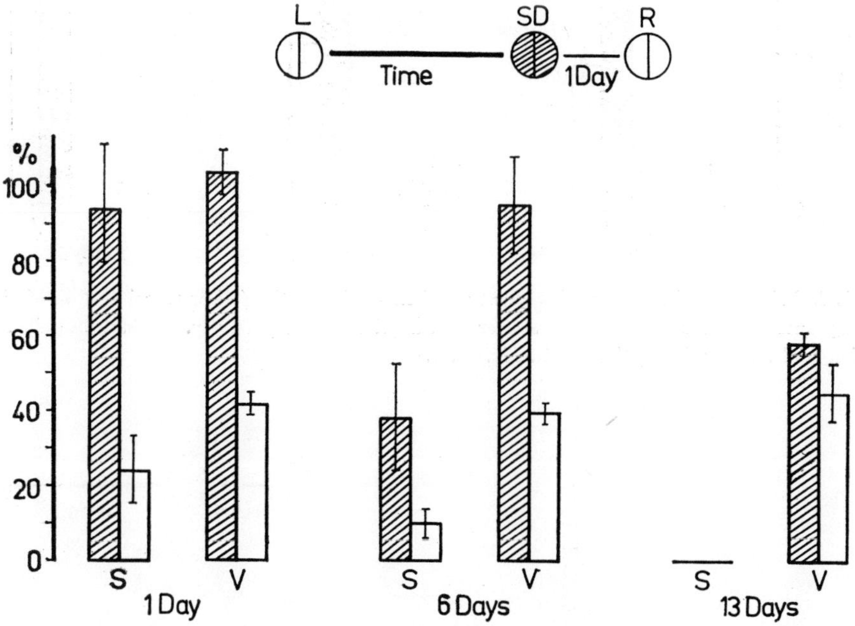

Fig. 11. 7. Effect of PCSD on retention of a spatial *(S)* or visual *(V)* discrimination habit consolidated to different extent (time allowed for consolidation before KCl application given below the columns). Other description as in Fig. 11. 6.

The interpretation of the above results is complicated by the proactive effects of the PCSD treatment. Acquisition of the T-maze habit by untrained rats subjected to PCSD was significantly slower during the following 3 days and recovered only after 7 days (Fig. 11.8). These proactive effects must be taken into account when evaluating the relearning data in experiments in which retention testing was performed 1 or 3 days after PCSD. Another interesting feature of PCSD amnesia is the transitory nature of its effect. When the retention test is performed 7 or 14 days after PCSD, retrieval of the impaired spatial discrimination is found to be considerably improved. Recovery of the visual discrimination is less conspicuous under similar conditions (Fig. 11.9). Engrams overtrained to different extents are differentially resistant to the PCSD treatment. This was most clearly demonstrated in experiments

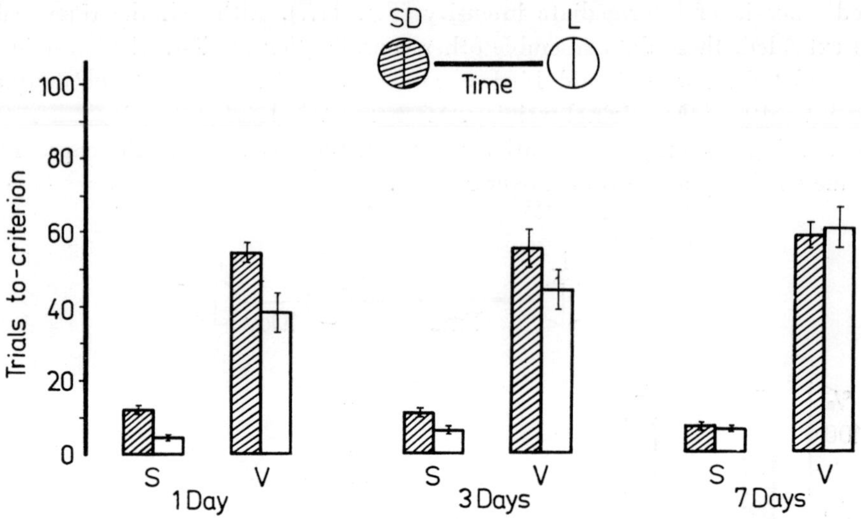

Fig. 11. 8. Effect of PCSD on the subsequent acquisition of a spatial *(S)* or visual *(V)* discrimination habit by untrained rats 1, 3, or 7 days after KCl application, respectively. Ordinate: number of to-criterion trials. Other descriptions as in Fig. 11. 6.

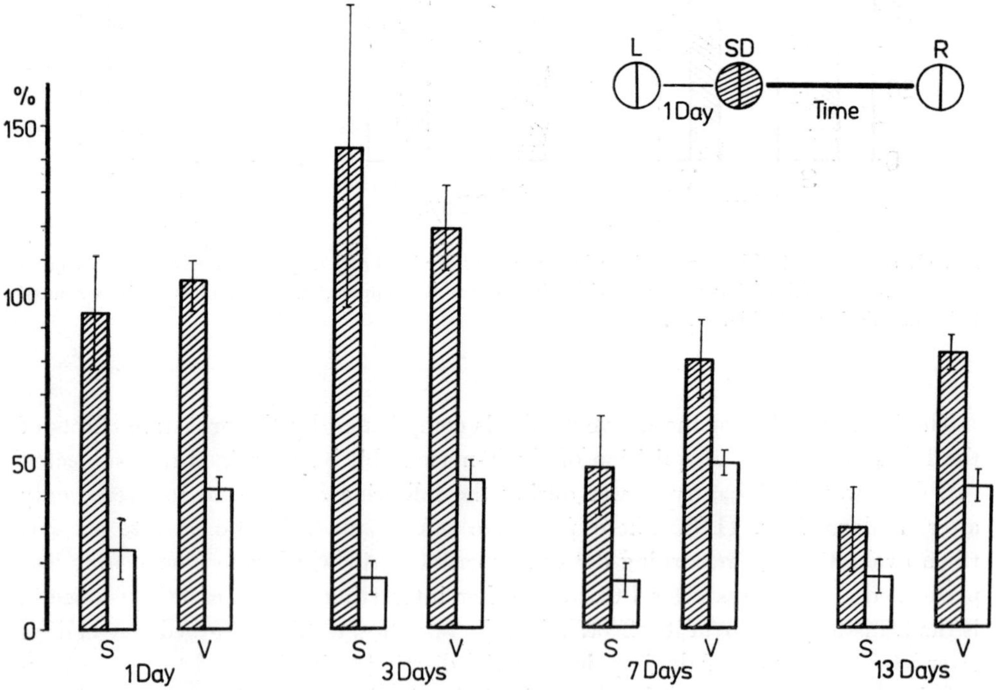

Fig. 11. 9. Recovery of PCSD amnesia of a spatial *(S)* or visual *(V)* discrimination habit after 1, 3, 7, or 13 days, respectively. Other description as in Fig. 11. 6.

in which rats were taught for 14 daily sessions a black-white discrimination and then trained in a single session on the fifteenth day the horizontal-vertical pattern discrimination. Prolonged CSD evoked on the sixteenth day did not affect the overtrained black-white discrimination habit but the recently acquired pattern discrimination was almost completely abolished (Fig. 11.10). Greater vulnerability of the more recent memories was convincingly demonstrated in ECS studies (Duncan 1948, Bureš and Burešová 1963) for shorter learning-interference intervals.

The possibility to interfere with later phases of consolidation was also reported by Avis and Carlton (1968), who used a simple conditioned emotional reaction and bilateral hippocampal injection of 5 to 12 μl of 25 % KCl (see p. 310). The time required for completing 110 licks at a water spout was measured in rats that had been water deprived for 24 hours. Four days later the animals were given four 15-sec tone-footshock pairings in the same apparatus with the water tube removed. Bilateral hippocampal injection of 25 % KCl or of saline followed 24 hours after learning and retention was tested 4 days later. The deprived animal was allowed to perform 100 licks, then the tone was switched on, and the time required for the next 10 licks was measured. Good retention was found in the saline-injected rats who took more than 300 sec for the 10 licks, which were completed in about 1 min or less by 70 % of the KCl injected animals.

Hughes (1969) confirmed the above results with the same technique. He found, however, that the hippocampal KCl injection impaired retention even if applied 3, 7, and 21 days after learning. In another series of experiments he used a constant learning-injection interval of 24 hours and varied the injection-retrieval interval. Impaired retention was found at each interval, but retrieval was significantly better at 21 days than at 4 or 7 days after training. These results cannot be due to a proactive effect of KCl since according to Avis and Carlton (1968) rats given hippocampal injections 3 days before training and tested on the next day show perfect retention. This suggests that hippocampal KCl injection does not produce any prolonged inability to inhibit the on-going responses and that the above results are due to some interference with memory storage rather than to performance deficits.

Hughes' experiments were replicated with better controlled hippocampal depression by Kapp and Schneider (1971). Hippocampal SD induced immediately after training caused amnesia which did not improve during the 3 week acquisition-retention interval. When the hippocampal SD was evoked 24 hr after training, retention was poor 4 days later but improved almost to the control level after 3 weeks.

Also the retrograde amnesia induced in the interhemispheric transfer paradigm (see p. 276) by unilateral CSD in the recipient hemisphere recovers over 15 days, the recovery being proportional to the interval separating the transfer trial from the disruption treatment (Mayes 1973).

The hypothetical consolidation process can be affected by CSD by two different mechanisms, the relative importance of which changes with the duration of the depression. The initial effect, which is the same with a single CSD wave as with

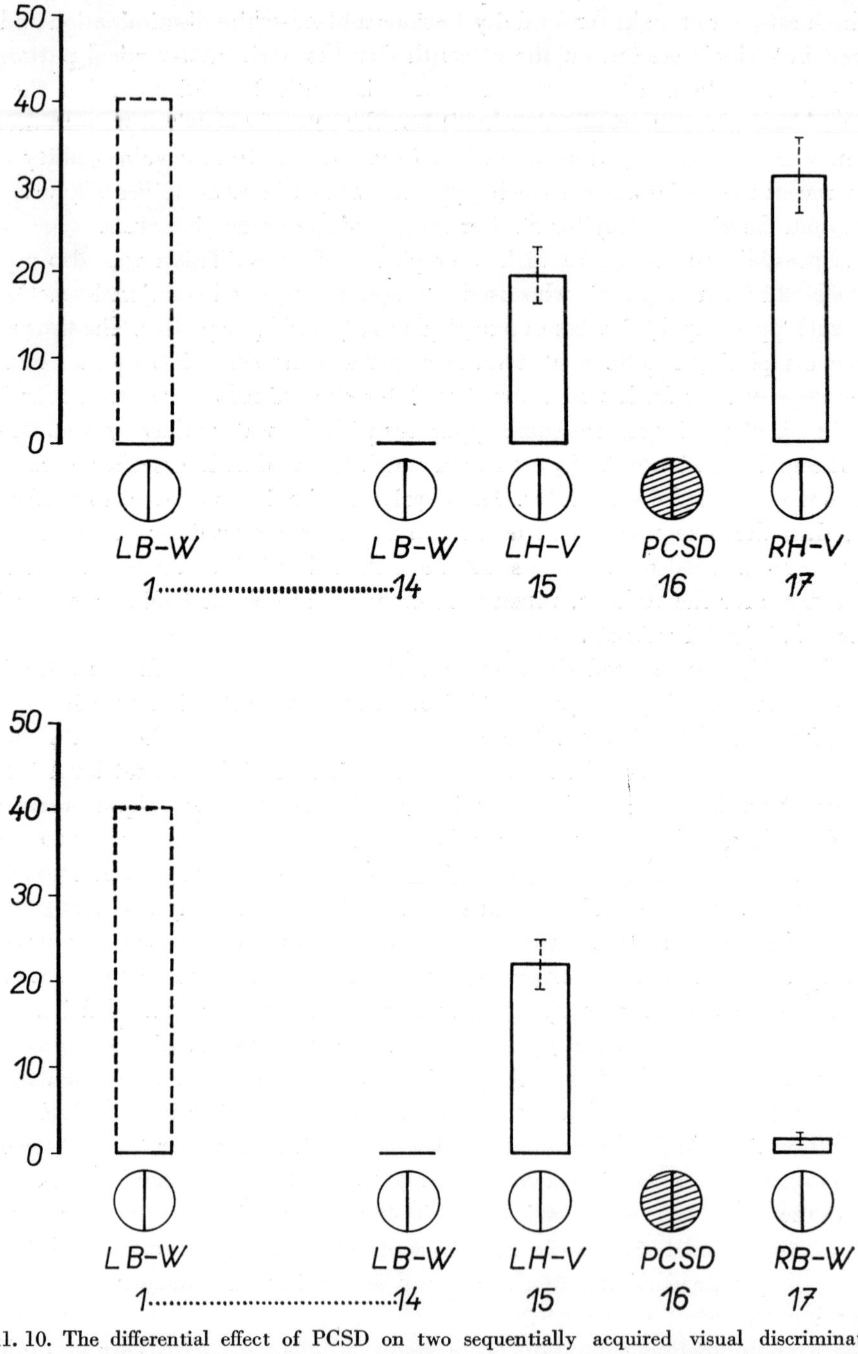

Fig. 11. 10. The differential effect of PCSD on two sequentially acquired visual discriminations. *B—W* indicates black-white; *H—V* indicates horizontal - vertical discrimination. Ordinate: number of to-criterion trials during learning *(L)* and retention testing *(R)*. Experimental paradigm indicated under the respective columns. Numbers correspond to days (Burešová and Bureš 1971a)

PCSD, is due to a temporary blockade of a large mass of neural elements. This impairment of on-going neural activity, which may interfere with the earliest phases of engram formation, smoothly changes into the later continuous depression of EEG activity caused by a deep disorganization and exhaustion of metabolic processes. In particular the decrease in protein synthesis reported by Křivánek (1969a, 1970) may resemble in some way the memory-disturbing effects of inhibition of protein metabolism described by Flexner, Flexner, and Roberts (1967), Agranoff (1967), and Barondes and Cohen (1963).

Since PCSD may affect both late consolidation stages and retrieval processes, it is difficult to appreciate the relevance of these experiments for consolidation studies. The main facts, that is, that PCSD affects differentially the retrieval of engrams of different strength and age and that this deficit is reversible, suggest the existence of a very prolonged, metabolically maintained consolidation phase lasting for days. Prolonged CSD applied during this phase reduces the engram to an irretrievable template, but does not annihilate the memory trace altogether. If enough time is allowed for recovery, the complete engram regenerates from the template again at a rate similar to the slow consolidation process.

The same findings can also be interpreted as a result of impaired retrieval. An obvious consequence of this explanation is that well consolidated engrams are more easily retrievable than recent memories and that consolidation positively correlates with retrievability.

Short-Term Memory

With the conventional methods for studying short-term memory (delayed responses, delayed alternation) it is almost impossible to insert CSD into the stimulus-response interval without interfering with the response. New experimental possibilities were opened by the analysis of the conditioned taste aversion produced by association of the flavor of consumed food with symptoms of subsequent poisoning (for review see Garcia and Ervin 1968 and Rozin and Kalat 1971). Aversion develops even when the intoxication follows several hours after the gustatory experience. This feature is of great biological importance, since it allows the animal to establish a causal link between a particular food and the late consequences of its ingestion. Storage of the initially indifferent gustatory trace during the long CS-UCS interval represents a unique model of short-term memory, well suited for experimental analysis.

Davis and Bureš (1972) evoked saccharin aversion in rats which were allowed to drink 0.1 % saccharin for 10 min and were intoxicated by intraperitoneal injection of lithium chloride (0.14 M, 2 ml/100 g) five hours later. Saccharin aversion was not prevented by bilateral CSD evoked 5 min after or 15 min before LiCl injection. On the other hand, CSD evoked in the middle of the 5-hr CS-UCS interval caused a marked reduction of the saccharin aversion. As pointed out in Chapter 9 (see p. 247), conditioned taste aversion develops even when the poison is administered under bilateral CSD, provided that the taste stimulus has been applied to intact animal. It seems that the gustatory experience is stored both at the cortical and subcortical levels and that the subcortical engram can survive for some time even in absence of normal cortical function. This notion was supported by further experiments (Burešová and Bureš 1973) in which bilateral CSD was evoked 15 min after saccharin drinking and maintained for the rest of the CS-UCS interval which was varied from thirty minutes to 5 hours. With short CS-UCS delays (30 min, 1 hr) functional decortication did not reduce the taste aversion in comparison with untreated controls. With longer CS-UCS delays the gustatory trace decayed more rapidly under bilateral CSD than in control rats.

3. Cortical Spreading Depression and Electrical Manifestations of Conditioning

Although SD is an essentially electrophysiological phenomenon, it was only infrequently used in studies concerned with direct electrophysiological analysis of conditioning. This is due not only to the technical difficulties connected with simultaneous use of SD and the particular electrophysiological technique applied for conditioning but also to the different background experience of the investigators. Whereas the ultimate goal of most SD experiments is to find out which brain regions are indispensable for a definite behavioral pattern, electrophysiology searches for changes of electrical activity meaningfully related to this behavior. In a wide sense the two approaches are complementary, but they are usually incompatible in one study. The use of CSD remained nearly exclusively limited therefore to the most obvious application, that is, to establishing the role of the cerebral cortex in the mechanism of electrical manifestations of conditioning in subcortical structures.

One of the simplest instances of electrophysiologically established plasticity is habituation of evoked responses to repeated sensory stimuli (for other forms of habituation see p. 269). This phenomenon described by Galambos, Sheatz, and Vernier (1956) and by Hernandez-Peón and Scherrer (1955) has been studied in detail by many investigators (for example, Garcia-Austt, Bogacz, and Vanzulli 1961, Fernandez-Guardiola, Roldán, Fanjul, and Castells 1961). It is characterized by a gradual decrease of responses to the repetitively applied stimulus but not to other stimuli of the same modality. The amplitude of the habituated response can be increased to the initial level by various "dishabituation" procedures, for example, by a brief interruption of the train of stimuli, by introducing an intense novel stimulus, by associating the habituated stimulus with pain or food, and so on. Although habituation occurs even at the level of receptors and in the lower relay nuclei of sensory pathways, its selectivity suggests participation of a discrimination process, controlled by higher brain centers. In order to check the possible role of the cerebral cortex in habituation Weiss (1962) studied the effect of bilateral CSD on habituation of acoustic evoked responses in the inferior colliculus of unanesthetized freely moving rats. Click stimuli applied at regular 2-sec intervals for up to 6 hours elicited lowering of the collicular response only in 1 out of 12 control experiments. Bilateral CSD caused no initial changes of shape or amplitude of the evoked potential, but prolonged (4 to 5 hours) repetition of clicks resulted in a decrease of amplitude in 10 out of 14 experiments. The habituated responses could often be dishabituated by external stimuli such as opening of the sound-proof box. These results indicate in agreement with surgical decortication studies (Sharpless and Jasper 1956) that habituation of evoked responses can proceed without participation of the cortex. Acute functional ablation even seems to facilitate habituation, but this conclusion must be accepted with caution. Since evoked potentials in different subcortical locations are influenced by overall excitability changes, which might become important after several hours of CSD, the specificity of the habituation process must be carefully checked under such conditions. The effect of unilateral CSD on the habituation of visual evoked responses in the rabbit was described by Koreli and Brožek (1972). One or two CSD waves considerably accelerated habituation of evoked responses in the ipsilateral visual cortex, probably by enhancing the depression of synaptic inputs to this region. Such results support Horn's (1967) hypothesis that habituation is due to self-generated decrease of sensitivity rather than to active gating.

A more important role is ascribed to the cerebral cortex in the mechanism of conditioning. Electrical changes recorded at some subcortical level during learning may either be a manifestation of local plasticity or a consequence of the plastic change occurring elsewhere. A decision between these two possibilities is important for the interpretation of most electrophysiological findings in conditioning. In two studies CSD was applied with just such a purpose in mind.

Burešová and Bureš (1965a, also Bureš and Burešová 1965, 1968) used in rats the classical conditioning of reticular units originally described by Yoshii and Ogura (1960) in cats. Experiments were performed in unanaesthetized curarized animals fixed in a stereotaxic apparatus. The microelectrode was slowly inserted into the pontobulbar reticular formation until a well-isolated and stable unit was found. Its response to sound (CS) and to sciatic nerve stimulation (UCS) was tested with the poststimulation histogram technique. Only units showing a clear-cut reaction to the unconditioned stimulus (decrease or increase of spontaneous firing) but not reacting to the CS were used for conditioning which consisted of pairing a 2-sec acoustic signal (200 or 2000/sec) with an immediately following sciatic shock at 1-min intertrial intervals (Fig.11.11). Under control conditions the acoustic stimulus started to elicit a statistically significant change of spontaneous firing rate after a few tens of reinforced trials in about 50 % of examined units (Fig. 11.12A). The conditioned reactions usually imitated the response evoked by the UCS, but in approximately 20 % of cases conditioning resulted in an opposite change that probably anticipated the UCS effect. In a group of 18 units, conditioning was performed under bilateral CSD, that was checked by disappearance of cortical primary responses

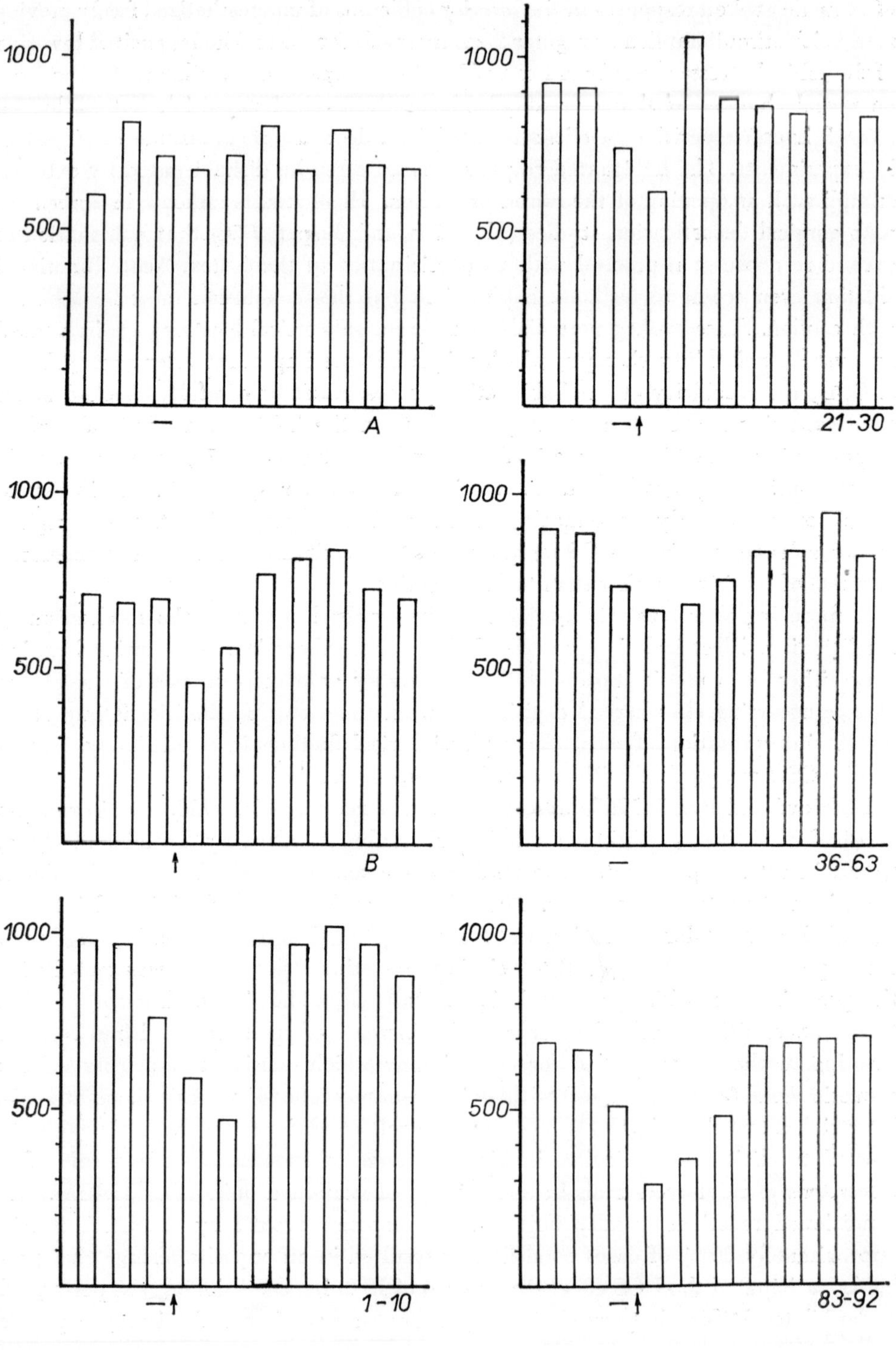
1000
500
A
1000
500
21-30
1000
500
B
1000
500
36-63
1000
500
1-10
1000
500
83-92

to sciatic nerve stimulation. In spite of suppression of cortical functions, conditioning was again successful in 50 % of the units, although the incidence of conditioned reactions in the first 50 reinforced trials was less frequent than in intact animals (20 % as compared with 45 % — Fig. 11.12B). Only imitatory conditioned reactions were found in the functionally decorticated animals. The difference between normal and functionally decorticated animals was best expressed when the result of conditioning was tested by omitting the unconditioned stimulus in 10 consecutive trials (Fig. 11.12C). No conditioned reactions were found under these conditions in the SD group, while in the control group more than 50 % of the units persisted in displaying conditioned reactions even in extinction trials.

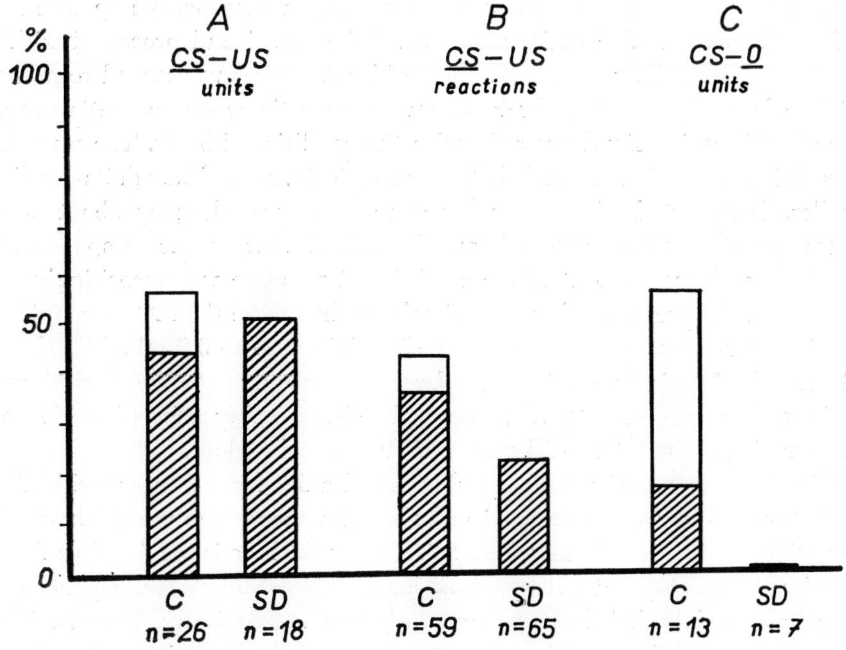

Fig. 11. 12. The effect of functional decortication on conditioning of reticular units. Incidence of conditioned reactions in the third (*CS—US*) and fourth interval (*CS—0*). Imitatory reactions are the shaded parts of the columns; inverse reactions are the empty parts of the columns; *C* is the control group; *SD* is the spreading depression group. For details see text (Burešová and Bureš 1965a).

Fig. 11. 11. Poststimulation histogram of reactions of a reticular unit to an acoustic conditioned stimulus (horizontal bar, *A*), to a nociceptive unconditioned stimulus (arrow, *B*), or to combinations of both stimuli. Serial numbers of the integrated trials are given below the histograms. Number of spikes accumulated in the individual intervals is given on the ordinate. The histogram from trials 36 to 63 was obtained by integrating every third trial in which the unconditioned stimulus was omitted (Burešová and Bureš 1965a).

Changes of unit activity observed in the above experiments are manifestations of conditioned emotional reaction, accompanied in freely moving animals by various vegetative and somatic symptoms. As shown in Chap. 9. Sec. 4., such conditioning can proceed even under bilateral CSD. It is not surprising therefore that the same applies to the electrophysiological counterpart of the conditioned emotional reaction. The analogy between electrophysiological and behavioral findings can be pursued still further; in both cases the conditioned reactions in functionally decorticated animals develop slower, are less variable, and more susceptible to extinction.

More specific effects of CSD were recently reported by Woody and Brožek (1969a, b) for the conditoned eye blink in cats. Mechanical stimulation of glabella (glabella tap) served as the UCS, a loud click as the CS. The CS-UCS interval was either 20 or 400 msec. Electrical responses were recorded with chronically implanted electrodes from the region of the trigeminal and facial nuclei and processed with the averaging technique. Whereas a click alone did not elicit any marked response in the facial nucleus, after 600 to 900 reinforcements acoustic evoked potentials started to appear in this region simultaneously with the conditioned blink. The waveshape of the conditioned reaction resembled the unconditioned one, although its amplitude was smaller. It consisted of an early low component, preceding by about 2 msec the electromyogram of the orbicularis muscle, and of a larger late component. The latency of the early component of the conditioned response was surprisingly brief, 17 ± 3 msec on the average. After the animals reached more than 90 % conditioned reactions in several consecutive sessions of 150 trials, 0.05 to 0.2 ml 25 % KCl was applied through chronically implanted polyethylene cannulas to the frontal motor areas. The rather large volume of the applied fluid probably affected a wide area, and SD extended the effect to still more remote cortical regions.

Immediately after injection the animal assumed a fixed vacant stare with dilated pupils. Postural tonus was maintained and the cat responded to pin prick and loud auditory stimuli with the pinna reflex. Blinking could be elicited by touching the cornea or by glabella tap but not by a loud hand clap. Although the response to the UCS was preserved both behaviorally and electrophysiologically, the conditioned eye blink was lost and the conditioned evoked potentials in the facial nucleus decreased to or below the level seen in the untrained animal. They reappeared 30 min to several hours later, depending on the amount of KCl injected (Fig. 11.13).

The above results indicate that subcortical centers are not blocked by functional elimination of the anterior frontal cortex and perhaps of the more posterior cortical areas. Functional decortication may interfere, however, with cortical elements directly participating in the conditioned reaction. In spite of the extremely brief latency of the conditioned eye blink, the times required for conduction of nerve impulses from the ear to the auditory and motor areas and to the facial nucleus are well within admissible limits. This interpretation postulates a direct "in series" connection of the cerebral cortex in the reflex arc of the conditioned eye blink. The cerebral cortex may control conditioned eye blink also in a different way, by exerting a tonic excitatory influence on an essentially subcortical conditioned reflex. Although in this case the cerebral cortex is connected in parallel, it represents an important auxilliary mechanism, the elimination of which can impair the conditioned reaction completely. Further experiments are needed to decide between these possibilities.

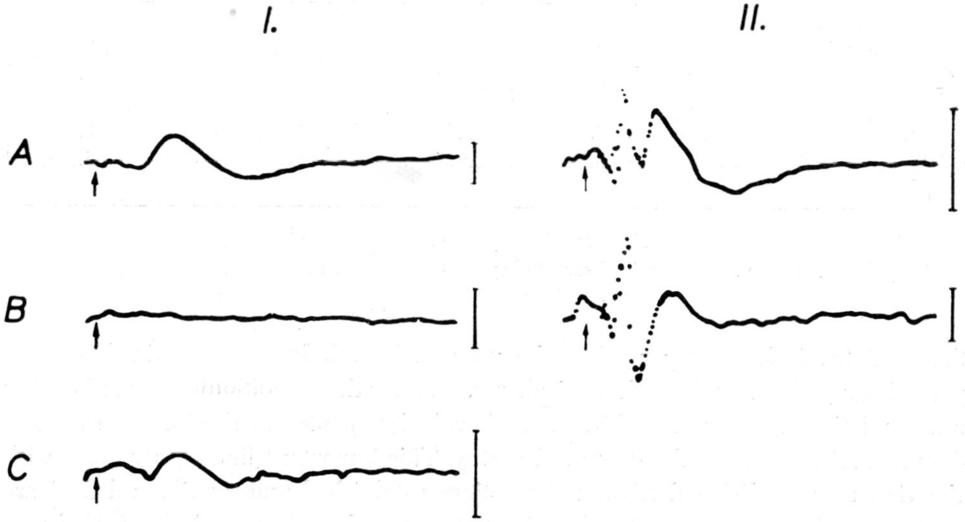

Fig. 11. 13. Effect of KCl application to frontoparietal cortex on conditioned (I) and unconditioned (II) blink responses recorded from the facial nucleus of a cat. Averaged waveforms ($n = 128$). *(A)* Before KCl. *(B)* After KCl during presumed depression of cortex. *(C)* Recovery of conditioned response. Calibration: 50 μV. Response lengths 102 msec. I and II are from different animals (Woody and Brožek 1969a).

Another interesting application of CSD in the electrophysiology of conditioning was attempted by Travis (1964b). In rats with implanted electrodes in the visual cortices evoked responses to light flashes were recorded before and after 2 to 3 days of habituation. Cortical SD was then elicited in the left hemispheres by 25 % KCl. The conditioning procedure, started during unilateral CSD, consisted of 60 unavoidable shocks each following a series of six flashes (1/1.5 sec) applied with a 40-sec intertrial interval. After a recovery period of 10 to 12 hours, visual evoked responses were again recorded from both hemispheres. The same procedure was used in a control group, but no conditioning was applied during left CSD. The results are illustrated in Table 11.4. The amplitude of the visual evoked response declined during habituation in both experimental and control animals. Left CSD further decreased the evoked responses in the left hemisphere, while evoked responses in the right hemisphere were unchanged or slightly increased. Conditioning did not cause an immediate increase of evoked responses in the intact hemisphere, but its effect became apparent later. Evoked potentials from the previously depressed left hemisphere remained low whereas in

Table 11.4.

Combined Average Evoked Potential Amplitude Changes (Travis 1964b)

	Electrode Placement	Untrained	Habituated	Left CSD	Postconditioning	
					Left CSD	After CSD
Experimental Subjects (n = 4)	Left	4.32	2.60*	2.09*	2.34**	2.24*
	Right	3.59	2.37**	2.40*	2.54	3.52
Control Subjects (n = 4)	Left	3.48	2.14**	1.94**	—	2.46**
	Right	3.29	1.84*	2.59**	—	2.32*

* Significant change from untrained sample beyond 0.05 level of confidence.
** Significant change from untrained sample beyond 0.01 level of confidence.

the right hemisphere they reached the untrained level. In control animals evoked potentials remained low in both hemispheres. It seems that conditioning applied during unilateral CSD counteracts habituation of evoked responses in the intact cortex but does not influence it in the depressed cortex. This important finding contrasts with the view that conditioned emotional reactions established under unilateral CSD are poorly lateralized (see p. 269) and easily transfer to the other hemisphere. Unfortunately only small groups of animals (four experimental and four controls) were used by Travis (1964b) and his averaging technique was not described in detail. A replication of this study would be most desirable.

4. Effects of Cortical Spreading Depression on Complex Subcortical Functions

Although functional decortication does not interfere with the basic functions of lower brain centers (see Chap. 8) a more thorough analysis reveals substantial modifications of complex reactions integrated at the subcortical level. The present section reviews the available evidence.

Food and Water Intake

As pointed out by Burešová (1956) rats under bilateral CSD are aphagic and adipsic. Teiltelbaum and Cytawa (1965) and Cytawa and Teiltelbaum (1967) analyzed the impairment of feeding behavior caused by application of 14 mg KCl onto each hemicortex in more detail. During the first hour after KCl application, the animals occasionally licked smooth surfaces or gnawed the rough ends of Purina pellets, but made no active attempts to find food or water. After 2 to 3 hours the rats began to eat a liquid diet, but they did not eat pellets or drink water 6 to 8 hours after CSD onset. It is interesting to note that the recovery after CSD resembles on a condensed time scale, recovery of feeding after bilateral lesions of the hypothalamic feeding centers or postnatal development of feeding: eating of wet and palatable food appears first, then eating of dry food, and last drinking of water (Teitelbaum 1971).

Levitt and Krikstone (1968) confirmed that rats on 24 hours water deprivation do not drink under bilateral CSD even when water was dropped on their face and mouth region. Cortical SD also blocked drinking induced by carbachol (1 to 3 μg) injected into the lateral septal nucleus. This effect was obviously not specific to cholinergic mechanisms, but probably was due according to these authors "to cortical deactivation and withdrawal of cortical facilitating or maintaining influences". Schneider (1965) also found that bilateral CSD greatly reduced water intake. The inhibition of drinking seemed to be less pronounced in his experiments, probably because a slightly different technique was used to induce CSD (4 days elapsed between preparing the trephine openings and eliciting CSD).

Freedman, Ferguson, and Wilson (1972) examined consumption of 16 % glucose during the first hour of bilateral CSD. Adipsia was complete after 12-hour deprivation but the number of licks increased to approximately 40 % of the control value in animals deprived for 48 hours. Normal rats offered 4 glucose concentrations (4, 8, 16, and 32 %) preferred the 8 % solution whereas the bilaterally depressed animals licked most frequently the 32 % solution. These results indicate that some regulation of food and water intake remains preserved even during functional decortication.

The aphagic effects of CSD are still more pronounced in animals with bilateral lesions in the lateral hypothalamus (Teitelbaum and Cytawa 1965, Cytawa and Teitelbaum 1967). Cortical SD elicited in these animals 35 to 45 days after lesions and 15 days after complete recovery caused a much longer impairment of food and water intake than in normal animals. The rats did not eat or drink anything for at least 24 hours, then took a liquid diet. Water and dry food intake was renewed only the third day after CSD, and in some animals still later. It was concluded that CSD reinstated the lateral hypothalamic syndrome, probably by removing the facilitatory influence of the cerebral cortex on the hypothalamic tissue adjacent to the lesion which during the recovery period gradually takes over the lost functions. Similar results were obtained for compensation of behavioral consequences of septal lesions (Cytawa and Teitelbaum 1967, 1968, Teitelbaum 1971). Cortical SD evoked several weeks after the lesion reinstates the septal syndrome of hyperemotionality. The remarkable ability of the central nervous system to compensate for tissue loss by using alternate routes and developing vicarious functions is perhaps an example of learning (Lucco and Aranda 1964), which takes place in mammals with considerable participation of the cerebral cortex. The general validity of this explanation is doubtful, however, since Weiss and Fifková (1963) were not able to impair the compensation of circling movements induced by lateralized caudate lesions, with CSD. Also Glass and Thomas (1970) were not able to reinstate the septal syndrome by bilateral CSD but they examined the reactivity of their rats only during the first three hours of functional decortication, whereas Cytawa and Teitelbaum (1967) reported the maximum reactivity increase 5 to 10 hours after KCl application.

The hypothesis about cortical participation in the recovery of lost hypothalamic functions was not confirmed by Wampler and Rehovsky (1973), who studied the effect of bilateral CSD in rats with ventromedial hypothalamic lesions. Functional decortication not only failed to reinstate in the static obese rats the voracious eating typical for the "dynamic" stage of hyperphagia, but even caused a longlasting (14 days) decrease of food intake. The authors suggest that CSD suppresses eating by increasing activity of ventromedial hypothalamus and that this effect is prolonged in lesioned animals.

In a repeat of the experiments of Teitelbaum and Cytawa (1965), Balinska, Burešová, and Fifková (1967) investigated the effect of bilateral CSD on feeding behavior and alimentary conditioning in normal rats and in rats recovered from bilateral lesions of the feeding centers in the lateral hypothalamus. A prolonged impairment of food intake was only obtained in the short-recovery group, in which KCl application immediately followed complete restitution of normal feeding (usually 3 weeks after the lesions). This effect cannot be regarded as strictly specific, however, since other functions, for example cortical postural reflexes, were also suppressed for a longer time in the operated than in the unoperated control group. Consequences of the hypothalamic lesions (starvation, degeneration) probably decrease the resistance of the central nervous system to noxious stimuli. In animals allowed another 3 weeks for recovery, CSD evoked by 25 % KCl caused the same impairment as in unoperated controls. A difference between operated and unoperated rats could be revealed even after a long recovery by application of 1 % KCl, which suppressed feeding for 40 to 50 min in the latter but for 160 to 180 min in the former group (Fig. 11.14). This finding indicates that elimination of cortical functions induces a transitory impairment of subcortical compensatory mechanisms, the duration of which is inversely proportional to the duration of postoperational recovery and which may outlast for several hours or days the actual cortical depression. Restitution of compensation proceeds independently of the continuing CSD and with 25 % KCl it is completed before cortical function has recovered. Thus suppression of feeding coincides with the impairment of other cortical functions. With 1 % KCl the subcortical impairment outlasts the releasing cortical depression, and food intake or alimentary conditioned reactions are suppressed for longer periods than cortical postural reflexes or avoidance responses. Although CSD caused a deeper impairment of feeding in the lesioned than in normal animals, the difference was by no means as spectacular as that obtained in Teitelbaum's laboratory. Strain and age may account for the discrepancy between the results of the two studies, but the main cause probably must be sought in the intensity of the CSD treatment. Balinska,

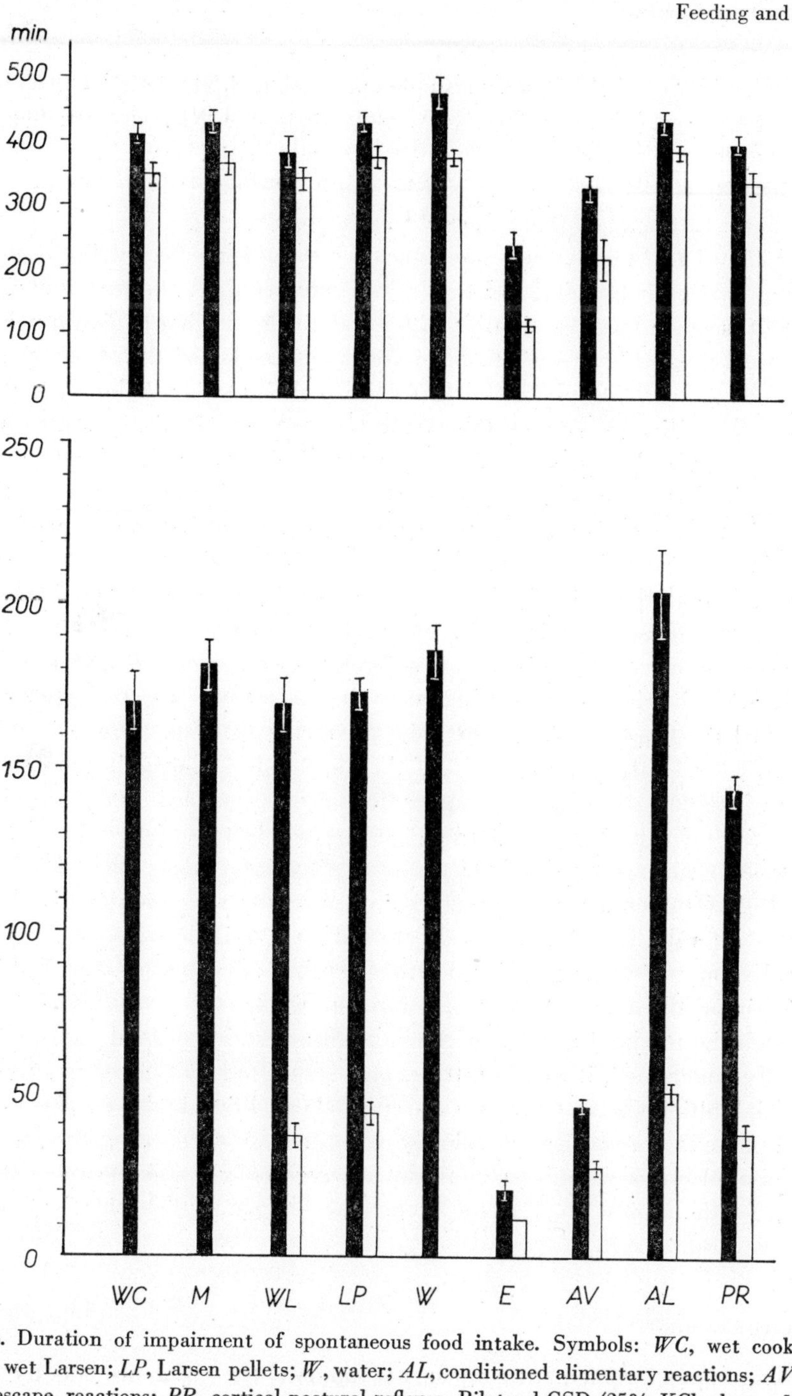

Fig. 11. 14. Duration of impairment of spontaneous food intake. Symbols: *WC*, wet cookies; *M*, milk; *WL*, wet Larsen; *LP*, Larsen pellets; *W*, water; *AL*, conditioned alimentary reactions; *AV*, avoidance; *E*, escape reactions; *PR*, cortical postural reflexes. Bilateral CSD (25% KCl above, 1% KCl below) induced in rats recovered from bilateral hypothalamic lesions (long recovery). Black columns indicate experimental animals; white columns indicate unoperated controls (Balinska, Burešová, and Fifková 1967).

Burešová, and Fifková (1967) used a single application of 2 to 3 mg KCl, while Teitelbaum and Cytawa (1965) applied 14 mg of crystalline KCl on each hemisphere. The latter method resembles prolonged CSD treatment (see p. 324) which elicits a deep impairment of engram consolidation and interferes with retrieval of consolidated engrams. Some of the amnesic effects are reversible, the restitution being complete after 1 to 2 weeks. Such results are in general agreement with the suggestion that compensation is learning and that as a newly acquired and less overtrained experience, it is much more susceptible to CSD than the feeding habits in normal animals. Balinska, Burešová, and Fifková (1967) also reported the effects of thalamic SD on feeding. Injection of 1 µl 25 % KCl into the anterior thalamus impaired an alimentary conditioned reaction (magazine feeding) for 25 min in control rats and for 65 min in animals recovered from a bilateral lesion of the hypothalamic feeding center. As the impairment of avoidance and escape reactions was longer in the operated than in the unoperated rats, the results must be regarded as nonspecific.

Whereas the repeated waves of CSD cause inhibition of consummatory behavior, single waves of unilateral CSD are accompanied by an activation of feeding and drinking (Huston and Bureš 1970). Single waves of CSD were elicited from the occipital cortex of rats by microelectrophoretic injection of K^+ and the SPC was recorded with implanted Ag-AgCl electrodes. After the negative slow potential had reached the frontal cortex most animals started to drink from a drinking tube (Fig. 11.15). Probability distribution of the onset times of drinking measured from the peak of the slow potential wave under the rostral electrode is plotted in Fig. 11.16. The duration of drinking varied from a few seconds to several minutes. Elicited eating was seen in most animals in the same time interval as elicited drinking. In a later study (Huston and Brožek 1971) similar results were obtained in the rabbit. During unilateral CSD most animals started to eat in a stereotyped aggressive manner. In contrast with rats, elicited eating in rabbits began soon after KCl injection (after 4 min on the average), that is, before the whole cortex was invaded by CSD.

Although the mechanism of the CSD induced activation of food and water intake is not fully understood, it can be interpreted as an aftereffect of the preceding motivational inhibition. With CSD waves repeated at brief intervals the excitatory rebound phase is obscured or completely absent. Also when eating and/or drinking is elicited by electrical stimulation of the lateral hypothalamus, single waves of bilateral CSD induce the typical block of the evoked consummatory behavior for 5 to 10 min (Huston and Bureš 1973).

Thermoregulation

Impairment of thermoregulation during bilateral CSD was described by Burešová (1957c). Functionally decorticated rats or mice exposed to a low ambient temperature cooled off more rapidly than control animals with brain intact. Thus immersion into a cool bath (13 °C) decreased colonic temperature in 30 min from 38 to 30

Fig. 11. 15. Drinking elicited by single CSD waves in the left (*LSD*), right (*RSD*), or in both (BSD) hemispheres. *D* indicates cumulative recording of licking; *L, R* indicate SPC recordings from the left and right hemispheres, respectively. Arrows indicate electrophoretic injection of K^+ into occipital cortex (Huston and Bureš 1970).

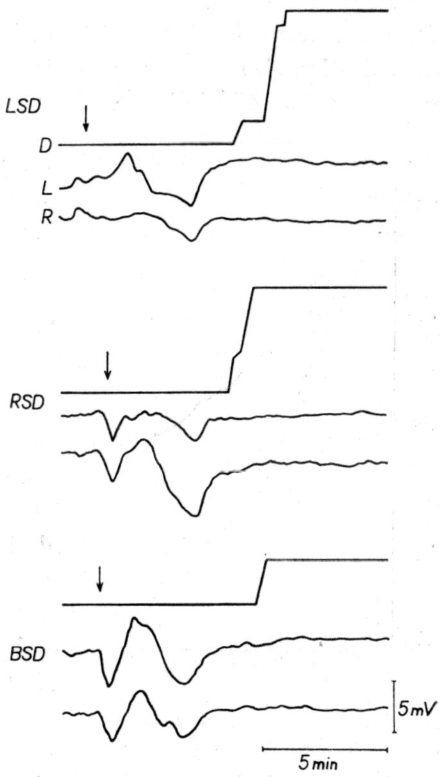

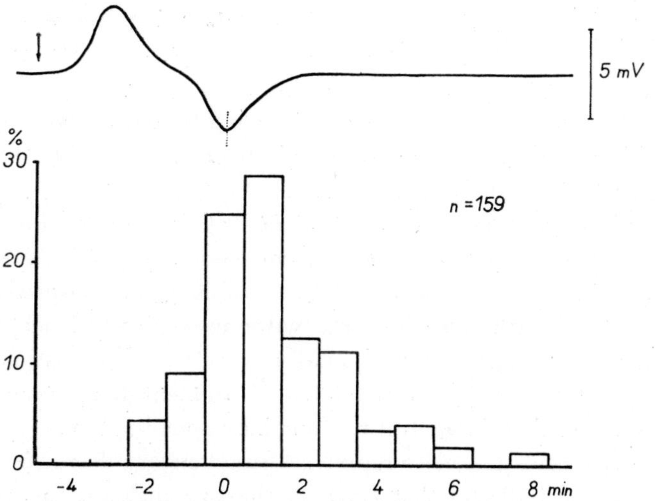

Fig. 11. 16. Drinking elicited by single waves of CSD. (Above) Typical SPC recording. Upward deflection corresponds to the passage of the SPC elicited from occipital cortex under the electrode at the level of bregma, downward deflection to the SPC reaching the frontal pole of the hemisphere. (Below) Percentage of cases when drinking started at different intervals before (negative values) or after (positive values) SPC reached maximum negativity under the rostral electrode (Huston and Bureš 1970).

degrees in normal animals and to 22 degrees in CSD rats (Fig. 11.17). Functional decortication also reduced the resistance of rats to high temperatures; decorticated rats exposed to 45 °C died considerably earlier than undepressed control animals.

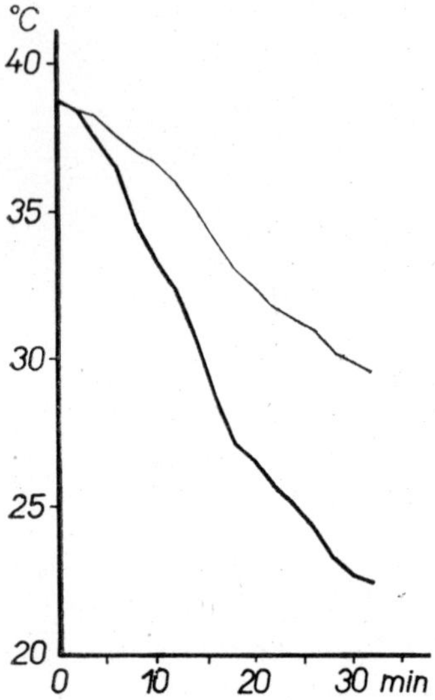

Fig. 11. 17. Time course of body cooling in normal (thin line) and functionally decorticate rat (heavy line) immersed in ice water. Ordinate: colonic temperature in degrees centigrade. Abscissa: time in minutes (Burešová 1957c)

The impaired ability to maintain body temperature in bilaterally depressed animals was confirmed by Cytawa and Teitelbaum (1965, 1967). These authors compared the effect of CSD on normal rats and on rats with extensive anterior hypothalamic lesions, which initially caused a severe impairment of thermoregulation that slowly improved over a period of several weeks or months. Under bilateral CSD fully recovered animals exposed for 2 hours to an ambient temperature of 0 °C dropped their body temperature from 38 to 31 degrees, as compared to 36 degrees in normal rats. The thermoregulation of the lesioned animals remained impaired for several days after CSD. Similarly as in rats recovered from the bilateral damage of the hypothalamic feeding center (see p. 337) in this case CSD also reinstates the original syndrome, probably by disrupting labile compensation. In an attempt to analyse the mechanism of the CSD effect, Burešová (1957c) measured O_2 consumption in restrained rats using the technique described by Bargeton and Krumm-Heller (1949). While CSD did not elicit significant changes of O_2 consumption in rats exposed to 29 or 36 °C, it considerably reduced both body temperature and O_2 uptake in animals exposed to an ambient temperature of 10 °C.

The changes in oxygen consumption evoked by CSD were studied in more detail by Dybowski and Ewert (1966). Under normothermic conditions, KCl application elicits an immediate increase of O_2 uptake to 120 % of the predepression value (probably associated with shivering and motor unrest), which slowly decays over the following hour. The authors found, in agreement with Burešová (1957c), that the increase of O_2 uptake caused by reduction of ambient temperature to 22 °C was lower in decorticated than in control rats and correspondingly that the body temperature of decorticated rats fell more rapidly. A simultaneous decrease in body temperature and O_2 uptake indicates that CSD set the hypothalamic thermostat to a new value. This conclusion is also supported by the experiments of Rüdiger and Seyer (1965, see p. 301) that demonstrated an impairment of the hypothalamic thermoceptive mechanisms during ipsilateral CSD.

Dybowski and Rüdiger (1967) subjected the initial increase of heat production induced by CSD to further analysis. They established that these effects are not due to the pain caused by KCl contact with the skin wound or with dural receptors. The O_2 uptake increases even when KCl is applied in a solution of a local anaesthetic that effectively eliminates dural sensitivity. They suggest that CSD affects thermoregulation in two phases, an early short-lasting excitatory phase corresponding to the cortical burst of unit activity immediately preceding the actual cortical depression, and a late prolonged phase, characterized by deep inhibition of hypothalamic functions. It seems, however, that the increased O_2 uptake is longer (20 to 30 min) than would be compatible with the above explanation. Other factors (circulation, neurosecretion) must be considered therefore in further research.

Endocrine Functions

Close connections between the hypothalamus and hypophysis, as well as hypothalamic neurosecretion raise the question of how these functions are influenced by CSD that affects other forms of hypothalamic activity.

Marked changes of water metabolism caused by CSD were demonstrated by Burešová (1957b) (Fig. 11.18). Rats given an intragastric water load of 5 % body weight excreted over a 2-hour period under normal conditions 43 % of the injected water but only 12 % when 25 % KCl was applied onto both hemispheres simultaneously

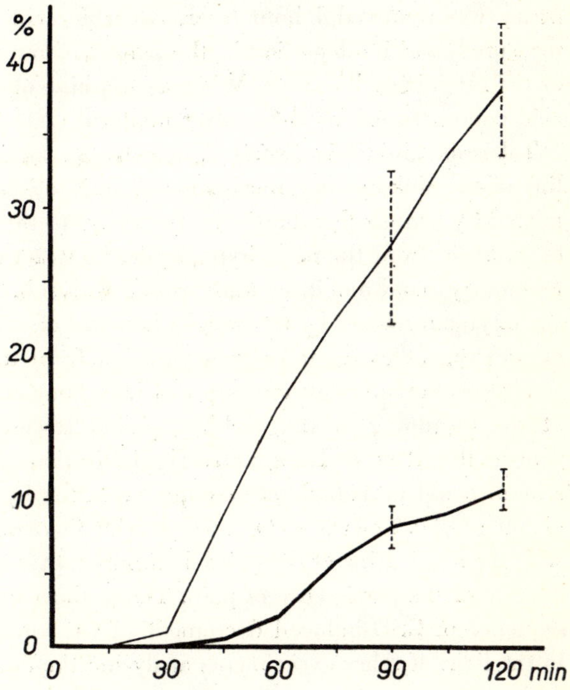

Fig. 11. 18. The effect of CSD on water metabolism. Ordinate: cumulative percentage of excreted water load in 13 control rats (thin line) and in 16 CSD rats (25 % KCl, heavy line). The dashed vertical lines indicate the standard error of the mean. The difference between the amount of excreted water load in the control and experimental animals is statistically significant for $P = 0.01$ after 90 min. The origin of the time axis corresponds to the initiation of CSD and to the administration of 5% water load (Burešová 1957c).

with the administration of water. As water retention in experimental animals may by due either to decreased glomerular filtration or to increased tubular reabsorbtion, estimation of creatinine clearance was used to decide between these two mechanisms. The results indicated that the filtration rate was not significantly affected by CSD (the creatinine clearance values being 19 $\pm$ 3 ml/hour and 16 $\pm$ 2 ml/hour for the control and experimental animals, respectively), but that the concentrating power of kidneys was considerably increased by functional decortication, the ratio of creatinine concentration in urine and plasma rising from 12 in control rats to 37 in experimental animals. The above findings suggest that the CSD effects on diuresis are mediated through a humoral link represented by increased production of antidiuretic hormone. Increased neurosecretion contrasts with the electrophysiological signs of decreased activity of most hypothalamic neurons (see p. 176). Further research is required to decide whether CSD affects the neurosecretory cells in a different way than the majority of hypothalamic neurons, or whether in the same cell neurosecretion is independent of the spike-generating mechanism.

A more general conclusion is that the cerebral cortex exerts a tonic inhibitory effect on hormone secretion, the enhancement of which by CSD can be interpreted as a release phenomenon. This interpretation was supported by results obtained for other endocrine functions. Taleisnik and Caligaris (1962) reported that CSD induces a release of luteinizing hormone. In their experiments one ovary was removed under ether anesthesia, at the same time trephine openings were made over the occipital cortex and CSD was elicited by 25 % KCl in the experimental animals. The second ovary was removed 1 hour later. Ascorbic acid concentration in both ovaries was measured, and its depletion in the second ovary was taken as an index of liberation of the luteinizing hormone. Whereas trephine openings alone decreased the ascorbic acid concentration by 3 %, after bilateral CSD the depletion was 19 %.

Taleisnik and Deis (1964) demonstrated an influence of CSD on the humoral link of the milk-ejection mechanism. Tactile stimuli generated by suckling are transmitted by lemniscal and reticular pathways to the hypothalamus and provoke release of oxytocin from the neurohypophysis. Contraction of the myoepithelial cells of the mammary gland mobilizes milk from the alveoli. Taleisnik and Deis (1964) measured the oxytocin release by the weight increase of a litter of 9-day old rats over 1 hour of suckling following 9 hours separation from the mother. Whereas under control conditions the milk ejection rate was 5.0 g/hour, painful stimuli applied to the mother at the beginning of the suckling period (trephine openings) reduced the weight gain of the litter to 1.1 g/hour. The inhibition of milk ejection caused by stressful stimuli could be completely compensated for by intraperitoneal oxytocin injection of 200 mU/kg. The same effect was attained by eliciting bilateral CSD simultaneously with the application of the painful stimulus; that is, the weight gain remained normal in spite of the persistence of pain. The authors interpret the above results as a consequence of CSD-induced decrement of the animals' reactivity to painful stimuli. In the light of other experiments analyzing the decreased pain sensitivity of functionally decorticated animals in a quantitative way (Thompson and Enter 1967, see p. 256), this explanation can hardly account for a complete blockade of oxytocin inhibition. An alternative possibility is that CSD causes release of oxytocin by a similar mechanism as in the case of antidiuretic and luteinizing hormones.

Graul (1968) studied the effect of CSD on the changes of blood glucose and plasma hydroxycorticosteroid level induced by stressful stimuli. Three levels of stress were used: (a) restraining the rat in a small cage, (b) fixing it to an operation table with subsequent intravenous injection of saline, or (c) of 1 IU of insulin. Blood sugar was raised by procedure (b) and lowered by procedure (c) as compared with the control level (a). Neither this control level nor the stress-induced changes of blood glucose were significantly modified by CSD, although a slight tendency to hyperglycemia was manifest in most CSD groups. Similar finding suggestive of CSD-induced hyperglycemia were also reported by Burešová (1955). On the other hand, Kulikova (1964) found in rabbits pronounced hypoglycemia developing during 30 min of bilateral CSD. The plasma level of 17-hydroxycorticosteroids increased proportionally to the intensity of stress in intact rats. Bilateral CSD eliminated this reaction completely and decreased the 17-hydroxycorticosteroids in plasma instead. The decrease was most marked in the maximum stress group (c), in which the 17-hydroxycorticosteroid level in plasma reached about 70 μg/100 ml in intact rats but only 35 μg/100 ml in functionally decorticated animals. On the other hand Jonec (1964) was not able to find any difference in the ascorbic acid or corticosterone content of the adrenal glands and in the plasma corticosterone level between sham CSD rats and functionally decorticated rats subjected to short-term cold stress.

Somewhat related to the problem of stress is the development of gastric ulcers in rats restrained in small cages (Rossi, Bonfilis, and Lieffoghe 1956). As shown by Malecki, Borkowska, Krzywosinski, and Malinowska (1968) animals immobilized during bilateral CSD develop within 24 hours 2.5 times more ulcers than intact animals exposed to the same stress. Correspondingly the area of the ulcerated gastric mucosa increases from 46 mm^2 in the control group to 114 mm^2 in the CSD group. In a similar way functional decortication also affects ulcers evoked by single injection of 5 mg/kg of reserpine. On the contrary massive ulceration by ligation of the pylorus is considerably decreased (by approximately 50 %) in CSD animals. Interpretation of the above results is difficult. Although increased ulceration in depressed animals may reflect their lower resistance to immobilization stress or their higher sensitivity to noradrenaline, the reverse effect of CSD on the ulcers evoked by pylorus ligation can be due either to a slow and continuous action of the latter stimulus or to the different mechanism of its effect.

Less attention has been paid to the CSD effects on the brain reactivity to hormones. Malyshenko (1969) attempted to influence by unilateral functional decortication the EEG changes evoked by administration of estradiol to ovariectomized rats, but these results are rather inconclusive.

Sexual Behavior

Mating behavior represents a complex system of instinctive reactions controlled by different levels of the central nervous system. According to Beach (1940, 1944) surgical decortication abolishes sexual activity in male but not in female rats. Larsson (1962) repeated Beach's experiments using the functional decortication technique. Bilateral application of 25 % KCl on the cerebral cortex completely inhibited the copulatory activity of male rats for approximately 2 hours. The animals spent most of the time in a corner of the observation cage and responded to the approaches of the female by weak squealing. When the rats finally started to copulate, ejaculation was attained after a lower number of intromissions than normally. The passive components of the female sexual response (ear wiggling, lordosis, acceptance of male) were inhibited by CSD only in some rats and their recovery was rapid. The female's active pursuing of and presentation to the male was lost, however, for periods comparable to the duration of inhibition in males. It was concluded that CSD eliminates in both males and females the active components of mating behavior without interfering seriously with the purely responsive components, which are sufficient to ensure passive admittance of the normal male by the decorticate female. Under certain conditions, the passive components can be even enhanced by CSD as shown by Clemens, Wallen, and Gorski (1967) for ovariectomized females treated with estrogen. The female was placed in a cage with a sexually active male and left there until the male mounted her 10 times or until 15 min elapsed. The number of lordosis posturings shown by the female was divided by the number of mounts. This ratio, called the lordosis quotient, increased during 1 hour after bilateral KCl application from the predepression value of 0.21 to 0.54. A similar increase of the lordosis quotient can be achieved by injection of 0.5 mg progesterone 4 hours before testing. The gradually developing facilitation of lordosis frequency by functional decortication may be due to a release of gonadotrophins, the secretion of which is normally inhibited by the intact cortex.

Single waves of unilateral CSD evoked by iontophoretic or pressure microinjection of K^+ are followed by penile errection in the rat (Huston, 1971). This seems to be a part of a more general syndrome of postdepression activation characterized by increased intake of food and water (see p. 340), stretching, and yawning.

Self-stimulation

Closely related to the effect of CSD on feeding, thermoregulation and other functions integrated at the hypothalamic level is the CSD-induced suppression of self-stimulation. Bureš, Burešová, Fifková, Olds, Olds and Travis (1961) found complete disappearence of self-stimulation with hypothalamic electrode placements under bilateral CSD. As pointed out by Olds (1962), the suppression is not due to a motor deficit since aversive tegmental stimulation evokes escape reactions of similar type (bar pressing) even in functionally decorticated rats. The assumption that reduced motivation level contributes to the blockade of operant or voluntary behavior under bilateral CSD is also supported by the experiments combining lateralized hypothalamic lesions or stimulation with functional hemidecortication (see p. 299).

Experimental Epilepsy

Whereas cortical and subcortical lesions have repeatedly been used for analyzing the anatomical substrate of different types of epileptic seizures (Servít 1963, 1966), CSD can be used for the same purpose with some advantage. Bureš and Burešová (1956d) investigated the effect of CSD on audiogenic epilepsy in mice (Fig. 11.19). In one experiment restrained mice were injected with 150 mg/kg metrazol and the epileptogenic stimulus was applied 2 min 30 sec later. Whereas in the control group seizures appeared in 77% of the cases, only 8% of experimental animals in which CSD was evoked by 1-min polarization of the cerebral cortex (3 mA) at the time of injection, displayed seizures. In another experiment audiogenic seizures were evoked in freely moving animals, the susceptibility of which was increased by 50 mg/kg metrazol injected 3 min prior to the application of the epileptogenic stimuluss Cortical SD was evoked 10 to 20 min before the intraperitoneal metrazol injection by bilateral application of 25% KCl to the exposed cortex. The incidence of seizures dropped from 57% in control animals to 35 % in functionally decorticate mice.

Essentially similar results were obtained by Chocholová (1962) in rats naturally susceptible to audiogenic siezures (Fig. 11.19). The epileptogenic stimulus was applied 20 min after bilateral CSD was elicited by 25% KCl. In a group of highly susceptible rats CSD decreased the incidence of seizures from 100 to 77%. In another group of rats with intermediate susceptibility the percentage of seizures dropped from 54 to 29%. In both groups seizures appearing under CSD were less severe on the average than under control conditions, although all main seizure types were observed, including the two-phase seizure (running-freezing-running-convulsions) considered by some authors (Krushinsky 1954) as a manifestation of cortical inhibitory influences.

Kesner, O'Kelly, and Thomas (1965) confirmed the above findings by using latencies of the running fit onset as a measure of the CSD effect. The latencies increased from a control level of 15 to 20 sec to 68 sec during bilateral CSD, and remained prolonged over 4 days after KCl application, suggesting some long-lasting consequences of the treatment. In other groups CSD was combined with metrazol (35 mg/kg, 4 min prior to sound onset) or phenobarbital (8 mg/kg, 15 min prior to sound). Wheras these drugs decreased or increased the latencies, respectively, CSD always increased them with respect to the new level. Slightly prolonged latencies of audiogenic seizures in functionally decorticated mice were also reported by Ward and Sinnett (1971). These authors made the interesting observation that mice under unilateral CSD develop asymmetrical convulsions with a marked tendency to fall to the side contralateral to the depressed hemisphere.

Myoclonic twitches evoked by the audiogenic stimulus in some rats either instead of or in addition to the seizure were completely suppressed during bilateral functional decortication (Semyokhina 1969). Cerebral cortex seems to be an obligatory link for mediating the myoclonic response.

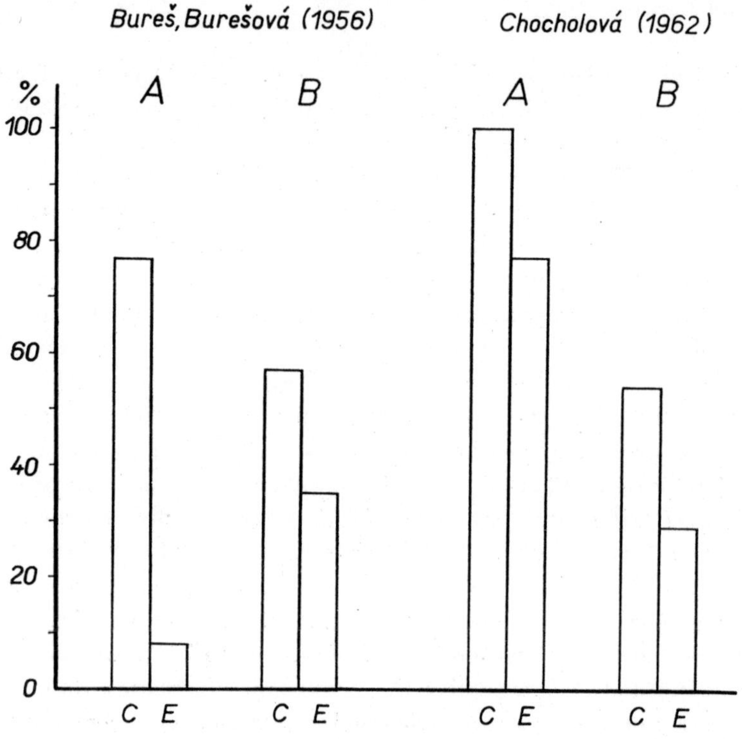

Fig. 11. 19. The decrease of audiogenic seizure susceptibility by CSD. Bureš and Burešová (1956d) used mice sensibilized by metrazol. (A) Restrained animals; CSD elicited by polarization. (B) Freely moving animals; CSD elicited by 25% KCl. Chocholová (1962) studied the effect of chemically induced CSD in rats naturally susceptible to audiogenic seizures. *(A)* Highly susceptible rats. *(B)* Rats with intermediate susceptibility. *(C)* Control animals. *(E)* Experimental animals with CSD elicited by topical application of 25 % KCl.

The decrease of audiogenic-seizure susceptibility caused by CSD is probably not due to blockade of the auditory pathways but rather to a slight general increase in seizure threshold, which could be demonstrated for other models of experimental epilepsy. Thus Bohdanecký, Bureš, Burešová, Nečina, and Weiss (1963) and Bohdanecký and Nečina (1963) injected mice intravenously with 1 % caffeine, 0.25 % metrazol, or 0.002 % strychnine at a rate of 0.3 ml/min until generalized convulsions appeared. Mice under bilateral CSD required a significantly higher threshold dose for each drug than the undepressed controls. As the primary target structures of the three drugs are believed to be different (neocortex, brain stem, and spinal cord in the cases of caffeine, metrazol, and strychnine, respectively) the uniform results obtained under CSD seem to indicate that CSD affects the actual mechanism of seizure generalization to which all epileptogenic stimuli eventually converge.

Blockade of seizures produced by electroconvulsive shock in rats was reported by Thompson and Miller (1967). They used 200 msec, 50 mA ac current administered through alligator clips attached to the animal's pinnae, which consistently elicited full tonic-clonic seizures in normal or sham CSD animals. Thirty minutes after application of 25% KCl on both hemispheres the same ECS elicited only a violent jump but no convulsions or running fits. It seems that with the above ECS technique current density is maximum in the hypothalamic region. The excitability decrease caused in this area by functional decortication may therefore enhance the overall anticonvulsant effect of CSD. Electrophysiological manifestations of the antiepileptic effect of thalamic SD are described in Chap. 8 (p. 196).

Eye Movements

Participation of cerebral cortex in complex eye movement reflexes induced by vestibular or optic stimuli was studied by the surgical decortication technique. Buehler, Kohut, and King (1969) used application of 0.1 ml of 25 % KCl to the ectosylvian gyrus of one hemicortex in cats to influence caloric nystagmus evoked by irrigation of ears with 10°, 28°, or 48 C° water. First changes in the nystagmus occurred between 1 and 10 min after KCl application. Response in one direction (to the normal hemisphere in 75 % animals) was reduced whereas response in the other direction remained unchanged or was even increased. After this period of directional preponderance responses in both directions diminished. The electronystagmogram returned to the predepression pattern only after several hours or days. Recovery was sometimes preceded by the seizure activity in the EEG which could be precipitated by the caloric stimulation in some cases.

Hogberg (1968) studied optokinetic nystagmus in the painted turtle. The eye movement rate was measured during 15-sec periods at the beginning and end of a 15-min optokinetic stimulation. Drum rotation was then immediately reversed and eye movements were recorded for another 15 sec. Under control conditions the eye movement rate decreased during the 15-min stimulation (habituation) but increased over the initial level during the reversed direction test. Application of KCl to the chronically exposed forebrain changed neither the rate of eye movements at the outset of the optokinetic stimulation nor the amount of habituation. On the other hand the reflex rebound due to reverse drum rotation was decreased.

5. Applications of Cortical Spreading Depression in Psychopharmacology

The mechanism of drug action can be analyzed by comparing drug effects in intact and brain-lesioned animals. Elimination of the target structures may suppress the drug effect and thus indicate the site of the primary influence. Especially important in this context is the role of the cerebral cortex. Classical pharmacology even attempted to classify drugs into cortical and subcortical types (Pick 1937). With drugs diffusely affecting the entire brain, affinity to different neurons is determined more by their biochemical properties than by their location, but decortication may again enhance or suppress the drug effects by unbalancing the usual intercentral relationships and thus changing the conditions of drug action. Another approach compares the deficit caused by a lesion with the symptoms induced by drug administration. The following paragraphs review experiments in which CSD was applied instead of surgical decortication in psychopharmacological research.

Anesthetic Effects

In many experiments concerned with so-called electronarcosis application of rather intensive electric currents probably caused CSD, which participated in an uncontrollable manner in the overall effect. In fact such experiments, in which polarization of CNS in mice prolonged duration of barbiturate or chloral hydrate anesthesia (Servít, Bureš, Burešová, and Petráň 1953) served as the departure point for an analysis that established the narcotic action of CSD alone. In the original experiments current (1 to 3 mA, 5 min) was applied onto the cortex against an indifferent electrode on the belly immediately after injection of the anesthetic. In a later study (Bureš 1955) a much shorter current application (2 mA, 15 sec, anode on the cortex) was shown to prolong Evipan anesthesia (50 mg/kg) from 28 to 46 min provided it still evoked typical EEG depression. Polarization (2 mA, 1 min, anode on cortex) potentiated the narcotic effect of Evipan, even when applied up to 20 min before or 10 min after the injection of the drug to restrained animals. Since the effect of polarization applied 10 or 20 min before Evipan injection was suppressed by releasing the animal prior to drug administration, the immobilization stress seems to be important in this particular case. The narcotic effect cannot be ascribed to CSD only, however, since prolongation of Evipan anesthesia could also be achieved by polarization of the lower brain stem (Bureš and Burešová 1956a), which does not elicit any EEG changes, and in 4 to 8 day old mice with an immature cerebral cortex. Cortical SD evoked in mice by bilateral application of 25% KCl onto the exposed cerebral cortex (and thus uncomplicated by current spread) caused a clear-cut enhancement of the effect of Evipan injected up to 30 min after CSD onset.

Using the same technique Bohdanecký, Bureš, Burešová, Nečina and Weiss (1963) and Bohdanecký and Nečina (1963) showed that functionally decorticated mice anesthetized with Thiopental (33 mg/kg), Viadril (37 mg/kg) or ether (2 to 5 min exposure to saturated vapors) slept two to five times longer than intact controls. Not all types of anesthesia were influenced in the same way, however. Thus the magnesium sulphate (5 g/kg) anesthesia was considerably shortened by CSD (approximately four times in comparison with intact controls — Fig. 11.20). Cortical SD probably prolongs anesthesia by reducing the overall excitability of the brain in general and of the reticular formation in particular. Other possibilities must also be taken into account however, for example, increased penetration of the drug into the brain due to increased permeability of the blood-brain barrier and increased cortical blood flow (Burešová 1957a). The second explanation does not account for increased seizure threshold to various drugs (see p. 348), which is in agreement with the reduced excitability hypothesis. Prolongation of animal hypnosis by CSD (Bureš and Burešová 1956d; see p. 257) supports the same conclusion. Shortening of magnesium sulphate anesthesia cannot be explained by this mechanism and will require further analysis.

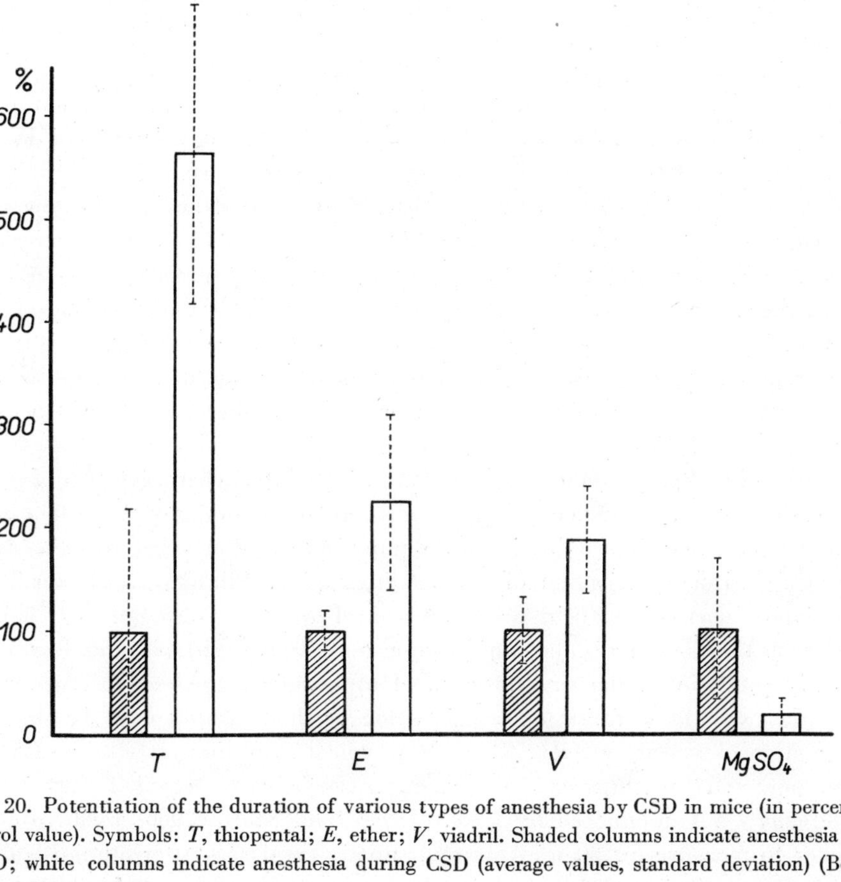

Fig. 11. 20. Potentiation of the duration of various types of anesthesia by CSD in mice (in percentage of control value). Symbols: *T*, thiopental; *E*, ether; *V*, viadril. Shaded columns indicate anesthesia without CSD; white columns indicate anesthesia during CSD (average values, standard deviation) (Bohdanecký and Nečina 1963).

Analgetic Effects

Slightly decreased cutaneous sensibility was demonstrated during CSD by Weiss and Bureš (1959) and by Thompson and Enter (1967). This effect is much better expressed in the potentiating influence of functional decortication on the effectiveness of different analgetics. Bohdanecký, Bureš, Burešová, Nečina, and Weiss (1963) used the squealing reaction evoked by electrical stimulation of the tail at 10-min intervals to assess the analgetic effects. The time during which this reaction was suppressed served as a measure of analgesia. Although functional decortication alone did not interfere with the squealing reaction, it prolonged the analgetic effect of phenylbutazon (100 mg/kg) and chlorpromazine (5 mg/kg) from 10 to 15 min to 90 to 100 min and that of pethidine (20 mg/kg) and morphine (5 mg/kg) from 80 to 90 min to 150 min. The mechanism of the CSD potentiation of analgetic effects is probably similar to the case of anesthesia. A prolonged analgetic effect of morphine in decorticated dogs was reported by Wikler (1952).

Effects on the Adrenergic and Cholinergic Systems

Bohdanecký and Nečina (1963) examined the effect of bilateral functional decortication on the so-called "aggregate toxicity" of amphetamine (Chance 1946); mice injected with amphetamine dosages sublethal for isolated animals (50 mg/kg) die if placed in groups of 10 animals in small glass containers. Contrary to expectation, CSD did not change the animals' behavior, the hyperactivity being apparently the same in the depressed and undepressed mice. During the 3-hour observation period, both decorticated and control groups lost about 78% of the animals. This indicates that the aggregate toxicity is not mediated by the cerebral cortex and that its mechanisms must be sought at the subcortical or even peripheral levels which are not markedly affected by CSD.

Mettler and Culler (1934) described potentiation of the mydriatic effect of atropine in decorticate dogs. Bohdanecký and Nečina (1963) used a microscope with a measuring ocular scale to estimate the size of the pupil in resting mice before and for 1 hour after intraperitoneal injection of 25 mg/kg atropine. Bilateral CSD was induced immediately after injection in the experimental animals. Although CSD alone did not change the diameter of the pupil (see also Burešová, Fifková, and Bureš 1966), it clearly potentiated the mydriatic effect of atropine, the pupil diameter being 50% larger and the duration of mydriasis longer than in undepressed animals.

Reduction of motor activity, which is a typical symptom of bilateral CSD, can be counteracted by drugs causing hyperactivity in rats, provided they influence brain regions not eliminated by CSD. Meyers and Stern (1966) used an activity chamber to measure for 30 min the motor activity of rats after administration of saline or scopolamine (0.2 mg/kg) in the presence or absence of bilateral CSD.

The usual depression of motor activity due to functional decortication could be partly counteracted by scopolamine, which caused a significant rise of activity in the last part of the measuring period. This result indicates that the anticholinergic effects of scopolamine may arouse hyperactivity even in decorticate animals. Bureš (1968) arrived at a similar conclusion using atropine. In his experiments rats learned a simple avoidance reaction (running from the electrifiable grid floor in one half of the runway to the wooden floor in the other half) either with brain intact or during bilateral CSD. The effects of physostigmine salicylate (1 mg/kg) and atropine sulphate (6 mg/kg) on learning were investigated under both conditions (Fig. 11.21).

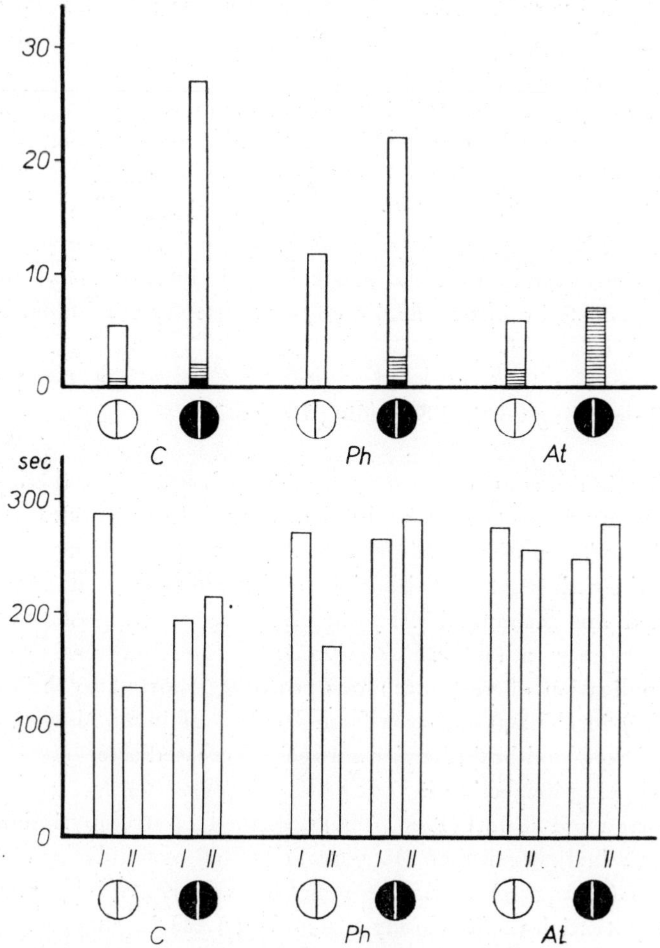

Fig. 11. 21. The effect of functional decortication and of physostigmine and atropine on learning of a simple avoidance reaction. (Above) Number of to-criterion trials (total columns) and of spontaneous return reactions (shaded part of columns). (Below) Time spent on the grid floor during the first (I) and second (II) exploratory test (Bureš 1968).

Learning the avoidance reaction was slower after physostigmine but not after atropine. Bilateral CSD caused the usual impairment of learning, most rats being able to reach the 9/10 criterion in less than 50 trials, however. Whereas physostigmine did not affect the learning ability of decorticated animals, atropinised CSD rats learned rapidly to run from start to goal, the avoidance criterion being attained with nearly the same speed as in normal animals. After reaching the goal, the rats often returned to the grid floor, however, where they received additional foot shocks. Spontaneous returning from the goal area to the electrified grid occurred in all CSD groups, but was most clear-cut in the atropinized animals. Thus the low number of the to-criterion trials after atropine does not indicate that the learning ability was improved, but rather that the overall activity of the animals was raised. This increased the probability of avoiding shocks as well as of receiving them by reaching or leaving the goal.

Atropine acts as a psychomotor stimulant in mice (Mennear 1965) and rats (Carlton and Didamo 1961) whereas cholinergic stimulants reduce spontaneous activity (Harris 1961) and decrease amphetamine toxicity (Mennear 1965). As the stimulating effect of atropine is considerably enhanced in functionally decorticated rats, its site of action must be sought mainly at the subcortical level. On the contrary the behavioral impairment due to CSD is not further increased by physostigmine, which probably affects brain regions directly or indirectly eliminated by CSD.

Drug Effects Resembling Cortical Spreading Depression

Systemic application of some drugs may cause depolarization of the cerebral cortex resembling in many respects sustained CSD. Very deep ether anesthesia, sublethal dose of cyanide and suprathreshold dosages of convulsants belong to this category. Unfortunately the rather extreme situations under which the CSD stage of the drug effect is reached are accompanied by anoxia, excessive hyperactivity, metabolic exhaustion and similar pathological conditions. The possibility of evoking CSD by intravenous application of glutamate was recently reported by Fifková and Van Harreveld (1970) in chicken embryos from 16 days of incubation up to hatching. Permeability of the blood-brain barrier abruptly decreased after hatching, the glutamate injections being ineffective in 5-day old chickens.

Recently Norton and Jewett (1966, 1967) described a pyrrolopyrimidine derivative BW 58-271 (2-methyl 4-benzyl-amino pyrrolo [2,3-d] pyrimidine) which caused in anesthetic doses (15 mg/kg) marked suppression of EEG activity accompanied by repeated slow potential waves closely resembling CSD in shape, amplitude (3 to 10 mV), duration (1 to 2 min), and repetition time (7 to 8 min). As these electrophysiological phenomena could not be explained by hypotension or anoxia, they seem to be a direct result of the drug effect. The assumption that the BW 58-271-induced anesthesia corresponds to prolonged CSD was supported by its behavioral consequences. Unlike other anesthetics (thiopental, ether), BW 58-271 partly disrupted short and long fixed-interval lever-pressing habits, that could be relearned to the control level within 3 weekly sessions. Also, BW 58-271 caused an increase of exploratory activity in rats previously habituated to experimental conditions. Thus the drug resembled CSD not only in the EEG response but also by its effects on consolidation or retrieval, which were in many respects similar to prolonged CSD evoked by repetitive application of 25% KCl onto the cortical surface (p. 324).

References

Adey W. R., Bystrom B. G., Costin A., Kado R.T., Tarby T. J., 1969: Divalent cations in cerebral impedance and cell membrane morphology. *Exp. Neurol.* **23**: 29—50.

Agranoff B. W., 1967: Memory and protein synthesis. *Sci. Am.* **216**:115—122.

Albert D. J., 1966a: The effect of spreading depression on the consolidation of learning. *Neuropsychologia* **4**:49—64.

Albert D. J., 1966b: The effects of polarizing current on the consolidation of learning. *Neuropsychologia* **4**:65—77.

Albert D. J., 1966c: Memory in mammals: Evidence for a system involving nuclear ribonucleic acid. *Neuropsychologia* **4**:79—92.

Ames A. III, 1956: Studies on water and electrolytes in nervous tissue. II. Effect of glutamate and glutamine. *J. Neurophysiol.* **19**:213—223.

Andjus R., 1951: Sur la possibilité de ranimer le rat adulte refroidi jusqu'a proximité du point de congélation. *C. R. Acad. Sci.* **232**:1591—1593.

Andjus R., Smith A. U., 1955: Reanimation of adult rats from body temperatures between 0 and +2 °C. *J. Physiol.* **128**:446—472.

Aquino-Cias J., Belcheva S., Bureš J., Fifková E., 1966: The influence of thalamic spreading depression on cortical and reticular unit activity in the rats. *Brain Res.* **1**:77—85.

Aquino-Cias J., Bureš J., 1966: The effect of thalamic spreading depression on the epileptic discharge in rats. In *Comparative and Cellular Pathophysiology of Epilepsy.* Servít Z. (ed.). Excerpta Medica Int. Congr. Ser. No 124, Amsterdam, pp. 258—269.

Aquino-Cias J., Bureš J., 1967: Seizure irradiation during functional elimination of the thalamus by spreading depresion in the rat. *Epilepsia* **8**:47—57.

Aquino-Cias J., Bureš J., Fifková E., Popova N. S., 1966: The effect of thalamic spreading depression on electric activity in the caudate nucleus and the hippocampus in rats. *Physiol. Bohemoslov.* **15**: 195—200

Aquino-Cias J., Harmony T., Guma E., 1967: Effect of strophantine and ouabain on cortical afterdischarges. *Arch. Int. Pharmacodyn. Thérap.* **168**:352—365.

Ashford C. A., Dixon K. C., 1935: The effect of potassium on the glucolysis of brain tissue with reference to the Pasteur effect. *J. Biochem.* **29**:159—168.

Atsev E., 1966: Dynamics of electrical manifestations of brain activity in cats and rabbits with an experimental epileptogenic focus (macro- and microelectrode investigations). In *Comparative and Cellular Pathophysiology of Epilepsy.* Servít Z. (ed.). Excerpta Medica Int. Congr. Ser. No 124, Amsterdam, pp. 221—234.

Avis H. H., Carlton P. L., 1968: Retrograde amnesia produced by hippocampal spreading depression. *Science* **161**:73—75.

Balinska H., Burešová O., Fifková E., 1967: The influence of cortical and thalamic spreading depression on feeding behavior of rats with lateral hypothalamic lesions. *Acta Biol. Exper.* (Warsaw) **27**:355—363.

Bao D. C., Ochs S., 1972: Incorporation of ^{3}H-leucine in rabbit cortex and transport into synaptosomes: Effect of spreading depression. *Federation Proc.* **31**: 304.

Bard P., Macht M. B., 1958: The behaviour of chronically decerebrate cats. *The Neurological Basis of Behavior,* G. E. W. Wolstenholme and C. M. O'Connor (eds.), Churchill, London, 55—75.

Bargeton D., Krumm-Heller C., 1949: Appareil pour la determination du metabolism des petits animaux par courts intervals de temps. *J. Physiol.* (Paris) **41**: 119.

Barlow H. B., 1953: Action potentials from frog retina. *J. Physiol.* **119**:58—68.

Barondes S. H., Cohen H. D., 1963: Puromycin effect on successive phases of memory storage. *Science* **151**:594—595.

Bassi M., Bernelli-Zazzera A., 1960: Effect of potassium ions on brain respiration and amino acid incorporation in brain proteins *in vitro*. *Experientia* **16**:430.

Beach F. A., 1940: Effects of cortical lesions upon the copulatory behavior of male rats. *J. Comp. Psychol.* **29**:193—245.

Beach F. A., 1944: Effects of injury to the cerebral cortex upon sexually receptive behavior in the female rats. *Psychosomatic Med.* **6**:41—53.

Beach F. A., 1966: Spreading depression and interhemispheric transfer of an avoidance response. *Psychon. Sci.* **5**:9—10.

Beck E. C., Doty R. W., 1957: Conditioned flexion reflexes acquired during combined catalepsy and de-efferentation. *J. Comp. Physiol. Psychol.* **50**:211—216.

Benešová O., Bureš J., Burešová O., 1957: Die Wirkung des Chlorpromazins und der Glykämie auf das elektrophysiologisch kontrollierte Überleben der Hirnrinde bei verschiedenen Körpertemperaturen. *Arch. Exp. Path. Pharmak.* **231**:550—561.

Benitez D., Pscheidt G. R., Stone W. E., 1954: Formation of ammonium ion in the cerebrum in fluoroacetate poisoning. *Am. J. Physiol.* **176**:488—492.

Benjamin R. M., Pfaffman C., 1955: Cortical localization of taste in albino rat. *J. Neurophysiol.* **18**: 56—64.

Bennett G. S., Edelman G. M., 1969: Amino acid incorporation into rat brain proteins during spreading cortical depression. *Science* **163**:393—395.

Beránek R., Fantiš A., Gutmann E., 1955: *Experimental Studies on Brain Edema* (in Czech.). NČSAV, Prague.

Beritoff I., 1926: Über die individuell erworbene Tätigkeit des Zentralnervensystems bei Tauben. *Pflügers Arch.* **213**:370—406.

Best P. J., 1972: Effects of shock intensity on transfer of shock avoidance under unilateral spreading depression. *Physiol. Behav.* **8**:279—282.

Best P., Hamburg M., 1969: Transfer of brightness discrimination under unilateral spreading depression. *Physiol. Behav.* **4**:805—808.

Best P. J., Zuckerman K., 1971: Subcortical mediation of learned taste aversion. *Physiol. Behav.* **7**: 317—320.

Bianki V. L., 1967: *Evolution of the Paired Function of Cerebral Hemispheres* (in Russian). LGU, Leningrad.

Bianki V. L., 1968a: Types and nature of interhemispheric relations (according to experiments with spreading depression) (in Russian). *Zh. Vyssh. Nerv. Deyat.* **18**:441—447.

Bianki V. L., 1968b: Influence of localization of a visual stimulus on the formation of a conditioned reflex to surroundings in each hemisphere (in Russian). *Zh. Vyssh. Nerv. Deyat.* **18**:598—607.

Bianki V. L., 1970: Dynamics of interhemispheric asymmetry (in Russian). *Biol. Nauki* **5**:37—41.

Bianki V. L., 1971: Interhemispheric synthesis and dominance. *Activitas nervosa superior* **13**: 131—139.

Bianki V. L., Makarova A. E., 1970: Functional asymmetry of the hemispheres caused by different localization of conditioning and testing stimuli (in Russian). *Zh. Vyssh. Nerv. Deyat.* **20**:50—58.

Bianki V. L., Pokrovskaya L. A., Voyevodenkova N. A., 1969: Interhemispheric synthesis of antagonistic conditioned reflexes (in Russian). *Zh. Vyssh. Nerv. Deyat.* **19**:928—935.

Bianki V. L., Trubacheva N. N., 1970: Functions of the different parts of corpus callosum in rats (in Russian). *Biol. Nauki* **2**:30—32.

Biersteker P. A., Collewijn H., Van Harreveld A., 1966: Asphyxial potentials of spinal gray matter, and of ventral and dorsal roots. *J. Physiol.* **185**:15—29.

Bindman L. J., Lippold O. C. J., Redfearn J. W. T., 1962: Long-lasting changes in the level of the electrical activity of the cerebral cortex produced by polarizing currents. *Nature* **196**: 584—585.

Bito L. Z., Myers R. E., 1972: On the physiological response of the cerebral cortex to acute stress (reversible asphyxia). *J. Physiol.* **221**: 349—370.

Bivens L. W., Ray O. S., 1965: Memory trace disruption by cortical spreading depression. *Psychol. Reports* **17**:175—178.

Black H., Suboski M. D., Freedman N. L., 1967: Effects of cortical spreading depression and ether following one-trial discriminated avoidance learning. *Psychon. Sci.* **9**:597—598.

Bloch-Rojas S., Toro A., Pinto-Hamuy T., 1964: Cardiac versus somatomotor conditioned responses in neodecorticate rats. *J. Comp. Physiol. Psychol.* **58**:233—236.

Bogen J. E., Bogen G. M., 1969: The other side of the brain III: The corpus callosum and creativity. *Bull. of the Los Angeles Neurol. Soc.* **34**:191—220.

Bohdanecká M., Bohdanecký Z., Jarvik M. E., 1967: Amnesic effects of small bilateral brain puncture in the mouse. *Science* **157**:334—336.

Bohdanecký Z., Bureš J., Burešová O., Nečina J., Weiss T., 1963: The use of spreading depression in neuropharmacology. In *Effects of Psychotropic Drugs on Higher Nervous Activity*, Pergamon Press, Oxford, pp. 191—196.

Bohdanecký Z., Nečina J., 1963: Course of some pharmacological tests in functionally decorticated animals. *Physiol. Bohemoslov.* **12**:55—61.

Bohdanecký Z., Weiss T., Fifková E., 1963: The influence of neocortical and hippocampal spreading depression on "theta rhythm" elicited by physostigmine. *Arch. int. Pharmacodyn.* **143**:23—33.

Bohdanecký Z., Weiss T., Fifková E., 1964: The effect of neocortical and hippocampal spreading depression on the slow wave EEG activity induced by atropine. *Arch. int. Pharmacodyn.* **148**:545—556.

Bondarenko T. T., 1964: Application of cortical spreading depression in chronic experiment (in Russian). *Biol. Nauki* **4**:61—64.

Bonnet V., Bremer F., 1937: Action du potassium, du calcium et de l'acétylcholine sur les activités électriques, spontanées et provoquées de l'écorce cérebrale. *C. R. Soc. Biol.* **126**:1271—1275.

Borenstein P., Buser P., 1960: Observations sur les projections du cortex dans la formation reticulée mésencéphalique chez le chat. *C. R. Soc. Biol.*, **154**:38—42.

Bradley P. B., Elkes J., 1957: The effects of some drugs on the electrical activity of the brain. *Brain* **80**:77—117.

Bremer F., 1958: Cerebral and cerebellar potentials. *Physiol. Rev.* **38**:357—388.

Brinley F. J., 1963: Ion fluxes in the central nervous system. *Int. Rev. Neurobiol.* **5**:183—242.

Brinley F. J., Kandel E. R., Marshall W. H., 1960: Potassium outflux from rabbit cortex during spreading depression. *J. Neurophysiol.* **23**:246—256.

Brooks M. C., Peck M. E., 1940: Effect of various cortical lesions on development of placing and hopping reactions in rats. *J. Neurophysiol.* **3**:66—73.

Brossard M., Quastel J. H., 1963: Studies of the cationic and acetylcholine stimulation of phosphate incorporation into phosholipids in rat brain cortex in vitro. *Can. J. Biochem. Physiol.* **41**:1243—1256.

Brožek G., 1966: Changes in the membrane potential of cortical cells during spreading depression. *Physiol. Bohemoslov.* **15**:98—103.

Brücke F., Petsche H., Pillat B., Deisenhammer E., 1959: Über Veränderungen des Hippocampus-Elektrencephalogrammes beim Kaninchen nach Novocaininjektion in die Septumregion. Naunyn-Schmiedeberg's *Arch. exp. Path. Pharmak.* **237**:276—284.

Buchwald N. A., Hull C. D., 1967: Some problems associated with interpretation of physiological and behavioral responses to stimulation of caudate and thalamic nuclei. *Brain Res.* **6**;1—11.

Buchwald N. A., Wyers E. J., Lamprecht C. W., Heuser G., 1961: The "caudate spindle". IV. A behavioral index of caudate-induced inhibition. *EEG Clin. Neurophysiol.* **13**:531—537.

Buehler B., Kohut R. I., King M. E., 1969: Repeatable alteration of vestibular responses by cortical depression. *Ann. Otol. Rhinol. Laryngol.* **78**:1234—1243.

Bureš J., 1954a: Electrotonic mechanisms in activity of central nervous system. Production of spreading depression of EEG activity by electrotonus. *Physiol. Bohemoslov.* **3**:272—287.

Bureš J., 1954b: Direct potential difference between cerebral hemispheres during depression of EEG activity in anesthetized and nonanesthetized rats. *Physiol. Bohemoslov.* **3**:288—295.

Bureš J., 1955: The relation between the depression of EEG activity brought about by electrotonus and the narcotic effect of a direct current. *Physiol. Bohemoslov.* **4**:98—107.

Bureš J., 1956: Some metabolic aspects of Leão's spreading depression. *J. Neurochem.* **1**:153—158.

Bureš J., 1957a: Ontogenetic development of steady potential differences in cerebral cortex in animals. *EEG Clin. Neurophysiol.* **9**:121—130.

Bureš J., 1957b: The effect of anoxia and asphyxia on spreading EEG depression. *Physiol. Bohemoslov.* **6**:444—453.

Bureš J., 1959: Reversible decortication and behavior. In *The Central Nervous System and Behavior*, Brazier M. A. B (ed.), Josiah Macy, Jr. Foundation, New York, pp. 207—248.

Bureš J., 1960: Block of Leão's spreading cortical depression by bivalent cations. *Physiol. Bohemoslov.* **9**:202—209.

Bureš J., 1962: *Spreading EEG Depression, Its Mechanism and Application* (in Czech). SZN, Prague.

Bureš J., 1964: Functional dissection of the mechanisms of learning. *Proc. XVII Int. Congr. Psychol. Washington*, North Holland, Amsterdam, pp. 349—350.

Bureš J., 1968: The effect of physostigmine and atropine on some behavioral and electrophysiological functions in rats. *Progress in Brain Res.* **28**:61—72.

Bureš J., Burešová O., 1956a: Zur Frage der Narkotischen Wirkung der Polarisation auf das Zentralnervensystem. *Physiol. Bohemoslov.* **5**:26—37.

Bureš J., Burešová O., 1956b: The question of ionic antagonism in spreading depression. *Physiol. Bohemoslov.* **5**:195—205.

Bureš J., Burešová O., 1956c: Metabolic nature and physiological manifestations of the spreading EEG depression of Leão. *Physiol. Bohemoslov.* **5**:Suppl. 4—6.

Bureš J., Burešová O., 1956d: The influencing of reflex acoustic epilepsy and reflex inhibition (animal hypnosis) by spreading EEG depression. *Physiol. Bohemoslov.* **5**:395—400.

Bureš J., Burešová O., 1957: Die anoxische Terminaldepolarisation als Indicator der Vulnerabilität der Grosshirnrinde bei Anoxie und Ischämie. *Pflügers Arch.* **264**:325—334.

Bureš J., Burešová O., 1959: The relationship between the localization of a focus of spreading EEG depression and the duration of conditioned reflex impairment evoked by depression. *Physiol. Bohemoslov.* **8**:333—338.

Bureš J., Burešová O., 1960a: Activation of latent foci of spreading cortical depression in rats. *J. Neurophysiol.* **23**:225—236.

Bureš J., Burešová O., 1960b: The use of Leão's spreading cortical depression in research on conditioned reflexes. *EEG Glin. Neurophysiol.* Suppl. **13**:359—376.

Bureš J., Burešová O., 1960c: The use of Leão's spreading depression in the study of interhemispheric transfer of memory traces. *J. Comp. Physiol. Psychol.* **53**:558—563.

Bureš J., Burešová O., 1962: La dépression envahissante comme instrument de récherche en neurophysiologie. *Actualités neurophysiologiques* **4**: 107—124.

Bureš J., Burešová O., 1963: Cortical spreading depression as a memory disturbing factor. *J. Comp. Physiol. Psychol.* **56**:268—272.

Bureš J., Burešová O., 1964: The effect of cortical spreading depression on evoked activity of reticular units. *Physiol. Bohemoslov.* **13**:584—593.

Bureš J., Burešová O., 1965: Spreading depression and cortico-subcortical interrelations in the mechanism of conditioned reflexes (in Russian). In *Refleksy golovnogo mozga,* Nauka, Moscow. pp. 55—63.

Bureš J., Burešová O., 1966a: Interhemispheric transfer of extinction of the passive avoidance reactions in the rats. *J. Comp. Physiol. Psychol.* **62**:459—461.

Bureš J., Burešová O., 1966b: The effect of independent storage of left and right discriminations in both hemispheres on subsequent reversal and alternation learning. *Activ. Nerv. Sup.* **8**:198—199.

Bureš J., Burešová O., 1968a: Spreading depression and cortico-subcortical interrelations in the mechanism of conditioned reflexes. In *Brain Reflexes,* Asratyan E. A. (ed.) *Progress in Brain Res.* **22**:378—387.

Bureš J., Burešová O., 1968b: The use of spreading depression in research into the functional organization of brain (in Russian). In *Cortical Regulation of Subcortical Activity*, Metsniereba, Tbilisi, pp. 116—131.

Bureš J., Burešová O., 1968c: Applications récentes de la dépression envahissante corticale à l'étude du comportement. *Actualités Neurophysiologiques* **8**:161—178.

Bureš J., Burešová O., 1970: The reunified split brain. In *The Neural Control of Behavior.* Whalen R. E., Thompson R. F., Verzeano M., Weinberger N. M. (eds.), Academic Press, New York, pp. 211—238.

Bureš J., Burešová O., 1972: Inducing cortical spreading depression. In *Methods in Psychobiology,* Vol. 2., Myers R. D. (ed.). Academic Press, New York, London, pp. 319—343.

Bureš J., Burešová O., Benešová O., Křivánek J., 1959: Cortical steady potentials during prolonged brain ischemia and following reanimation. *Proc. of XV Congr. Military Medicine and Pharm. Beograd —Opatija,* Beograd pp. 469—479.

Bureš J., Burešová O., Fifková E., 1961: The effect of cortical and hippocampal spreading depression on activity of bulbopontine reticular units in the rat. *Arch. Ital. Biol.* **99**:23—32.

Bureš J., Burešová O., Fifková E., 1964: Interhemispheric transfer of a passive avoidance reaction. *J. Comp. Physiol. Psychol.* **57**:326—330.

Bureš J., Burešová O., Fifková E., Olds J., Olds M. E., Travis R. P., 1961: Spreading depression and subcortical drive centers. *Physiol. Bohemoslov.* **10**:321—331.

Bureš J., Burešová O., Fifková E., Rabending G., 1965: Reversible deafferentation of cerebral cortex by thalamic spreading depression. *Exp. Neurol.* **12**:55—67.

Bureš J., Burešová O., Fifková E., Rabending G., 1966: Reversible deafferentation of cerebral cortex by thalamic spreading depression in rats. In *Corticosubcortical Relationship in Sensory Regulation,* Gonzales Martin D. and Guma E. (eds.). Academy of Sciences, Havana, pp. 1—13.

Bureš J., Burešová O., Janebová M., 1968: The effect of spreading depression in the thalamus, corpus striatum and hippocampus on the activity of a chemically induced focus of paroxysmal activity in the rat cerebral cortex. *Physiol. Bohemoslov.* **17**:533—549.

Bureš J., Burešová O., Křivánek J., 1960: Some metabolic aspects of Leão's spreading cortical depression. In *Structure and Function of the Cerebral Cortex,* Tower D. B. and Schadé J. P. (eds.). Proc. Sec. Int. Meeting of Neurobiologists, Elsevier, Amsterdam, pp. 257—265.

Bureš J., Burešová O., Weiss T., 1960: Functional consequences of hippocampal spreading depression. *Physiol. Bohemoslov.* **9**:219—227.

Bureš J., Burešová O., Weiss T., Fifková E., 1963: Excitability changes in nonspecific thalamic nuclei during cortical spreading depression in the rat. *EEG Clin. Neurophysiol.* **15**:73—83.

Bureš J., Burešová O., Weiss T., Fifková E., Bohdanecký Z., 1962: Experimental study of the role of hippocampus in conditioning and memory functions. In *Physiologie de l'hippocampe,* CNRS, pp. 241—256.

Bureš J., Burešová O., Záhorová A., 1958: Conditioned reflexes and Leão's spreading cortical depression. *J. Comp. Physiol. Psychol.* **51**:263—268.

Bureš J., Burešová O., Zacharová D., 1957: Effect of changes in body temperature on spreading EEG depression. *Physiol. Bohemoslov.* **6**:454—461.

Bureš J., Fifková E., 1968: The effect of potassium liberated from nerve structures invaded by spreading depression on conduction in fibers of the adjacent white matter. *Physiol. Bohemoslov.* **17**:405—410

Bureš J., Fifková E., Mareš P., 1964: Spreading depression and maturation of some forebrain structures in rats. In *Neurological and Electroencephalographic Correlative Studies in Infancy,* Kellaway P., Petersen I. (eds.), Grune and Stratton, New York, pp. 27—36.

Bureš J., Fifková E., Maršala J., 1960: Leão's spreading depression in pigeons. *J. Comp. Neurol.* **114**:1—10.

Bureš J., Hartman G., 1967: Conduction block in capsula interna fibers caused by striate spreading depression in rats. *Experientia* **23**:736—738.

Bureš J., Hartman G., Lukyanova L. D., 1967: Blockade of thalamocortical and pyramidal pathways by striatal spreading depression in rats. *Exp. Neurol.* **18**:404—415.

Bureš J., Koshtoyants Kh. S., 1955: The role of the tissue SH-bonds in the initiation of spreading depression of the electrical activity of the cerebral cortex (in Russian). *DAN SSSR* **105**:1118—1120.

Bureš J., Kozlovskaya I. B., Fifková E., 1964: Excitability changes in nonspecific thalamic nuclei during striatal depression in the rat. *Arch. int. Physiol. Bioch.* **72**:776—786.

Bureš J., Křivánek J., 1958: Washing of brain surface by epidural fistula — a method for the study of brain electrolytes in vivo. *Zweites Int. Symp. Über den Mechanismus der Erregung.* VEB Deutscher Verlag der Wissenschaften, Berlin, pp. 1—3.

Bureš J., Křivánek J., 1960: Ionic movements in the brain as studied with the aid of washing the cortical surface with an epidural cannula. *Physiol. Bohemoslov.* **9**:488—493.

Bureš J., Křivánek J., 1962: Über die Rolle einiger Aminosäuren im Mechanismus der sich verbreitenden EEG-Depression. In *Struktur und biologische Funktion der Eiweisse.* III Humboldt Symposium über Grundfragen der Biologie, Gustav Fischer Verlag, Berlin, pp. 181—184.

Bureš J., Petráň M., Zachar J., 1960: *Electrophysiological Methods in Biological Research.* Academia, Prague.

Burešová O., 1955: *Physiological Consequences of Direct Stimulation of the Central Nervous System by Electric Current and by Potassium Ions* (in Czech). Thesis, Institute of Physiology, Czechoslovak Academy of Sciences, Prague.

Burešová O., 1956: The influence of spreading cortical depression on unconditioned and conditioned alimentary reflexes (in Russian). *Physiol. Bohemoslov.* **5**:350—358.

Burešová O., 1957a: Changes in cerebral circulation in rats during spreading EEG depression. *Physiol. Bohemoslov.* **6**:1—11.

Burešová O., 1957b: Influencing water metabolism by spreading EEG depression. *Physiol. Bohemoslov.* **6**:12—20.

Burešová O., 1957c: Disturbance in thermoregulation and metabolism as result of prolonged EEG depression. *Physiol. Bohemoslov.* **6**:369—375.

Burešová O., 1966: To the specificity of the chemical transfer of the memory traces by brain extracts. Proceedings of the Vth Int. Congr. CINP. Excerpta Medica, Amsterdam, pp. 236—237.

Burešová O., Bureš J., 1958: Electrical indicators of irreversible ischaemic changes in cerebral cortex of the rat (in Czech). *Čs. Fysiol.* **7**:438—439.

Burešová O., Bureš J., 1960: The use of partial functional decortication in the study of the localization of conditioned reflexes. *Physiol. Bohemoslov.* **9**:210—218.

Burešová O., Bureš J., 1965a: Classical conditioning and reticular units. *Acta Physiol. Acad. Sci. Hung.* **26**:55—57.

Burešová O., Bureš J., 1965b: Interhemispheric synthesis of memory traces. *J. Comp. Physiol. Psychol.* **59**:211—214.

Burešová O., Bureš J., 1968: The role of the transmitting and receiving hemispheres in the interhemispheric transfer of T-maze alternation acquired during unilateral cortical spreading depression in rats. *Comm. Behav. Biol.*, Part A, 1:115—119.

Burešová O., Bureš J., 1969a: Can the brain be improved? *Endeavour* **28:** 139—145.

Burešová O., Bureš J., 1969b: The effect of prolonged cortical spreading depression on learning and memory in rats. *J. Neurobiol.* **1**:135—146.

Burešová O., Bureš J., 1970: The amnesic effect of cortical spreading depression. *Activitas Nervosa Superior* **12**:168—169.

Burešová O., Bureš J., 1971a: The effect of prolonged cortical spreading depression on consolidation of visual engrams in rats. *Psychopharmacologia* **20**:57—65.

Burešová O., Bureš J., 1971b: Interocular and interhemispheric transfer of visual engrams in callosotomized rats. *Physiol. Bohemoslov.* **20**:557—563.

Burešová O., Bureš J., 1971c: The significance of the crossed and uncrossed projections for the acquisition and retrieval of visual engrams in hooded and albino rats. *Psychologische Forschung* **35**:46—56.

Burešová O., Bureš J., 1971d: Drug induced facilitation of the transcommissural information flow in rats. XXV Int. Congr. Physiol. Sci., Munich, Abstr. of Comm. p. 90.

Burešová O., Bureš J., 1972: Determinants of successful interhemispheric transfer of pattern discrimination in rats. *Activ. nerv. sup.* **14**:18—23.

Burešová O., Bureš J., 1973: Cortical and subcortical components of the conditioned saccharin aversion in rats. *Acta Biol. Exp.* (Warsaw), in Press.

Burešová O., Bureš J., Beran V., 1958: A contribution to the problem of the "dominant" hemisphere in rats. *Physiol. Bohemoslov.* **7**:29—37.

Burešová O., Bureš J., Fifková E., 1962: Analysis of the effect of cortical spreading depression on the activity of reticular neurons. *Physiol. Bohemoslov.* **11**:375—382.

Burešová O., Bureš J., Fifková E., Vinogradova O., Weiss T., 1962: Functional significance of corticohippocampal connections. *Exp. Neurol.* **6**:161—172.

Burešová O., Bureš J., Gerbrandt L. K., 1968: The effect of an electroconvulsive shock on retention of a spatial discrimination or its reversal. *Physiol. Behav.* **3**:155—159.

Burešová O., Bureš J., Křivánek J., 1960: Activation of subthreshold foci of cortical spreading depression by asphyxia or hypoglycemia (in Czech). *Čs. Fysiol.* **9**:220.

Burešová O., Bureš J., Lukaszewska I., 1966: Strain differences in retrieval of unilateral and bilateral engrams. *Physiol. Behav.* **1**:331—333.

Burešová O., Bureš J., Rustová M., 1971: Conditions for interhemispheric transfer of initially lateralized visual engrams in rats. *J. Comp. physiol. Psychol.* **75**:200—206.

Burešová O., Bureš J., Weiss T., Fifková E., 1961: The use of spreading depression as a neuronographic method. Vth Int. Congr. EEG Clin. Neurophysiol., Rome, Abstracts of Communications.

Burešová O., Fifková E., Bureš J., 1966: Pupillary paralysis evoked by thalamic spreading depression in rats. *Exp. Brain Res.* **2**:168—175.

Burešová O., Fifková E., Ross R. B., 1965: The effect of thalamic spreading depression on acquisition and consolidation of the passive avoidance reaction in rats. *Activitas Nervosa Superior* **7**:162—163.

Burešová O., Goldowitz D., 1971: Time labelling of independently acquired lateralized engrams. XXV Int. Congr. Physiol. Sci., Munich, Abstr. of Comm. p. 91.

Burešová O., Kozlovskaya I. B., Fifková E., Weiss T., 1961: Combined anatomical and functional elimination of the cerebral cortex and subcortical structures as a method for studying the mechanism of conditioned reflexes. *Physiol. Bohemoslov.* **10**:237—248.

Burešová O., Lukaszewska I., Bureš J., 1966: Interhemispheric synthesis of goal alternation and jumping escape reaction. *J. Comp. Physiol. Psychol.* **62**:90—94.

Burešová O., Marusyeva A. M., Bureš J., Fifková E., 1964: The influence of cortical spreading depression on unit activity in the colliculus inferior of the rat. *Physiol. Bohemoslov.* **13**:227—235.

Burešová O., Nadel L., 1970: Interhemispheric transfer in the rat. *Physiol. Behav.* **5**:849—853.

Burešová O., Poupa O., 1959: Effect of adrenalectomy and substitution of corticoids on spreading depression. *Physiol. Bohemoslov.* **8**:202—210.

Burešová O., Rüdiger W., Bureš J., Fiková E., 1962: The role of the hypothalamic drinking center in unconditioned and conditioned control of water intake. *Physiol. Bohemoslov.* **11**:492—496.

Burešová O., Shima I., Bureš J., Fifková E., 1963: Unit activity in regions affected by the spreading depression. *Physiol. Bohemoslov.* **12**:488—494.

Burešová O., Votava J., Bureš J., 1966: Interhemispheric synthesis of competing and complementing experiences. *Physiol. Behav.* **1**:59—63.

Burgoyne L., Pote R., Freedman N., 1967: Conditioned cardiac acceleration under spreading cortical depression. *Psychon. Sci.* **9**:417—418.

Burns B. D., Grafstein B., 1953: Spreading depression in isolated cerebral cortex. XIXth Int. Physiol. Congr. Montreal, Abstr. of Comm., pp. 251—252.

Buser P., Bruner J., Sindberg R., 1963: Influences of the visual cortex upon posteromedial thalamus in the cat. *J. Neurophysiol.* **26**:677—691.

Buser P., Richard D., Lescop J., 1969: Controle par le cortex sensorimoteur de la réactivité de cellules réticulaires mésencephaliques chez le chat. *Exp. Brain Res.* **9**:83—95.

Bykov K. M., 1924: Experiments concerning the paired cooperation of cerebral hemispheres (in Russian). *Russ. Fiz. Zh.* **7**:294—295.

Campbell B. A., Campbell E. H., 1962: Retention and extinction of learned fear in infant and adult rats. *J. Comp. Physiol. Psychol.* **55**:1—8.

Carew T. J., Crow T. J., Petrinovich L. F., 1970: Lack of coincidence between neural and behavioral manifestations of cortical spreading depression. *Science* **169**:1339—1342.

Carlson K., 1966: Aspects of Avoidance Learning Stored Subcortically. Paper presented at Eastern Psychol. Assoc., New York.

Carlson K. R., 1967: Cortical spreading depression and subcortical memory storage. *J. Comp. Physiol. Psychol.* **64**:422—430.

Carlton P. L., Didamo P., 1961: Augmentation of the behavioral effects of amphetamine by atropine. *J. Pharmacol. Exp. Therap.* **132**:91—96.

Caspers H., Schütz E., Speckmann E. J., 1963: Gleichspannungsveränderungen an der Hirnrinde bei Sauerstoffmangel. *Z. Biol.* **114**:112—126.

Caspers H., Simmich W., 1966: Cortical d-c shifts associated with seizure activity. In *Comparative and Cellular Pathophysiology of Epilepsy*. Servít Z. (ed.) Excerpta Medica, Int. Congr. Ser. No 124, Amsterdam, pp. 151—163.

Castelluci V. F., Goldring S., 1970: Contribution to steady potential shifts of slow depolarization in cells presumed to be glia. *EEG Clin. Neurophysiol.* **28**:109—118.

Cerf J. A., 1963: L'action physiologique et pharmacologique des ions alcalino-terreux sur les fibres nerveuses. *Handb. Exp. Pharmak.* **17**,Teil I, 164—285.

Chamberlain T. J., Halick P., Gerard R. W., 1963: A fixation of experience in the rat spinal cord. *J. Neurophysiol.* **26**:662—673.

Chance M. R. A., 1946: Aggregation as a factor influencing toxicity of sympathomimetic amines in mice. *J. Pharmacol.* **87**:214.

Chang H., T. 1950: The repetitive discharge of corticothalamic reverberating circuit. *J. Neurophysiol.* **13**:235—258.

Chang H. T., 1955: Cortical response to stimulation of medullary pyramid in rabbit. *J. Neurophysiol.* **18**:332—352.

Chatfield P. O., Lyman C. P., 1954: Subcortical electrical activity in the golden hamster during arousal from hibernation. *EEG Clin. Neurophysiol.* **6**:403—408.

Chocholová L., 1962: The role of the cerebral cortex in audiogenic seizure in rat. *Physiol. Bohemoslov.* **11**:452—457.

Clemens L. G., Wallen K., Gorski R. A., 1967: Mating behavior: Facilitation in the female rat after cortical application of potassium chloride. *Science* **157**:1208—1209.

Cofoid D. A., 1965: Interhemispheric spread and graded response in spreading cortical depression. *Psychon. Sci.* **2**:343—344.

Cole K. S., 1949: Dynamic electrical characteristic of the squid axon membrane. *Arch. Sci. Physiol.* **3**:253—258.

Collewijn H., Schadé J. P., 1962a: Potassium movements in the cerebral cortex during asphyxia. *Arch. Morph. Neerl. Scand.* **5**:11—17.

Collewijn H., Schadé J. P., 1962b: Cerebral impedance changes in hypothermia. *Arch. Int. Physiol. Bioch.* **70**:200—210.

Collewijn H., Schadé J. P., 1964a: Conductivity of the cerebral cortex after circulatory arrest at body temperatures from 37 to 18 °C. *Arch. Int. Physiol. Bioch.* **72**:181—193.

Collewijn H., Schadé J. P., 1964b: Chloride, potassium, and water content of apical dendrites and their changes after circulatory arrest, at body temperatures from 37 to 20 °C. *Arch. Int. Physiol. Bioch.* **72**:194—210.

Collewijn H., Van Harreveld A., 1966: Membrane potential of cerebral cortical cells during spreading depression and asphyxia. *Exp. Neurol.* **15**:425—436.

Coons E. E., Miller N. E., 1960: Conflict versus consolidation of memory traces to explain "retrograde amnesia" produced by ECS. *J. Comp. Physiol. Psychol.* **53**:524—531.

Crain S. M., 1952: Development of electrical activity in the cerebral cortex of the albino rat. *Proc. Soc. Biol. Med.* **81**:49—51.

Creutzfeldt O. D., Watanabe S., Lux H. D., 1966a: Relations between EEG phenomena and potentials of single cortical cells. I. Evoked responses after thalamic and epicortical stimulation. *EEG Clin. Neurophysiol.* **20**:1—18.

Creutzfeldt O. D., Watanabe S., Lux H. D., 1966b: Relations between EEG phenomena and potentials of single cortical cells. II. Spontaneous and convulsoid activity. *EEG Clin. Neurophysiol.* **20**:19—37.

Crow T. J., Petrinovich L., Carew T. J., 1973: Electrophysiological correlates of cortical spreading depression. *Behav. Biol.* **8**: 219—226.

Cummins J. T., McIlwain H., 1961: Electrical pulses and the potassium and other ions of isolated cerebral tissues. *Biochem. J.* **79**:330—341.

Curatolo A., Marchetti M., Salleo A., Brancati A., 1967: Azione degli amino-acidi-dicarbossilici sull'attivita elettrica spontanea della corteccia cerebrale di gatto. *Arch. Sci. biol.* **51**:89—97.

Curtis D. R., 1964: Microelectrophoresis. In *Physical Techniques in Biological Research. Vol. V.* Nastuk W. L. (ed.) Electrophysiological Methods, Part A. pp. 144—192, Academic Press, New York-London.

Curtis D. R., Phillis J. W., Watkins J. C., 1959: The depression of spinal neurones by γ-aminobutyric acid and β-alanine. *J. Physiol.* **146**:185—203.

Curtis D. R., Phillis J. W., Watkins J. C., 1960: The chemical excitation of spinal neurones by certain acidic amino acids. *J. Physiol.* **150**:656—682.

Curtis D. R., Watkins J. C., 1963: Acidic amino acids with strong excitatory actions on mammalian neurones. *J. Physiol.* **166**:1—14.

Cytawa J., Teitelbaum P., 1965: Spreading cortical depression and recovery from subcortical damage. XXIII Int. Congr. Physiol. Sci. Tokyo, Abstr. of Papers, p. 475.

Cytawa J., Teitelbaum P., 1967: Spreading depression and recovery of subcortical function. *Acta Biol. Exper.* (Warsaw) **27**:345—353.

Cytawa J., Teitelbaum P., 1968: Spreading depression and recovery from septal hyperemotionality. *Folia Biologica* **16**:459—468.

Davis J. L., Bureš J., 1972: Disruption of saccharin aversion learning by cortical spreading depression in the CS-UCS interval. *J. Comp. Physiol. Psychol.* **8**:398—402.

Demetrescu M., Demetrescu M. 1962: Ascending inhibition and activation from the lower brain stem: The influence of pontine reticular stimulation on thalamocortical evoked potentials in cat. *EEG Clin. Neurophysiol.* **14**:602—620.

Deutsch J. A., 1969: The physiological basis of memory. *Ann. Rev. Psychol.* **131**:85—104.

De Valois J. C., 1966: *An Electrophysiological Study of Cerebral Anoxia.* Academisch proefschrift, Amsterdam.

Deza L., Eidelberg E., 1967: Development of cortical electrical activity in the rat. *Exp. Neurol.* **17**: 425—438.

Diamond J. M., Wright E. M., 1969: Biological membranes: The physical basis of ion and nonelectrolyte selectivity. *Ann. Rev. Physiol.* **31**:581—646.

Dickens F., Greville G. D. B., 1935: The metabolism of normal and tumor tissue. *Biochem. J.* **29**:1468—1483.

Do Carmo R. J., Leão A. A. P., 1972: On the relation of glutamic acid and some allied compounds to cortical spreading depression. *Brain Research* **39**:515—518.

Dondey M., Albe-Fessard D., Le Beau J., 1962: Premières applications neurophysiologiques d'une méthode permettante le blockade electif et reversible des structures centrales par réfrigération localisée. *EEG Clin. Neurophysiol.* **14**:758—763.

Donoso A. O., Stefano Z. J. E., 1966: Cerebral changes in the noradrenaline content during cortical spreading depression in the rat. *Acta Physiol. Latino-Amer.* **16**:22—25.

Doolittle J. H., Thompson C. W., 1966: Retroactive effects of topical applications of potassium chloride, pentylenetetrazol, and strychnine on the acquisition of a maze habit in rats *Psychon. Sci.* **5**:265—266.

Dorfman C. J., Bohdanecká M., Bohdanecký Z., Jarvik M. E., 1969: Retrograde amnesia produced by small cortical stab wounds in the mouse. *J. Comp. Physiol. Psychol.* **69**:324—328.

Dorfman L. J., 1963: Interhemispheric transfer of an avoidance response. Undergraduate Res. Project in Psychol. 5:22—35.

Druckman R., 1952: A critique of "suppression" with additional observations in the cat. *Brain* **75**:226—243.

Dubner R., Brown F. J., 1968: Response of cells to restricted visual stimuli in an association area of cat cerebral cortex. *Exp. Neurol.* **20**:70—86.

Duda P., Ruščák M., Zachar J., 1958: Brain metabolism during depolarization evoked by asphyxia and spreading depression (in Slovak) *Čs. Fysiol.* **7**:446—447.

Duda P., Ruščák M., Zachar J., 1961: Spreading cortical depression and the polarization gradient of the cerebral cortex. *Physiol. Bohemoslov.* **10**:438—447.

Duda P., Zachar J., Ruščák M., 1958: The time course of terminal anoxic depolarization following spreading depression (in Slovak) *Čs. Fysiol.* **7**:448—449.

Duncan C. P., 1948: Habit reversal induced by electroshock in the rat. *J. Comp. Physiol. Psychol.* **41**:11—16.

Duncan C. P., 1949: The retroactive effect of electroshock on learning. *J. Comp. Physiol. Psychol.* **42**:32—44.

Durinian R. A., Rabin A. G., 1963: Mechanisms of interaction of the specific and nonspecific brain structures. *DAN SSSR* **153**:1213—1215.

Dusser de Barenne J. G., Mc Culloch W. S., 1936a: Some effects of local strychninization on action potentials of the cerebral cortex of the monkey. *Trans. Am. Neurol. Assoc.* **62**:171.

Dusser de Barenne J. G., McCulloch W. S., 1936b: Functional boundaries in the sensory motor cortex of the monkey. *Proc. Soc. Exp. Biol. N. Y.* **35**:329—331.

Dusser de Barenne J. G., McCulloch W. S., 1938a: Functional organization in the sensory cortex of the monkey (*Macaca mulatta*). *J. Neurophysiol.* **1**:69—85.

Dusser de Barenne J. G., McCulloch W. S., 1938b: Sensory motor cortex, nucleus caudatus, and thalamus opticus. *J. Neurophysiol.* **1**:364—377.

Dusser de Barenne J. G., McCulloch W. S., 1941: Suppression of motor response obtained from area 4 by stimulation of areas 4S. *J. Neurophysiol.* **4**:311—323.

Dybowski G., Ewert A., 1966: Zur Wirkung der funktionellen Dekortikation auf die Temperaturregulation der Ratte. *Acta Biol. Med. German.* **17**:170—177.

Dybowski G., Rüdiger W., 1967: Zur Steigerung der Wärmeproduktion der Ratte bei epiduraler Applikation von KCl-Lösung. *Acta Biol. Med. German.* **18**:209—217.

Eayrs J. T., Goodhead B., 1959: Postnatal development of the cerebral cortex in the rat. *J. Anat.* **93**:385—401.

Eccles J. C., 1953: *The Neurophysiological Basis of Mind: the Principles of Neurophysiology.* Oxford Univ. Press (Clarendon), Oxford.

Eccles J. C., 1957: *The Physiology of Nerve Cells.* Johns Hopkins Press, Baltimore.

Eccles J. C., 1964: *The Physiology of Synapses.* Springer Verlag, Berlin—Göttingen—Heidelberg.

Egorov Yu. V., Kuznetsova G. D., 1972: Regional changes of electrical impedance in the cerebral tissue in the site of excitation of spreading depression. IV International Biophysics Congress, Moscow Abstracts of contributed papers. Vol. 3, p. 333.

Eidelberg E., Kolmodin G. M., Meyerson B. A., 1965: Ontogenesis of steady potential and direct cortical response in fetal sheep brain. *Exp. Neurol.* **12**:198—214.

Eidelberg E., Kolmodin G. M., Meyerson B. A., 1967: Effect of asphyxia on the cortical steady potential in adult and fetal sheep. *Acta Physiol. Scand.* **69**:257—261.

Ellen P., 1963: Spreading depression and position responses during conflict. *Am. Psychologist* **18**:431.

Encabo H., Buser P., 1964: Influence des aires primaires néocorticales sur les réponses sensorielles visuelles et acoustiques de la tête du noyau caudé. *EEG Clin. Neurophysiol.* **17**:144—153.

Esquibel M. A., 1956: Alteração da impedancia elétrica durante a depressão alastrante em pombos. *Ann. Acad. Brasil. Ci.* **28**:XLIII.

Essig C. F., Adkins F. J., Barnard G. L., 1953: Electrocorticographic effects of acetylcholine in monkeys and cats. *Proc. Soc. Exper. Biol. Med.* **82**:551—553.

Essig C. F., Marshall W. H., 1950: Enhancement of spreading cortical depression by a dialyzing technique. *Proc. Soc. Exp. Biol. Med.* **75**:429—432.

Estes W. K., 1955a: Statistical theory of spontaneous recovery and regression. *Psychol. Rev.* **62**:145—154.

Estes W. K., 1955b: Statistical theory of distributional phenomena in learning. *Psychol. Rev.* **62**:369—377.

Feldberg W., Sherwood S. L., 1957: Effects of calcium and potassium injected into the cerebral ventricles of the cat. *J. Physiol.* **137**:408—416.

Fernandez-Guardiola A., Roldán E. R., Fanjul M. L., Castells C., 1961: Role of the pupillary mechanism in the process of habituation of the visual pathways. *EEG Clin. Neurophysiol.* **13**:564—567.

Fertziger A. P., Ranck J. B. Jr., 1970: Potassium accumulation in interstitial space during epileptiform seizures. *Exp. Neurol.* **20**:571—585.

Fifková E., 1964a: Spreading depression in the neo-, paleo-, and archicortical structures of the brain of the rat. *Physiol. Bohemoslov.* **13**:1—15.

Fifková E., 1964b: Leão's spreading depression in the thalamic nuclei of rat. *Experientia* **20**:635—637.

Fifková E., 1964c: Development of spreading depression during ontogenesis in the rat. *Physiol. Bohemoslov.* **13**:263—267.

Fifková E., 1966a: Thalamic spreading depression in the rat. *EEG Clin. Neurophysiol.* **20**:68—76.

Fifková E., 1966b: Spreading depression in subcortical structures in rabbit. *Brain Res.* **2**:61—70.

Fifková E., 1966c: Anatomical limits of spreading depression in the cerebral cortex, hippocampus, caudate nucleus and thalamus (in Russian). In *Neural Mechanisms of motor activity.* Asratyan E. A. (ed.). Nauka, Moscow, pp.: 303—310.

Fifková E., Bureš J., 1964: Spreading depression in the mammalian striatum. *Arch. Int. Physiol. Bioch.* **72**:171—179.

Fifková E., Bureš J., 1966: The effect of thalamic spreading depression on conduction in the visual and auditory pathways. *Physiol. Bohemoslov.* **15**:344—352.

Fifková E., Bureš J., Koshtoyants O. Kh., Křivánek J., Weiss T., 1961: Leão's spreading depression in the cerebellum of rat. *Experientia* **17**:1—5.

Fifková E., Křivánek J., 1965: Some nonelectrical indicators of spreading depression (in Czech). Čs. Fysiol. **14**:265—266.

Fifková E., Maršala J., 1967: Stereotaxic atlases for the cat, rabbit, and rat. In *Electrophysiological Methods in Biological Research* Bureš J., Petráň M., Zachar J. (eds.), Publ. House Czech. Acad. Sci., Prague, pp. 653—731.

Fifková E., Syka J., 1964: Relationships between cortical and striatal spreading depression in rat. *Exp. Neurol.* **9**:355—366.

Fifková E., Van Harreveld A., 1970: Glutamate effects in the developing chicken. *Exp. Neurol.* **28**:286—298.

Findlay W., Magee W. L., Rossiter R. J., 1954: Incorporation of radioactive phosphate into lipids and pentosonucleic acid of cat brain slices. The effect of inorganic ions. *J. Biochem.* **58**:236—243.

Finney D. J., 1950: *Probit Analysis*. Cambridge University Press, London.

Flexner L. B., 1952: The development of the cerebral cortex: A cytological functional and biochemical approach. *Harvey Lect.* **47**:156—179.

Flexner L. B., Flexner J. B., Roberts R. B., 1967: Memory in mice analyzed with antibiotics. *Science* **155**:1377—1383.

Folbergerová J., 1961: The effect of potassium and some other factors upon the incorporation of ^{35}S-methionine into protein of brain cortex slices. *Physiol. Bohemoslov.* **10**:130—138.

Fonyó A., Kovách A. G. B., Makláy E., Leszkowsky G., Mészáros J., 1958: The effect of potassium ions and glutamate on the incorporation of ^{32}P into nucleotides and phosphocreatine in brain slices. *Acta Physiol. Acad. Sci. Hung.* **14**:305—307.

Forman D., Ward J. W., 1957: Responses to electrical stimulation of caudate nucleus in rats in chronic experiments. *J. Neurophysiol.* **20**:230—244.

Frankenhaeuser B., 1951: Limitations of method of strychnine neuronography. *J. Neurophysiol.* **14**: 73—79.

Frankenhäuser B., Hodgkin A. L., 1957: The action of calcium on the electrical properties of squid axon. *J. Physiol.* **137**:218—247.

Frankenhäuser B., Meves H., 1958: The effect of magnesium and calcium on the frog myelinated nerve fiber. *J. Physiol.* **142**:360—365.

Freedman N., 1969: Recurrent behavioral recovery during spreading depression. *J. Comp. Physiol. Psychol.* **68**:210—214.

Freedman N. L., Bureš J., 1972: Conditions of phasic impairment of avoidance responding during bilateral spreading depression. *J. Comp. Physiol. Psychol.* **78**:433—441.

Freedman N. L., Ferguson D. G., Wilson D., 1972: Regulatory and nonregulatory effects of functional decortication on eating in rats. *J. Comp. Physiol. Psychol.* **81**:233—242.

Freedman N., Lash L., 1966: Conditioned avoidance decrement under spreading depression. *Psychon. Sci.* **5**:411—412.

Freedman N., Pote R., 1969: Activity impairment with circumscribed frontal spreading depression and ablation. *Psychol. Reports* **24**:623—625.

Freedman N., Pote R., Butcher R., Suboski M. D., 1968: Learning and motor activity under spreading depression depending on EEG amplitude. *Physiol. Behav.* **3**:373—376.

Freygang W. H. Jr., Landau W. M., 1955: Some relations between resistivity and electrical activity in cerebral cortex of cat. *J. Cell. Comp. Physiol.* **45**:377—392.

Freygang W. H. Jr., Landau W. M., Marshal W. H., 1954: Changes in resistance and electric potential in the cortex. *Fed. Proc.* **13**:48.

Fuster J. M., Alexander G. E., 1970: Delayed response deficit by cryogenic depression of frontal cortex. *Brain Res.* **20**:85—90.

Gaete Avaria L., Křivánek J., 1973: Double labelling study of the spreading depression effect on the incorporation of labelled leucine into the proteins of the brain mitochondrial subfractions. *J. Neurochem.* **20**:905—908.

Galambos R., 1961: A glia—neural theory of brain function. *Proc. Nat. Acad. Sci.* **47**:129—136.

Galambos R., Sheatz G., Vernier V. B., 1956: Electrophysiological correlates of a conditioned response in cats. *Science* **123**:376—377.

García-Austt E., Bogacz J., Vanzulli A., 1961: Significance of photic stimulus on the evoked response in man. In *Brain Mechanism and Learning*. Delafresnaye J. F. (ed.) Blackwell, Oxford, pp. 603—623.

Garcia J., Ervin F. R., 1968: Gustatory-visceral and telereceptor-cutaneous conditioning:adaptation in internal and external milieus. *Commun. Behav. Biol.*, Part A, **1**:389—415.

Garcia Ramos J., Pradáč J., 1968: Electrochemistry of the fine indium-platinized electrodes used in biology. *Currents in Modern Biol.* **2**:165—170.

Gartside I. B., 1968: Mechanisms of sustained increases of firing rate of neurons in the rat cerebral cortex after polarization: Reverberating circuits or modification of synaptic conductance? *Nature* **220**:382—383.

Gartside I. B., 1971: Interhemispheric transfer of long term increases of cortical activity. *J. Physiol.* **216**:1—2P.

Gazzaniga M. S., 1963: Effect of commissurotomy on preoperatively learned visual discrimination. *Exp. Neurol.* **8**:14—19.

Gedevani D. M., 1943: The remote effects of stimulation of cortical foci on EEG (in Russian). *Tr. Inst. Fiziol. Tbilisi* **5**:263.

Gerbrandt L. K., Burešová O., Bureš J., 1968: Discrimination and reversal learning followed by a single electroconvulsive shock. *Physiol. Behav.* **3**:149—153.

Giammanco S., Paderni M. A., 1967: Modificazioni dell'attivita bioelettrica spontanea del nucleo caudato indotte dall'applicazione locale di KCl sulla corteccia cerebrale, nel gatto. *Bol. Soc. Ital. Biol. Sper.* **43**:1688—1691.

Gibson I. M., Mc Ilwain H., 1965: Continuous recording of changes in membrane potential in mammalian cerebral tissues in vitro; recovery after depolarization by added substances. *J. Physiol.* **176**:216—283

Giurgea C., 1970: *UCB 6215 Piracetam.* Research Report of the UCB—DIPHA. Liège.

Giurgea C., 1972: Vers une pharmacologie de l'activité intégrative du cerveau. Tentative du concept nootrope en psychopharmacologie. *Actualités Pharmacologiques* **25**:115—156.

Glass J. D., Thomas G. J., 1970: Effects of cortical ablations upon recovery from the septal syndrome in hooded rats. *Physiol. Behav.* **5**:879—882.

Goldensohn E., Escueta A., Runk L., 1967: Unit membrane shifts and firing patterns during spreading depression. *EEG Clin. Neurophysiol.* **23**:77—97.

Goldensohn E. S., Schoenfeld R. L., Hoefer P. F. A., 1951: The slowly changing voltage of the brain and the electrocorticogram. *EEG Clin. Neurophysiol.* **3**:231—236.

Goldensohn E. S., Walsh G., 1968: Sequential functional changes in single cortical neurons during spreading depression. *EEG Clin. Neurophysiol.* **24**:290—291.

Goldman D. E., 1943: Potential, impedance, and rectification in membranes. *J. Gen. Physiol.* **27**:37—60.

Goldner A. M., Cassidy M. M., Tidball C. S., 1967: Nonspecifity of the divalent cations capable of restoring normal intestinal permeability after chelation depletion. *Proc. Soc. Exp. Biol. Med.* **124**:884—887.

Goldowitz D., Burešová O., Bureš J., 1972: Time labelling of independently acquired lateralized engrams in rats. *Physiol. Behav.* **9**:699—704.

Goldowitz D., Burešová O., Bureš J., 1973: Forgetting of lateralized engrams studied by interhemispheric conflict in rats. *Behav. Biol.* **8**:183—192

Goldring S., O'Leary J. L., 1951: Experimentally derived correlates between EEG and steady cortical potential. *J. Neurophysiol.* **14**:275—288.

Goldring S., O'Leary J. L., 1954: Correlation between steady transcortical poteniial and evoked response. I. Alterations in somatic receiving area induced by veratrine, strychnine, KCl and novocaine. *EEG Clin. Neurophysiol.* **6**:189—200.

Goldring S., O'Leary J. L., Lam R., 1953: Effect of malonitrile upon the electrocorticogram of the rabbit. *EEG Clin. Neurophysiol.* **5**:395—400.

Gollander M., Ochs S., 1963: Evaluation of EEG depression as an index of spreading depression in chronic preparations. *Amer. Psychologist* **18**:431.

Gorman A. L. F., 1967: Surface versus intracellular polarization of cortical cells. *Nature* **216**:288—289.

Gouras P., 1958: Spreading depression of activity in amphibian retina. *Am. J. Physiol.* **195**:28—32.

Grafstein B., 1956a: Mechanism of spreading cortical depression. *J. Neurophysiol.* **19**:154—171.

Grafstein B., 1956b: Locus of propagation of spreading cortical depression. *J. Neurophysiol.* **19**:308—316.

Grafstein B., 1963: Neuronal release of potassium during spreading depression. In *Brain Function,* Vol. 1, Brazier M. A. B. (ed.). Univ. of California Press, Berkeley, pp. 87—116.

Grafstein B., Sastry P. B., 1957: Some preliminary electrophysiological studies on chronic neuronally isolated cerebral cortex. *EEG Clin. Neurophysiol.* **9**:723—725.

Graul C., 1968: Zum Einfluss der „spreading depression" auf Blutzucker und Plasma-11-Hydroxykortikosteroide der Ratte bei unterschiedlicher Belastung. *Acta Biol. Med. Germ.* **20**:523—526.

Greene E., 1971: Comparison of hippocampal depression and hippocampal lesion. *Exp. Neurol.* **31**: 313—325.

Grossman S. P., Mountford H., 1964: Learning and extinction during chemically induced disturbance of hippocampal functions. *Am. J. Physiol.* **207**:1387—1393.

Gustson P. P., 1963: The effect of cortical depression on evoked responses of the lateral geniculate body (in Russian). *DAN SSSR,* **150**:945—948.

Gutmann W., Brožek G., Bureš J., 1972: Cortical representation of conditioned eye blink in the rabbit studied by a functional ablation technique. *Brain Research* **40**:203—213.

Hall T. L., Thompson R. W., 1971: Interhemispheric transfer as a function of light intensity discrimination difficulty. *J. Comp. Physiol. Psychol.* **77**:166—170.

Hamburg M. D., Best P. J., Cholewiak R. W., 1968: Cortical lesions resulting from chemically induced spreading depression. *J. Comp. Physiol. Psychol.* **66**:492—494.

Hanawa I., Kuge K., Matsumura K., 1967a: Effects of some common ions on the transretinal d-c potential and electroretinogram of the isolated frog retina. *Jap. J. Physiol.* **17**:1—20.

Hanawa I., Kuge K., Matsumura K., 1967b: Studies of the slow depressive potential of the isolated frog retina. *Jap. J. Physiol.* **17**:321—334.

Hanawa I., Kuge K., Matsumura K., 1968: Mechanism of the slow depressive potential production in the isolated frog retina. *Jap. J. Physiol.* **18**:59—70.

Harmony T., 1969: *Caracteristicas Electrofisiologicas y Metabolicas del Foco Epileptico Cortical.* Thesis. Centro Nacional de Investigaciones cientificas, Habana, Cuba.

Harmony T., Fernandez-Bouzas A., Toro A., Szava S., 1973: The epileptogenic effect of disodiumacetate (Na_2 EDTA) topical treatment of rat cerebral cortex. *Physiol. Bohemoslov.* **22**:

Harris L. S., 1961: The effect of various anticholinergic drugs on spontaneous activity of mice. *Fed. Proc.* **20**:395.

Hart J. B., Geyer M. A., 1971: Selective block of reversal memory by physostigmine injection, hippocampal depression, or cortical spreading depression. *Fed. Proc.* **30**:389.

Heald P. J., 1954: Rapid changes in creatine phosphate level in cerebral cortex slices. *Biochem. J.* **57**: 673—679.

Hendrickson C. W., Pinto-Hamuy T., 1967: Nonretention of a visual conditioned heart-rate response under neocortical spreading depression. *J. Comp. Physiol. Psychol.* **64**:510—513.

Hernandez Peon R., Scherrer H., 1955: Habituation to acoustic stimuli in cochlear nucleus. *Fed. Proc.* **14**:71.

Hertz L., 1965: Possible role of neuroglia: A potassium-mediated neuronal-neuroglial-neuronal impulse transmission system. *Nature* **206**:1091.

Hertz L., 1966: Neuroglia localization of potassium and sodium effects on respiration in brain. *J. Neurochem.* **13**:1373—1387.

Hertz L., 1968: Potassium effect on ion transport in brain slices. *J. Neurochem.* **15**:1—16.

Hertz L., Clausen T., 1963: Effect of potassium and sodium on respiration: their specificity in slices from certain brain regions. *J. Biochem.* **89**:526—533.

Herz A., Zieglgänsberger W., Färber G., 1969: Microelectrophoretic studies concerning the spread of glutamic acid and GABA in brain tissue. *Exp. Brain Res.* **9**:221—235.

Hestrin S., 1949: The reaction of acetylcholine and other carboxylic acid derivatives with puroxylamine and its analytical application. *J. Biol. Chem.* **180**:249—256.

Heuser G., Buchwald N. A., Wyers E. J., 1961: The "caudate spindle". II. Facilitatory and inhibitory caudate—cortical pathways. *EEG Clin. Neurophysiol.* **13**:519—524.

Higashida H., Miyake A., Tarao M., Watanabe S., 1971: Membrane potential changes of neuroglial cells during spreading depression in the rabbit. *Brain Research* **32**:207—211.

Hillman H. H., Campbell W. J., McIlwain H., 1963: Membrane potentials in isolated and electrically stimulated mammalian cerebral cortex. Effects of chlorpromazine, cocaine, phenobarbitone, and protamine on the tissue's electrical and chemical responses to stimulation. *J. Neurochem.* **10**:325—339.

Hillman H. H., McIlwain H., 1961: Membrane potentials in mammalian cerebral tissues in vitro: Dependence on ionic environment. *J. Physiol.* **157**:263—278.

Hines M., 1936: The anterior border of monkey's *(Macaca mulatta)* motor cortex and the production of spasticity. *Am. J. Physiol.* **116**:78.

Hirsch H., Scholl H., Dickmans H. A., Eisolt J., Gaehtgens P., Mann H., Krankenhagen B., 1968: Die corticale Gleichspannung des Hundegehirns bei Veränderung des arteriellen pO_2 und pCO_2. *Pflügers Arch.* **301**:344—350.

Hirsch H., Scholl H., Dickmans H. A., Eisolt J., Mann H., Krankenhagen B., 1968: Über die corticale Gleichspannung nach Überschreiten der Wiederbelebungszeit des Gehirns. *Pflügers Arch.* **301**:351—357.

Hirsch H., Scholl H., Paschke K. G., Schmid-Schönbein H., 1968: Die Veränderung der corticalen Gleichspannung bei kompletter und inkompletter Ischämie des Gehirns. *Pflügers Arch.* **301**:334—343.

Hjelle L. A., Thompson R. W., 1965: Retention of an avoidance response learned under bilateral spreading depression. *Psychol. Reports* **16**:1153—1156.

Höber R., 1945: *Physical Chemistry of Cells and Tissues.* Blakiston, Philadelphia.

Hodgkin A. L., 1958: Ionic movements and electrical activity in giant nerve fibers, *Proc. Roy. Soc. B.* **148**:1—37.

Hodgkin A. L., 1963: quoted by Grafstein (1963).

Hodgkin A. L., Katz B., 1949: The effect of sodium ions on the electrical activity of the giant axon of the squid. *J. Physiol.* **108**:37—77.

Hodgkin A. L., Keynes R. P., 1955: Active transport of cations in giant axons from *Sepia* and *Loligo*. *J. Physiol.* **128**:28—60.

Hodgkin A. L., Rushton W. A. H., 1964: The electrical constants of a crustacean nerve fiber. *Proc. Roy. Soc. B.* **133**:444—479.

Hogberg D. K., 1968: The effects of cortical spreading depression, tectal and cortical lesions and caffeine on optokinetic nystagmus habituation and reflex rebound in the painted turtle. *Diss. Abstr.* **29**:786.

Holdstock T., Schwartzbaum J., 1965: Classical conditioning of heart rate and GSR in the rat. *Psychophysiol.* **2**:25—38.

Holmgren B., 1966: Drug-dependent conditioned reflexes. In *Cortico-Subcortical Relationships in Sensory Regulation.* Gonzalez Martin D. and Guma E. (eds.). Acad. Sci., Havana pp. 342—355.

Holubář J., Fischer J., 1967: Electrophysiological properties of the epileptogenic cortical foci produced by a new cobalt-gelatine method in rats. An attempt to correlate the electrophysiological, histological and histochemical data. *Physiol. Bohemoslov.* **16**:278—284.

Horn G., 1967: Neuronal mechanisms of habituation. *Nature* **215**:707—711.

Horridge G. A., 1956: The nerves and muscles of medusae. V. Double innervation in Scyphozoa. *J. Exp. Biol.* **33**:366—383.

Hossman K. A., 1971: Cortical steady potential, impedance and excitability changes during and after total ischemia of cat brain. *Exp. Neurol.* **32**:163—175.

Hugelin A., Bonvallet M., 1957a: Tonus cortical et controle de la facilitation motrice d'origin réticulaire. *J. Physiol.* (Paris) **49**:1171—1200.

Hugelin A., Bonvallet M., 1957b: Interrelations réticulo—corticales. *J. Physiol.* (Paris) **49**:1201—1223.

Hughes R. A., 1969: Retrograde amnesia in rats produced by hippocampal injections of potassium chloride: Gradient of effect and recovery. *J. Comp. Physiol. Psychol.* **68**:637—644.

Huizar Sánchez P., Garcia Ramos J., 1969: Spreading redox potentials in the cat's cortex. *Acta Physiol. Latino-Amer.* **19**:30—42.

Hull C., Buchwald N., 1968: Effects of subcortically induced spreading depression on behavior. *Anat. Rec.* **160**:368—369.

Hull C. D., Buchwald N. A., Ling G., 1967: Effects of direct cholinergic stimulation of forebrain structures. *Brain Res.* **6**:22—35.

Hull C. D., Buchwald N. A., Vieth J. B., 1967: Cortical intracellular analyses of responses to inhibitory and desinhibitory stimuli. *Brain Res.* **6**:12—21.

Hull C. D., Van Harreveld A., 1964: Absence of conduction of spreading depression through cortical regions damaged by asphyxiation. *Am. J. Physiol.* **207**:921—924.

Huston J., 1971: Yawning and penile erection induced in rats by cortical spreading depression. *Nature* **232**:274—275.

Huston J. P., Brožek G., 1971: Arousal of consummatory behaviour in rabbits by single waves of cortical spreading depression. *Physiol. Behav.* **7**:595—599.

Huston J. P., Bureš J., 1970: Drinking and eating elicited by cortical spreading depression. *Science* **169**:702—704.

Huston J. P., Bureš J., 1973: Effects of cortical spreading depression on behaviors elicited by hypothalamic stimulation in rats. *Physiol. Behav.* **10**:775—780

Hydén H., 1959: Biochemical changes in glial cells and nerve cells of varying activity. *Proc. IV Int. Congr. Biochem.*, Symp. III, Brücke F., (ed.), Pergamon Press, New York p. 64.

Hydén H., Egyházi E., 1963: Glial RNA changes during a learning experiment in rats. *Proc. Nat. Acad. Sci.* **49**:618—624.

Ichijo M., Ochs S., 1967: Effect of spreading depression on the N-wave DCR and on Betz cells. *Physiologist* **10**:209.

Ichijo M., Ochs S., 1970: Spreading depression of negative wave of direct cortical response and pyramidal tract response. *Brain Res.* **23**:41—56.

Ito K., 1960: Metabolic relationship of succinate and pyruvate in brain tissue with special reference to the potassium effect. *Jap. J. Exp. Med.* **30**:261—277.

Janebová M., 1967: Cortical spreading depression as a means of analyzing the role of the thalamic gustatory area in taste discrimination in rats. *Physiol. Bohemoslov.* **16**:18—22.

Janebová M., 1971: Initiation of Leão's spreading depression by electrophoretic application of threshold dosages of potassium ions. *Physiol. Bohemoslov.* **20**:447—451.

Jasper H., Stefanis G., 1965: Intracellular oscillatory rhythms in pyramidal tract neurones in the cat. *EEG Clin. Neurophysiol.* **18**:541—553.

Jílek L., Trojan S., 1968: *Ontogenesis of the Brain.* Proc. Int. Symp. Univ. Karlova, Praha.

John E. R., Tschirgi R. D., Wenzel B. M., 1959: Effects of injections of cations into the cerebral ventricles on conditioned responses in the cat. *J. Physiol.* **146**:550—563.

Johnson J. D., Gazzaniga M. S., 1970: Interhemispheric imitation in split brain monkeys. *Exp. Neurol.* **27**:206—212.

Johnson J. D., Gazzaniga M. S., 1971: Reversal behavior in split-brain monkeys. *Physiol. Behav.* **6**: 707—709.

Johnson W. L., Goldring S., O'Leary J. L., 1965: Behavioral, unit and slow potential changes in methionine sulfoximine seizures. *EEG Clin. Neurophysiol.* **18**:229—238.

Jonec V., 1964: Spreading depression and adrenocortical function in the adaptation of the organism to repeated short-term stress. *Activitas Nerv. Sup.* **6**:32—33.

Jouvet M., 1962: Recherches sur les structures nerveuses et les mécanismes responsables des differentes phases du sommeil physiologique. *Arch. Ital. Biol.* **100**:125—206.

Kapp B. S., Schneider A. M., 1971: Selective recovery from retrograde amnesia produced by hippocampal spreading depression. *Science* **173**:1149—1151.

Karahashi Y., Goldring S., 1966: Intracellular potentials form "idle" cells in cerebral cortex of cat. *EEG Clin. Neurophysiol.* **20**:600—607.

Kato G., Somjen G. G., 1969: Effects of microiontophoretic administration of magnesium and calcium on neurons in the central nervous system of cats. *J. Neurobiol.* **1**:181—195.

Katzman R., Leiderman P. H., 1953: Brain potassium exchange in normal adult and immature rats. *Am. J. Physiol.* **175**:263—270.

Kellaway P., Petersen I., 1964: *Neurological and Electroencephalographic Correlative Studies in Infancy.* Grune and Stratton, New York.

Keller H. H., Bartholini G., Pieri L., Pletscher A., 1972: Effect of spreading depression on the turnover of cerebral dopamine. *Europ. J. Pharmacol.* **20**:287—290.

Kelly J. S., Krnjevič K., Somjen G., 1969: Divalent cations and electrical properties of cortical cells. *J. Neurobiol.* **1**:197—208.

Kempinsky W. H., 1954: Steady potential gradients in experimental cerebral vascular occlusion. *EEG Clin. Neurophysiol.* **6**:375—388.

Kerr S. E., Ghantus M., 1936: The carbohydrate metabolism of brain. II. The effect of varying the carbohydrate and insulin supply on the glycogen, free sugar, and lactic acid in mammalian brain. *J. Biochem. Chem.* **116**:9—20.

Kesner R. P., O'Kelly L. I., Thomas G. J., 1965: Effects of cortical spreading depression and drugs upon audiogenic seizures in rats. *J. Comp. Physiol. Psychol.* **59**:280—282.

Kety S. S., 1960: Measurement of local blood flow by the exchange of an inert, diffusible substance. *Met. Med. Res.* **8**:228—236.

King F. A., Marchiava P. L., Moruzzi G., 1963: The time course of the mydriatic response to darkness in the midpontine pretrigeminal cat. *Arch. Ital. Biol.* **101**:545—551.

Kini M. M., Quastel J. H., 1959: Carbohydrate—amino-acid interrelationship in brain cortex in vitro. *Nature* **184**:252—256.

Kinosita H., 1937: Entrapped circuit wave. *Zool. Mag.* (Tokyo) **49**:437—455.

Klee M. R., Lux H. D., 1962: Intracelluläre Untersuchungen über den Einfluss hemmender Potentiale im motorischen Cortex. II. Die Wirkungen elektrischer Reizung des Nucleus caudatus. *Arch. Psychiat. Nervenkr.* **203**:667—689.

Kleinzeller A., Rybová R., 1957: Glycogen synthesis in brain cortex slices and some factors affecting it. *J. Neurochem.* **2**:45—57.

Kohn B., 1967: Spreading depression and stimulus control of interhemispheric transfer. *Neuropsychologia* **5**:275—286.

Koppmann J. W., O'Kelly L. I., 1966: Unilateral cortical spreading depression: A determiner of behavior at a choice point. *J. Comp. Physiol. Psychol.* **62**:237—242.

Korányi L., Endröczi E., Lissák K., 1965: Disinhibition of extinguished conditioned reflex under spreading depression. *Acta Physiol. Ac. Sci. Hung.* **27**:353—357.

Koreli A., Brožek G., 1972: Influence of cortical spreading depression on the habituation of visual evoked responses in the rabbit cortex and hippocampus. *Physiol. bohemoslov.* **21**:90.

Koroleva V. I., 1970: Use of dynamic diagrams in the analysis of the properties of spreading depression (in Russian). *Zh. Vyssh. Nerv. Deyat.* **20**:1295—1297.

Koroleva V. I., Kuznetsova G. D., 1971: Neuronal activity in the focus of cortical spreading depression (in Russian). *Zh. Vyssh. Nerv. Deyat.* **21**:1316—1318.

Koroleva V. I., Kuznetsova G. D., 1972: Properties of spreading depression elicited from two KCl foci in the cerebral cortex of rats. In *Electrical Activity of Brain and Formation of Simple Temporary Connections* (in Russian). Rusinov V. S. (ed.). Nauka, Moscow, pp. 130—144.

Krauthamer G., Albe-Fessard D., 1965: Inhibition of nonspecific sensory activities following striopallidal and capsular stimulation. *J. Neurophysiol.* **28**:100—124.

Křivánek J., 1958: Changes of brain glycogen in the spreading EEG depression of Leão. *J. Neurochem.* **2**:337—343.

Křivánek J., 1959: Incorporation of ^{32}P into the phosphate fractions of the rat brain during spreading EEG depression (in Czech). *Čs. Fysiol.* **8**:417—418.

Křivánek J., 1960: *On the Metabolic Background of the Spreading Cortical Depression* (in Czech). Thesis. Inst. of Physiol., Czechoslovak Acad. Sci., Prague.

Křivánek J., 1961: Some metabolic changes accompanying Leão's spreading cortical depression in the rat. *J. Neurochem.* **6**:183—189.

Křivánek J., 1962: Concerning the dynamics of the metabolic changes accompanying cortical spreading depression. *Physiol. Bohemoslov.* **11**:383—391.

Křivánek J., 1968: Changes in the metabolism of protein, water, and potassium in the course of repeated spreading cortical depression (in Czech). *Čs. Fysiol.* **17**:221.

Kiřvánek J., 1969a: Changes in protein, electrolyte, and water metabolism caused by prolonged spreading cortical depression in rats. *J. Neurobiol.* **1**:147—154.

Křivánek J., 1969b: Concerning the mechanism of potassium ions effect onto incorporation of ^{14}C-leucine into protein of the brain cortex in vivo (in Czech). *Summaries of Vth Natl. Biochem. Cong.*, Brno 1969, p. 6—17.

Křivánek J., 1970: Effect of spreading cortical depression on the incorporation of ^{14}C-leucine into rat brain protein. *J. Neurochem.* **17**:531—538.

Křivánek J., 1972a: Spreading cortical depression and acetylcholinesterase activity in rat cerebral cortex. *Physiol. bohemoslov.* **21**:163—169.

Křivánek J., 1972b: Incorporation of ^{14}C from glucose into glycogen and some amino acids of the cerebral cortex under influence of potassium ions in vivo. *Physiol. bohemoslov.* **21**:615—612.

Křivánek J., Bureš J., 1960: Ion shifts during Leão's spreading cortical depression. *Physiol. Bohemoslov.* **9**:494—503.

Křivánek J., Bureš J., Burešová O., 1958: Evidence for a relationship between creatine phosphate level and polarity of the cerebral cortex. *Nature* **182**:1799.

Křivánek J., Bureš J., Burešová O., 1959: The relationship between the level of certain brain metabolites and the degree of cortical polarity following temporary ischemia of the brain in rats. *Physiol. Bohemoslov.* **8**:195—202.

Křivánek J., Fifková E., 1965: The value of ultramicroanalysis of lactic acid in tracing the penetration of Leão's cortical spreading depression. *J. Neurol. Sci.* **2**:385—392.

Krnjević K., 1965: Action of drugs on single neurons in the cerebral cortex. *Brit. Med. Bull.* **21**:10—14.

Krnjević K., Mitchell J. F., 1960: Diffusion of acetylcholine in agar gels and in the isolated rat diaphragm. *J. Physiol.* **153**:562—572.

Krnjević K., Phillis J. W., 1963: Iontophoretic studies of neurons in the mammalian cerebral cortex. *J. Physiol.* **165**:274—304.

Krnjevič K., Randič M., 1965: Cortical inhibition and spreading depression. *Abstr. XXIII Int. Congr. Physiol. Sci. Tokyo*, p. 395.

Krnjevič K., Randič M., Straughan D. W., 1966: An inhibitory process in the cerebral cortex. *J. Physiol.* **184**:16—48.

Krushinsky L. V., 1954: Studies on interrelationship between excitation and inhibition in normal and pathological conditions by the method of acoustic stimulation (in Russian). *Uspekhi Sovr. Biol.* **37**: 74—93.

Kuffler S. W., 1967: Neuroglial cells: Physiological properties and potassium mediated effect of neuronal activity on the glial membrane potential. *Proc. Roy. Soc. B.* **168**:1—21.

Kukleta M., 1965a: Les liaisons temporaires localisées sous le cortex de cerveau. *Arch. Int. Physiol. Biochem.* **73**:696—703.

Kukleta M., 1965b: Preuve de localisation sous-corticale des traces de mémoire dans le cerveau du rat. *Scripta medica* **38**:19—31.

Kukleta M., 1966: Application de la dépression envahissante à l'étude de la localisation des traces de mémoire. *Physiol. Behav.* **1**:229—232.

Kukleta M., 1967: The use of unilateral cortical spreading depression in the study of subcortical storage of memory traces in rats. *Physiol. Behav.* **2**:301—304.

Kukleta M., 1968a: Memory components of shock escape reaction in rat. *Physiol. Behav.* **3**:773—776.

Kukleta M., 1968b: Active avoidance behaviour of rats under unilateral cortical spreading depression. *Scripta medica* **41**:259—264.

Kukleta M., Libouban S., 1967: Acquisition du conditionnement instrumental chez les rats fonctionnellement décortiqués. *J. Physiol.* (Paris) **59**:442.

Kulikova V. S., 1964: *The Role of Cerebral Cortex in the Unconditioned Control of Blood Sugar Level* (in Russian). Dissertation, Pavlov's Institute of Physiology, Academy of Sciences, Leningrad.

Kunc L., 1964: The effect of unilateral cortical spreading depression on feeding behavior in rats (in Czech). *Čs. Fysiol.* **13**:217.

Kunc L., 1971: Asymmetry of hemispheres studied by means of unilateral cortical spreading depression in rats. *Activitas Nervosa Superior* **13**:13—17.

Kunc L., Kukleta M., 1965: Functional asymmetry in the effect of unilateral spreading depression in rats. *Activitas Nervosa Superior* **7**:163—164.

Kupferman I., 1965: Failure of spreading depression to produce retrograde amnesia. *Psychon. Sci.* **3**:43—44.

Kupferman I., 1966: Is the retrograde amnesia that follows cortical spreading depression due to subcortical spread? *J. Comp. Physiol. Psychol.* **6**:466—467.

Kurayev G. A., 1967: On the inhibitory effect of neostriatal bodies on conditioned reflexes in lower monkeys (in Russian). *Zh. Vyssh. Nerv. Deyat.* **17**:747—749.

Laget P., Neverlée H. de, 1962: Évolution de la dépression envahissante et du potential stable dans l'éveil cortical. *J. Physiol.* (Paris) **54**:362—363.

Laget P., Neverlée H. de, 1963: Étude du potential stable et de la dépression envahissante chez le lapin en cours de développement. *J. Physiol.* (Paris) **55**:278—279.

La Grutta V., Abbadessa S., Avelone S., Commare A. F., 1966: Les réponses évoquées de noyau caudé à la suite modifications de l'excitabilité de l'aire auditive primaire. *Arch. Int. Physiol. Bioch.* **74**:837—844.

Langford A., Freedman N., Whitman D., 1971: Further determinants of interhemispheric transfer under spreading depression. *Physiol. Behav.* **7**:65—71.

Larsson K., 1962: Spreading cortical depression and the mating behavior in male and female rats. *Zeitschrift für Tierpsychologie* **19**:321—331.

Lashley K. S., 1929: *Brain Mechanisms and Intelligence.* Univ. Chicago Press, Chicago.

Lashley K. S., 1950: In search of the engram. *Symp. Soc. Exptl. Biol.* **4**:454—482.

Laursen A. M., 1963: Corpus striatum. *Acta Physiol. Scand.*, Suppl. 211

Leão A. A. P., 1944a: Spreading depression of activity in the cerebral cortex. *J. Neurophysiol.* **7**: 359—390.

Leão A. A. P., 1944b: Pial circulation and spreading depression of activity in cerebral cortex. *J. Neurophysiol.* **7**:391—396.

Leão A. A. P., 1947: Further observations on the spreading depression of activity in the cerebral cortex. *J. Neurophysiol.* **10**:409—419.

Leão A. A. P., 1951: The slow voltage variation of cortical spreading depression of activity. *EEG Clin. Neurophysiol.* **3**:315—321.

Leão A. A. P., 1954: Circulação na pia-mater e depressão alastrante da atividade do córtex cerebral. *An. Acad. Brasil. Ci.* **26**:XXII—XXIII.

Leão A. A. P., 1961: Composição iônica extracelular a depressão alastrante. *An. Acad. Brasil Ci.* **33**: XXXVIII—XXXIX.

Leão A. A. P., 1963: On the spread of spreading depression. In *Brain Function,* Vol. 1, M. A. B. Brazier (ed.) Univ. California Press, Berkeley, pp. 78—85.

Leão A. A. P., Martins-Ferreira H. M., 1953: Alteração da impedancia elétrica no decurso da depressão alastrante da atividade do córtex cerebral. *An. Acad. Brasil. Ci.* **25**:259—266.

Leão A. A. P., Martins-Ferreira H. M., 1954: Iniciaçao da depressão alastrante da atividade do córtex cerebral por aplicaçao local de agentes quimicos. *An. Acad. Brasil. Ci.* **26**:XVII.

Leão A. A. P., Martins-Ferreira H. M., 1956: Condições necessárias para a ocorrência da depressão alastrante. *An. Acad. Brasil. Ci.* **28**:XV.

Leão A. A. P., Martins-Ferreira H., 1958: Nota sôbre a ocorrência da depressão alastrante no hippocampo e no corpo estriado. *An. Acad. Brasil. Ci.* **30**:I.

Leão A. A. P., Martins-Ferreira H., 1959: The negative voltage variation of spreading depression and circulatory arrest. XXI Int. Congr. Physiol. Sci. Buenos Aires, Abstr. of Comm. p. 160.

Leão A. A. P., Martins-Ferreira H., 1961: Nota acêrca da depressão alastrante no cerebelo, tubérculo quadrigemino anterior e bulbo olfativo. *An. Acad. Bras. Ci.* **33**:XXXIX—XL.

Leão A. A. P., Martins-Ferreira H., 1963: Nota acêrca de variação lenta de voltagem da depressão alastrante no bulbo olfativo. *An. Acad. Brasil. Ci.* **35**:I—II.

Leão A. A. P., Martins-Ferreira H., 1965: Efeito do potássio sobre a variação lenta de voltagem da depressão alastrante. *Ciencia e Cultura* **17**:279—280.

Leão A. A. P., Morrison R. S., 1945: Propagation of spreading cortical depression. *J. Neurophysiol.* **8**:33—45.

Levitt R. A., Krikstone B. J., 1968: Cortical spreading depression and thirst. *Physiol. Behav.* **3**:421—423.

Li C. L., McIlwain H., 1957: Maintenance of resting membrane potentials in slices of mammalian cerebral cortex and other tissues in vitro. *J. Physiol.* **139**:178—190.

Li C. L., Salmoiraghi G. C., 1963: Cortical steady potential changes: Extracellular microelectrode investigations. *Nature* **198**:858—859.

Libet B., Gerard R. W., 1938: Chemical control of potentials of the isolated frog brain. *Am. J. Physiol.* **123**:128.

Libet B., Gerard R. W., 1941: Steady potential fields and neuron activity. *J. Neurophysiol.* **4**:438—455.

Lipsett M. N., Crescitelli F., 1950: The effects of increased potassium concentration on the metabolism of cat cerebral cortical slices. *Arch. Biochem.* **28**:329—337.

Lishman W. A., Eayrs J. T., 1966: Localization of a memory trace in the intact rat. *Physiol. Behav.* **1**:161—166.

Lowry O. H., Passouneau J., 1964: The relation between substrates and enzymes of glycolysis in brain. *J. Biol. Chem.* **239**:31—42.

Lowry O. H., Roberts N. R., Leiner K. Y., Wu M.-L., Farr A. L., Albers R. W., 1954: The quantitative histochemistry of brain. III. Ammon's horn. *Biol. Chem.* **207**:39—49.

Lucco J. V., Aranda L. C., 1964: An electrical correlate to the process of learning. *Acta Physiol. Latino-Amer.* **14**:274—288.

Lukyanova L. D., Bureš J., 1967: Changes in pO_2 due to spreading depression in the cortex and nucleus caudatus of the rat. *Physiol. Bohemoslov.* **16**:449—455.

Lund R. D., 1965: Uncrossed visual pathways of hooded and albino rats. *Science* **149**:1506—1507.

Lux H. D., Klee M. R., 1962: Untersuchungen über den Einfluss hemmender Potentiale im motorischen Cortex. 1. Die Wirkung elektrischer Reizung unspezifischer Thalamuskerne. *Arch. Psychiat. Nervenkr.* **203**:648—666.

Machek J., Saier J., Desplan C., Naquet R., 1963: Étude de la crise cardiazolique après thalamectomie. *J. Physiol.* (Paris) **55**:290—291.

MacLean P. D., 1958: Contrasting functions of limbic and neocortical systems of the brain and their relevance to psychophysiological aspects of medicine. *Am. J. Med.* **25**:611—626.

Magni F., Moruzzi G., Rossi G. F., Zanchetti A., 1959: EEG arousal following inactivation of the lower brain stem by selective injection of barbiturate into lower brain stem circulation. *Arch. Ital. Biol.* **97**:33—46.

Magun R., Ross J., 1954: Untersuchungen über die fortschreitende Reduktion ("spreading depression") der corticalen Spontanaktivität. *Dtsch. Nervenheilk.* **171**:403—415.

Malakhovskaya D. B., 1972: The effect of cortical spreading depression on the conditioned cleaning reflex in young rabbits (in Russian) *Zh. Vyssh. Nerv. Deyat.* **22**:89—95.

Malecki J., Borkowska B., Krzywosinski L., Malinowska O., 1968: The influence of cortical spreading depression on development of experimental gastric ulcers in rats. *Acta Physiol. Polonica* **19**:273—278.

Malliani A., Purpura D. P., 1967: Intracellular studies of the corpus striatum. II. Patterns of synaptic activities in lenticular and entopeduncular neurons. *Brain Res.* **6**:341—354.

Malyshenko N. M., 1969: The use of spreading depression for studying the effect of estrogen on the bioelectrical activity of the brain of intact and ovariectomized albino rat (in Russian). *Probl. Endokr.* **15**:99—104.

Mareš P., 1964: Ontogenetic development of membrane potentials in telencephalic structures in the rat. *Physiol. Bohemoslov.* **13**:256—262.

Marshall W. H., 1950: Relation of dehydration of brain to spreading depression of Leão. *EEG Clin. Neurophysiol.* **2**:177—185.

Marshall W. H., 1952: Conditions for recording spreading depression. *EEG Clin. Neurophysiol.* **4**:223—224.

Marshall W. H., 1959: Spreading cortical depression of Leão. *Physiol. Rev.* **39**:239—279.

Marshall W. H., 1965: Quelques problèmes de neurophysiologie générale du cerveau. *Actualités Neurophysiologiques* **6**:43—54.

Marshall W. H., Essig C. F., 1951: Relation of air exposure of cortex to spreading depression of Leão. *J. Neurophysiol.* **14**:265—273.

Marshall W. H., Essig C. F., Dubroff S. J., 1951: Relation of temperature of cerebral cortex to spreading depression of Leão. *J. Neurophysiol.* **14**:153—166.

Marshall W. H., Essig C. F., Witkin L. B., 1951: Spreading depression. *Am. J. Physiol.* **167**:808.

Martins-Ferreira H., 1954: Variações lentas de voltagem do cortex cerebral. Thesis. Instituto de Biofisica, Rio de Janeiro.

Martins-Ferreira H., 1955a: Variações lentas de voltagem do córtex cerebral por aplicação local de substancia químicas. *An. Acad. Brasil. Ci.* **27**:24.

Martins-Ferreira H., 1955b: Variações lentas de voltagem durante a depressão alastrante. *An. Acad. Brasil. Ci.* **27**:24—25.

Martins-Ferreira H., 1962: Depressão alastrante na retina. *An. Acad. Brasil. Ci.* **34**:XLIV.

Martins-Ferreira H., Leão A. A. P., 1958: Nota sôbre o estudo da depressão alastrante em répteis. *An. Acad. Brasil. Ci.* **30**:I.

Martins-Ferreira H., de Oliveira Castro G., 1964: Variações de luz difundida na retina durante a depressão alastrante. *An. Acad. Brasil. Ci.* **36**:243.

Martins-Ferreira H., de Oliveira Castro G., 1965: Alteração da impedancia elétrica da retina durante a depressão alastrante. *An. Acad. Brasil. Ci.* **37**:364.

Martins-Ferreira H., de Oliveira Castro G., 1966: Light-scattering changes accompanying spreading depression in isolated retina. *J. Neurophysiol.* **29**:715—726.

Martins-Ferreira H., de Oliveira Castro G. 1969: Electric impedance changes accompanying spreading depression in isolated retina. *An. Acad. Brasil. Ci.* **41**:4.

Mase K., Takahashi U., Ogata K., 1962: The incorporation of (^{14}C) glycine into the protein of guinea-pig brain cortex slices. *J. Neurochem.* **9**:281—288.

Massion J., Meulders M., 1961: Les potentiels évoqués visuels et auditifs du centre médian et leurs modifications après décortication. *Arch. Int. Physiol. Bioch.* **69**:26—29.

Matsuura T., Bureš J., 1971: The minimum volume of depolarized neural tissue required for triggering cortical spreading depression in rat. *Exp. Brain Res.* **12**:238—249.

Mayes A. R., 1973: Disruption of the interhemispheric transfer of active avoidance learnt during unilateral cortical spreading depression. *Behavioral Biology* **8**:207—217.

Mayes A. R., Cowey A., 1973: The interhemispheric transfer of avoidance learning: an examination of the stimulus control hypothesis. *Behavioral Biology* **8**:193—205.

McGaugh J. L., Madsen M. C., 1964: Amnesic and punishing effects of electroconvulsive shock. *Science* **144**:182—183.

McIlwain H., 1954: Electrically excited metabolism of separated mammalian cerebral tissues. *EEG Clin. Neurophysiol.* **6**:93—101.

Megirian D., Bureš J., 1970: Unilateral cortical spreading depression and conditioned eyeblink responses in the rabbit. *Exp. Neurol.* **27**:34—45.

Meikle T. H., Sechzer J. A., 1960: Interocular transfer of brightness discrimination in "split brain" cats. *Science* **132**:734—735.

Meikle T. H., Sechzer J. A., Stellar E., 1962: Interhemispheric transfer of tactile conditioned responses in corpus callosum sectioned cats. *J. Neurophysiol.* **25**:530—543.

Mello A. C. de, Silva M. G. da, 1960: Nota sôbre a variação lenta de voltagem da depressão alastrante no neocortex em condições de hipoglicemia. *An. Acad. Brasil Ci.* **32**:XXVI.

Mennear J. H., 1965: Interactions between central cholinergic agents and amphetamine in mice. *Psychopharmacol.* **7**:107—114.

Meschersky R. M., Gustson P. P., 1964: Cortical modulation of primary responses in lateral geniculate body. *Physiol. Bohemoslov.* **13**:236—241.

Mettler F. A., Culler E., 1934: Action of drugs on the chronic decorticated preparation. *J. Pharmacol.* **52**:366.

Meyer D. R., Isaac W., Maher B., 1958: The role of stimulation in spontaneous reorganization of visual habits. *J. Comp. Physiol. Psychol.* **51**:546—548.

Meyer J. S., Denny-Brown D., 1955: Studies of cerebral circulation in brain injury. II. Cerebral concussion. *EEG Clin. Neurophysiol.* **7**:529—544.

Meyer J. S., Gotoh F., Tazaki Y., 1961: Inhibitory action of carbone dioxide and acetazolamide in seizure activity. *EEG Clin. Neurophysiol.* **13**:762—775.

Meyers B., Stern W. C., 1966: Effect of bilateral spreading depression and scopolamine on motor activity in rats. *Psychol. Reports* **18**:267—270.

Mogenson G. J., 1965: Effect of spreading cortical depression on avoidance responses conditioned to peripheral or central stimulation. *EEG Clin. Neurophysiol.* **18**:663—669.

Mogenson G. J., Peterson R. J., 1966: Effects of spreading cortical depression on cardiac and somatomotor conditioned responses. *Can. J. Physiol. Pharmacol.* **44**:39—45.

Monakhov K. K., Fifková E., Bureš J., 1962a: Vertical distribution of the slow potential change of spreading depression in the cerebral cortex of the rat. *Physiol. Bohemoslov.* **11**:269—276.

Monakhov K. K., Fifková E., Bureš J., 1962b: Steady potential field of hippocampal spreading depression. *J. Cell. Comp. Physiol.* **59**:155—161.

Montemurro D. G., Stevenson J. A. F., 1957: Adipsia produced by hypothalamic lesions in the rat. *Can. J. Biochem. Physiol.* **35**:31—37.

Morlock N. L., Mori K., Ward A. A. Jr., 1964: A study of single cortical neurons during spreading depression. *J. Neurophysiol.* **27**:1192—1198.

Morrison R. S., Dempsey E. W., 1942: A study of thalamocortical relations. *Am. J. Physiol.* **135**:281—292.

Muñoz-Martínez E. J., 1968: Effect of spreading depression on the activation of corticospinal tract. *Proc. Int. Union. Physiol. Sci.* **7**:308.

Muñoz-Martínez E. J., 1970: Facilitation of cortical cell activity during spreading depression. *J. Neurobiol.* **2**:47—60.

Myers R. E., 1957: Corpus callosum and interhemispheric communication: Enduring memory effects. *Fed. Proc.* **16**:398.

Myers R. E., Sperry R. W., 1958: Interhemispheric communication through the corpus callosum. *Arch. Neurol. Psychiat.* **80**:298—303.

Myslivečk J., Hassmannová J., Springer V., 1962: An attempt to analyze the higher nervous activity with eliminated cerebral cortex. *Activitas Nerv. Sup.* **4**:125—126.

Myslivecek J., Hassmannová J., Springer V., 1964: Experimental analysis of the higher nervous activity in rats with bilateral and unilateral elimination of cerebral hemispheres (spreading depression) (in Czech). *Čas. Lék. Čes.* **103**:140—146.

Nadel L., 1966: Cortical spreading depression and habituation. *Psychon. Sci.* **5**:119—120.

Nadel L., 1971: Interhemispheric transfer: monocular input and varied sensory conditions. *Physiol. Behav.* **6**:655—661.

Nadel L., Burešová O., 1968: Monocular input and interhemispheric transfer in the reversible split brain. *Nature* **220**:914—915.

Nadel L., Burešová O., 1969: Interocular transfer in the hooded rat. *Physiol. Behav.* **4**:613—619.

Nadel L., Burešová O., 1970: Monocular input and interhemispheric transfer: Reversed transfer trials. *Commun. Behav. Biology.* Part A. **5**:63—66.

Narahashi T., Moore J. W., Scott W. R., 1964: Tetrodotoxin blockage of sodium conductance increase in lobster giant axons. *J. Gen. Physiol.* **47**:965—974.

Narikashvili S. P., 1963: Cortico—subcortical interaction in the activity of analyzers (in Russian). *Fiz. Zh. SSSR* **49**:1303—1309.

Néverlée H. de, 1966: Modifications des potentiels évoqués somatique et visuel durant la "spreading depression" corticale chez le lapin en cours de dévelopment. *J. Physiol.* (Paris) **58**:573.

Néverlée H. de, Laget P., 1965: Propagation de la "dépression envahissante" (spreading depression) et maturation corticale régionale chez le jeune lapin. *C. R. Soc. Biol.* **159**:1332—1337.

Néverlée H. de, Laget P., 1966: Sensibilité des différentes aires corticales à la dépression envahissante (spreading depression) au cours de la maturation chez le jeune lapin. *J. Physiol.* (Paris) **58**:574.

Néverlée H. de, Laget P., 1967: Depression envahissante homo - et contralatérale au cours de la maturation corticale; effets de l'abaissement de la température. *C. R. Soc. Biol.* **161**:237—244

Noble D., Hall A. E., 1963: The conditions for initiating "all-or-nothing" repolarization in cardiac muscle. *Biophysical J.* **3**:261—273.

Norton S., Jewett R. E., 1966: A pyrrolopyrimidine with depressant actions on the CNS. *J. Pharmacol. Exptl. Ther.* **154**:152—160.

Norton S., Jewett R. E., 1967: Effects of prolonged EEG suppression by a pyrrolopyrimidine on learned behavior. *Physiol. Behav.* **2**:317—322.

Ochs S., 1958: Effects of spreading depression on direct cortical response studied with an island technique. *J. Neurophysiol.* **21**:159—170.

Ochs S., 1962: The nature of spreading depression in neural networks. *Int. Rev. Neurobiol.* **4**:1—69.

Ochs S., Hunt K., 1960: Apical dendrites and propagation of spreading depression in cerebral cortex. *J. Neurophysiol.* **23**:432—444.

Ochs S., Hunt K., Booker H., 1961: Spreading depression using chronically implanted electrodes. *Am. J. Physiol.* **200**:1211—1214.

Olds J., 1962: Spreading depression and hypothalamic behavior mechanisms. *Fed. Proc.* **21**:648—658.

Okamoto K., Quastel J. H., 1970: Tetrodotoxin-sensitive uptake of ions and water by slices of rat brain in vitro. *Biochem. J.* **120**:37—47.

Oliveira Castro G. de, 1966: Branching pattern of amacrine cell processes. *Nature* **212**:832—834.

Oliveira Castro G. de, Martins-Ferreira H., 1968: Deformações e variações de espessura da retina durante a depressão alastrante. An. Acad. brasil. Ci. **40**:3

Oliveira Castro G. de, Martins-Ferreira H., 1970: Deformations and thickness variations accompanying spreading depression in the retina. *J. Neurophysiol.* **33**:891—900.

Ookawa T., Bureš J., 1969: Spreading depression in the striatum and optic lobes of the chicken. *Brain Res.* **13**:119—128.

Ookawa T., Gotoh J., 1964: Spreading EEG depression in chickens. *Poultry Sci.* **43**:1294—1296.

Opitz E., Thorn W., 1949: Überlebenszeit und Erholungszeit des Warmblütergehirns unter dem Einfluss der Höhenanpassung. *Pflügers Arch.* **251**:369—387.

Orkand R. K., Nicholls J. G., Kuffler S. W., 1966: The effect of nerve impulses on the membrane potential of glial cells in the central nervous system in amphibia. *J. Neurophysiol.* **29**:788—806.

Overton D. A., 1964: State dependent or "dissociated" learning with pentobarbital. *J. Comp. Physiol. Psychol.* **57**:3—12.

Paderni M. A., Giammanco S., 1967: L'importanza dell' area somestesica nelle risposte evocate dal nucleo caudato per stimulazione del nervo sciatico controlaterale, nel gatto. *Boll. Soc. Ital. Biol. Sper.* **43**:1283—1286.

Paderni M. A., Giammanco S., 1968: Le correlazioni tra corteccia cerebrale e nucleo caudato studiate con l'impiego della "spreading depression" de Leão. *Arch. Fisiol.* **66**:19—41.

Paolino R. M., Levy H. M., 1970: A cannula assembly for inducing cortical spreading depression in free-moving animals. *Physiol. Behav.* **5**:1499—1500.

Paolino R. M., Levy H. M., 1971: Amnesia produced by spreading depression and ECS: Evidence for time-dependent memory trace localization. *Science* **172**:746—749.

Pape L. G., Katzman R., 1972a: K^{42} distribution in brain during simultaneous ventriculocisternal and subarachnoid perfusion. *Brain Research* **38**:49—69.

Pape L. G., Katzman R., 1972b: Response of glia in cat sensorimotor cortex to increased extracellular potassium. *Brain Research* **38**:71—92.

Papez J. W., 1937: A proposed mechanism of emotion. *Arch. Neurol. Psychiat.* **38**:725—743.

Pearlman Ch. A., Jarvik M. E., 1961: Retrograde amnesia produced by spreading cortical depression. *Fed. Proc.* **20,** Part I.:340

Pearlman Ch. A. Jr., 1966: Similar retrograde amnesic effects of ether and spreading cortical depression. *J. Comp. Physiol. Psychol.* **61**:306—308.

Peterson G. M., Devine J. V., 1963: Transfer in handedness in the rat resulting from small cortical lesions after limited forced practice. *J. Comp. Physiol. Psychol.* **56**:752—756.

Petsche H., Stumpf C., Gogolák G., 1962: The significance of the rabbit's septum as a relay station between midbrain and the hippocampus. I. Control of hippocampus arousal activity by septum cells. *EEG Clin. Neurophysiol.* **14**:202—211.

Phillis J. W., Ochs S., 1971: Excitation and depression of cortical neurones during spreading depression. *Exp. Brain Research* **12**:132—149.

Pick E. P., 1937: Über Änderung energetischer Vorgänge im Gehirn durch Schlaf und Erregungsmittel und deren örtliche Begrenzung. *Kl. Wochenschrift* **43**:1481.

Plotkin H. C., 1967: Role of the neocortex in acquisition of avoidance conditioning. *Nature* **213**:1053—1054.

Plotkin H. C., Russell I. S., 1969a: The hemidecorticate learning deficit :Evidence for a quantitative impairment. *Physiol. Behav.* **4**:49—55.

Plotkin H. C., Russell I. S., 1969b: Quantitative adjustment in magnitude of the hemidecorticate learning deficit by CS duration manipulation. *Physiol. Behav.* **4**:709—721.

Plotkin H. C., Russell I. S., 1969c: Unilateral cortical spreading depression and escape learning. *Physiol. Bohemoslov.* **18**:395—399.

Poggio G. F., Vierenstein L. J., 1964: Time series analysis of impulse sequences of thalamic somatic sensory neurons. *J. Neurophysiol.* **27**:517—545.

Potter R. L., Van Harreveld A., 1962: The effect of metrazol on the glutamate metabolism of cerebral cortex. *J. Neurochem.* **9**:105—112.

Prince D. A., Lux H. D., Neher E., 1973: Measurement of extracellular potassium activity in cat cortex. *Brain Research* **50**:489—495.

Purpura D. P., McMurtry J. G., 1965: Intracellular activities and evoked potential changes during polarization of motor cortex. *J. Neurophysiol.* **28**:165—166.

Quarton G. C., 1967: The enhancement of learning by drugs and the transfer of learning by macromolecules. In *The Neurosciences*. Quarton G. C., Melnechuk T., Schmitt F. O. (eds.). Rockefeller University Press, New York, pp. 744—755.

Rabedeau R. G., 1966: Retrograde amnesia due to spreading cortical depression: Paradoxical effect of shock-SD interval. *Psychon. Sci* **5**:113—114.

Rabin A. G., 1964: Cortical regulation of the reticular nucleus of thalamus (in Russian). *DAN SSSR* **156**:478—480.

Rabin A. G., 1965: Selective cortical control of the evoked activity of the reticular structures (in Russian). *Fiz. Zh. SSSR* **51**:159—163.

Ranck J. B., 1964: Specific impedance of cerebral cortex during spreading depression and an analysis of neuronal, neuroglial, and interstitial contributions. *Exp. Neurol.* **9**:1—16.

Rapoport J. L., Marshall W. H., 1964: Measurement of cortical pH in spreading cortical depression. *Am. J. Physiol.* **206**:1177—1180.

Ray O. S., Emley G., 1964: Time factors in interhemispheric transfer of learning. *Science* **144**:76—78.

Ray O. S., Emley G., 1965: Interhemispheric transfer of learning. *Life Sci.* **4**:271—279.

Rebert C. S., 1970: Spreading depression in squirrel monkey lissencephalic cortex. *Physiol. Behav.* **5**:239—241.

Reed V. G., Trowill J. A., 1969: Stimulus control value of spreading depression demonstrated without shifting depressed hemispheres. *J. Comp. Physiol. Psychol.* **69**:40—43.

Rhoton A., Goldring S., O'Leary J. L., 1960: Comparison of direct cerebral and cerebellar responses. *Am. J. Physiol.* **199**:677—682.

Robertson A. D. J., Evans C. R., 1965: Single unit activity in the cat's visual cortex: Modification after an intensive light flash. *Science* **147**:303—304.

Roitbak A. I., 1955: *Bioelectrical Phenomena in the Cerebral Cortex* (in Russian). Izd. AN GSSR, Tbilisi.

Roldán E., Weiss T., Fifková E., 1963: Excitability changes during the sleep cycle of the rat. *EEG Clin. Neurophysiol.* **15**:775—785.

Rolleston F. C., Newsholme E. A., 1967: Control of glycolysis in cerebral cortex slices. *Biochem. J.* **104**:524—533.

Roodyn D. B., Reis P. J., Work T. S., 1961: Protein synthesis in mitochondria. Requirements for the incorporation of radioactive amino acids into mitochondrial protein. *J. Biochem.* **80**:9—21.

Roper S., Bourassa Ch. M., 1972: Photic responses in rat cerebellum. *Brain Research* **39**:251—254.

Rose J. E., Woolsey C. N., 1948: Structure and relations of limbic cortex and anterior thalamic nuclei in rabbit and cat. *J. Comp. Neurol.* **89**:279—347.

Rosenblueth A., García-Ramos J., 1966: Some phenomena usually associated with spreading depression. *Acta Physiol. Latino-amer.* **15**:142—179.

Rosenblueth A., Garcia Ramos J., Nims L. F., 1967: The relation between the impedance and the e. m. f. changes in the cerebral cortex. *Acta physiol. Latino-amer.* **17**:76—87.

Ross R. B., Russell I. S., 1964: Lateralization and one-trial interhemispheric transfer of avoidance conditioning. *Nature* **204**:909—910.

Ross R. B., Russell I. S., 1967: Subcortical storage of classical conditioning. *Nature* **214**:210—211.

Rossi G., Bonfilis S., Lieffoghe F., 1956: Technique nouvelle pour produire des ulcérations gastriques chez le rat blanc: l'ulcère de contrainte. *C. R. Soc. Biol.* **150**:2124.

Rounds H. D., 1967: KCl-induced spreading depression in the cockroach. *J. Insect Physiol.* **11**:869—873.

Rounds H. D., 1968: KCl-induced "spreading depression" and ventilation in the cockroach. *Comp. Biochem. Physiol.* **24**:653—655.

Routtenberg A., 1972: Intracranial chemical injection and behavior: a critical review. *Behav. Biol.* **7**:601—641.

Rozin P., Kalat J., 1971: Specific hungers and poison avoidance as adaptive specializations of learning. *Psychological Review* **78**:459—486.

Rüdiger W., 1962: Interfering subcortical stimulations and cortical spreading depression. *Physiol. Bohemoslov.* **11**:392—398.

Rüdiger W., Bureš J., 1962: Cortical spreading depression and tegmental and hypothalamic threshold stimulation producing locomotor flight. *Physiol. Bohemoslov.* **11**:399—403.

Rüdiger W., Burešová O., Fifková E., 1962: Die Wirkung der sich verbreitenden Aktivitätsdepression (Phänomen von Leão) in der Grosshirnrinde auf die Entladungsaktivität von Einzelneuronen im Dienzephalon der Ratte. *Acta Biol. Med. Germ.* **9**:371—385.

Rüdiger W., Fifková E., 1963: Operant behavior and subcortical drive during spreading depression. *J. Comp. Physiol. Psychol.* **56**:375—379.

Rüdiger W., Seyer G., 1965: On the lateralization of corticohypothalamic relations as revealed by thermosensitive behavior in the rat. *Physiol. Bohemoslov.* **14**:515—522.

Rüdiger W., Weiss T., Fifková E., 1962: Threshold for eliciting the hippocampal theta rhythm by electrical stimulation in tegmentum and hypothalamus during cortical spreading depression in rats. *Experientia* **18**:22—24.

Ruščák M., 1961: Changes in amino nitrogen during EEG depression. *J. Neurochem.* **7**:305—307.

Ruščák M., 1962a: Influence of various stimuli on lactic acid, alanine and gamma-aminobutyric acid levels in rat brain. *Nature* **195**:290—292.

Ruščák M., 1962b: Changes in the level of γ-aminobutyric acid (GABA) in the ischemic brain of rats following application of some stimuli evoking EEG depression. *Physiol. Bohemoslov.* **11**:192—198.

Ruščák M., 1964: Incorporation of ^{35}S-methionine into proteins of the cerebral cortex in situ in rats during spreading EEG depression. *Physiol. Bohemoslov.* **13**:16—20.

Ruščák M., Duda P., 1959: Brain metabolism during EEG depression and cerebral anemia (in Slovak). *Čs. Fysiol.* **8**:429—430.

Ruščák M., Ruščáková D., 1971: *Metabolism of the Nerve Tissue in Relation to Ion Movements in Vitro and in Situ.* University Park Press, Baltimore-London-Tokyo.

Ruščáková D., 1964a: Effect of potassium ions on the morphological picture of cells of the cerebral cortex. *Physiol. Bohemoslov.* **13**:161—166.

Ruščáková D., 1964b: Recovery processes in cells of the cerebral cortex after the application of potassium ions. *Physiol. Bohemoslov.* **13**:167—171.

Rusinov V. S., 1965: Dominant and its role in the formation of temporal connections. *Proc. Int. Union Physiol. Sci.* **4**:613—617, XXIII Int. Congr. Tokyo.

Russell I. S., 1969: Cortical mechanisms and learning. In *Animal Discrimination Learning.* Gilbert R. M. and Sutherland N. S. (eds.) Academic Press, London, New York, pp. 335—356.

Russell I. S., Kleinman D., Plotkin H. C., Ross R. B., 1969: The role of the cortex in acquisition and retention of a classically conditioned passive avoidance response. *Physiol. Behav.* **4**:575—581.

Russell I. S., Ochs S., 1961: One-trial interhemispheric transfer of learning engram. *Science* **133**: 1077—1078.

Russell I. S., Ochs S., 1963: Localization of a memory trace in one cortical hemisphere and transfer to the other hemisphere. *Brain* **86**:37—54.

Russell I. S., Plotkin H. C., Kleinman D., 1968: Cortical spreading depression and the problem of motor impairment. *Physiol. Behav.* **3**:849—855.

Russell I. S., Plotkin H. C., Kleinman D., 1970: Task difficulty and lateralization of learning in the functional split brain rat. *Physiol. Behav.* **5**:469—478.

Rybová R., 1959: Effect of cations on γ-aminobutyric acid level in slices of brain cortex. *Nature* **185**:542—543.

Santibañez H. G., Espinoza S., 1968: Cortico-hypothalamic interaction in cats. *Acta Biol. Exp.* (Warsaw) **28**:83—92.

Sattin A., Rall T. W., 1967: The effect of brain extracts on the accumulation of cyclic 3',5' -AMP in slices of guinea pig cerebral cortex. *Federation Proc.* **26**:707.

Schadé J. P., 1957: *Electro-area-grafie van de Cortex Cerebri.* F. V. Rossen, Amsterdam.

Schadé J. P., 1959: Maturational aspects of EEG and of spreading depression in rabbit. *J. Neurophysiol.* **22**:245—257.

Schadé J. P., 1964: On the contribution of neuroglia to the function of the cerebral cortex. In: *Neurological and Electroencephalographic Correlative Studies in Infancy*, Kellaway P., Petersen I. (eds.) Grune and Stratton, New York, pp. 37—51.

Schadé J. P., Collewijn H., 1962: Slow potential and unit activity in the optic system of cephalopods. *Proc. Int. Un. Physiol. Sci.* **2**, Abstr. No. 1161.

Schadé J. P., Collewijn H., 1964: Neurobiological studies on cephalopods. I. Spreading depression and impedance changes in the retina. *Neth. J. Sea Res.* **2**:123—144.

Schneider A. M., 1965: Effects of unilateral and bilateral spreading depression on water intake. *Psychon. Sci.* **3**:287—288.

Schneider A. M., 1966: Retention under spreading depression: A generalization-decrement phenomenon. *J. Comp. Physiol. Psychol.* **62**:317—319.

Schneider A. M., 1967: Control of memory by spreading cortical depression: A case for stimulus control. *Psychol. Rev.* **74**:201—215.

Schneider A. M., 1968: Stimulus control and spreading cortical depression: Some problems reconsidered. *Psychol. Rev.* **75**:353—358.

Schneider A. M., 1972: Retrograde amnesic effects of unilateral spreading depression. *Physiol. Behav.* **9**:97—99.

Schneider A. M., Behar M., 1964: A chronic preparation for spreading cortical depression. *J. Exp. Anal. Behav.* **7**:350.

Schneider A. M., Ebbesen E., 1967: Interhemispheric transfer of lever pressing as stimulus generalization of the effect of spreading depression. *J. Exp. Anal. Behav.* **10**:193—197.

Schneider A. M., Hamburg M., 1966: Interhemispheric transfer with spreading depression: A memory transfer or stimulus generalization phenomenon? *J. Comp. Physiol. Psychol.* **62**:133—136.

Schneider A. M., Kay H., 1968: Spreading depression as a discriminative stimulus for lever pressing. *J. Comp. Physiol. Psychol.* **65**:149—151.

Schneider M., 1956: Die Wirkung der Hypothermie auf das ZNS, besonders auf seine Wiederbelebungszeit. *XX Int. Physiol. Congr.*, Abstracts of Reviews, Brussels, pp. 98—103.

Schwartzbaum J. S., Kreinick C. J., Mello W. F., 1972: Cortical evoked potentials and synchronization of electrocortical activity during consummatory behavior in rats. *Brain Research* **36**:171—182.

Sedláček J., 1964: Effect of EEG depression on the temporary connection in chick embryos. *Physiol. Bohemoslov.* **13**:510—515.

Sedláček J., 1966: Development of the steady potential of the brain of chick embryos. *Physiol. Bohemoslov.* **15**:111—116.

Sedláček J., 1967a: The effect of K^+ and g-strophantin upon cortical steady potential in guinea-pig embryos. *Physiol. Bohemoslov.* **16**:342—349.

Sedláček J., 1967b: Development of the effect of K^+ and g-strophantin, and metabolic inhibitors upon the steady potential and impedance of the brain tissue in chick embryos. *Physiol. Bohemoslov.* **16**:350—357.

Sedláček J., 1969: Kinetics of substances in the developing cerebral tissue of chick embryos (in Czech). *Sborník Lékařský* **71**:37—43.

Sedláček J., Macek O., 1965: DC potential and high-frequency impedance of the cerebral hemispheres in guinea-pig fetuses in the perinatal period. *Physiol. Bohemoslov.* **14**:371—378.

Sedláček J., Macek O., 1966a: Development of the steady potential and high-frequency impedance of the cerebral cortex in guinea-pig embryos. *Physiol. Bohemoslov.* **15**:52—61.

Sedláček J., Macek O., 1966b: The development of brain impedance in chick embryos. *Physiol. Bohemoslov.* **15**:104—110.

Sedláček J., Macek O., 1968: The effect of potassium, ouabaine, and sodium fluoride on the development of cell potentials in the tissue of the cerebral hemispheres of chick embryos. *Physiol. Bohemoslov.* **17**:553—562.

Selfridge O., 1948: Studies on flutter and fibrillation. V. Some notes on the theory of flutter. *Arch. Inst. Cardiol. Mex.* **18**:177—187.

Semyokhina A. F., 1969: Cortico-subcortical relationships under conditions of spreading depression of the neocortex. *Zh. Vyssh. Nerv. Deyat.* **19**:143—148.

Servít Z., 1963: *Reflex Mechanisms in the Genesis of Epilepsy*. Proceedings of a symposium held in Prague and Liblice, Elsevier, Amsterdam.

Servít Z., 1966: Comparative and cellular pathology as a method of research in the pathogenesis of epilepsy. In *Comparative and Cellular Pathophysiology of Epilepsy*. Servít Z. (ed.) Excerpta Medica, Int. Congr. Ser. No 124, Amsterdam, pp. 7—15.

Servít Z., Bureš J., Burešová O., Petráň M., 1953: Beitrag zur Frage der Elektronarkose (in Russian). *Physiol. Bohemoslov.* **2**:337—346.

Seylaz J., Molnar L., 1966: Observations récentes sur les corrélations entre le débit cérébral et la dépression envahissante. *C. R. Soc. Biol.* **160**:294—298.

Schanberg S. M., Schildkraut J. J., Kopin I. J., 1967: The effects of pentobarbital on the fate of intracisternally administered norepinephrine -^{3}H. *J. Pharmacol. Exp. Therap.* **157**:311—318.

Schanberg S. M., Schildkraut J. J., Křivánek J., Kopin I. J., 1968: Effect of cortical spreading depression on norepinephrine -^{3}H metabolism in brain stem. *Experientia* **24**:909—910.

Shanes A. M., 1958: Electrochemical aspects of physiological and pharmacological action in excitable cells. *Pharmacol. Rev.* **10**:165—273.

Sharpless S., Jasper H., 1956: Habituation of the arousal reaction. *Brain* **79**:655—680.

Sheridan C. L., 1965: Interocular transfer of brightness and pattern discrimination in normal and corpus callosum sectioned rats. *J. Comp. Physiol. Psychol.* **59**:292—294.

Shibata M., Bureš J., 1971: Entrapped wave of spreading cortical depression in the rat. XXV Int. Congr. Physiol. Sci., Munich, Abstr. of Comm. p. 511.

Shibata M., Bureš J., 1972: Reverberation of cortical spreading depression along closed-loop pathways in rat cerebral cortex. *J. Neurophysiol.* **35**:381—388.

Shibata M., Bureš J., 1973: Methods of stopping the reverberating cortical spreading depression in the rat. *Activitas Nerv. Sup.* **16**:2—3.

Shima I., 1964: Behavioral consequences of striatal spreading depression in pigeons. *J. Comp. Physiol. Psychol.* **57**:37—41.

Shima I., Fifková E., 1963: Remote effects of striatal spreading depression in pigeon brain. *Jap. J. Physiol.* **13**:630—640.

Shima I., Fifková E., Bureš J., 1963: Limits of spreading depression in pigeon striatum. *J. Comp. Neurol.* **121**:485—492.

Shimizu H., Creveling C. R., Daly J. W., 1970: Cyclic adenosine 3', 5'-monophosphate formation in brain slices: stimulation by batrachotoxin, ouabaine, veratridine, and potassium ions. *Mol. Pharmacol.* **6**:184—188.

Shirane Y., 1961: Biochemical studies on Leão's phenomenon (in Japanese). *Fukuoka Med. Acta* **52**: 135—147.

Sloan N., Jasper H., 1950: Identity of spreading depression and "supression". *EEG Clin. Neurophysiol.* **2**:59—78.

Sokolov V. B., Bureš J., Fifková E., 1966: Unit activity of thalamic and hypothalamic neurons during thalamic spreading depression in rats. *Arch. Int. Physiol. Bioch.* **74**:498—508.

Solomon R. L., Turner L. H., 1962: Discriminative classical conditioning in dogs paralyzed by curare can later control discriminative avoidance responses in the normal state. *Psychol. Bull.* **69**:202—219.

Somjen G. G., Kato G., 1968: Effects of magnesium and calcium on neurons in the central nervous system. *Brain Res.* **9**:161—164.

Sonnenschein R. R., Walker R. M., 1956: Local cerebral blood flow in spreading cortical depression. *Fed. Proc.* **15**:175.

Speckmann E. J., Caspers H., 1963: Verschiebungen des corticalen Bestandpotentials bei Atemstillstand. *Pflügers Arch.* **278**:76.

Speckmann E. J., Caspers H., 1966: Die sogenannte anoxische Terminal-depolarisation und ihre Beziehung zur Wiederbelebungszeit des Gehirns. *Pflügers Arch.* **289**:R1—2.

Speckmann E. J., Caspers H., 1967: Les modifications du potentiel continu cortical pendant l'arrêt respiratoire. *Rev. Neurol.* (Paris) **177**:5—19.

Spehlmann R., Creutzfeldt O. D., Jung R., 1960: Neuronale Hemmung im motorischen Cortex nach elektrischer Reizung des Caudatum. *Arch. Psychiat. Nervenkr.* **201**:332.

Sperry R. W., 1959: Preservation of high-order function in isolated somatic cortex in callosum-sectioned cat. *J. Neurophysiol.* **22**:78—87.

Sperry R. W., 1961: Cerebral organization and behavior. *Science* **133**:1749—1757.

Sperry R. W., 1964: The great cerebral commissure. *Sci. Am.* **210**:42—52.

Sperry R. W., 1967: Split-brain approach to learning problems. In *The Neurosciences,* Quarton G. C., Melnechuk T., Schmitt F. O. (eds.). Rockefeller Univ. Press, New York pp. 714—722.

Spies G., 1967: A study of learning and retroactive inhibition under unilateral cortical depression. *Psychon. Sci.* **7**:377—378.

Squire L. R., 1966: Transfer of habituation using spreading depression. *Psychon. Sci.* **5**:261—262.

Squire L. R., Liss P. M., 1968: Control of memory by spreading cortical depression: A critique of stimulus control. *Psychol. Rev.* **75**:347—352.

Starzl T. E., Niemer W. T., Dell M., Forgrave P. R., 1953: Cortical and subcortical electrical activity in experimental seizures induced by metrazol. *J. Neuropath. Exp. Neurol.* **12**:262—276.

Stille G., 1971a: Zur Pharmakologie katatonigener Stoffe. 2. Mitteilung: Ausschaltung des N. caudatus und die katatonigene Wirkung der Neuroleptika. *Arzneimittel-Forschung* **21**:386—390.

Stille G., 1971b: Zur Pharmakologie katatonigener Stoffe. 6. Mitteilung: Schluss. *Arzneimittel-Forschung* **21**:997—1003.

Stille G., Sayers A., 1969: Effect of a striatal spreading depression on the pharmacogenic catatonia. *Int. J. Neuropharm.* **8**:181—189.

Stumpf C., Petsche H., Gogolák G., 1962: The significance of the rabbit's septum as a relay station between midbrain and the hippocampus. II. Differential influence of drugs upon both the septal cell firing pattern and the hippocampus theta activity. *EEG Clin. Neurophysiol.* **14**:212—219.

Sugawara H., Wada E., 1957: Effect of potassium and malonate on the content of labile phosphate in the brain tissue. *Sci. Paper Coll. Gen. Ed. Univ. Tokyo* **7**:121—130.

Sugaya D., Takato M., Noda Y., 1971: Spreading depression under the effect of tetrodotoxin. *J. Physiol. Soc. Japan* **33**:591—592.

Sunenshine H., Schwartz M., 1969: Spreading depression vs. lesion effects of KCl on classical conditioning in the rabbit. *Psychon. Sci.* **17**:315—316.

Suzuki H., Uneoka K., 1966: Effect of cortical spreading depression on operant behavior in the rabbit. *Physiol. Behav.* **1**:301—304.

Swenson L. C., Goldowitz D., 1972: Learning of instrumental avoidance responses under conditions of bilateral spreading depression in rats. *Psychon. Sci.* **29**:43—45.

Takagaki G., 1968: Control of aerobic glycolysis and pyruvate-kinase activity in cerebral cortex slices. *J. Neurochem.* **15**:903—916.

Taleisnik S., Caligaris L., 1962: Release of luteinizing hormon by cerebral cortex spreading depression. *Experientia* **18**:578.

Taleisnik S., Deis R. P., 1964: Influence of cerebral cortex on inhibition of oxytocin release induced by stressful stimuli. *Am. J. Physiol.* **207**:1394—1398.

Tapp J. T., 1962: Reversible cortical depression and avoidance in the rat. *J. Comp. Physiol. Psychol.* **55**:306—308.

Tarby T. J., Costin A., Adey W. R., 1966: Effects of tetrodotoxin on impedance in normal and asphyxiated cerebral tissue. *Exp. Neurol.* **22**:517—531.

Tasaki I., Singer I., Takenaka T., 1965: Effects of internal and external ionic environment on excitability of squid giant axon. *J. Gen. Physiol.* **48**:1095—1123.

Teitelbaum P., 1971: The encephalization of hunger. *Progress in Physiological Psychology* **4**:319—350.

Teitelbaum P., Cytawa J., 1965: Spreading depression and recovery from lateral hypothalamic damage. *Science* **147**:61—63.

Thompson R., 1965: Centrencephalic theory and interhemispheric transfer of visual habits. *Psychol. Rev.* **72**:385—398.

Thompson R. W., 1964: Transfer of avoidance learning between normal and functionally decorticate states. *J. Comp. Physiol. Psychol.* **57**:321—325.

Thompson R. W., 1965: Effect of intertrial interval on avoidance learning in rats trained under bilateral spreading depression. *Psychol. Reports* **16**:472—474.

Thompson R. W., Enter R., 1967: Shock level and unconditioned responding in rats under sham, unilateral, or bilateral spreading depression. *J. Comp. Physiol. Psychol.* **63**:521—523.

Thompson R. W., Hjelle L. A., 1965: Effects of stimulus and response complexity on learning under bilateral spreading depression. *J. Comp. Physiol. Psychol.* **59**:122—124.

Thompson R. W., Miller J. E., 1967: Spreading cortical depression blockade of seizures produced by electroconvulsive shock. *Psychon. Sci.* **9**:69—70.

Tolkunov B. F., 1969: Changes in evoked unit activity of the cerebral cortex and the reticular formation in rats after functional elimination of the caudate nucleus (in Russian). *Zh. Vyssh. Nerv. Deyat.* **19**: 488—494.

Tolkunov B. F., 1970: Corticostriatal interrelationships in mammals (in Russian). In *Electrophysiological Studies on the Central Nervous System of Vertebrates.* Karamyan A. I. (ed.). Nauka, Leningrad, pp. 14—22.

Tolkunov B., Burešová O., Bureš J., Kuznetsova G., Fifková E., 1965: Use of spreading depression in study of relationships between the cerebral cortex and the striatum in rats. *Physiol. Bohemoslov.* **14**:253—260.

Tolkunov B. F., Fifková E., 1964: Spreading depression in the telencephalon of turtle (in Czech). *Čs. Fysiol.* **13**:509.

Trachtenberg M. C., Hull C. D., Buchwald N. A., 1970: Electrophysiological concomitants of spreading depression in caudate and thalamic nuclei of the cat. *Brain Res.* **20**:219—231.

Travis R. P., 1964a: The role of spreading cortical depression in relating the amount of avoidance training to interhemispheric transfer. *J. Comp. Physiol. Psychol.* **57**:42—46.

Travis R. P., 1964b: Amplitude changes in evoked potentials during conditioning with unilateral spreading depression. *J. Neurophysiol.* **5**:495—501.

Travis R. P., Sparks D. L., 1963: The influence of unilateral and bilateral spreading depression during learning upon subsequent relearning. *J. Comp. Physiol. Psychol.* **56**:56—59.

Trevarthen C. B., 1962: Double visual learning in split brain monkeys. *Science* **136**:258—259.

Tsai L., Maurer S., 1930: Righthandedness in white rats. *Science* **72**:436.

Tschirgi R. D., Inanaga K., Taylor J. L., Walker, M., Sonnenschein R. R., 1957: Changes in cortical pH and blood flow accompanying spreading cortical depression and convulsion. *Am. J. Physiol.* **190**:557—562.

Tschirgi R. D., Taylor J. L., 1958: Slowly changing bioelectric potentials associated with the blood-brain barrier. *Am. J. Physiol.* **195**:7—22.

Tsukada Y., Takagaki G., Hirano S., 1958: Incorporation of radioactive phosphate into protein-bound phosphorus fractions of brain slices in reference to its relation to the metabolic activity. *J. Biochem.* (Tokyo) **45**:489—501.

Tuge H., Kanayama Y., Chang H. Y., 1960: Comparative studies on the development of EEG. *Jap. J. Physiol.* **10**:211—220.

Tuge H., Shima I., 1959: Defensive conditioned reflex after destruction of the forebrain in pigeons. *J. Comp. Neurol.* **111**:427—446.

Udvarhelyi G. B., Walker A. E., 1965: Dissemination of acute focal seizures in the monkey. Part 1 (From cortical foci). *Arch. Neurol.* **12**:333—356.

Van Harreveld A., 1957: Changes in volume of cortical neuronal elements during asphyxiation. *Am. J. Physiol.* **191**:233—242.

Van Harreveld A., 1958: Changes in diameter of apical dendrites during spreading depression. *Am. J. Physiol.* **192**:457—463.

Van Harreveld A., 1959: Components in brain extracts causing spreading depression of cerebral cortical activity and contraction of crustacean muscle. *J. Neurochem.* **3**:300—315.

Van Harreveld A., 1961: Asphyxial changes in the cerebellar cortex. *J. Cell. Comp. Physiol.* **57**:101—110.

Van Hareveld A., 1966: *Brain Tissue Electrolytes.* Butterworths, Washington, D. C.

Van Harreveld A., Biber M. P., 1962: Conductivity changes in some organs after circulatory arrest. *Am. J. Physiol.* **203**:609—614.

Van Harreveld A., Biersteker P. A., 1964: Acute asphyxiation of the spinal cord and of other sections of the nervous system. *Am. J. Physiol.* **206**:8—14.

Van Harreveld A., Bogen J. E., 1956: Regional differences in propagation of spreading cortical depression in the rabbit. *Proc. Soc. Exp. Biol.* **91**:297—302.

Van Harreveld A., Dafny N., Khattab F. I., 1971: Effects of calcium on the electrical resistance and the extracellular space of cerebral cortex. *Exp. Neurol.* **31**:358—367.

Van Harreveld A., Fifková E., 1969: Glutamate release from the retina during spreading depression. *Sec. Int. Meeting. Int. Soc. Neurochem.* Milan. Abstr. of Comm., p. 208.

Van Harreveld A., Fifková E., 1970: Glutamate release from the retina during spreading depression. *J. Neurobiol.* **2**:13—29.

Van Harreveld A., Fifková E., 1971a: Light- and electron-microscopic changes in central nervous tissue after electrophoretic injection of glutamate. *Exp. Mol. Pathol.* **15**:61—81.

Van Harreveld A., Fifková E., 1971b: Effects of glutamate and other amino acids on the retina. *J. Neurochem.* **18**:2145—2154.

Van Harreveld A., Fifková E., 1972: Effects of metabolic inhibitors on the release of glutamate from the retina. *J. Neurochem.* **19**:1439—1450.

Van Harreveld A., Hawes R. C., 1946: Asphyxial depolarization in the spinal cord. *Am. J. Physiol.* **147**:669—684.

Van Harreveld A., Khattab F. I., 1967: Changes in cortical extracellular space during spreading depression investigated with the electron microscope. *J. Neurophysiol.* **30**:911—929.

Van Harreveld A., Kooiman M., 1965: Amino acid release from the cerebral cortex during spreading depression and asphyxiation. *J. Neurochem.* **12**:431—439.

Van Harreveld A., Malhotra S. K., 1966: Demonstration of extracellular space by freeze-drying in the cerebellar molecular layer. *J. Cell. Sci.* **1**:223—278.

Van Harreveld A., Malhotra S. K., 1967: Extracellular space in the cerebral cortex of the mouse. *J. Anat.* **101**:197—207.

Van Harreveld A., Ochs S., 1956: Cerebral impedance changes after circulatory arrest. *Am. J. Physiol.* **187**:180—192.

Van Harreveld A., Ochs S., 1957: Electrical and vascular concomitants of spreading depression. *Am. J. Physiol.* **189**:159—166.

Van Harreveld A., Schadé J. P., 1959: Chloride movements in cerebral cortex after circulatory arrest and during spreading depression. *J. Cell. Comp. Physiol.* **54**:65—84.

Van Harreveld A., Schadé J. P., 1960: On distribution and movement of water and electrolytes in the cerebral cortex. In *Structure and Function of the Cerebral Cortex.* Tower D. B., Schadé J. P., (eds.), Elsevier, Amsterdam, pp. 239—254.

Van Harreveld A., Stamm J. S., 1951: Conditions for recording of Leão's spreading depression. *EEG Clin. Neurophysiol.* **3**:323—328.

Van Harreveld A., Stamm J. S., 1952: Vascular concomitants of spreading cortical depression. *J. Neurophysiol.* **15**:487—496.

Van Harreveld A., Stamm J. S., 1953a: Effect of pentobarbital and ether in the spreading cortical depression. *Am. J. Physiol.* **173**:164—170.

Van Harreveld A., Stamm J. S., 1953b: Cerebral asphyxiation and spreading cortical depression. *Am. J. Physiol.* **173**:171—175.

Van Harreveld A., Stamm J. S., 1953c: Spreading cortical convulsions and depressions. *J. Neurophysiol.* **26**:352—366.

Van Harreveld A., Stamm J. S., 1954a: Relation between asphyxial damage to the cortex and the spreading depression. *Am. J. Physiol.* **178**:117—122.

Van Harreveld A., Stamm J. S., 1954b: Consequences of cortical convulsive activity in rabbit. *J. Neurophysiol.* **17**:505—520.

Van Harreveld A., Stamm J. S., 1955: Cortical responses to Metrazol and sensory stimulation in the rabbit. *EEG Clin. Neurophysiol.* **7**:363—370.

Van Harreveld A., Stamm J. S., Christensen E., 1956: Spreading depression in rabbit, cat and monkey. *Am. J. Physiol.* **184**:312—320.

Van Harreveld A., Steiner A., 1970: Extracellular space in frozen and ethanol substituted central nervous tissue. *Anat. Rec.* **166**:117—130.

Van Harreveld A., Tachibana S., 1962: Recovery of cerebral cortex from asphyxiation. *Am. J. Physiol.* **202**:59—65.

Van Harreveld A., Terres B., Dernburg E. A., 1956: Cortical discontinuity and propagation of spreading depression. *Am. J. Physiol.* **184**:233—238.

Vernadakis A., Woodbury D. M., 1965: Cellular and extracellular spaces in developing rat brain. *Arch. Neurol.* **12**:284—293.

Vyskočil F., Kříž N., Bureš J., 1972: Potassium-selective microelectrodes used for measuring the extracellular brain potassium during spreading depression and anoxic depolarization in rats. *Brain Research* **39**:255—259.

Walker A. E., Udvarhelyi G. B., 1965a: Dissemination of acute focal seizures in the monkey, Part 2 (From subcortical foci). *Arch. Neurol.* **12**:357—380.

Walker A. E., Udvarhelyi G. B., 1965b: The generalization of a seizure. *J. Nerv. Ment. Dis.* **140**:252.

Walker F. D., Hild W. J., 1972: Spreading depression in tissue culture. *J. Neurobiol.* **3**:223—235.

Walker J.L. Jr., 1971: Ion-specific liquid ion-exchanger microelectrodes. *Analytical chemistry* **43**: 89A—92A.

Waller H. J., Feldman S. F., 1967: Somatosensory thalamic neurons: Effect of cortical depression. *Science* **157**:1074—1077.

Wampler R. S., Rehovsky D. A., 1973: Decrease in food intake following cortical spreading depression in static obese rats with ventromedial hypothalamic lesions. *J. Comp. Physiol. Psychol.* **82**:23—29.

Ward R., Sinnett E. E., 1971: Spreading cortical depression and audiogenic seizures in mice. *Exp. Neurol.* **31**:437—443.

Watanabe S., Creutzfeldt O. D., 1966: Spontane postsynaptische Potentiale von Nervenzellen des motorischen Cortex der Katze. *Exp. Brain Res.* **1**:48—64.

Weil C. S., 1952: Tables for convenient calculation of median effective dose (LD_{50} or ED_{50}) and instructions in their use. *Biometrics* **8**:249—263.

Weiss T., 1960: *The Application of Cortical Spreading Depression in Analysis of the Intercentral (Particularly Cortico—Subcortical) Relationships* (in Czech). Dissertation. Inst. of Physiol., Czechoslovak Acad. Sci., Prague.

Weiss T., 1961a: Short-lasting cortical desynchronization in the course of the propagation of spreading EEG depression in one hemisphere. *Physiol. Bohemoslov.* **10**:27—35.

Weiss T., 1961b: The spontaneous EEG activity of the mesencephalic reticular formation during cortical spreading depression. *Physiol. Bohemoslov.* **10**:108—116.

Weiss T., 1962: Acoustic collicular evoked responses during cortical spreading depression in freely moving unanesthetized rats. *Experientia* **18**:417—418.

Weiss T., Bohdanecký Z., 1963: Influence of drugs and neocortical spreading depression on hippocampal "arousal reaction". *Experientia* **19**:127—128.

Weiss T., Bureš J., 1959: The arousal reaction during unilateral EEG spreading depression. *Physiol. Bohemoslov.* **8**:393—399.

Weiss T., Fifková E., 1960: The use of spreading EEG depression to analyze the mutual relationship between the neocortex and hippocampus. *EEG Clin. Neurophysiol.* **12**:841—850.

Weiss T., Fifková E., 1961a: The effect of spreading cortical depression on activity of subcortical relay nuclei of specific afferent pathways. *Arch. Int. Physiol. Bioch.* **69**:69—78.

Weiss T., Fifková E., 1961b: Bioelectric activity in the thalamus and hypothalamus of rats during cortical spreading EEG depression. *EEG Clin. Neurophysiol.* **13**:734—744.

Weiss T., Fifková E., 1961c: Evoked responses in the mesencaphalic tegmentum during cortical spreading depression. *Physiol. Bohemoslov.* **10**:117—121.

Weiss T., Fifková E., 1963: The effect of neocortical and caudatal spreading depression on "circling movements" induced from the caudate nucleus. *Physiol. Bohemoslov.* **12**:332—338.

Weiss T. R., Kado R. T., Adey W. R., 1966: Impedance and d-c potential shifts during cortical spreading depression. *Activ. Nerv. Sup.* **8**:194—195.

Weiss T., Roldán E., Bohdanecký Z., Fifková E., 1964: Electroencephalographic signs of anesthesia and sleep during neocortical spreading depression in rats. *EEG Clin. Neurophysiol.* **16**:429—437.

Wendell-Smith C. P., Blunt M. J., 1965: Possible role of neuroglia. *Nature* **208**:600—602.

Whieldon J. A., Van Harreveld A., 1950: Cumulative effects of minimal cortical stimulation. *EEG Clin. Neurophysiol.* **2**:49—57.

White R. P., Himwich H. E., 1954: Ablation studies on the mechanism of forced circling in rabbits. *Am. J. Physiol.* **179**:684—

Wiener N., Rosenblueth A., 1946: The mathematical formulation of the problem of conduction of impulses in a network of connected excitable elements, specifically in cardiac muscle. *Arch. Inst. Cardiol. Mex.* **16**:205—265.

Wikler A., 1952: Pharmacologic dissociation of behavior and EEG "sleep patterns" in dogs: Morphine, n-allylnormorphine, and atropine. *Proc. Soc. Exp. Biol. N. Y.* **79**:261—265.

Winokur G., 1965: Bilateral spreading depression and avoidance learning in rats. *Psychon. Sci.* **3**:107—108.

Winokur G. L., Trufant S. A., King R. B., O'Leary J. L., 1950: Thalamocortical activity during spreading depression. *EEG Clin. Neurophysiol.* **2**:79—90.

Wollenberger A., 1947: Metabolic action of the cardiac glycosides. *J. Pharmacol.* **91**:39—51.

Wong E. K., Jr., 1969: Changes in impedance and phase angle in the cerebral cortex during spreading depression. *Acta Physiol. Latino-amer.* **19**:63—66.

Woody C. D., Brožek G., 1969a: Conditioned eye blink in the cat: Evoked responses of short latency. *Brain Res.* **12**:257—260.

Woody C., Brožek G., 1969b: Changes in evoked responses from facial nucleus of cat with conditioning and extinction of an eye blink. *J. Neurophysiol.* **32**:717—726.

Yoshida H., Quastel J. H., 1962: Effects of metabolic inhibitors on potassium and acetylcholine-stimulated incorporation of phosphate into phospholipids of rat brain cortex slices. *Biochim. Biophys. Acta* **57**:67—72.

Yoshii N., Ogura H., 1960: Studies on the unit discharge of brain-stem reticular formation in the cat. I. Changes of reticular unit discharge following coditioning procedure. *Med. J. Osaka Univ.* **11**:1—17.

Zachar J., Ruščák M., 1958: Brain metabolism during spreading depression (in Slovak). *Čs. Fysiol.* **7**:191—192.

Zachar J., Zacharová D., 1961a: The refractory phase of Leão's spreading cortical depression. *Physiol. Bohemoslov.* **10**:341—348.

Zachar J., Zacharová D., 1961b: Subthreshold changes at the site of initiation of spreading cortical depression by mechanical stimuli. *EEG Clin. Neurophysiol.* **13**:896—904.

Zachar J., Zacharová D., 1962: The release thresholds of the spreading depression in the lissencephalic brain of some phylogenetic species (in Slovak). *Bratislavské Lékařské Listy* **42**:602—610.

Zachar J., Zacharová D., 1963: *Initiation of Spreading Cortical Depression* (in Slovak). VSAV, Bratislava.

Zacharová D., Zachar J., 1961: Initiation of spreading cortical depression by local cooling of the cerebral cortex. *Physiol. Bohemoslov.* **10**:332—340.

Zacharová D., Zachar J., 1966: Comparative aspects of spreading cortical depression (in Slovak). *Biologia* **21**:794—800.

Recent SD publications which came to our attention during proof reading.

Kow L. M., Van Harreveld A., 1972: Ion and water movements in isolated retinas during spreading depression. *Neurobiology* **2**:61—69.

Lehr P. P., Nachman M., 1973: Lateralization of learned taste aversion by cortical spreading depression. *Physiol. Behav.* **10**:79—83.

Lux D. H., Neher E., 1973: The equilibration time course of $[K^+]_o$ in cerebral cortex. *Exp. Brain Res.* **17**:190—205.

Pieri L., Bartholini G., Keller H. H., Pletscher A., 1973: Effect of spreading depression on electrical activity and dopamine turnover in the striatum of rats. *Experientia* **29**:452—454.

Plotkin H. C., Russell I. S., 1973: Compensation of a hemidecorticate learning deficit by manipulation of input redundancy. *Physiol. Behav.* **10**:601—606.

Prado—Alcala R. A., Grinberg—Zylberbaum J., Alvarez—Leefmans J., Brust—Carmona H., 1973: Suppression of motor conditioning by the injection of 3M KCL in the caudate nuclei of cats. *Physiol. Behav.* **10**:59—64.

Rosenthal M., Somjen G., 1973: Spreading depression, sustained potential shifts and metabolic activity of cerebral cortex of cats. *J. Neurophysiol.* **36**:739—749.

Ross W. J., Gorski R. A., 1973: Effect of potassium chloride on sexual behavior and the cortical EEG in the ovariectomized rat. *Physiol. Behav.* **10**:643—646.

Russell I. S., 1971: Neurological basis of complex learning. *British Medical Bulletin* **27**:278—285.

Schneider A. M., 1973: Spreading depression: a behavioral analysis. In *The Physiological basis of memory* Deutsch J. A. (ed.). Academic Press, New York and London, pp. 269—303.

Sugaya E., Takato M., Noda Y., 1971: Glial membrane potential during spreading depression under the effect of tetrodotoxine. *J. Physiol. Soc. Japan* **33**:654—655.

Van Harreveld A., Fifková E., 1973: Effect of amino acids on the isolated chicken retina, and on its response to glutamate stimulation. *J. Neurochem.* **20**:947—962.

Author index

L

M

N

O

T

Subject index

O

P